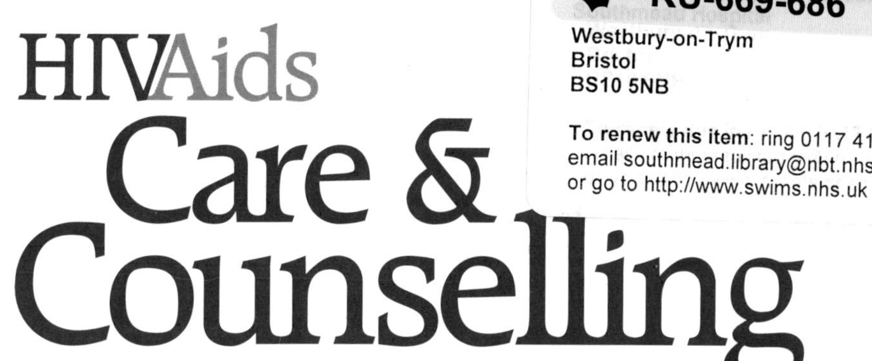

HIV/Aids Care & Counselling

A MULTIDISCIPLINARY APPROACH

THIRD EDITION

I dedicate this book to everyone who is infected with and affected by HIV and Aids.

Your courage, determination, compassion and hope inspire us all.

Pearson Education South Africa
Forest Drive, Pinelands, Cape Town

First published 1999
Third Edition 2005

ISBN 1 86891 366 X

Published by Alison Paulin
Editorial management by Lisa Compton
Edited by Gawie du Toit and Emma Buchanan
Proofread by Emma Buchanan
Book design and typesetting by Zebra Publications
Cover design by designworx and Sharon Mayers
Artwork by Karlie Hadingham and Gawie du Toit

Material in chapters 14 and 17 credited to Muchiru and Fröhlich, 2001 is reprinted with permission of Macmillan Botswana from *HIV/AIDS: Home-based care, a guide for caregivers*, by Muchiru, S. and Fröhlich, J.

Printed and bound by Creda Communications

Preface

We have seen many changes in the HIV/Aids field since the first edition of this book in 1999. Much more is known about the HI virus and its consequences; antiretroviral therapy is more advanced and more available; vaccine development is in different trial phases in various parts of the world; diagnostic tests have been refined to give more reliable results in a much shorter time; the advent of rapid testing has brought HIV management to the doorstep of many people in remote rural areas; and the general management of HIV infection and opportunistic infections is more effective. We can now truly say that HIV/AIDS has become a chronic treatable disease rather than a progressive fatal disease.

But amidst medical and scientific advances, we also saw human tragedy escalating – especially in sub-Saharan Africa. Infection rates are still on the increase – it is estimated that in 2003 alone, three million people in sub-Saharan Africa became infected with HIV. The rising death rate is immobilising the economies, education and health services of many countries; Africa is facing an orphan crisis unprecedented in human memory; grandmothers are denied a peaceful old age by having to bury their children and care for their grandchildren; stigma and prejudice remain rife, making HIV infection and Aids an unspeakable disease not to be named or talked about; and the rights of women and children are widely disregarded – leaving them disempowered and unable to protect themselves from HIV and Aids.

The medical and scientific advances so evident in the First World are often not implemented in Africa – not because of a lack of *know-how*, but because of a lack of political *will-power* and *commitment*. Examples are the unavailability of antiretroviral medication; or, where it is available, the lack of access to the poor. Prevention of mother-to-child transmission and

The Raka metaphor

Each chapter of this book is prefaced by a short quotation from the poetic drama *Raka*, written in 1941 by the Afrikaans poet N.P. van Wyk Louw (1906–1970). I have used Raka as a metaphor for HIV/AIDS and the destruction and havoc it inflicts on individuals and the community.

Raka, half-human and half-ape, appears without warning near the village of Koki and his people. Raka uses primitive cunning, guile and brute strength to undermine the culture and very existence of the community. Everybody except Koki is afraid to resist Raka, and some of the villagers are even attracted and drawn to the beast's insidious primitive sensuality and power. The hero Koki, aware of the deadly challenge posed by Raka, ventures into the dark forest to confront him.

The quotes from *Raka* are translations of freely selected (and sometimes slightly adapted) passages from the poem. *Raka* has a tragic ending, and the work warns that beasts of unknown origin may at any time attack and destroy our culture, our integrity, our hopes, our community and our very lives. That is why I think *Raka* is an appropriate metaphor for the threats and challenges of the HIV/AIDS pandemic.

PEET VAN DYK

voluntary counselling and testing services are non-existent in many of the hardest-hit countries; national orphan policies do not exist; and many countries still do not have prevention programmes in place.

But human tragedy always gives rise to the emergence of extraordinary people. And the true heroes of the Aids epidemic are the caregivers: lay, professional as well as family caregivers. Many of these caregivers have been kind enough to share their experiences with me. Their compassion, care and commitment to ease the pain of those infected and affected by HIV is truly commendable. Many innovative ideas included in this book originated from them, including memory projects, orphan care programmes, garden and food schemes for poor communities, educational programmes to change harmful behaviour, outreach projects for the youth, and more.

In the third edition of *HIV/Aids Care and Counselling* I have tried to capture the recent changes and advances in the field of HIV/AIDS. I am sincerely grateful to everyone who supported me during the preparation of this edition. Special thanks to my soulmate and husband, Peet, for your unconditional love and support. And to my children Jaco, Marlene and Ewald – who were still at school when the first edition saw the light, and who are now three beautiful young adults – I hope that, by the time your grandchildren are born, Aids will be a distant memory, only to be read about in history books . . .

> Aids is likely to be with us for a very long time, but how far it spreads and how much damage it does is entirely up to us.
>
> (Peter Piot, UNAIDS, 2004:9)

ALTA VAN DYK
October 2004

Contents

Part 2

Prevention and Empowerment in the HIV/Aids Context

Part 3

HIV/Aids Counselling

List of Illustrations

List of Tables

part 1

Fundamental Facts about HIV/Aids

INTRODUCTION TO PART 1

Aids counsellors must be very well informed about all aspects of HIV infection and Aids, and they must have the resources and motivation to keep up with developments. No matter whether a counsellor's function is psychological, spiritual, medical, marriage guidance, educational or social, he or she will *always* be asked very basic questions about HIV/Aids. Most of the care and counselling needs of HIV-positive clients involve the effect of the virus on their lives. Part 1 of this book will answer most of the questions that you or your clients might have about HIV and Aids.

Chapter 1 offers a definition of HIV and Aids and looks at the history of the HIV/Aids pandemic. It explains the unique characteristics of the HI virus and how it affects the human immune system, and explores the latest developments in the search for a vaccine.

Chapter 2 examines how the virus is transmitted via sexual intercourse and contaminated blood, and how it may be transmitted from mother to baby. It also explores important issues such as why it is difficult for disempowered women to avoid HIV infection, and how poverty and other social problems contribute to the spread of HIV. This chapter also discusses some of the latest developments in the continuing debate about breastfeeding and formula feeding.

Chapter 3 describes and discusses the symptoms of HIV infection, Aids and Aids-related illnesses in adults and children. The important relationship between the CD4 cell count, the viral load and disease progression is also explored. Because tuberculosis (TB) is the most serious and most commonly occurring oppor-

Learning outcomes

After completing Part 1 you should be able to develop and present an HIV/Aids awareness programme that conveys the following information to a target group:*

- the normal functioning of the immune system
- the effects of HIV on the immune system
- the ways in which HIV is transmitted
- the clinical symptoms of HIV infection and Aids
- the relationship between CD4 cells, the HI virus and phases of infection
- the diagnosis of HIV infection
- the management and treatment of HIV, including the use of antiretroviral therapy

*The people in a target group may have very different backgrounds, interests, concerns and education. For example, a target group may include schoolchildren, caregivers in home-based care programmes, lay counsellors, social workers, nurses, specialist interest groups, ordinary members of the community, and so on.

tunistic infection in HIV-positive individuals in Africa, this chapter devotes special attention to the diagnosis and treatment of TB. Chapter 3 also emphasises that it is important for health care professionals who work in Africa to recognise and treat the symptoms of other sexually transmitted infections (STIs).

Chapter 4 describes the diagnosis of HIV. Methods of testing for HIV are discussed in some detail in this chapter, and additional material is provided for health care professionals who have no access to HIV antibody tests. Suggestions are made as to how they might diagnose HIV infection and Aids in adults and children by recognising the symptoms specific to this disease in Africa. This chapter also describes the various HIV tests such as the ELISA (enzyme-linked immunosorbent assay) antibody test, rapid tests and p24 antigen and PCR tests, and basic concepts such as the 'window period'.

Chapter 5 looks at the management of HIV infection and Aids. It discusses how you can find out what the condition of the immune system is (for example by establishing the CD4 cell count and the viral load in the bloodstream), and what the methods of treatment are (such as antiretroviral therapy). The use of antiretroviral drugs for the prophylactic treatment of rape survivors, the prevention of mother-to-child transmission, and the management of hazardous occupational exposure to HIV (by needle-stick injuries, for example) are also addressed in this chapter.

chapter

1 HIV and the Immune System

The coming of Raka

From across the water he stepped out, among the broken reeds . . .
and he laughed silently with white teeth showing – crouching, waiting . . .
and the great beast emerged suddenly and quietly from the warm slime.
And finally Koki's heart recognised that he had come to a boundary –
that he was enclosed by something dark and dull and strong.

A few decades ago, a terrible disease, previously unknown to the human race, began to kill people in the most alarming and terrifying circumstances. It was as though a dreadful beast had entered the bloodstream of the human race. Wherever this microscopic beast appeared, it produced panic, fear, guilt, hysteria, accusations, terrible suffering and always, in the end, death.

Now the beast has a name: HIV/Aids. It is known to be a virus, but it is unlike any virus previously known. Its deadly effects are felt all over the world, but nowhere more tragically than in sub-Saharan Africa, where most of the infections in the world occur.

HIV/Aids has become one of the most destructive plagues in history. It is a monster that threatens to destroy our society because it is changing the rules by which we live. But we cannot despair just because we feel defenceless against it – we have to take decisive and practical steps to defend ourselves against it. And there is no room for complacency: the statistics are frightening, and time is running out.

1.1 THE DEFINITION OF AIDS

Aids is short for Acquired Immune Deficiency Syndrome. We say that this disease is *acquired* because it is not a disease that is inherited. It is caused by a virus (the human immunodeficiency virus or HIV) that enters the body from outside. *Immunity* is the body's natural ability to defend itself against infection and disease. A *deficiency* is a shortcoming – the weakening of the immune system so that it can no longer defend itself against passing infections. A *syndrome* is a medical term for a collection of specific signs and symptoms that occur together and that are characteristic of a particular condition.

Although we use the term 'disease' when we talk about it, Aids is *not a specific illness*. It is really a *collection of many different conditions* that manifest in the body (or specific parts of the body) because the HI virus has so weakened the body's immune system that it can no longer fight the disease-causing agents that are constantly attacking it. It is therefore more accurate to define Aids as a *syndrome* of opportunistic diseases, infections and certain cancers – each or all of which has the ability to kill the infected person in the final stages of the disease.

1.2 HISTORICAL BACKGROUND TO AIDS

The first recognised cases of Aids occurred in the USA in 1981 when a very rare form of pneumonia (caused by a parasite called *Pneumocystis carinii*), cytomegalovirus infections, thrush and Kaposi's sarcoma (a rare form of skin cancer) suddenly appeared simultaneously in several patients. These patients had a number of characteristics in common: they were all young homosexual men with compromised (damaged) immune systems (Adler, 1988). Soon afterwards a new disease, which undermined the immune system and caused diarrhoea and weight loss, was identified in central Africa in heterosexual people.

Initially, scientists and doctors were baffled because the causes and the modes of transmission of this new disease (called 'slim disease' in Africa) could not immediately be identified. Only in 1983 was it discovered that the disease was caused by a virus, known at that stage as LAV (lymphadenopathy-associated virus) and HTLV-III (human T cell lymphotropic virus type III). In May 1986 the virus causing this condition was renamed HIV (human immunodeficiency virus).

Two viruses are now associated with Aids: HIV-1 and HIV-2. HIV-1 is associated with infections in Central, East and southern Africa, North and South America, Europe and the rest of the world. HIV-2 was discovered in West Africa (Cape Verde Islands, Guinea-Bissau and Senegal) in 1986 and it is mostly restricted to West Africa. HIV-2 is structurally similar to HIV-1, but HIV-2 is less pathogenic than HIV-1, and HIV-2 infections have a longer latency period with slower progression to disease, lower viral counts and lower rates of transmission.

The history of the discovery of the HI virus is both interesting and controversial. Dr Luc Montagnier of the Louis Pasteur Institute in Paris, France, discovered HIV-1 in 1983. A year later Dr Robert Gallo of the United States claimed that *he* had been the first to discover the virus. What followed was a protracted court case about the alleged 'theft' by Gallo of Montagnier's virus, which had been sent to Gallo in good faith for research purposes. The bipartisan feelings aroused by this court case were so intense that they threatened to undermine the 1987 bilateral talks between the French prime minister, Jacques Chirac, and the American president, Ronald Reagan. The issue was eventually resolved by a last-minute compromise which permitted both Montagnier and Gallo to be officially recognised as co-discoverers of the virus (Connor & Kingman, 1988).

However, the bitter dispute was renewed in 1990 when Pasteur Institute scientists decided to analyse the genetic structure of Gallo's virus and compare it with Montagnier's initial isolate of the virus (Schoub, 1999:10). They found that the two viruses were so similar that it was very unlikely that they were not one and the same (taking into account natural changes in genetic structure that would be expected to occur between different virus isolates). It was found that in September 1983 Montagnier had, in fact, as a courteous scientist would be expected to, sent his original isolates of the virus to Gallo, soon after he had made his first isolation. Before a scandal again threatened to shake the scientific world, the dispute was quashed when Montagnier's laboratory admitted that there had been contamination of strains, and that the Frenchman had inadvertently contaminated Gallo's strains. It has now finally been accepted that credit should be shared between the two: Montagnier for the original isolation of the HI virus, and Gallo for being able to propagate the virus in cell culture. Gallo also was the first person to develop the critically needed diagnostic tests for HIV.

The frightening new disease and the dispute between the two countries' scientists grabbed the public attention. A journalist, Randy Shilts (who later died of Aids), wrote a book about it (*And the band played on*) which in 1993 was made into a film with an all-star cast (many of whom agreed to work for reduced fees).

1.3 THEORIES OF THE ORIGINS OF HIV/AIDS

No other disease has ever fired the imagination of the world as much as HIV and Aids have done. The following questions are always asked: Where did Aids come from? Is it a new or an old disease? Where did HIV originate? These are difficult questions, and we may never find out the answers. According to Schoub (1999:13), little is known about the origins of any human virus, let alone HIV. He says the following about the origin of Aids:

> Various scenarios of the birth and development of the epidemic have been built around pieces of knowledge recruited from a number of sources. At present the answers to both the origin of the disease as well as to the ancestry of the virus remain as unresolved as when the questions were first posed.

Is Aids a centuries-old disease of Africa?

There are two main theories about the origin of the Aids epidemic.

One theory is as follows: Aids is not a new disease, but has been present for centuries in central Africa. It remained undetected only because of the lack of diagnostic facilities. The clinical symptoms of Aids (such as fever and pneumonia) were ascribed to malaria and TB. The spread of HIV/Aids was limited because there was little contact with outsiders, and it was introduced to the Western world only when international travel became more common.

One of the arguments against this theory is that modern testing of archived blood samples from Africa rarely shows any signs of HIV infection before the 1980s (Schoub, 1999:14). In tests carried out on these frozen blood samples, the earliest sample shown to be positive for HIV antibodies was taken in 1959 in Kinshasa in the then Belgian Congo. Also, doctors with many years of clinical experience in Africa deny that before the 1980s they ever saw diseases resembling the very obvious characteristics of Aids. It seems that Aids is indeed a new disease and that HIV was introduced into the human population in the 1950s.

Did HIV cross the species barrier?

The second theory about the origin of Aids is that HIV crossed the species barrier from primates to humans at some time during the twentieth century (Korber, 2000). HIV is related to a virus called SIV or simian immunodeficiency virus, which is found in primates. There are a number of SIV strains and each strain is specific to the monkey species that it infects. For example, SIVagm infects the African green monkey, SIVmnd infects the mandrill ape, and SIVsm the sooty mangabey monkey (Schoub, 1999). Under natural conditions, each strain will infect only its own specific species of monkey and it will also not infect humans. HIV also cannot infect any animal other than humans, except under experimental laboratory conditions where infection can be induced in chimpanzees. Immunodeficiency viruses occur in other animals too, for example in cats, cattle, horses, sheep and goats, but natural infections with these viruses are also species-specific and will not spread to animals from other species.

Within the SIV group of viruses, SIVsm (the sooty mangabey virus) shows the closest relationship to an HIV strain, and specifically to HIV-2. It is interesting to note that HIV-2 is confined mostly to West Africa, which is also the natural habitat of the sooty mangabey monkey. However, the link between HIV-1 and SIV is not so clear. According to Schoub (1999:15)

> . . . this missing link may have been discovered by the isolation of a virus from a captive chimpanzee in Gabon in 1989. This virus (called SIVcpz) is far more closely related to HIV-1 than any other immuno-deficiency virus, and it is also the only virus that possesses the same set of genes as HIV-1.

Scientists still treat this finding with some reserve. This chimpanzee was a captive animal, and it is therefore possible that SIVcpz could be a human virus which for some unknown reason infected that particular chimpanzee.

The question still remains how simian viruses could have been transmitted from monkeys to humans. It is believed that the virus probably crossed from primates to humans when contaminated animal blood entered cuts on the hands of people who were butchering SIV-infected animals for food. Another possibility is that chimpanzee and monkey blood, which was used for malaria research long ago, could have been the conduit into the human species.

There is also a theory that incriminates early oral polio vaccines as the source of SIV infection of humans with its subsequent mutation to HIV (Hooper, 1999). Early trials of oral polio vaccines in the late 1950s were carried out by spraying prototype vaccines into the mouths and throats of several hundred thousand people in Rwanda, Zaire and Burundi, precisely the early epicentre of the Aids epidemic in Africa. Oral polio vaccines, which contain a suspension of live vaccine strains of the polio virus, are produced on cell cultures derived from the kidneys of African green monkeys. It is believed by some that the vaccines could have been contaminated by SIVagm from the monkey kidneys at a time when vaccines were not tested for contaminating simian viruses. Schoub believes that theories like this may cause untold harm to immunisation programmes such as the global effort to eradicate polio.

In summary it can be said that the Aids epidemic began in humans in the late seventies and early eighties, and that there were only a few isolated cases of Aids-like diseases before then. Although the virus probably crossed the species barrier from primates to humans, it is impossible to say exactly how or when that happened. The initial spread of HIV was probably limited to isolated communities in Africa who had little contact with the outside world, but various factors, such as migration, improved transportation networks, tourism, socio-economic instability, multiple sexual partners, injecting drug use and an exchange of blood products, ultimately caused the virus to spread all over the world.

Enrichment

How is HIV prevalence measured?

National estimates of HIV prevalence in countries with HIV/Aids epidemics are based on data about pregnant women tested for HIV at antenatal clinics (UNAIDS, 2003:6). This assumes that HIV prevalence among pregnant women is similar to that of the rest of the adult population (aged 15 to 49).

This assumption was tested in studies conducted in a number of African countries. HIV prevalence among pregnant women at antenatal clinics was compared with the prevalence detected by voluntary HIV testing surveys among the adult population (men and non-pregnant women) in the same community.

These studies confirmed the assumption that HIV prevalence among pregnant women is roughly equivalent to the prevalence among the adult population in urban and in rural areas. Both sources of data (pregnant women and voluntary testing surveys) have advantages and disadvantages, and there is no absolute standard for HIV surveillance. All HIV estimates need to be assessed critically, whether they are based on a national survey or on sentinel surveillance data (on pregnant women).

Data from antenatal clinics are especially useful for assessing HIV trends, and national surveys help to fill out the picture of the epidemic. Such surveys, conducted every three to five years, can be valuable components of surveillance systems and can help improve estimates of the levels and trends in HIV prevalence.

1.4 THE HIV/AIDS EPIDEMIC: A GRIM PICTURE

By the end of 2003 there were approximately 37.8 million people in the world living with HIV/Aids. (Estimates range from 34.6 to 42.3 million.) Of these, about 35.7 million were adults, and 2.1 million were children younger than 15 (UNAIDS, 2004). The global epidemic has already killed more than 3 million people, and it is estimated that in 2003 alone, a further 5 million people acquired HIV.

Sub-Saharan Africa remains by far the region worst affected by HIV/Aids. According to the UNAIDS epidemic update (UNAIDS, 2004) the epidemic in sub-Saharan Africa remains rampant, with 23.1 to 27.9 million adults and children living with HIV/Aids.

How long it will stay like this will depend on the vigour, scale and effectiveness of prevention, treat-

> ment and care programmes. Urgent and dramatic headway is required on all these fronts, and in unison. Anything less will spell failure.
>
> (UNAIDS, 2003:4)

HIV prevalence varies considerably across the continent. It ranges from less than 1% in Mauritania to almost 40% in Botswana and Swaziland. Although southern Africa has less than 2% of the world's population, it is home to about 30% of the world's people living with HIV/Aids. More than one in five pregnant women are HIV positive in most countries in southern Africa.

A trend analysis of antenatal clinic sites in eight countries (between 1997 and 2002) shows HIV prevalence among pregnant women levelling off at almost 40% in Gaborone (Botswana) and Manzini (Swaziland), and at almost 16% in Blantyre (Malawi) and 20% in Lusaka (Zambia). Prevalence exceeded 30% in South Africa's mainly urban Gauteng province, and in Maputo (Mozambique) it was 18% in 2002.

In South Africa, 2002 surveillance data show that, countrywide, the average rate of HIV prevalence in pregnant women attending antenatal clinics has remained roughly at the same high levels since 1998 – ranging between 22% and 23% in 1998–1999 and then shifting even higher to around 25% in 2000–2002. A slight decline in prevalence among pregnant teenagers has been offset by consistently high HIV levels among pregnant women aged 20–24, and rising levels among those aged 25–34 (see Figure 1.1 on page 8).

In five of South Africa's nine provinces, including those with the biggest populations, at least 25% of pregnant women are now HIV positive. The epidemic varies within South Africa: in KwaZulu-Natal HIV prevalence among those who attend antenatal clinics is almost 37%, about three times higher than in the Western Cape, the province with the lowest prevalence.

Based on surveillance of antenatal clinics, it is estimated that 5.3 million South Africans were living with HIV at the end of 2003. The epidemic started only relatively recently in South Africa, and current trends indicate that Aids deaths will continue to increase rapidly over the next five years at least.

> In short, the worst still lies ahead. Only a speedily realised national antiretroviral programme could significantly cushion the country against the impact.
>
> (UNAIDS, 2003:8–9)

In 12 years, HIV prevalence in people between the ages of 15 and 49 rose from less than 1% to about 21.5% in South Africa.

In four neighbouring countries – Botswana, Lesotho, Namibia and Swaziland – the epidemic has assumed devastating proportions. HIV prevalence has reached extremely high levels in these countries without showing any signs of levelling off. In 2003, national HIV prevalence in Swaziland and in Botswana was almost 39%. Just a decade earlier, both had stood at 4%. Neither in Botswana nor in Swaziland is there any sign of a significant decline in HIV prevalence among young pregnant women aged 15–24. HIV prevalence in antenatal sites in Namibia rose to over 21% in 2003, while Lesotho's 2003 data show an increase among antenatal clinic attendees to an infection rate of 30% (UNAIDS, 2003:9).

The HIV infection rate in Zimbabwe is about 24.6%, with no real signs of decline. There are signs that the epidemic has levelled off in Zambia, where the national HIV prevalence has remained stable since the mid-1990s at almost 16% of the age group 15–49 years. In Mozambique, median HIV prevalence ranged from 8% among pregnant women in the north to 15% and 17% respectively in the centre and south. Angola gives cause for concern despite the comparatively low HIV levels of 3.9% detected to date. After almost four decades of war, huge population movements are under way. Millions of people have been able to leave the cities and towns they had been trapped in; internal and cross-border trading movements are resuming; and an estimated 450 000 refugees are returning (many from neighbouring countries with high HIV prevalence rates). Such conditions could prime a sudden eruption of the epidemic (UNAIDS, 2003:10). (See Figure 1.2 on page 8 for HIV prevalence among adults aged 15–49 in southern African countries at the end of 2003.)

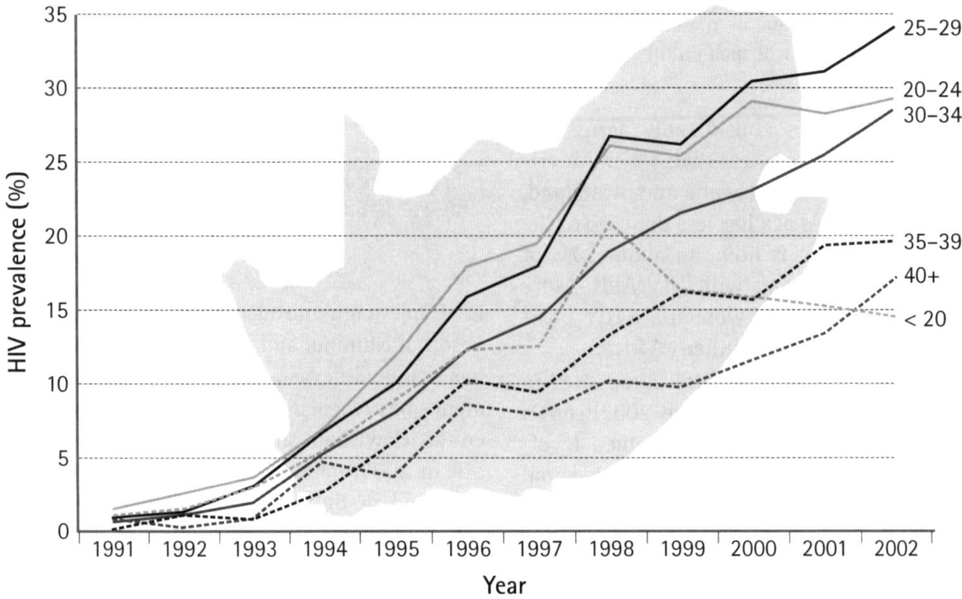

Figure 1.1

HIV prevalence among pregnant women at antenatal clinics in South Africa, by age group: 1991–2002

(Source: Department of Health, South Africa)

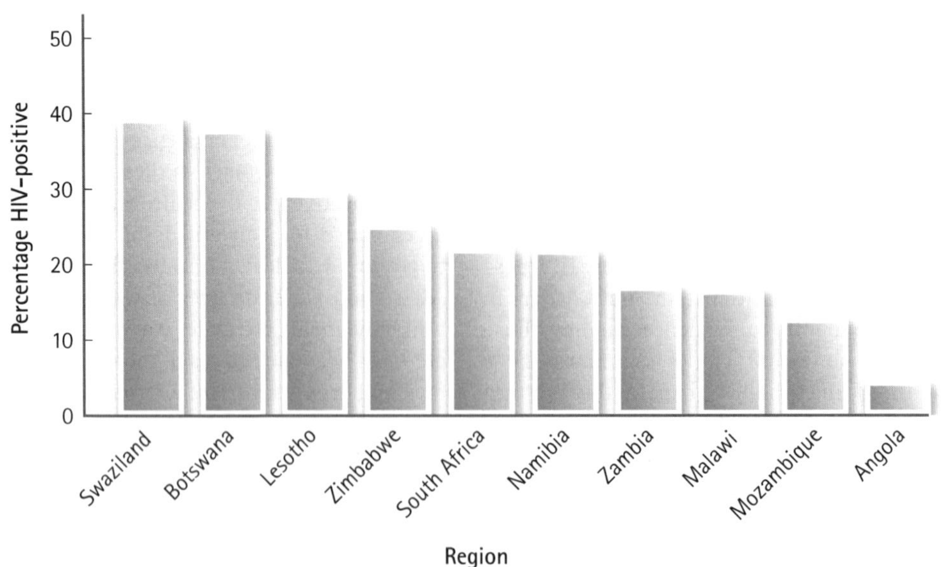

Figure 1.2

HIV prevalence among adults (15–49) in southern African countries at the end of 2003

A distinct picture emerges in East Africa and parts of Central Africa where the HIV prevalence continues to recede. In Kampala, Uganda, HIV prevalence fell to 8% in 2002 – a remarkable feat considering that the HIV prevalence among pregnant women in two urban antenatal clinics in the city stood at 30% a decade ago. To date, no other country has matched this achievement. HIV prevalence among pregnant women also showed a modest decline in Rwanda, Ethiopia, Kenya and parts of the Democratic Republic of the Congo. In West Africa the prevalence varies from around 1% in Senegal to the much graver situation in Cote d'Ivoire, where more than 10% of pregnant women are HIV positive.

Although there has been an upsurge of political support, stronger policy formulation, boosted funding and moves towards cushioning societies against the impact of the Aids epidemic, much more has to be done if the epidemic is to be reversed in Africa. National reports tracking progress towards implementation of HIV/Aids prevention programmes show that many countries have no national orphan policies in place; voluntary counselling and testing coverage is threadbare; and prevention of mother-to-child transmission is virtually non-existent in many of the hardest-hit countries (UNAIDS, 2003:13). Over 70% of countries reporting from Africa on efforts to reduce HIV transmission to infants and young children have virtually no programmes to administer prophylactic antiretroviral therapy to women during childbirth and to newborns. Almost half the African countries reporting have not adopted legislation to prevent discrimination against people living with HIV/Aids. Only one in four countries reports that at least 50% of patients with other sexually transmitted infections (co-factors for HIV infection) are being diagnosed, counselled and treated.

Antiretroviral treatment coverage remains low in low- and middle-income countries. The World Health Organization estimated that only 400 000 people had access to antiretroviral drugs in 2003, while 5–6 million people in these countries need ART immediately. Some countries such as Botswana, Cameroon, Eritrea, Nigeria, Uganda and recently South Africa have made serious efforts to increase access to antiretroviral drugs through both the public and private sectors.

Enrichment

The HIV epidemic – where to get the picture

If you want to obtain the most up-to-date information about HIV/Aids in Africa as well as in the rest of the world, visit the UNAIDS website: http:/www.unaids.org. If you don't have access to the Internet, read your local papers, visit your local HIV/Aids prevention centres, and get information from your government's health department. The *Mail & Guardian's* Aids barometer is an example of where to get the latest statistics.

1.5 WHAT IS A VIRUS?

Before discussing the HI virus in particular, we will look at the characteristics of viruses in general. A virus is a very small organism, and unlike other life forms (e.g. human cells) they cannot replicate themselves (or make copies of themselves) within their own cores, because they do not have the chemical 'machinery' to do so. Viruses are parasites in the sense that they need to use the biochemical facilities of living cells (such as human cells) to reproduce. Outside a living cell, viruses are nothing but inactive, lifeless and harmless chemicals. Viruses transport their own genetic material into living cells, and then use the 'machinery' of the cells to make more copies of themselves.

Viruses (like all living cells) have genes necessary for their replication. Genes hold the master code of an organism and determine what the organism is and how it functions. Like human cells, most viruses contain DNA in their cores. However, some viruses (such as HIV) have RNA instead of DNA in their cores, and these are called retroviruses. Retroviruses are the only living organisms with RNA in their nuclei.

All viruses consist of two main parts:

- The *core* houses the genetic material or genes (DNA or RNA).
- The *capsule* or shell protects the core and forms the outer layer of the virus. It acts as a vehicle to transfer the virus from cell to cell and from person to person. This capsule is composed of protein projections (or glycoprotein projections) that look like spikes. The virus uses these spikes to attach itself to the

specific receptors (or binding sites) of a host cell that it will infect. The protein projections on the virus and the receptor sites on the cell can be compared to a lock and key. The key on the virus (glycoprotein projection) will fit only into a specific lock (the receptor or binding site on the capsule of the host cell).

Some viruses (such as HIV) also have a third component called a *lipid envelope*, which is a loose, fragile membrane covering the capsule (Schoub, 1999:57). In the case of HIV, the glycoproteins are embedded in the envelope.

One of the characteristic features of viruses is that they infect only specific cells. A specific virus can also only attach to a very specific receptor site on the host cell (the key-and-lock interaction as described above). The protective function of the immune system is based on this specificity of viruses. It produces antibodies that attach themselves to the outermost proteins of the virus. An antibody acts as a shield between the virus and the host cell, and so prevents the virus from attaching to the cell's receptor sites. But if the structure of the antigen (or foreign substance) changes, the antibody cannot attach to it, and then the host's immune protection system cannot function. (See enrichment box 'The definition of an antigen' below.)

1.6 HIV: THE HUMAN IMMUNODEFICIENCY VIRUS

Aids is caused by the human immunodeficiency virus. HIV was the first member of the retrovirus family to occur in humans (Schoub, 1999). Before the mid-1970s, retroviruses occurred primarily in the animal kingdom. Retroviruses are usually very simple viruses, but HIV is very complex. HIV can change itself so quickly that different variants of the virus can be found in a single infected individual. HIV also has the extraordinary ability to evade the immune system of the host.

The HI virus is roughly circular in shape (see Figure 1.3 on page 11). The inner core of the virus is cone-shaped, and this is the chief feature by which the HI virus is recognised through an electron microscope. The genetic material of the virus (two copies of single-stranded RNA) as well as the reverse transcriptase enzyme are housed in the core of the virus. The main protein of the core of the virus is called p24, and it plays an important role in diagnosing HIV infection.

The core of the virus is surrounded by an envelope (the outer layer of the virus). Two very important viral proteins or antigens (called glycoproteins) are anchored into the outer surface of the envelope. The first envelope protein is a knob-like protein called gp120, and the other is a smaller spike-like protein called gp41. These proteins play a critical role in the initial steps of infection (attachment and penetration into the cell) as well as in the production of antibodies that neutralise the virus. The gp120 makes contact with the cells to be infected, and binds to the CD4 receptors. (These are described further on.) The gp41 fuses the envelope of the virus to the membrane of the host cell, thus allowing the entry of the virus into the cell for the further steps of replication.

Like other viruses, HIV can reproduce itself only by becoming a 'parasite' inside a living cell. It cannot live and multiply outside human cells. But this is true of *all* viruses, so what makes HIV so dangerous? The answer is that the HI virus does something that no other known virus has ever done: it directly attacks and hijacks the most important defensive cells of the human

Enrichment

The definition of an antigen

An antigen is any foreign (or invading) substance which, when introduced into the body, elicits an immune response such as, for example, the production of antibodies that react specifically with these antigens. Antigens are almost always composed of proteins, and they are usually present on the surface of viruses or bacteria. When antibodies react to antigens, they can either destroy or de-activate the antigens.

Activity

Devise a series of transparencies to explain what Aids is, what the HI virus looks like, and where it comes from (historical background). Try to make use of descriptive pictures rather than words.

immune system, the CD4 or T helper cells. As it does this, it slowly reduces the total number of healthy CD4 cells in the body – thereby progressively weakening the ability of the human immune system to defend itself against attack from outside.

What makes HIV so effective in destroying human lives is that, as far as we know, *the defenders of our immune systems (the CD4 or T helper cells) have no way of defending us against the HI virus.*

To understand fully how HIV attacks the immune system, it is necessary first of all to understand how a healthy immune system functions. We will now look at how the immune system successfully defends the body against attack by *other* bacteria or viruses – viruses such as the well-known influenza or 'flu' virus (Evian, 2000; Gayton, 1971; Jaret, 1986; Mader, 1998; Selwyn, 1986; Weber & Weiss, 1988). When we understand the differences between how HIV and an ordinary virus (such as the flu virus) attacks the immune system, we will understand:

- exactly how HIV is different from other viruses; and
- why the human body is ultimately defenceless against HIV invasion.

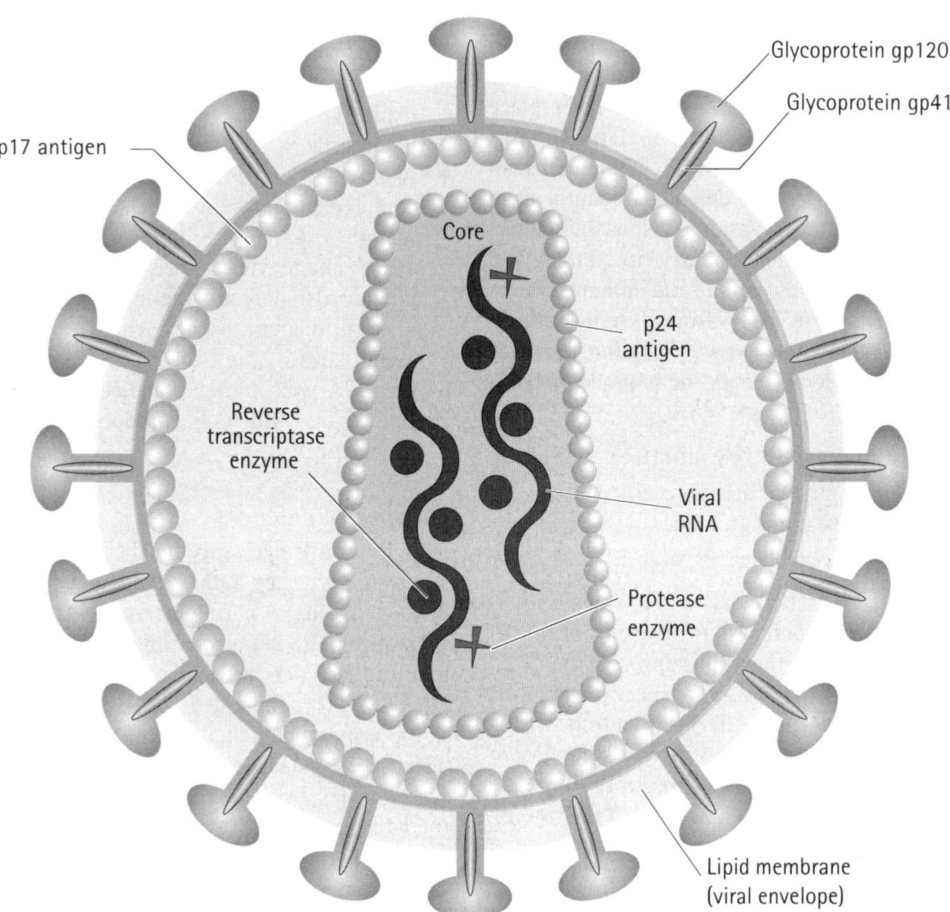

Figure 1.3
A model of the structure of the HI virus

1.7 HOW A HEALTHY IMMUNE SYSTEM FUNCTIONS

Immunity is the ability of the body to defend itself against infectious agents, foreign cells and even abnormal body cells such as cancer cells. The body must have an efficient immune system to avoid being taken over by parasites, bacteria, viruses and toxins. The body's immune system is a complex system of blood proteins and white blood cells that work together to repel attacks by invading organisms. The lymphatic system, especially the lymph nodes, the spleen, the thymus gland and the bone marrow, plays an important role in the development of these blood proteins and white blood cells.

The war within us

The best way to understand the immune system is to imagine a microscopic *war* that takes place inside the body (Jaret, 1986). In terms of this metaphor, we can characterise the immune system as the *defence force* that defends a country from external threats and invasions. Just as the soldiers of an army defend their country from attack and invasion, the various parts of the immune system defend the human body from external attack. Before we explore the war within us further, let us meet the key role players of the immune system.

Key role players in the immune system

The defences of the immune system can be divided into two main groups:

- the *non-specific defences*; and
- the *specific defences.*

The non-specific defences form the front line of the body's army. If they fail to protect the body, the full force of the army, the specific defences, are called in to fight off the invading organisms. Figure 1.4 on page 13 gives a summary of the most important role players in the immune system. Use this summary to follow the discussion on the defences of the immune system.

The non-specific defences

Three types of non-specific defences are effective in protecting the body against many types of infectious agents. These non-specific defences are: barriers to entry, the inflammatory reaction, and protective proteins.

- The skin and the mucous membranes lining the respiratory, digestive and urinary tracts serve as mechanical *barriers to entry* by microbes.
- Any minor injury that breaks the skin causes an *inflammatory reaction*, characterised by redness, pain, swelling and heat. Such a break in the skin allows microbes to enter the body, and the resulting inflammatory reaction is a call-up for phagocytic white blood cells (e.g. *macrophages*) to the site of bacterial invasion to devour or eat the bacteria. Some tissues in the body have resident macrophages, which routinely act as scavengers, devouring old blood cells, bits of dead tissue and other debris. Macrophages can also stimulate the immune response by bringing about an explosive increase in the number of white blood cells.
- A number of *plasma proteins*, also called complement proteins, are activated when microbes enter the body. These proteins attract phagocytes to the scene of infection to phagocytise (devour) the microbes. They can also kill bacteria by attacking the walls and membranes of the bacteria, making holes in them. (A well-known complement protein is interferon, which is produced by virus-infected cells.)

The specific defences

Sometimes it is necessary for the body to rely on a *specific defence* rather than a non-specific defence against a particular antigen (or foreign substance). The main role players in the specific immune defence are the *lymphocytes*. Lymphocytes are subdivided into two main functional groups, namely *T lymphocytes* (so called because they mature in the *t*hymus gland) and *B lymphocytes* (so called because they mature in the *b*one marrow.)

The T lymphocytes are themselves subdivided into various subtypes, mainly on functional grounds. The two most prominent lymphocyte subtypes are the *CD4 lymphocytes* (also called the T helper lymphocytes) and the *CD8 lymphocytes* (also called the suppressor

T lymphocytes). The CD4 lymphocytes are the main regulatory cells of the immune system because they enhance the response of other immune cells. The CD8 or suppressor T lymphocyte has the opposing effect to the CD4 lymphocyte and acts to balance it. Suppressor T cells, for example, regulate the immune response by suppressing further development of CD4 cells. Under normal circumstances there are approximately four times as many CD4 lymphocytes as there are CD8 lymphocytes.

T lymphocytes can be subdivided further into *killer T lymphocytes* (or cytotoxic T lymphocytes) and *memory T lymphocytes*. When activated as part of the immune response the killer T cells will kill cells infected by a particular micro-organism such as a virus, as one way of eliminating the intruding organism. Killer T cells also attack viruses by producing soluble proteins that inhibit the replication of viruses inside infected cells (Schoub, 1999:79). A population of memory T cells usually persists, perhaps for life, after suppression of the immune response by the suppressor T cells. These memory T cells can stimulate macrophages and B cells whenever the same antigen re-enters the body.

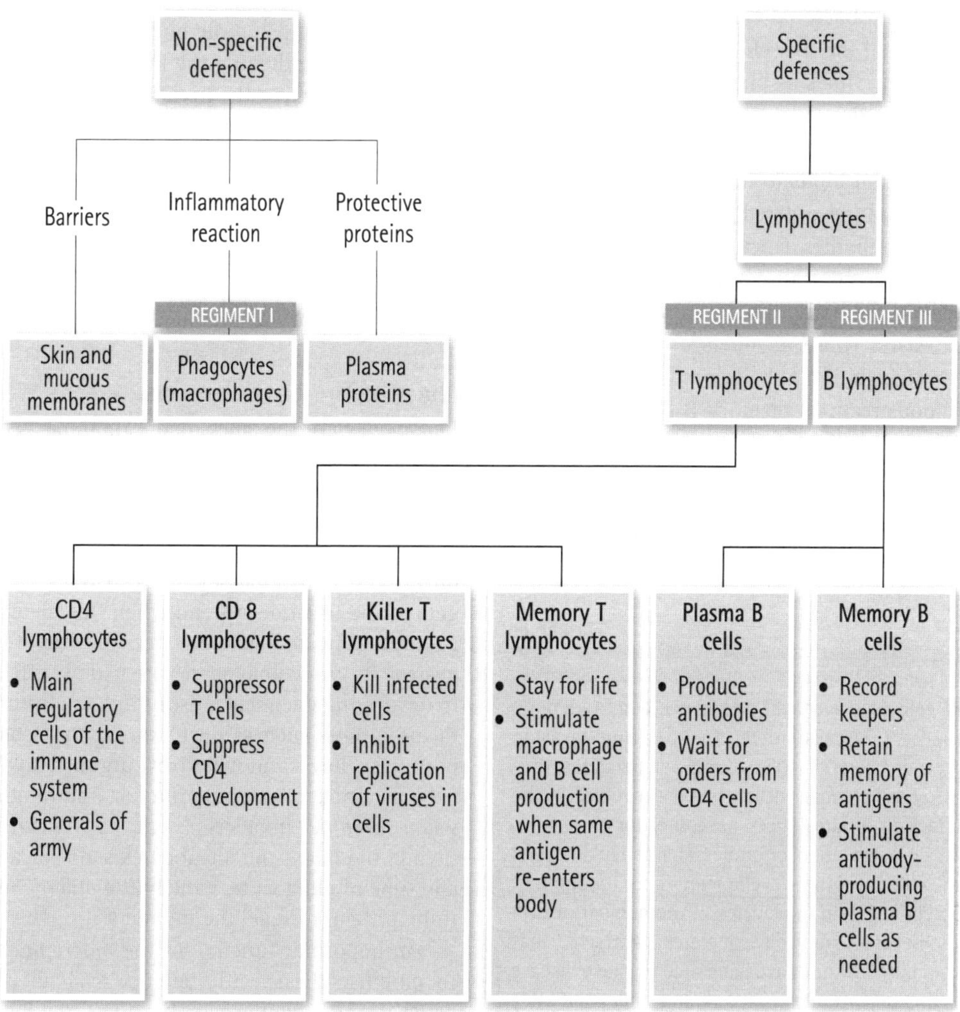

Figure 1.4
The key role players in the immune system

B lymphocytes (or B cells) give rise to *plasma B cells* and *memory B cells*. Plasma B cells produce antibodies, while memory B cells – the record keepers of the immune system – retain a 'memory' of antigens they have experienced for a more rapid response on re-exposure to the same antigen. Each type of B cell makes an antibody specially equipped to recognise the specific shape of a particular antigen. This means that our immune systems produce up to a billion different antibody types to combat all the microbes we are likely to encounter. When a B cell with its specific antibody (receptor) on its surface encounters a bacterial cell bearing an appropriate antigen, the B cell becomes activated to divide many times as plasma cells to mass-produce antibodies against that specific antigen. Note that a B cell does not clone until its antigen is present and binds to its receptors, and until it is stimulated (or 'ordered') by CD4 cells to mass-produce antibodies. Once antibody production is sufficient to neutralise the amount of antigen present in the body, the development of plasma cells ceases. Those members of a clone that do not participate in antibody production remain in the bloodstream as memory B cells. If the same antigen enters the system again, memory B cells quickly divide and give rise to new antibody-producing plasma cells. Memory B and memory T cells are the means by which active, long-term immunity is possible.

Enrichment

Role of CD4 cells in the body's immune response

CD4 cells play a crucial role in the body's immune response. CD4 cells protect the body from invasion by certain bacteria, viruses, fungi and parasites; they destroy some cancer cells; they are involved in the production of substances necessary for the body's defence, such as interferon and interleukins; and they influence the development and function of macrophages and monocytes. If the number of CD4 cells becomes radically depleted, antigens that would normally not have been able to cause disease use this opportunity to attack and infect the body (Evian, 2000). That is why such infections are called *opportunistic infections*.

The soldiers of the immune system at war

We will now look at how the white blood cells ('soldiers') work together to protect the body against invading organisms.

The white blood cells can be divided into *three regiments*: (1) the phagocytes (including macrophages), (2) the T lymphocytes, and (3) the B lymphocytes (see Figure 1.4). Each of these regiments has its own mission and defence strategy, but they all have the same objective: to identify and destroy all invasive substances or organisms that might be harmful to the body.

There are *four phases* in each immune response the body makes:

Phase I: Recognising the enemy
Phase II: Strengthening the body's defence
Phase III: Attacking the invader
Phase IV: Halting the attack once the battle has been won

The function of each 'regiment' (phagocytes, T cells and B cells) during the four phases of immune response is illustrated in Figure 1.5 on page 15. (In the explanation that follows, the numbers refer to the numbers in the illustration.)

Phase I: The battle begins

Phagocytes are the spies of the immune system, constantly patrolling the whole body (the bloodstream, tissue and lymphatic system). Their purpose is to identify any substance, object or organism that is foreign (and potentially dangerous) to the body. Phagocytes are also the scavengers of the immune system: when they detect an enemy, they immediately try to engulf and destroy it. While phagocytes are usually effective in destroying chemical poisons and environmental pollutants such as dust, smoke and asbestos particles, they cannot destroy organic invaders such as viruses, bacteria, protozoa and fungi. So, when *organic* invaders (such as flu viruses) invade the body, the phagocytes send for a special type of phagocyte, namely the *macrophages*, to help them to repel the invaders.

An important function of the *macrophages* is to mobilise the specific defence system, which consists of the *lymphocytes* (i.e. the T and B cells). The macrophage achieves this defensive mobilisation by surrounding the virus and capturing a specific particle, called an *antigen*, from the invading virus. The macrophage then displays this antigen on its own cell surface as a 'captured banner or flag of war' (Jaret, 1986). This flag (the antigen) plays a critical role in the immune system's response: it alerts the next 'regiment', namely the *T cells*, to attack the invaders. (See encircled part in Phase I in Figure 1.5.)

T cells are preprogrammed in the thymus to recognise the antigen (the 'flag' carried by the macrophage) by its shape. The antigens on the surface of the virus fit exactly into the receptors of T cells (like pieces of a puzzle). In the thymus, the T cells 'learn' to recognise all the antigens (puzzle pieces) that nature may create – and these occur in millions of different forms. Thus, for example, one T cell may learn to recognise (or fit) the antigen of the hepatitis virus, while another may recognise a certain type of flu antigen. There are even T cells that can recognise artificial antigens manufactured in laboratories – antigens that the body has never encountered in millions of years of evolution.

The type of T cell that recognises the antigen (or the 'banner' displayed by the macrophage) is the *CD4 cell* (or *T helper cell*). The CD4 cells are the most important cells in the immune system – they are the generals or commanders of the body's defensive army. After the macrophages present their banners of war (antigens) to the CD4 cells, the CD4 cells combine forces with the macrophages and so the next phase of the war begins (see enrichment box 'Macrophages as antigen-presenting cells' on page 17).

Phase II: The forces multiply

Once the CD4 cells have combined with the macrophages, they activate the remaining components of the defence system in order to mobilise

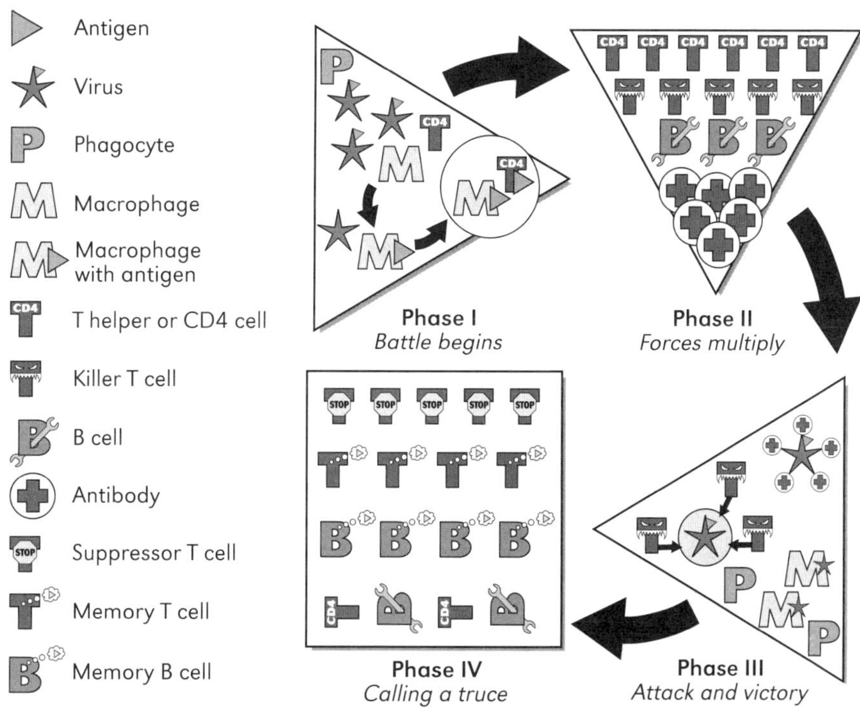

Figure 1.5
How the immune system functions
(Source: Adapted from Jaret, 1986:708–709)

Enrichment

Explaining the immune system to children

Just like a country, the body has to be protected from nasty invaders who want to harm it. So, like a country, the body needs a defence force. Meet the body's defence force!

The *Phagocytes* (a type of white blood cell) are on security patrol. While on their usual rounds looking for intruders, they spot a real nasty customer – a member of the Flu Virus terror gang. The Phagocytes immediately ask headquarters to send *Macrophages* to come and check out the situation. The Macrophages (type of white blood cell) confiscate the invader's identity document (an *antigen*) and decide that they'll have to call in the big guys: the *CD4* Division – T Cells or *T Helper Cells* who help protect the body against dangerous outside forces.

General CD4 takes one look at the invading virus's ID document and immediately recognises the invader as a Flu Virus. She realises that the body is in trouble, and straight away gives the command to attack. The CD4 cells join the Macrophages and together they activate the body's defence system. They call in more CD4 cells and Phagocytes and they send messages to the crack troops, the *B Cells* and *Killer T Cells,* to join them.

Meanwhile the Flu Viruses are hiding in the body's cells where they try to multiply their forces as quickly as they can. But the Killer T Cells, with the help of some of the CD4 Cells, drive the Flu Viruses out of their hiding places by destroying these hiding places (the cells). While this is happening, the B Cells are working very hard to manufacture *antibodies.* These antibodies now grab the exposed Flu Viruses, cling to them, slow them down and make them easy targets for the Phagocytes to attack and destroy. When all the invaders have been killed, the body can slowly begin to return to normal once again.

The last stage is in the hands of the peacemaking corps, the *Suppressor T Cells.* When the situation is under control, they order the B Cells to stop making antibodies, and the Killer T Cells to stop their attack. Phagocytes clean up the litter of dead cells and other substances, and the body begins to heal.

But this incident will not be forgotten: the *Memory T* and *Memory B Cells* in the records department, will always remember the Flu Viruses. If they ever again try to invade, they will be recognised immediately and stopped in their tracks – the body is now immune to attacks by the Flu Virus gang.

its full capacity. Thus, as the CD4 cells begin to multiply, they activate more phagocytes and send chemical messages ('orders') to the *B cells* and *killer T cells* – which are sensitive to the invading virus – to multiply. (See Phase II in Figure 1.5.)

These *B cells* (or the third 'regiment') are located in the lymph nodes, and we may compare them to small munitions factories. The B cells then multiply and divide into two groups: *plasma B cells* and *memory B cells.* The plasma B cells manufacture antibodies that render invading organisms harmless by neutralising them or by clinging to their surfaces (thus preventing them from performing their function).

Phase III: The attack and victory

While the immune system prepares its forces, the viruses will already have penetrated some of the cells in the body. When they are ready, the *killer T cells* (with the aid of certain CD4 cells) destroy these infected cells by chemically piercing their membranes so that the contents spill out. This 'spilling out' interrupts the multiplication cycle of the virus (see Phase III in Figure 1.5). Once the contents of an infected cell have spilled out, *antibodies* neutralise the viruses by attaching themselves to the viruses' surfaces, thereby preventing them from attacking other cells. This slows the progress of the invading organisms and makes them easy victims for the *phagocytes* or the macrophages, which then come to 'digest' them. Antibodies also produce chemical reactions that can kill infected cells. When all the invaders have been destroyed, the war is won and all that remains to be done is 'demobilisation'.

Phase IV: The cessation of hostility

Once the attackers have been vanquished, a third member of the T cell family takes control: the *suppressor T* or peacemaker (see Phase IV in Figure 1.5). Suppressor T cells release a substance that stops B cells from doing their work (namely the manufacture of antibodies). They also 'order' the killer T cells to stop attacking and the CD4 cells to stop their work.

Memory T and *B cells* 'remember' the specific invader (antigen) and they remain in the blood and lymphatic system – ready to act defensively should the same virus once again invade the body. At this point, the 'war' has been won and the person will in future be immune to this particular virus. (See enrichment box 'Explaining the immune system to children' on page 16.)

It usually takes from a week to a few months to develop effective immunity against invading agents. When we are first exposed to a disease, we may become very ill because we have not yet developed immunity, but later, when again exposed to the same invading agent, our immune systems will quickly counter it before any damage can be done. So, if we are exposed to very small doses (not enough to make us really ill) of some types of dangerous invading agents such as tetanus toxin, we will develop immunity against that agent. This immunity is so effective that we will later be able to withstand 100 000 times the normally lethal dose of that toxin without any ill effects. This example illustrates how extremely efficient the body can be in developing the kind of immunity it needs to protect itself against foreign invasive agents (Gayton, 1971:118).

Enrichment

Macrophages as antigen-presenting cells

CD4 cells (as well as killer T cells) are unable to recognise an antigen (or foreign substance) that is present in lymph or blood. They have to rely on an *antigen-presenting cell* (or APC) to present the antigen ('banner of war') to them. When an APC, usually a macrophage, engulfs a microbe, the microbe is broken down into antigen fragments. These antigen fragments are linked to certain proteins, and only then can they be presented to a T cell. Once a macrophage presents an antigen to a CD4 cell, the CD4 cell multiplies and stimulates the production of memory T cells which can recognise this same antigen. Once a killer T cell recognises an antigen, it attacks and destroys any cell that is infected with the same virus. Antigen-presenting cells are found throughout the body but especially in the bloodstream, in the lymph nodes and in mucous membranes. In the mucous membranes, these cells are called Langerhans cells and they have direct implications for HIV infection, as they are important vehicles for transporting HIV from the mucous membranes of the genital tract to the lymph nodes (Schoub, 1999:76).

1.8 THE EFFECT OF HIV ON THE IMMUNE SYSTEM

If the body is so efficient in protecting itself against invading organisms, why can it not protect itself against HIV? What makes HIV different from other viruses such as the flu virus? How does HIV elude the immune system?

When HIV invades the body, the macrophages attempt to do their usual job by capturing a particle (an antigen) from HIV. *But it is when the macrophages attempt to make contact with the CD4 cells to warn them about the invasion that the real problem begins. The HI viruses attack the CD4 cells directly – the unique response that makes HIV so dangerous (and ultimately fatal) to human beings.* Figure 1.6 on page 18 illustrates the life cycle of the HI virus and shows how HIV 'hijacks' the CD4 cell and forces it to channel its activities into manufacturing more viruses. We will now explain exactly how HIV invades CD4 cells. Have a look at Figure 1.6 to follow the process.

The glycoprotein projections on the virus's outer layer (gp120) attach themselves firmly to the outer layer of the CD4 cell (onto a CD4 receptor). (See Step 1 in Figure 1.6.) After attachment, the gp120 protein splits open to expose the gp41 protein, which is otherwise covered by the gp120. The gp41 now causes fusion to take place between the viral envelope and the cell membrane (see Step 2 in Figure 1.6).

The virus then sheds its outer layer and enters the CD4 cell. The core protein capsule of the virus breaks open, releasing two copies of single-stranded viral RNA as well as the reverse transcriptase enzyme (Step 3). In order to use the CD4 cell to manufacture more viruses, the HIV's viral RNA must be changed (reverse transcribed) to viral DNA. The HIV itself carries with it an enzyme called *reverse transcriptase* which it then uses to transform its viral RNA into double-stranded proviral DNA (Step 4).

The proviral DNA then fuses with the host cell's own DNA in the nucleus of the cell with the help of the viral enzyme, integrase (Step 5), and makes numerous copies of viral RNA and viral proteins (Step 6). The enzyme protease enables this new viral RNA and the viral proteins to assemble into new viral particles which are released from the cell as fully functional HI viruses (Step 7). As the new HI viruses bud from the cell, they kill the hijacked cell in the process. They then move out into the bloodstream or surrounding tissue to infect more cells – and repeat the whole process over again.

Although all viruses live and multiply solely in cells, HIV hijacks the most important defensive cells in the immune system, the CD4 cells, and turns them into efficient virus factories to manufacture perfect replicas of themselves (the viruses). When this happens, the CD4 cells are unable to do what they would normally do when confronted by an alien virus, that is, orchestrate and coordinate the body's defences *against* the HI viruses. Instead, they themselves are captured and forcibly turned into small factories to *manufacture* HI viruses, the very carriers of death against which they are supposed to defend the body.

Although several antibodies are formed during this process, they are completely powerless to protect the body against the long-term destructive effects of the HI virus. The body is left defenceless. The soldiers cannot function effectively without any orders from their generals.

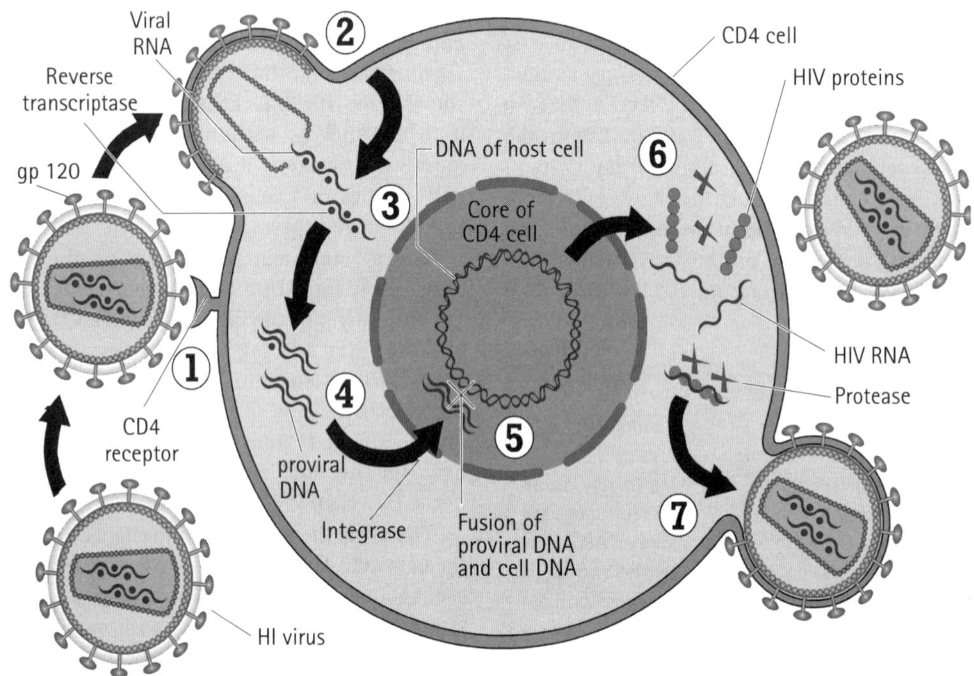

Step 1: The HI virus attaches to the CD4 cell's receptors.
Step 2: The CD4 cell and HI virus join membranes.
Step 3: The HI virus injects its RNA (as well as reverse transcriptase) into the CD4 cell.
Step 4: Viral RNA is changed into proviral DNA through a process called reverse transcription.
Step 5: The proviral DNA joins with the cell's DNA in the core of the cell, causing it to produce more viral RNA and viral proteins.
Step 6: The viral RNA and viral proteins assemble into more HI viruses.
Step 7: The new viruses break free from the cell, killing it and infecting more cells.

Figure 1.6
How the HI virus invades a CD4 cell

Why is it important to understand the replication process of the HI virus?

An understanding of the replication process helps us understand why HIV eludes the immune system. Also, each stage in the replication cycle may provide an opportunity for the design of an effective antiretroviral drug (Schoub, 1999).

Does HIV infect only CD4 cells?

Not only CD4 cells are infected by HIV. The glycoprotein projections (gp120) on the virus's outer layer attach themselves to *CD4 receptors*, which are present on various types of cells such as monocytes (a large phagocytic white blood cell), macrophages, the Langerhans cells found in the skin and in the mucous membranes of the body, and certain brain cells. Scientists were initially astonished by the presence of the virus in the brain because the blood–brain barrier usually prevents *all* foreign substances such as viruses from entering the brain. Because monocytes are among the few cells that move through the blood–brain barrier, researchers deduced that HIV enters the brain by hiding in these very cells in a Trojan-horse fashion (Levy, 1990; Schoub, 1999). Monocytes constantly circulate to the central nervous system where they change into microglial cells which are the macrophage equivalents in the brain.

Enrichment

HIV is a retrovirus. What is a retrovirus?

'Retro' indicates that HIV does the 'reverse' of what other viruses do. The normal transcription of genetic information in cells is *from DNA to RNA to proteins.* But the genetic information of HIV (and other retroviruses) is contained in RNA (rather than in the DNA – as in ordinary viruses). All retroviruses (including HIV) contain a unique enzyme (reverse transcriptase) which the virus uses to transform its viral RNA into viral DNA in order to produce more viruses.

1.9 VARIABILITY AND SUBTYPES OF HIV

One of the most important properties of HIV is its variability. HIV can mutate (change) very rapidly. The immune system relies heavily on its ability to recognise micro-organisms from their outer protein layer. Because HIV changes its outer layer so rapidly, it is extremely difficult to detect any similarity between the outer layer of one HI virus and another. Because of this rapid mutation, the body cannot defend itself against its enemy because its enemy is constantly changing its identity. This peculiarity of HIV (the fact that it rapidly changes its 'identity') is one of the reasons why it is so difficult to develop an HIV vaccine.

The variability of HIV is due mainly to the inaccuracy of its genetic copying mechanism and the tendency of this mechanism to make errors. During each replication cycle of the virus, about 10 to 20 mistakes are made. RNA viruses tend to be more variable than DNA viruses, because the RNA replication mechanism does not have a facility to repair mistakes (as the DNA mechanism does). In addition to this, the reverse transcriptase enzyme also tends to make mistakes when it makes a DNA copy of the RNA viral template. Errors may therefore creep in at any of the stages of RNA replication, and this may lead to variability in the end product of the virus. This rapidity of change in HIV is the reason why, over time, different strains of the HI virus can be found in one HIV-positive person. These strains may vary significantly in terms of their rate of growth, their virulence in killing cells, their sensitivity to antibodies produced by the host and their ability to evade the host's immune response (Schoub, 1999:66).

In addition to these variations of the virus, there are a number of different subtypes (clades) of HIV-1, each predominating in a different part of the world (Peeters, 2000; Schoub, 1999:67). Various genetic subtypes of HIV-1 have been identified to date, and these are named A, B, C, D, F, G, H, J and K. Some of these subtypes also

Activity

Explain the effect of HIV on the immune system to children. Expand on the story in the enrichment box 'Explaining the immune system to children' on page 16 about the flu virus's attack on the body. Explain to children what will happen to the body when it is attacked by an HI virus instead of a flu virus.

recombine to form circulating recombinant forms. This means, for example, that subtype A may combine with subtype C to form a new subtype of the virus.

HIV-1 subtype B is the predominant subtype in Europe, North America, Japan and Australia. Subtype C is the predominant subtype in southern Africa and India. Knowing the predominant subtype in a specific part of the world is important for vaccine development. A vaccine developed against HIV-1 subtype B will probably have no effect in southern Africa, where HIV-1 subtype C is the predominant subtype. HIV-2 is classified into genetic subtypes A to G. Most HIV-2 infections are caused by subtypes A and B.

HIV-1 subtype C is a very virulent subtype. The following characteristics of subtype C were identified by scientists at the International Aids Conference in Barcelona (2002):

- Subtype C has a very high prevalence (20–40%). (This means that when subtype C is prevalent in a country, the infection rate is usually between 20% and 40%.)
- Subtype C infection is more likely to be transmitted from mother to baby.
- Subtype C infection is characterised by high viral loads in the blood.
- Subtype C is more diverse or variable.
- Subtype C mutates very readily.
- Subtype C spreads faster than any of the other subtypes.

 Enrichment

HIV hides out in the memory T cells

HI viruses have the ability to hide in the memory T cells where they build up a supply of viruses that lie quietly in waiting until they get active at a later stage. This inactive supply of HI viruses in memory T cells is called a 'latent reservoir' of viruses, and it is one of the reasons why HIV cannot be eradicated completely by drugs. Latent cells can live for more than 44 months.

1.10 HIV VACCINES

What is a vaccine and how does it work?

A vaccine is a substance given to stimulate the immune system to protect the person from infection by a specific micro-organism (Schoub, 1999:186). We can say that a vaccine is a substance that teaches the body to recognise and defend itself against bacteria and viruses that cause disease. The development of vaccines relies on the principle that the immune system is specifically activated by the *protein components* of an organism. The body does not have to be exposed to the dangers of the organism itself: the immune response (that is, the development of antibodies and/or killer T cells) can be activated by administering only the relevant *proteins* of the organism. A successful vaccine will enable the body to stop or immobilise an invading virus. It is important to note that a vaccine is not a cure. It prevents infection or slows disease progression.

Brief history of vaccines

Vaccines have been around for thousands of years. One of the earliest examples of a vaccine comes from the Mano people of Liberia, who used to take fluid from a smallpox sore and scratch it into the skin of an uninfected person using a thorn (*Introducing HIV/Aids vaccines*, 2002). The first modern vaccine was developed much later in 1796 when Edward Jenner used matter from cowpox pustules to protect individuals from smallpox – a similar but more dangerous version of the disease. (The word 'vaccine' is derived from the Latin word for 'cow'.) By the end of the nineteenth century Louis Pasteur succeeded in producing vaccines for cholera, anthrax and rabies. Because of vaccines, diseases such as tetanus, polio, smallpox, diphtheria, mumps, measles, pertussis (whooping cough) and rubella (German measles) have decreased rapidly, and millions of lives are saved annually. Vaccines are also available for influenza, chickenpox, hepatitis A and B, and TB.

How is a vaccine developed?

As was seen earlier, the *protein component* of an organism is needed to stimulate an immune response. Viral vaccines are therefore prepared from purified proteins. Some methods use the whole virus particle after it has been 'killed' or inactivated by chemicals or heat (as is the case with influenza vaccine). There is no danger that these kinds of vaccines will produce the diseases associated with that specific virus. An alternative method is to keep the virus alive, but to alter it genetically so that it will be able to stimulate the host's immune response without causing disease. This method is far too dangerous to use in the production of HIV vaccines, because live vaccine strains may still produce illness on very rare occasions.

A vaccine for HIV

Because of safety concerns, HIV vaccines are not developed from live, weakened or inactivated viruses. The majority of HIV vaccine developments investigate the use of various antigens (or proteins) of the virus, such as the surface glycoproteins of HIV, namely gp120, gp160 or gp140 or a combination of glycoproteins (see Figure 1.3 on page 11 for the position of the surface glycoproteins). Because they are the outermost proteins on the virus surface, they would be the proteins most likely to set off a protective immune response.

The problem with these surface proteins is that they are also the most variable of the antigens. They mutate and change their identifiable characteristics very rapidly and so confuse the immune system. It was reported at the Aids Conference in Bangkok (2004) that all the vaccine trials using surface proteins have failed. Some vaccine trials therefore concentrate instead on those proteins of the virus that show the least variation between strains, such as the gp41 glycoprotein and the gag gene (core proteins). These are internal proteins, not situated on the surface of the virus. (See Figure 1.3 for the position of gp41 and the p24 antigen, a product of the gag gene.)

South African vaccine researchers use the gag gene from HIV-1 subtype C – the predominant virus circulating in South Africa – to develop a vaccine that will work specifically in South Africa. There is no possibility that this vaccine will cause HIV infection. The vaccine contains only a copy of a small section of genetic material from HIV (the gag gene), and it does not include the genetic elements needed to reconstitute live HIV.

A vaccine vector (a biological delivery system) is needed to deliver the vaccine into the body. South African researchers use an artificial virus-like particle, a Venezuelan equine encephalitis (VEE) vaccine replicon particle as a vector (or carrier) for the HIV gene (Galloway, 2003:5). In making this vaccine, the genetic material of the VEE virus is removed and replaced with a gene or genes cloned from the HI virus. Instead of producing its own structural proteins, the VEE vector is used like a machine to produce large amounts of HIV protein in the person who has been vaccinated. (Note that neither the VEE vector nor the HIV vaccine can cause VEE or HIV infection in the vaccinated person.) It is hoped that the HIV protein will set off immune responses protective against HIV infection. The process has several layers of safety features, and rigorous safety testing of each vaccine batch ensures that vaccine preparations are safe.

Vaccine clinical trials

Before an HIV vaccine can be registered and licensed for general public use, it has to pass three phases of human clinical trials. A number of HIV vaccine trials are being carried out all over the world.

- *Phase 1* assesses the safety of the vaccine, and the immune system's responses to it. The trials aim to confirm that the test vaccine does not produce significant side-effects in human volunteers. Trials are carried out on 40–120 healthy, HIV-negative, low-risk, adult (over 18) volunteers who are willing and able to give informed consent. The duration of phase 1 trials is usually about 18 months to 2 years.
- *Phase 2* further assesses safety and immune response, and investigates the best way of giving the vaccine (for example by injection under the skin, or injection into the muscle), and when, how much and how often to give it. Participants will be hundreds of healthy, HIV-negative, low- to high-risk adult volunteers per trial. The duration of phase 2 trials is about 2 years.
- *Phase 3* trials assess efficacy (whether the vaccine will prevent HIV infection, or slow down or prevent disease progression). Thou-

sands of healthy, HIV-negative, high-risk adult participants will be used in each trial. The duration of phase 3 trials is usually 3 to 4 years or more.

The South African Medicines Control Council approved the first human phase 1 HIV vaccine trial in South Africa at the end of 2003. The volunteers were closely monitored over a 12-month period. They were supplied with detailed information about the candidate vaccine and underwent intensive risk-reduction counselling. They were monitored on an ongoing basis throughout the trial to ensure their safety and that they did not expose themselves to unnecessary risk. The test vaccine has already been extensively tested in laboratory and animal studies (Galloway, 2003).

How effective will an HIV vaccine be?

There are various obstacles in the development of an HIV vaccine. HIV is a very complex virus and the development of an effective and safe vaccine is hampered by factors such as the genetic diversity of HIV, the different strains of HIV, and the ability of HIV subtypes to recombine to form new subtypes.

It is not yet clear whether an HIV vaccine can be developed that will *prevent* HIV infection. For now, vaccine researchers hope that they will be able to develop a vaccine that might at least have an effect on the following:

- *Susceptibility.* The vaccinated person is less susceptible to HIV infection.
- *Disease progression.* A vaccinated person who does get infected will stay healthy in spite of the infection.
- *Infectiousness.* A vaccinated person who does get infected with HIV will be less infectious to sex partners than an HIV-positive person who was not vaccinated.

1.11 THE BODY'S RESPONSE TO HIV INFECTION

Different people (for reasons not yet fully understood) respond differently to HIV infection. Some people remain healthy and active for as long as 10 to 15 years with few or no signs of immune depression, while other people deteriorate rapidly and develop full-blown Aids within 5 to 7 years, or even sooner. There are many known reasons why HIV infection may progress more rapidly in some individuals than in others. Some of the reasons why people respond differently are:

- There are different strains of HIV (some are more virulent or active).
- When people are infected, they receive different 'dosages' of the virus, and this results in higher or lower viral counts in the blood.
- Different human bodies respond differently to the virus.
- The general health of the person concerned affects the course of the disease.

People who are already chronically ill with illnesses such as malaria or TB, and whose health status is poor because of malnutrition, poverty, recurrent infections, repeated pregnancies or anaemia, will experience a much more rapid deterioration than relatively healthy individuals who become infected with HIV (Evian, 2000).

1.12 CONCLUSION

Scientists now have a clear and precise understanding of how HIV destroys the body's immune system, but so far all attempts to eliminate the virus completely from the body, or to make the human body immune to the virus, have failed. *At this stage the only way to stop Aids is to prevent transmission of the virus.* This is only possible when one has a proper understanding of exactly how the virus is transmitted from one person to another. The transmission of HIV from one person to another is the theme of the next chapter.

chapter

2 The Transmission of HIV

Raka wants to enter

But now Raka kept close to the homestead, like a dog.
Around the kraal he sneaked with a sound like the rustling of small night animals.
A woman would sometimes turn in her sleep – restlessly,
and then suddenly cry out from lust and fear.
Because only half awake,
she knew that the beast was naked and prowling around in the dark.

HIV infection is transmitted primarily:

- by sexual intercourse;
- by HIV-infected blood passing directly into the body of another person; and
- by a mother to her baby during pregnancy or childbirth, or as a result of breastfeeding.

HIV has been identified in various body fluids, but it is especially highly concentrated in blood, semen and vaginal fluids. Although HIV is present in saliva, tears, sweat and urine, the concentration of the virus in these fluids is too low for successful transmission.

For infection with HIV to occur, two things must happen:

- the virus must find a way to enter the bloodstream; and
- the virus must 'take hold'.

This is more likely to happen if:

- the virus is present in *sufficient quantities* (in the semen, vaginal fluid, blood or breast milk);
- the virus gets *access into the bloodstream*; and
- the *duration of exposure* is long enough. The risk of infection increases with the length of time a person is exposed to the virus (Brouard et al., 2004:5).

This chapter will concentrate primarily on the transmission of HIV. The prevention of HIV will be discussed throughout the book where relevant.

2.1 SEXUAL TRANSMISSION OF HIV INFECTION

HIV infection is sexually transmitted primarily through *unprotected* (that is, without a condom), *penetrative* vaginal or anal intercourse, and through oral sexual contact under certain conditions. HIV is transmitted when the virus enters a person's bloodstream via the body fluids of an infected individual. In order to gain entry into the body, the HI virus needs to connect to CD4 receptors, which are found on various types of cells such as macrophages and CD4 cells. Because many of the cells in the linings of the genital and anal tract have just such receptors, HIV can easily gain entrance into these cells (Evian, 2000). The mucous membranes of the genital tract also have an abundance of antigen-presenting cells such as Langerhans cells that are ready and waiting to transport the HI antigens to the waiting CD4 cells (see enrichment box).

Enrichment

Langerhans cells: 'Taxi cells' for HIV

Langerhans cells are found in the skin and in the mucous membranes of the body, and there are large numbers of them in the mucous membranes of the female and male genitalia. Langerhans cells are antigen-presenting cells, which means that they present foreign antigens to the immune system. The Langerhans cells circulate continually between the peripheral mucous membranes and the CD4 lymphocytes found in the lymph nodes and other lymphoid tissue. According to Schoub (1999:83), the Langerhans cells may well be the key to understanding how HIV is transmitted across an intact genital mucous membrane – in other words, when there are no breaks in the mucous membranes – during sexual intercourse. (Observations of HIV transmission by artificial insemination have established that sexual transmission of HIV could occur across an intact mucous membrane.) It is believed that once the Langerhans cell is infected by HIV in the mucous membrane, its natural migration route transports it to the CD4 cells in the lymphoid tissue where it functions as an antigen-presenting cell, presenting the HIV antigen directly into the waiting hands (or CD4 receptors) of the CD4 cell. Langerhans cells can therefore be called the 'taxi cells' of the immune system.

Because the membrane linings of body cavities – especially in the anal-rectal area and to a lesser extent in the vagina – are very delicate, they can be torn as a result of friction generated during sexual intercourse. Such (often microscopic) tears make it easy for the virus to enter the sex partner's bloodstream – either through the tears or by mixing with blood from larger tears.

Women are more likely than men to become infected with HIV during unprotected vaginal intercourse, although HIV-positive women are highly infectious during menstruation because of the presence of HIV-infected blood. The recipient of semen in anal sex (the passive partner) runs a greater risk of infection than the active partner because of the inflexibility of the mucous membrane in the anus. The mucous membrane that lines the anal-rectal area is easily torn during anal intercourse.

Individuals who have other sexually transmitted infections (STIs) such as syphilis, gonorrhoea, chancroid and chlamydia are particularly prone to HIV infection. Research has shown that an untreated STI in either partner increases the risk of HIV transmission during unprotected intercourse tenfold (World Health Organization [WHO], 2000a). Individuals with genital herpes or genital ulcers or sores are especially susceptible to HIV infection because these conditions create openings in the mucous membranes through which HIV can move.

As we noted in chapter 1, HIV is attracted to the *immune cells* of the body. STIs cause genital inflammation and the inflammation attracts numerous immune cells with CD4 receptors to the site of infection. This of course creates ideal conditions for the HI virus to latch onto the CD4 receptors in and around the genital tract. Because of this relationship between genital infections and immune cells, it is so much easier for HIV to enter the body cells of people with STIs. The discharges produced by many STIs contain a very high concentration of HIV if that person is also HIV positive.

Why are women more easily infected by HIV than men?

The risk of becoming infected with HIV during unprotected vaginal intercourse is two to four times higher for women than it is for men (WHO, 2000a). One of the reasons why women are more susceptible to HIV infection than men is that women, as the recipients of semen, are exposed to semen for a longer time. While semen remains in the body of a woman for a few hours, a man is exposed to the body fluids of a woman for only a short time. Because there may also be a higher concentration of HIV in semen than in vaginal fluids, transmission to a woman is more likely. A woman also has a larger surface area of mucosa (the thin lining of the vagina and cervix) exposed to the partner's secretions during sexual intercourse.

In addition, many women may be unaware that they have cervical or vaginal conditions (such as STIs, erosions, open sores and infections) that facilitate the transmission of HIV. These conditions often go undetected because many are painless and not outwardly conspicuous, being hidden inside the vagina or cervix.

Apart from STIs, infection or damage to the vaginal walls is often caused by the use of herbal and other substances for the practice of 'dry sex' (see 'The dangerous practice of "dry sex"' on page 138). Spermicidal (i.e. sperm-killing) preparations used by women, such as creams containing nonoxynol-9, may also cause allergies, irritation and inflammation of the vaginal walls.

Transmission of HIV is more likely to occur just before, during or immediately after menstruation because of the large, raw area of the inner uterine lining that is exposed (Evian, 2000). Younger women are especially vulnerable to HIV infection because their genital tracts are not yet fully mature, their vaginal secretions are not so copious, and they are more prone to lacerations of the vaginal mucosa (UNAIDS, 2000c). There is evidence to suggest that women once again become more vulnerable to HIV infection after menopause (WHO, 2000a). Rape, rough sex, previous genital mutilation (female circumcision) and anal sex (which is often practised to preserve virginity and to prevent pregnancy) can cause tearing and bleeding and this further increases the risk of HIV transmission.

Apart from their biological vulnerability, women become more vulnerable in societies in which they are seen as having lower status than men. This makes women dangerously vulnerable in sexual relationships because they do not have the authority to express or enforce their needs. Because of their low status, most women from poor (socio-economically depressed) communities have little or no control over their sex lives. They are not in a position to negotiate safer sex practices because they fear violence and abandonment should they try to do so. The husbands of women from poor communities often have casual sex when they have to leave their families behind to find work in the cities. Sometimes dire poverty and need drive women from such communities to prostitution because (ironically) this is the only way they feel they can survive. Their low self-image and lack of personal authority also make such women particularly vulnerable to rape. Young girls especially are often coerced, raped or enticed into sex by someone older, stronger or richer than themselves. It is well known that older 'sugar daddies' often offer schoolgirls gifts or money in return for sex.

A shocking report by the Medical Research Council of South Africa indicated that the majority of women in their study who reported that they had been raped were raped between the ages of 10 and 14 years of age, and that schoolteachers were the perpetrators in 33% of these cases. In many cases, the teachers threatened to fail the girls in their examinations if they did not have sex with them. Schools, which should be a safe haven, become a place of terror for many girls (Galloway, 2002b).

The assertion that women are more susceptible to HIV than men, and statistics showing that in some countries twice as many women are infected with HIV, should not be interpreted to mean that men are safe from HIV. It means only that the risk for women is even higher than for men, and where other STIs are present, men lose this advantage and are as vulnerable as women.

Activity

Develop a government programme that will educate women to make themselves less vulnerable to HIV infection. Start by listing the reasons why women are particularly vulnerable to HIV infection, then suggest how each of these factors can be neutralised.

What is a vaginal microbicide?

Many women are simply not in a position to insist that their partners use condoms because they fear rejection or a violent reaction from their partners if they do so. What these women ideally need is a non-barrier method, which they themselves can apply and control without their partners' knowledge. A microbicide in the form of a vaginal cream might be the answer and may turn out to be a major factor in controlling the spread of HIV.

But what is a microbicide? A *microbicide* is a substance that kills microscopic organisms such as bacteria, viruses and parasites. Researchers are currently developing microbicides that can be inserted into the vagina (or into the rectum) with the aim of destroying infection-causing organisms including HIV (Galloway, 2002a:16). In other words, microbicides could be used to prevent the sexual transmission of HIV and other STIs.

A microbicide could be produced in the form of a gel, cream, suppository, film or lubricant, or in the form of a sponge or vaginal ring that slowly releases the active ingredient over time. As a female-controlled prevention method, microbicides would empower women to take control over their own sexual health. Women who cannot insist on condom use would now be able to protect themselves without the partner's knowledge.

Unfortunately microbicides are not yet available. South Africa is one of the countries in the forefront of microbicide research, and scientists are currently testing many substances which they hope will prevent HIV and other STIs by:

Enrichment

Male circumcision and HIV infection

Several studies have indicated that circumcised men are less likely to become infected with HIV than uncircumcised men (if they are not practising safe sex). One of the reasons for this may be that the skin of the glans penis usually thickens after circumcision.

A review of 27 published studies on the association between HIV and male circumcision in Africa found that, on average, circumcised men were half as likely to be infected with HIV as uncircumcised men. A study in Kenya among the Luo group found that while 25% of uncircumcised men were infected with HIV, just under 10% of circumcised men were infected. A study of over 6 800 men in rural Uganda has suggested that the *timing* of circumcision is an important factor affecting rates of infection: HIV infection was found in 16% of men who were circumcised after the age of 21 and in only 7% of those circumcised before puberty.

Although it seems that circumcision (especially if it is done before puberty or before boys become sexually active) does provide some degree of protection against HIV infection, the practical implications for Aids prevention are not obvious or straightforward. Circumcision in Africa is part of various ethnic, religious and adult initiation traditions, and if the same blade is used without sterilisation between circumcisions on a number of boys, HIV-infected blood could pass from one boy to another. The high prevalence rate of other sexually transmitted infections in Africa may also contribute to HIV infection, regardless of whether the male is circumcised or not. The direction of the protective effect of circumcision is also not clear yet. Although it may lower female to male transmission to a certain degree, we do not know for certain if it also works the other way around, and protects the female sex partner.

Circumcision should definitely *NOT* be promoted as a way of preventing HIV infection, because circumcision does *NOT* prevent infection. In addition, the belief that it is a way of preventing infection may cause ignorant people to abandon safer sex practices such as using condoms. Rumours already exist in many African countries that circumcision acts as a 'natural condom'. While circumcision may slightly reduce the probability of HIV infection, it certainly does not eliminate it. In one South African study, it was found that two out of five circumcised men were infected with HIV, compared with three out of five uncircumcised men. Relying on circumcision for protection against HIV would, under such circumstances, be a bit like 'playing Russian roulette with two bullets in the gun rather than three' (UNAIDS, 2000c:70–71).

- killing or immobilising the pathogens;
- blocking infection by creating a barrier between the pathogen and the mucous membranes; and
- preventing the infection from taking hold after it has entered the body.

Some microbicides will also include spermicidal substances (to prevent pregnancy). Women will therefore have a choice between microbicides with or without contraceptive properties. Although a microbicide may be the only option open to some women, it does not eliminate the need for condoms. When used consistently and correctly, condoms are likely to provide better protection against HIV and other STIs than microbicides (Caesar, 2002). Researchers doubt whether a microbicide will ever be able to provide 100% protection against HIV.

How many sexual contacts with an HIV-positive person are necessary before one becomes infected oneself?

It is impossible to say how many sexual contacts with an infected partner or partners are necessary before an HIV-negative person becomes HIV positive. Research on married couples where one partner was HIV positive has shown that there is no correlation at all between the number of sexual contacts and the infection rate. While some partners may become infected after one sexual contact, others may remain uninfected after several hundred contacts. Several factors may contribute to the chances of contracting HIV infection after a single sexual act. Some of these factors are multiple sex partners, the presence of other STIs, the viral concentration (or 'load') in the semen or vaginal fluids of the infected sex partner, trauma (or bleeding) during sex, and menstruation. In spite of all this, one should always keep in mind that *one single unprotected sexual contact* with an HIV-positive partner may lead to infection with HIV, especially when the viral load in the partner's blood is high.

Can one be infected with HIV through having oral sex?

Oral sex (stimulation of the genitals with the mouth) may cause a person to become infected with HIV if the lining of the mouth is exposed to infected seminal fluid or vaginal and rectal mucus – especially if the person providing the oral stimulation has sores, bleeding gums or inflammation in his or her mouth. (See 'Is oral sex safe?' on page 137 for methods of making oral sex safe.)

When is an HIV-positive person most infectious to other people?

Although it is possible for HIV to be transmitted at any time during the course of the disease, HIV-positive people are considered most infectious soon after becoming infected with the virus (in the first 4–8 weeks during seroconversion*) *and* during the final phase of Aids when severe symptoms of Aids appear. HIV-positive people are more infectious during these phases because the viral load in their blood is very high at these times. Some studies found that the viral load in semen peaks 3 weeks after infection, and that during this stage HIV is 20 times more transmissible per sex act (International Aids Conference, 2002).

The prevention of sexual transmission of HIV will be discussed in Chapter 8.

2.2 TRANSMITTING HIV THROUGH CONTAMINATED BLOOD

The HI virus can be transmitted from one person to another when a person receives HIV-contaminated blood in a blood transfusion; when he or she uses needles that are contaminated with HIV-infected blood to inject drugs; or when he or she is injured with blood-contaminated needles, syringes, razor blades or other sharp instruments.

* Seroconversion is the point at which a person's HIV status changes from being negative to positive. After seroconversion an HIV test will be positive. Seroconversion usually occurs 4–8 weeks after infection with the HI virus.

The re-use of instruments in traditional African healing or in cultural practices such as circumcision and scarification also poses the risk of HIV transmission.

Blood transfusions and blood products

According to the World Health Organization (WHO, 2000a), there is a 90–95% chance that someone receiving blood from an HIV-positive donor will become infected with HIV themselves. All donated blood should therefore be screened for HIV antibodies, and blood that is found to be infected should be destroyed. The WHO states that all blood transfusion services throughout the world should observe the following three essential guidelines to ensure a safe blood supply:

1. All national blood transfusion services should be organised on a non-profit basis.
2. While there should be a policy of excluding all paid or professional donors, voluntary (non-paid) donors who fall into the category of *low risk* as far as infection is concerned should be encouraged to come back regularly.
3. All donated blood must be screened for HIV, as well as for hepatitis B and syphilis (and, if possible, also for hepatitis C).

Blood products such as factor VIII (proteins promoting the clotting of blood, which are used for haemophiliacs) are heated to 60 °C and this heating process destroys the virus. It is unfortunately not possible to render whole blood safe by means of heating because red blood cells disintegrate at high temperatures.

Although blood is currently far safer than it was in the past, the 'window period' (the period *after* infection but *before* antibodies are formed) still creates problems for blood transfusion services. Because infected blood donated during the window period does not test positive for HIV antibodies, it slips through the net and is therefore not destroyed. Blood transfusion services use *antibody* tests such as the ELISA (enzyme-linked immunosorbent assay) test to test donor blood. *Antigen or virus* tests, such as the PCR test with its much shorter window period, are far too expensive for general use by blood banks.

Although the risk of HIV infection through a blood transfusion is very low, there is, unfortunately, no such thing as 'no-risk blood'. It is therefore the moral and ethical responsibility of people who engage in high-risk sexual activities and high-risk drug-using activities not to donate blood. Blood transfusions should be given to patients only when it is essential in order to save their lives. Under certain circumstances it is possible for patients to donate their own blood for storage and later use during and after a scheduled operation.

The HI virus is also present in the organs, tissue and semen of infected donors. All donor products are therefore tested for HIV antibodies. HIV-positive people should be encouraged not to carry donor cards.

Enrichment

Is it safe to receive immunoglobulin preparations?

Immunoglobulin preparations (e.g. gamma globulin injections) are safe and do not carry a major risk of HIV infection. Immunoglobulins are antibodies that are prepared from the serum of individuals who have recovered from illnesses. This preparation is then given to a patient who has been unexpectedly exposed to an infectious disease (such as hepatitis B) to create passive immunity and to prevent illness. Although immunoglobulin preparations are made from the serum of many individuals, they are safe because the immunoglobulin proteins are freed from any contaminating viruses in the blood during the preparation process (Schoub, 1999).

Injecting drug users

People who share syringes and needles to inject drugs run a very high risk of being infected with HIV. In many countries outside Africa, drug injection is called the 'second epidemic that drives the virus'. In some countries (such as Georgia, Italy, Portugal, Spain and Yugoslavia) over half of all Aids cases have been attributed to the use of contaminated needles used to inject drugs (UNAIDS, 2000c:74).

HIV is easily transmitted when needles are shared because drug users usually inject drugs directly into their bloodstreams. In order to ensure that the needle has struck a vein, drug users first draw blood into the syringe before they inject the drug. Small amounts of blood always remain in the needle and it is this drop that is injected directly into the bloodstream of the next user. Because the virus is highly concentrated in blood, these tiny 'blood transfusions' of HIV-infected blood between drug users using the same infected needle constitute an ideal method for passing on the virus.

People who inject drugs not only put themselves at risk; they also put their sex partners at risk. It is estimated that nine out of ten cases of transmission of HIV among heterosexuals in New York City can be traced back to having sex with a drug user who takes drugs intravenously (UNAIDS, 2000c:75). The problem of HIV transmission is aggravated by the fact that many people who inject drugs resort to prostitution to obtain the money they need to support their drug habit.

Although Africa (relatively speaking) does not yet have a very large number of people who use syringes for the self-administration of drugs, the authorities should not wait until it is too late before educating people about how easy it is to transmit HIV by sharing infected needles. Some African countries with less stringent border and harbour regulations than South Africa are very popular as points of entry for drug traffickers. South Africa itself is increasingly becoming a destination and transit point for drug traffickers, and we may therefore expect that intravenously injected drugs will become a very serious problem in this country. (See 'Prevention of HIV in injecting drug users' on page 142.)

Blood-contaminated needles, syringes and other sharp instruments

HIV can be transmitted through contaminated needles and sharp instruments in hospitals or clinics where medical hygiene is poor, or through accidental exposure to contaminated needles or other sharp instruments. It can also be transmitted through tattooing, ear piercing, contact with infected blood at the scene of an accident, and ritual circumcision or scarification. Those who carry out tattooing and ear piercing, and traditional healers and their clients, should be educated about the importance of using clean instruments to save lives.

How great is the risk of HIV transmission when a person has been accidentally exposed to the blood of an infected person?

Nurses and other people who care for HIV-positive people are often concerned about the risk of contracting HIV. All known cases of HIV transmission in health care settings have occurred in the context of *accidents*, i.e. occasions when a health care professional has been accidentally

Enrichment

Hepatitis B and HIV: which is more infectious?

While many health care professionals are afraid of HIV infection, some may be unaware of the risks posed by hepatitis B. Hepatitis B is a blood-borne viral infection of the liver which is caused by the hepatitis B virus (HBV). HBV is transmitted in the same way as HIV, namely through sexual contact, needle-sharing, the infection of a baby by its mother, and contaminated blood or blood products. Like HIV, HBV is not transmitted by casual contact such as shaking hands, sharing eating utensils, and so on.

In thc case of both HIV and HBV the occupational risk of infection is directly proportional to the degree of contact that a health care professional has had with infected blood or blood products. However, given similar exposure to a similar volume of infected blood, the risk of transmission is much greater for hepatitis B than it is for HIV: the chance of becoming infected by a single exposure to HIV-infected blood after being pricked by an HIV-contaminated needle is 0.37%, whereas the danger of HBV transmission under similar circumstances ranges from 20 to 40%.

Although most people recover from hepatitis B in about six months, others may continue to suffer from chronic infections or develop severe liver problems, or develop cirrhosis, cancer or even acute fatal liver failure. Health care professionals should therefore be extremely cautious when they handle body fluids to avoid being infected by either HIV or HBV.

One of the important differences between HIV infection and hepatitis B is that hepatitis B is preventable through vaccination. Health care professionals who work in situations in which they are exposed to blood and body fluids should insist on being vaccinated against hepatitis B. (Three doses of Engerix-B confer protection lasting 3–5 years. This vaccine is readily available at most pharmacies.)

exposed to infected blood and/or other body fluids in a way that permits transmission of the virus. Examples of such accidents are:

- when a person is accidentally pierced with a needle containing blood from an infected patient (a needle-stick injury);
- when a person is cut by a scalpel, glass or other sharp instrument that is contaminated with infected blood;
- when a person makes prolonged contact with an infected person's blood without the use of gloves;
- when a person whose skin is chapped, has abrasions, or is affected by dermatitis is exposed to large amounts of HIV-infected blood; and
- when HIV-infected blood accidentally splashes into the eyes or mouth of the caregiver.

The average risk of HIV infection following exposure through the skin to HIV-infected blood is 0.3% (or approximately one chance in 300). The risk of HIV infection after being pricked by an HIV-contaminated *hollow-bore* needle is approximately 0.37%. The risk of infection is lower after a prick from a solid needle (such as a suture needle) or after being cut by a scalpel blade than after a prick from a hollow-bore needle. Splashes of blood or body fluids contaminated with blood, semen, or vaginal fluids in the eyes or mouth of the caregiver carry a considerably lower risk, about 0.1% or less (Schoub, 1997a, 1999; 'Update', 1996). While these statistics show that accidental exposure to HIV-infected blood does not necessarily lead to infection, it is understandable that such statistics are not reassuring to people who have been exposed to the virus in any of these ways.

The risk of HIV transmission may be higher if an injury involves large volumes of blood (for example in the case of a deeply penetrating wound); if the needle has been in the vein or artery of the HIV-positive person; or if the viral load in the blood is high (as is the case in pre-terminal Aids patients or during acute seroconversion illness). Post-exposure prophylaxis in the form of antiretroviral medication should be made available to all health care professionals who have sustained needle-stick injuries or other accidents with HIV-infected blood. (See 'Using antiretroviral therapy to manage occupational exposure' on page 83.)

Health care personnel should note that any serous fluid (the yellowish protein-rich liquid that separates from coagulated blood), amniotic (pregnancy) fluid, cerebrospinal fluid and pleural (chest) fluid, as well as fluid from the abdomen, heart and joints, are all as infectious as HIV-infected blood when a person is HIV positive.

What quantity of infected blood needs to be present before HIV is transmitted?

It is impossible to say exactly how much blood is required to transmit HIV. The risk of infection is directly proportionate to the concentration of HIV (the viral load) in the blood. Recently infected individuals with acute seroconversion illness, and patients in the final stage of infection (Aids), usually have very high viral levels in their blood. The higher the concentration of HIV in the blood, the lower the quantity of blood required to transmit the virus. Because it is impossible to tell just by looking at a person how high the concentration of HIV is in his or her blood, or indeed even whether a person is infected or not, one should always follow the golden rule:

> Always take proper precautions when handling blood and any other body fluids to which universal precautions apply.

For how long can the virus survive outside the body?

We should distinguish between the lifespan of HIV when it is outside the body *and* outside body fluids, and when it is outside the body but still present in body fluids such as blood. As soon as the HI virus is no longer in a body fluid, it becomes extremely fragile and dies – especially when it is exposed to oxygen, heat and dryness in the atmosphere. While HIV cannot survive outside body fluids for very long, it can probably live outside the body for many hours *so long as it remains in some or other body fluid such as blood.* Body fluid spills should always be handled with extreme care. One should always take proper precautions when handling blood or body fluids that contain visible blood. (See page 290 for methods of cleaning up body fluid spills.)

2.3 MOTHER-TO-CHILD TRANSMISSION OF HIV

Mother-to-child transmission (MTCT) or vertical transmission of HIV is one of the major causes of HIV infection in children. It is estimated that about 600 000 children are infected in this way each year, and this figure accounts for 90% of HIV infections in children (WHO, 2000a). Unless preventive measures are taken, 20–40% of children born to HIV-positive women are infected. HIV can be transmitted from an infected mother to her baby via the placenta during pregnancy, through blood contamination during childbirth, or through breastfeeding.

A mother is more likely to pass the HI virus to her baby during pregnancy, childbirth or breastfeeding if:

- she becomes infected with HIV just before the pregnancy, during the pregnancy or during the breastfeeding period (because she will have a high viral load in her blood or breastmilk during seroconversion); and if
- she has advanced, symptomatic HIV disease with
  - a high viral load (> 50 000 viral particles/ml);
  - a low CD4 cell count (< 200 cells/mm^3);
  - symptoms of Aids.

If the mother has a low viral load during pregnancy, childbirth or breastfeeding (< 1 000 viral particles/ml), the likelihood of transmitting the virus to her baby is low (Evian, 2003).

Pregnancy

Although most mother-to-child transmissions occur close to the time of delivery or during the birth process, it is estimated by some researchers that up to 23% of transmissions occur *in utero* even as early as the first trimester of pregnancy (Schoub, 1999). As has been explained, a woman is more likely to transmit the virus to her fetus during pregnancy if she becomes infected just before or during pregnancy, or if she has an HIV-related illness or Aids (the last phase of the infection). This is because at these times the viral load is usually very high and the CD4 cell count low. Any situation that may result in an increase in the viral load (e.g. an infection such as tuberculosis) will add to the risk of transmitting the virus to the baby.

Pregnancy itself does not seem to have any significant effect on the progress of HIV disease if the mother is in the early asymptomatic phase of infection. In women who have more advanced HIV disease pregnancy may cause more rapid progress to Aids. Generally, HIV seems not to have a serious effect on pregnancy, but there are indications from some parts of Africa that HIV infection may cause an increased likelihood of intra-uterine growth retardation, prematurity, still births and congenital infections (Evian, 2003).

Mother-to-child transmission of HIV during pregnancy can be reduced in the following ways:

- Prevent new HIV infections. New infections during pregnancy may increase the viral load, which will increase the risk of mother-to-child transmission.
- Prevent and treat sexually transmitted infections. Genital infections and sexually transmitted infections may result in infections of the placenta.
- Give nutritional supplements such as iron, folate and multivitamins including vitamin A. These supplements have been shown to reduce the incidence of still birth, prematurity and low birth weight.
- Offer prophylactic antiretroviral therapy. This can reduce mother-to-child transmission by 50–60% when given during pregnancy and labour (see 'Using antiretroviral therapy to prevent mother-to-child transmission of HIV' on page 82).
- Encourage frequent follow-up visits to the clinic so that the mother's health can be monitored regularly.
- Perform fetal monitoring with non-invasive procedures.
- Offer counselling on safe sexual practices during pregnancy – preferably to both partners.

Enrichment

Re-infection with HIV should be avoided

HIV-positive individuals often think that they no longer have to protect themselves against infection by HIV. It is, however, very important for an HIV-positive person to protect himself or herself against re-infection with HIV. Each new infection can cause an increase in the viral load in the blood, and the person infected for a second or subsequent time may get a new strain of the virus. HIV-positive pregnant women should always use condoms to prevent re-infection. Any new HIV infection during pregnancy or breastfeeding is likely to result in an increase in the viral load, and this will increase the likelihood of mother-to-child transmission. Re-infection may also cause the mother's disease to progress more rapidly.

Childbirth

More than than 60% of cases of transmission of HIV infection from a mother to her baby occur during labour and delivery. The main reason for this is contact with the mother's blood and mucus in the birth canal during the birth process.

Mother-to-child transmission during labour can be reduced in the following ways (Evian, 2003):

- Give antiretroviral therapy to mother and baby (see 'Using antiretroviral therapy to prevent mother-to-child transmission of HIV' on page 82).
- Disinfect the birth canal with an antiseptic solution such as 0.25% chlorhexidine during vaginal examinations.
- Avoid unnecessary artificial rupture of the membranes. Rupture of the membranes for longer than four hours before delivery is associated with increases in mother-to-child transmission. Artificial rupture of the membranes should only be done if there are specific obstetric indications and then as late as possible.
- Avoid episiotomy (cutting the vulva to avoid lacerations of the perineum during labour) unless it is absolutely necessary.
- Minimise trauma to the baby by avoiding procedures such as fetal scalp monitoring, forceps delivery and vacuum extraction. These may cause minor skin lacerations.
- In women with very high viral loads, carry out elective caesarean sections if possible. Elective caesarean sections are not recommended as a routine measure, because they are costly and impractical in resource-constrained settings and pose the risk of post-operative complications.

Mother-to-child transmission after the birth can be reduced in the following ways:

- Avoid trauma to the newborn.
- Wipe away secretions from the baby's face.
- Avoid unnecessary suctioning, which may cause trauma to mucous membranes.
- Give the baby antiretroviral prophylaxis for the first 6 weeks.
- Consider alternatives to breastfeeding if possible.

Breastfeeding

About 20–30% of babies who are infected through mother-to-child transmission contract the virus through breastfeeding (WHO, 2000a). The baby may be at greater risk from breastfeeding if the mother was infected with HIV late in her pregnancy or in the months following birth because of the higher viral load during the seroconversion phase of infection. Women are also more infectious when they show symptoms of Aids. Mother-to-child transmission from breastfeeding can, however, occur at any time during the course of the mother's HIV infection, and HIV-infected cells are present in the breast milk of HIV-positive mothers throughout the breastfeeding period. What makes this risk even higher is that 80–90% of women in rural and remote areas in Africa breastfeed their babies for as long as two years. Some African studies have shown that breastfeeding increases the risk of infection by 12–43%.

Factors that may also affect mother-to-child transmission during breastfeeding are a vitamin A deficiency in the mother or child, breast diseases such as mastitis, cracked nipples, and diseases such as thrush and gastroenteritis in the infant.

The debate on breastfeeding versus bottle-feeding in Africa involves complex issues that include the following:

- Formula milk may not be readily available in poor communities.
- Mothers may not have access to clean and safe water supplies with which to prepare the feed.
- Mothers may not know how to sterilise bottles.
- Mothers may not know how to prepare the formula milk and what the correct powder-to-water ratio should be.
- Mothers may not know that they should use clean, boiled-and-cooled water for formula feeding.
- Mothers may not have access to fuel to boil water.
- Some mothers may also not realise that they will compromise the baby's health if they add more water (increase the water in the water-powder ratio) in an attempt to save money or to use the extra milk powder to feed other children in the family.

If a mother chooses to breastfeed her baby, antiretroviral therapy could be considered during the breastfeeding period.

Exclusive breastfeeding versus mixed feeding

Whether HIV-positive mothers should exclusively breastfeed their babies or combine breastfeeding with other fluids and foods has been extensively debated in recent years. It is now recommended that mothers who cannot afford formula milk, or who prefer breastfeeding for other reasons, should exclusively breastfeed their babies for three months or for six months. It should be kept in mind that the longer the mother breastfeeds her baby, the higher the chance that the baby might become infected because of longer exposure to the HI virus in the breast milk. It is therefore recommended that exclusive breastfeeding should be limited to three months, *IF* the mother has access to clean, running water as well as the means to sterilise bottles safely and to prepare formula milk when she changes to bottle feeding. If the mother does *NOT* have access to clean, running water and, for example, does not have a stove to sterilise bottles, exclusive breastfeeding for six months should be advised.

Exclusive breastfeeding means that the baby may not receive any other fluids or food to supplement the mother's breast milk. Studies have shown that the rate of HIV infection is significantly lower in babies who were exclusively breastfed than in babies who received mixed feeds. It is hypothesised that babies who are mixed-fed are more vulnerable to the HI virus because feeds other than breast milk may disturb the lining of the gastrointestinal tract (or gut), which facilitates the entry of the HI virus into the baby's system. It is further recommended that breastfeeding be abruptly and totally terminated after three or six months (without any weaning period). Babies of HIV-positive women should not be breastfed after six months because the positive effects of exclusive breastfeeding do not extend beyond six months, after which period the risk of infection rises again.

For various reasons exclusive breastfeeding is very difficult for some mothers. The personal circumstances of each individual mother should always be taken into account before giving her any advice about what she might do. If she cannot exclusively breastfeed her baby, the mother should be advised rather to feed her baby formula milk.

Expression and pasteurisation of breast milk

Mother-to-child transmission of HIV may also be prevented if breast milk is expressed and pasteurised. Researchers at Kalafong Hospital in South Africa investigated methods of pasteurising infected breast milk which would render the HI virus inactive. Pasteurisation usually occurs at temperatures of 56–62 °C. The HI virus is inactivated at these temperatures because its protein structure is broken down. To pasteurise the milk in hospitals, it should be heated to 62.5 °C for 30 minutes. At home it can be heated and then cooled immediately by putting it in a refrigerator or standing the container in cold water. Heat-treated breast milk should be put in a sterilised or very clean container and kept in a refrigerator or in a cool place before and after heat treatment to minimise contamination (Prevention of mother-to-child transmission, 2000).

The following method for pasteurising HIV-positive mother's milk at home was proposed by researchers at Kalafong Hospital. The mother boils 500 ml of water in an aluminium pot. After the water has reached boiling point, she takes the pot off the stove and places a glass container (for example a clean peanut-butter jar) containing her expressed milk into the pot. As soon as the glass container is placed into the water, the temperature of the water begins to cool down while the temperature of the milk begins to rise to about 60 °C – the ideal temperature for pasteurisation (Jeffery et al., 2000).

The World Health Organization's view on breastfeeding

The World Health Organization still recommends breastfeeding in poor countries to prevent babies dying from gastroenteritis and malnutrition. The health care professional should take all the circumstances of each mother into account before making a decision about whether to advise a mother to breastfeed or feed a breast-milk substitute from a bottle. She should also consider the health status of the other children in the area where the mother lives. If other children in the community are at risk of or already dying from infections (such as respiratory infections or diarrhoea) and suffering from poor nutrition, it is probably safer for the mother to breastfeed her baby.

The issue of bottle feeding should be handled very sensitively in Africa. Since mothers usually breastfeed in public, they are often stigmatised as being HIV positive when they do not breastfeed their babies.

The decision to breastfeed her baby or feed her baby with formula milk from a bottle should always be the mother's own decision. Health care professionals should give mothers all the information and advice they need to make their own informed choice. Never decide for other people what they should do: inform them as best you can and then trust them to make the right decision for their circumstances.

Enrichment

Birth control for HIV-positive women

Condoms are the best choice for contraception because they also prevent HIV transmission during sexual intercourse. Women who use other contraceptives (such as the pill) should be informed that these contraceptives do not prevent HIV infection and that they may infect their sexual partners if they do not use condoms as well. Intra-uterine contraceptive devices (IUCDs) are not recommended for HIV-positive women because they sometimes cause pelvic inflammation. The string of the IUCD may also cause minor abrasions to the partner's penis and this may facilitate HIV transmission to the partner. IUCDs may also increase menstrual blood flow and thus the chance of HIV transmission (Evian, 2000:208). HIV-positive mothers who breastfeed should be encouraged to use condoms to prevent re-infection with new strains of the virus, and to prevent an increase in their viral loads. In this way the use of condoms will reduce the chance of transmitting the virus to the baby through breast milk.

Activity

- Design a wall poster for a rural clinic to illustrate how HIV is transmitted. Take into account that 85% of the population served by this clinic cannot read.
- Advise an HIV-positive mother who lives in an informal settlement many kilometres from the nearest clinic on the best way to feed her newborn baby.

2.4 THE TRANSMISSION OF HIV INFECTION TO CHILDREN

HIV can infect the fetus in the uterus, or the infant during labour or after birth through breast milk. Infants and children may also be infected by the following practices or procedures that transmit HIV (WHO, 2000a:5-1):

- transfusion with HIV-contaminated blood or blood products;
- the use of non-sterile equipment in health care facilities;
- the use of non-sterile equipment by traditional healers (e.g. in surgeries or during the

processes of male and female circumcisions or scarification);
- sexual abuse or rape;
- needle sharing between drug addicts;
- sexual initiation practices involving sex workers; and
- child prostitution.

2.5 POVERTY AND DEPRESSED SOCIO-ECONOMIC CONDITIONS AS FACTORS CONTRIBUTING TO THE SPREAD OF HIV INFECTION

The devastating plagues of history (e.g. the bubonic plague or Black Death of the 14th century) usually emerged from specific social and economic environments that provided fertile grounds for the spread of infection. For example, in 1844 (during the industrial revolution in Europe) a doctor named Frederick Engels reported on the general health in England, saying that community vulnerability to sexually transmitted and other infections was due to 'social disorder and social chaos, and specifically to migration, uncontrolled and rapid urbanisation, prostitution, child labour, syphilis, TB, infant deaths, homelessness, poverty, and social and cultural transition'.

Similar socio-economic conditions exist today in Africa and other Third World countries. HIV/Aids and other sexually transmitted infections are often more common in communities living in depressed socio-economic conditions, and this is aggravated by the following factors:

- High unemployment forces men to migrate to cities. This disrupts family and social lives.
- Tradition accords a low status to women, and they are denied the authority to negotiate safe sex practices.
- Extreme poverty forces women to sell their bodies for sex.
- People live in extremely bad conditions and have limited or no access to health services.
- The prevalence of sexually transmitted infections is very high, and the use of contraceptives is low.
- There is widespread illiteracy and poor education.
- Alcohol abuse is common. This lowers thresholds of inhibition and compromises sensible decision making.
- The community is subject to famine, wars, conflict, crime and high levels of corruption. Traditional social and sexual morality is disintegrating. Old traditions that created cohesion and mutual help in communities have either been undermined or have disappeared altogether.

Prevention of HIV and reclaiming our world from Aids will take much more than distributing condoms. Upliftment of poor communities, improvement of working conditions, a decrease in unemployment, empowerment of women and a strong policy to protect women and children are all issues that will have to be addressed before an Aids-free society can become a reality.

2.6 MYTHS ABOUT THE TRANSMISSION OF HIV

Almost three decades of practical experience and research into the epidemic have shown that HIV is NOT transmitted through the following:

- Airborne routes such as coughing and sneezing. However, in the case of TB a mask should be worn when the sputum contains blood.
- Casual skin contact such as handshaking, hugging and touching. The virus cannot penetrate normal intact skin and does not readily enter through a healthy mouth or eye.
- Sharing food, water, plates, cups, spoons, toilet seats, showers or baths with an HIV-positive individual. The HI virus is not stable and does not survive for long periods outside the human body.
- Sharing clothing, towels and bed linen with an infected individual – provided that the linen is clean.
- Public swimming pools. Chlorine destroys and water dilutes the virus.
- Pets, or insects such as mosquitoes, bedbugs and moths. (See enrichment box 'Mosquitoes and Aids' on page 36.)
- Playing team sports, provided that there is no contact with blood.
- Restaurants and cafeterias. Exposure to heat, air and gastric juices destroys the HI virus.

- Sharing telephones, drinking fountains and public transport with HIV-positive people.
- Living with an Aids patient and sharing household equipment. Research shows that the people living with an Aids patient do not contract the disease if they take the necessary precautions, such as adhering to the rules of basic hygiene, not sharing razors and toothbrushes (a person may have bleeding gums), avoiding contact with body fluids and covering possible bloodspills with a bleach solution.
- Social contact between schoolchildren and sharing school facilities, provided that practices such as the mingling of blood by gang members are avoided.
- Kissing. The virus occurs in very low concentrations in saliva and kissing appears to be safe. However, people should be warned to avoid French or deep kissing if there are sores or punctures in the oral cavity, for example in a person who has bleeding gums.
- Donating blood. Although HIV can be transmitted through blood transfusions or through receiving infected blood, there is no way that a person can become infected through the process of *donating* or *giving* blood – provided that the instruments used during the process are clean.

There are some truly horrifying myths circulating in some communities about how to avoid HIV infection and Aids. These myths are extremely dangerous and should be counteracted in our society by means of intensive public education. For example, some people mistakenly believe that they will not get Aids (or that Aids can actually

Enrichment

Mosquitoes and Aids

The question: 'Why can mosquitoes not transmit the HI virus?' can be answered at various levels of complexity. The most straightforward answer is epidemiological (to do with the science of the transmission of disease). There is absolutely *no epidemiological evidence* that mosquitoes (or any other biting insect) play any role in HIV transmission (Schoub, 1999:122). It has been found that children who are sexually inactive and who live in mosquito-infested areas are NOT infected with HIV, even though they may regularly be infected by mosquito-borne diseases such as malaria and yellow fever. There is therefore no evidence that mosquitoes can also transmit HIV.

Why can mosquitoes transmit other diseases such as malaria, and not HIV? This question can best be answered by comparing mosquito-borne diseases with HIV. Arboviruses (e.g. yellow fever and dengue) and the malaria parasite can be transmitted by mosquitoes because they are adapted to multiply in the body of the mosquito before the mosquito infects a human. However, the HI virus cannot even survive the hostile environment of the mosquito's stomach, let alone multiply there. It is also important to emphasise that, during feeding, mosquitoes do not inject blood into their victim, but only their saliva (which is an anti-clogging agent).

But is it not possible for the HIV-infected blood to be *mechanically* transmitted by the proboscis (the needle-like feeding instrument) of mosquitoes?

The following facts show that this way of transmitting HIV is highly unlikely (if not impossible). The proboscis of a mosquito is many times smaller than the needle of a syringe. Even in the case of much larger needles the rate of transmission of HIV through needle-stick injuries is extremely low (0.37%). Far less blood can stick to the much smaller proboscis of the mosquito, making the chance of transmitting HIV even lower. A virus would need to be far more infectious than HIV before it could be transmitted by such a small quantity of blood. Although the evidence is not conclusive, this may indeed (in some rare cases) happen with the hepatitis B virus, which is many times more infectious than HIV (Schoub, 1999:122). The feeding behaviour of mosquitoes also makes it unlikely for the HI virus to be mechanically transmitted. Female mosquitoes usually take their blood meal from one person only. After drinking their fill, they sit for more than an hour, usually on a vertical surface like a wall, to get rid of all the excess fluids from the ingested blood, retaining only the high concentration of blood proteins which they need for the development of their eggs. After that they fly away, and it may be many days before they need another blood meal (Spielman & D'Antonio, 2002).

In conclusion, there is absolutely no scientific evidence that mosquitoes can transmit HIV. The fact that other diseases may be transmitted by mosquitoes is not evidence that they can also transmit HIV.

be cured) if they have sex with very fat women (who evidently don't have 'slim disease'), or with virgins, or with girls younger than 12 years of age, or with very young boys. Beliefs such as these can be the cause of abhorrent criminal behaviour and can also cause HIV infection to spread like wildfire. (See enrichment box 'Virgin cleansing and history'.)

It is unnecessarily stressful to live with countless unfounded fears about Aids. We must remember that the virus is transmitted ONLY when body fluids are exchanged in sexual intercourse, when a person is exposed to contact with HIV-contaminated blood, and from a pregnant or breastfeeding HIV-positive mother to her child.

Enrichment

Virgin cleansing and history

Virgin cleansing was once believed to be a way to cure venereal disease in Europe. English men in the 1800s believed that intercourse with a child virgin would cure syphilis. In the 1820s in Liverpool quack doctors kept special brothels to provide this cure. The girls used were often mentally impaired. A court case was reported in 1884 of a man with 'bad syphilis ulcers' who had raped a 14-year-old girl. His defence was that he had not intended to harm her, but only to cure himself. The similarities between 19th century Europe and 21st century Africa are intriguing but also very disturbing.

Activity

Organise a discussion group at work or in your community to discuss the following topics:

- The psychological function of myths and urban legends. Why do we share myths and urban legends with each other? How do they make us feel?
- Share a few generally believed myths or urban legends with each other. These myths may concern Aids or any other burning issue in your community.
- Discuss each myth or urban legend objectively and discuss why the myth is not true.

Read the article on the virgin cleansing myth: Leclerc-Madlala, S. (2002). On the virgin cleansing myth: gendered bodies, Aids and ethnomedicine. *African Journal of AIDS Research*, 1(2): 87–95.

2.7 CONCLUSION

Aids is a very serious disease that devastates individuals and societies alike. Fortunately we now know exactly how the virus is spread and what we can do to prevent and manage HIV infection. However, prevention is a complex issue, and if we are to control the epidemic we will need far more than condoms and antiretrovirals. Poverty, social injustice, disempowerment of women, neglect of children's rights, myths, negative attitudes and discrimination are all issues that must be tackled if we really want to win the battle against Aids.

chapter

3 Symptoms and Diseases Associated with HIV/Aids

Signs that Raka is nearby

At first he was not aware of the frightened wild animals
milling around in herds, and the small animals
gathering before his feet with anxious eyes.

Because of the unique way in which HIV attacks and disarms the immune system, all the body's defence mechanisms are disarmed. This means that the body can no longer protect itself against other diseases. As a result, all kinds of bacteria, fungi, protozoa and viruses can invade the body because they encounter no resistance. Even some kinds of cancer may take root and spread in the now defenceless HIV-infected body. The HI virus opens the body's protective gates (its immune system) and lets in all kinds of infections and diseases.

The health of an HIV-positive individual therefore depends on the condition of his or her immune system at any particular time. As we noted in chapter 1, the HI virus attacks and kills mainly the CD4 cells. If we measure the actual number of CD4 cells, we therefore have a very accurate indicator of the current status of the HIV-positive person's immune system. This count, called the CD4 cell count, is also the best predictor of how easily opportunistic infections will be able to take root in an HIV-positive person. However, counting the CD4 cells is an expensive and complex test and is therefore not always possible, so health care professionals often have to rely on an analysis of visible HIV-related symptoms to make an approximate diagnosis of the health status of an HIV-positive person.

3.1 THE RELATIONSHIP BETWEEN THE CD4 CELL COUNT, VIRAL LOAD AND PHASES OF HIV INFECTION

There is a very special relationship between the viral load and the CD4 cell count, and, if considered together, they can predict whether a person's journey towards the final phase of Aids will be rapid or slow. Viral load and CD4 cells have an inverse 'seesaw' relationship. This means that a *higher* viral load will go hand in hand with a *lower* CD4 cell count, because the virus destroys the CD4 cells. A *lower* viral load will go hand in hand with a *higher* CD4 cell count, because if there are fewer viruses in the blood, the immune system gets a chance to build up CD4 cells again. Disease progression (the extent to which an HIV-positive person gets sick with opportunistic diseases and infections) will depend on the viral load and on the CD4 cell count in the blood. The *higher the viral load*, and the *lower the CD4 cell count*, the easier it will be for all kinds of infections to attack the body. The progression to the final phase of Aids (and death) will therefore be much faster with a high viral load. On the other hand, an HIV-positive person with a *low viral load* and a *high CD4 count* can stay healthy for many years, because the immune system is strong enough to fight off infections.

The viral load value can be compared to the *speed* of a train on its journey towards Aids, while the CD4 cell count represents the *distance markers* on the way to the destination (i.e. Aids). The higher the viral load in the blood, the faster the train will move towards its destination. However, the journey to Aids will take much longer if the distance to the destination is longer (if the CD4 cell count is higher). To prolong an HIV-positive person's journey, it is imperative to keep the viral load (or the speed of the train) as low as possible, and to keep the CD4 cell count (the distance) as high as possible. The main purpose of any effort to manage the health of an HIV-positive person is to enhance the functioning of the immune system by lowering the viral load and increasing the CD4 cells as much as possible (Schoub, 1997b).

Figure 3.1 shows the relationship between a person's CD4 cell count, viral load and the phases of HIV infection. Note that the relationship between the CD4 cells, the viral load and phases of infection is not as definite and absolute as illustrated; they can vary from time to time. For example, the CD4 cell count can decrease in response to infections such as flu or herpes,

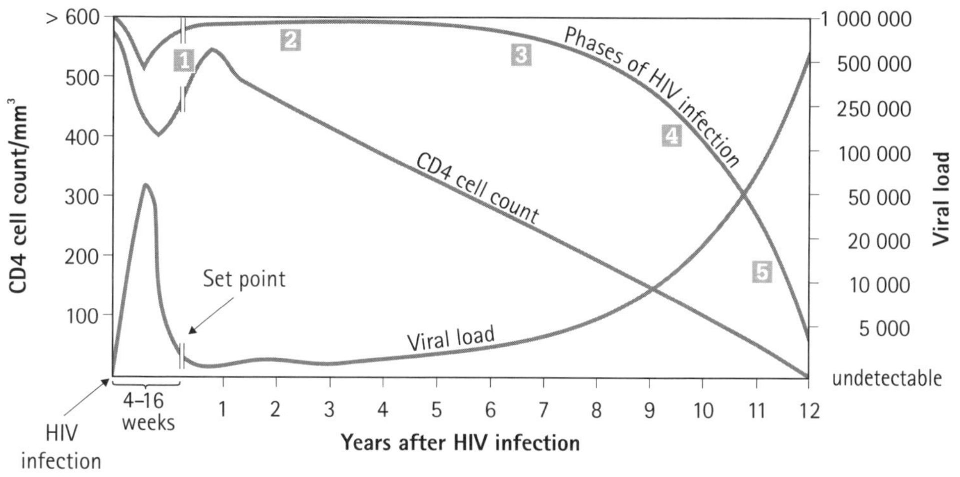

1 The primary HIV infection phase (or acute seroconversion illness)
2 The asymptomatic latent phase
3 The minor symptomatic phase
4 The major symptomatic phase with opportunistic diseases
5 The severe symptomatic phase: Aids-defining conditions

Note: This pattern may differ from individual to individual.

Figure 3.1
The relationship between a person's CD4 cell count, viral load and phases of HIV infection
(Source: Adapted from Evian, 2000:76)

stress, smoking or menstruation, and increase in response to exercise, positive living, antiretroviral therapy and something nice like taking a holiday. The viral load can also vary significantly. For example, infections such as flu or recent vaccinations can cause a temporary increase in viral load, while antiretroviral therapy will cause a decrease in viral load.

 Activity

Draw a picture to explain to a client the relationship between the viral load and the CD4 cell count. (Use the example of the train on its journey towards Aids if you cannot think of anything else.)

3.2 THE PHASES OF HIV INFECTION

Although HIV infection is *theoretically* divided into different phases, in *practice* these phases are not separate and distinct with easily identifiable boundaries. HIV-positive individuals also do not necessarily move in a distinct order from phase 1 to phase 5 of infection. At any time the development of HIV-related symptoms and opportunistic diseases will depend on the health of the immune system, in other words on the relationship between the CD4 cells and the viral load. There are many examples of people with severe immune depression (final phase of Aids) who 'moved back' to a minor symptomatic phase after starting antiretroviral treatment. It is nevertheless helpful to divide HIV infection into the following phases:

- the primary HIV infection phase (or acute seroconversion illness);
- the asymptomatic latent phase;
- the minor symptomatic phase;
- the major symptomatic phase; and
- the severe symptomatic phase, or Aids-defining conditions.

1. The primary HIV infection phase (or acute seroconversion illness)

The acute phase of HIV infection (also called acute seroconversion illness) begins as soon as seroconversion has taken place. Seroconversion means the point at which a person's HIV status *converts* or *changes* from being HIV negative to HIV positive. This usually coincides with the time when an HIV test will show that a person is HIV positive.

Seroconversion usually occurs about six weeks after infection with the HI virus. Approximately 30–60% of people infected with HIV will develop an illness similar to glandular fever at the time of seroconversion, and the symptoms of this fever will usually last a week or two. This seroconversion illness is often mistaken for a 'flu-like' viral infection, and it is characterised by symptoms such as a sore throat, headache, mild fever, fatigue or tiredness, muscle and joint pains, swelling of the lymph nodes, gastrointestinal symptoms, rash, and (occasionally) oral ulcers (Schoub, 1997b). According to Schoub (1999), acute seroconversion illness is seldom seen in children.

The HIV viral load is usually very high during the acute phase in the first weeks after infection (see Figure 3.1). This is due to very rapid multiplication and replication of the virus after infection. Or, to use our war metaphor: the enemy wants to send in as many of its soldiers as possible so as to overrun the local soldiers (CD4 cells) before being detected.

Because there are so many infectious HI viruses in the blood in the primary phase of infection, the HIV-positive individual is extremely infectious during this phase. However, it is not possible to say exactly at what point after exposure to the virus (or actual infection) the person becomes infectious to others. Remember that the viruses replicate at a tremendous rate before the immune system has had enough time to develop an immune response or to develop enough antibodies to be detected by HIV antibody tests (see 'The window period' on page 66).

The viral levels reach a steady state 16–24 weeks after infection. This is called the set point. A lower set point is usually an indication of a lowered viral burden in the body and a better outlook or prognosis for the patient. Some clinicians believe that immediate and aggressive treatment with antiretroviral therapy (HAART) for 9–12 months in the primary infection phase may be effective in reducing the viral load (SA HIV Clinicians Society, 2002a). However, this approach is still experimental, and evidence that it really works is limited. In any case, it is very difficult to tell whether a patient is in the primary or seroconversion phase.

Why does the viral load drop so dramatically after about 16 weeks of infection?

As can be seen in Figure 3.1, the viral load in the blood decreases dramatically 16–24 weeks after infection. This is because of the huge fight put up by the immune system, which has now had time to develop effective virus-specific immunity. A close look at Figure 3.1 will reveal that the CD4 cell count is increasing again at this point. But the immune system is facing a total and prolonged onslaught from the HI virus. It cannot keep up its defences indefinitely, and the virus will win in the end if the immune system does not receive help in the form of, for example, antiretroviral therapy.

What does it mean when we say that the viral load is 'undetectable' in the blood?

Viral loads can vary from 'undetectable' levels to values exceeding 2–3 million copies/ml of blood. Levels below 400 are considered 'undetectable' because they cannot be detected by the viral load test. An undetectable viral load does not mean that the person is no longer infected with HIV. The virus is still in the body, but at very low levels.

2. The asymptomatic latent phase of HIV disease

The second phase of HIV infection is the asymptomatic latent or silent phase. In this stage an infected person displays no symptoms. Infected individuals are often not even *aware* that they are carrying the HI virus in this stage, and may therefore unwittingly infect new sex partners. Even though the infected person may be ignorant of its presence, the virus nevertheless remains active in the body during this stage and it continues to damage and undermine the person's immune system (see enrichment box 'The titanic struggle in the so-called "silent phase"'). A positive HIV antibody test is often the only indication of HIV infection during this latent phase.

HIV-positive people can remain healthy for a long time, show no symptoms and carry on with their work in a normal way. Some people remain HIV positive for many years without any manifestation of clinical disease, while others may deteriorate rapidly, develop Aids and die within months. In some cases the only symptom during this phase is persistent generalised lymphadenopathy (swollen glands). The CD4 cell count usually decreases by 40–80 cells/mm^3 per year during the asymptomatic latent or silent phase (Evian, 2003:29).

The asymptomatic phase is usually associated with a CD4 cell count of between 500 and 800 cells/mm^3. (The normal CD4 cell count in healthy (non-infected) individuals is approximately 800–1 200 cells/mm^3.)

Performance scale 1: According to the World Health Organization staging system for HIV infection and disease, a person in the asymptomatic phase can be placed on *Performance scale 1*, which indicates *asymptomatic, normal* activity.

Enrichment

The titanic struggle in the so-called 'silent phase'

According to Schoub (1999:32) the clinical calmness of the latent phase deceptively conceals the titanic struggle that is taking place in the patient's body between rapidly replicating HIV and the frantic attempts of the CD4 population to replenish the vast number of cells destroyed by the virus. Studies of HIV-positive patients have demonstrated that in the clinically silent phase of infection, some 100 million virus particles are produced and destroyed daily while, at the same time, about 2 000 million CD4 lymphocytes, or 5% of the total population, are destroyed by the virus every day and need to be replaced by new cells. These findings illustrate not only the danger of the virus, but also the truly remarkable capacity of the body's immune system to be able to resist, even temporarily, this immense viral onslaught. After reaching very high levels in the first weeks after infection, the viral load usually reaches a steady state 4–6 months after infection. This steady state is due to the immune response, which helps to prevent HIV viral replication (Evian, 2003).

3. The minor symptomatic phase

In the third phase of infection, minor and early symptoms of HIV disease usually begin to manifest. This stage commences when people with HIV antibodies begin to present with one or more of the following symptoms:

- mild to moderate swelling of the lymph nodes in the neck, below the jaw, and in the armpits and groin;
- occasional fevers;
- herpes zoster or shingles;
- skin rashes, dermatitis, chronic itchy skin;
- fungal nail infections;
- recurrent oral ulcerations;
- recurrent upper respiratory tract infections;
- weight loss up to 10% of usual body weight; and
- malaise, fatigue and lethargy.

The minor symptomatic phase is usually associated with a CD4 cell count of between 350 and 500 cells/mm^3.

Performance scale 2: The individual in the minor symptomatic phase of HIV infection is usually able to carry on with his or her normal activities, despite being symptomatic.

What is shingles?

Shingles (or herpes zoster) is a viral infection caused by the same virus that causes chickenpox. In the days before the HIV/Aids pandemic, shingles used to be seen only in older people or in those who had weakened immune systems. Nowadays shingles is very common in people with HIV infection and Aids, and is regularly seen in young people. Shingles is often one of the first symptoms of HIV infection. It affects nerve cells and is characterised by an extremely painful skin rash (tiny blisters) on the face, limbs or body. It can also affect the eyes, causing pain and blurred vision. Shingles can be very severe in people with depressed immune systems.

4. The major symptomatic phase

Major symptoms and opportunistic diseases begin to appear as the immune system continues to deteriorate. At this point, the CD4 cell count becomes very low while the viral load becomes very high (see Figure 3.1). Signs of more severe HIV-related diseases begin to appear. These signs and symptoms are usually due to overgrowth of some of the body's natural flora with fungal infection and reactivation of old infections such as TB and herpes (Evian 2003:30). They are also caused by uncontrolled multiplication of HIV itself. More frequent and severe opportunistic diseases occur as the immune deficiency progresses. The following symptoms are usually an indication of advanced immune deficiency:

- persistent and recurrent oral and vaginal candida infections (or thrush): candida or thrush in the mouth is a common sign of immune deficiency and it does not usually occur unless the CD4 cell count is decreased – usually to < 350 cells/mm^3);
- recurrent herpes infections such as herpes simplex (cold sores);
- recurrent herpes zoster (or shingles);
- acne-like bacterial skin infections and skin rashes;
- intermittent or constant unexplained fever that lasts for more than a month;
- night sweats;
- persistent and intractable chronic diarrhoea that lasts for more than a month;
- significant and unexplained weight loss (more than 10% of the usual body weight);
- generalised lymphadenopathy (or, in some cases, the shrinking of previously enlarged lymph nodes);
- abdominal discomfort, headaches;
- oral hairy leukoplakia (thickened white patches on the tongue);
- persistent cough and reactivation of TB, especially in people from low socio-economic communities where TB is common; and
- opportunistic diseases of various kinds.

The onset of oral or vaginal candidiasis (thrush) and recurrent herpes infection, such as herpes simplex (cold sores) or herpes zoster (shingles), are commonly the first clinical signs of advanced immune deficiency.

The major symptomatic phase is usually associated with a CD4 cell count of between 200 and 350 cells/mm^3.

Performance scale 3: The person in the major symptomatic phase of HIV disease will usually have been bedridden for up to 50% of the day during the past month.

Enrichment

HIV and malaria

HIV-positive individuals are more prone to malaria than non-infected individuals. It has also been demonstrated that malaria causes a seven-fold increase in the HIV viral load of people with HIV infection. People with HIV infection should therefore take extra precautions when visiting malarial areas.

5. The severe symptomatic phase: Aids-defining conditions

Only when patients enter the last phase of HIV infection can they be said to have Aids. It usually takes about 18 months for the major symptomatic phase to develop into Aids.

Aids patients usually have a very high viral load and severe immune deficiency with a CD4 cell count below 200 cells/mm^3.

In the final stage of Aids, the symptoms of HIV disease become more acute: patients become infected by relatively rare and unusual organisms that do not respond to antibiotics; the immune system deteriorates exponentially (see Figure 3.1); and more persistent and untreatable opportunistic conditions and cancers begin to manifest. HIV-related organ damage is also common at this stage of Aids.

Performance scale 4: The Aids patient in the severe symptomatic phase will usually have been bedridden for more than 50% of the day during the past month. While people with Aids (the last phase of HIV disease) usually die within two years, antiretroviral therapy and the prevention and treatment of opportunistic infections may prolong this period.

Enrichment

A definition of opportunistic diseases

Opportunistic infections or diseases are caused by micro-organisms that do not normally become pathogenic in the presence of a healthy immune system (because a healthy immune system will kill them or render them inert). But when an immune system is unable to defend the body because it is being destroyed by HIV, opportunistic infections will 'take any opportunity' (hence the name) to attack the body successfully.

Symptoms of Aids

Any of the following symptoms, conditions or opportunistic infections can occur in the Aids patient:

- Because of continuous *diarrhoea, nausea and vomiting* (which may last for weeks or even for months), an Aids patient is usually thin and emaciated. Continuous diarrhoea is often caused by infections of the bowel.
- The patient is plagued by *oral manifestations* of HIV infection such as oral candidiasis, oral hairy leukoplakia, herpes simplex (cold sores), varicella zoster and bacterial periodontal conditions. Thrush in the mouth, throat or oesophagus may become so painful that the patient is no longer able to swallow or to eat.
- Persistent, recurrent *vaginal candidiasis* (yeast infection or thrush) is often the first sign of HIV infection in women. An increased incidence and severity of *cervical cancer* has also been reported in women with HIV infection. Studies indicate that amenorrhoea (absence of menstruation) in women of reproductive age, and severe pelvic infections with abscess formation, can also be associated with HIV infection in women (Friesen et al., 1997; Smeltzer & Bare, 1992).
- *Persistent generalised lymphadenopathy* (PGL) may be said to be present when lymph nodes are larger than one centimetre in diameter, in two or more sites other than the groin area, for a period of at least three months.
- Severe and recurrent *skin infections* such as warts, ringworm and folliculitis occur in some Aids patients. These conditions usually cause blisters and ulcerations.

- *Respiratory infections* may cause the patient to present with a persistent cough, chest pain and fever.
- Pneumonia, especially *Pneumocystis carinii pneumonia* (PCP), is often seen in patients with Aids. PCP is a parasitic infection of the lungs caused by a protozoan. PCP is characterised by a continual dry, non-productive cough, laboured and sometimes painful breathing, weight loss and fever. The disease is less common in black Africans.
- Wasting of the body tissues and marked *weight loss* are often seen in patients with Aids.
- Severe *herpes zoster* (or shingles) often occurs in people with depressed immune systems.
- The Aids patient is usually *fatigued and exhausted*, and this can promote multiple infections such as shingles, herpes, dermatitis or skin infections and ulcerative herpes simplex and PGL.
- *Peripheral neuropathy* (a disease of the peripheral nerves) often occurs in Aids patients. It is characterised by pains, numbness or pins and needles in the hands and feet.
- Aids patients sometimes suffer from *neurological abnormalities* such as HIV encephalopathy, which is characterised by symptoms such as memory loss, poor concentration, tremor, headache, confusion, loss of vision and seizures.
- Aids patients may develop *cryptococcal meningitis* (a fungal infection in the central nervous system) which causes fever, headache, malaise, nausea, vomiting, neck stiffness, mental status changes and seizures.
- *Toxoplasma encephalitis* (a protozoal infection of the brain that causes damage to the brain itself) can also occur. Cats are the major hosts of *Toxoplasma gondii*, the organism that causes the disease.

Table 3.1

Opportunistic infections, causing agents and cancers associated with Aids

	Causing agent/cancer	Opportunistic infection
Bacteria	• Mycobacterium tuberculosis • Group B streptococcus • *Haemophilus influenzae* • Pneumococci • *Salmonella* • Atypical mycobacterium	• Lungs, meninges • Lungs (usually in children) • Lungs (usually in children) • Lungs and bloodstream • Gastrointestinal tract and blood • Lung and other organs
Viruses	• Herpes simplex • Herpes zoster (shingles) • Cytomegalovirus	• Skin and nervous system • Skin and nervous system • Lungs, retina, brain, gastrointestinal tract, liver
Protozoa	• *Pneumocystis carinii* • Toxoplasmosis • Cryptosporidium	• Lungs • Meninges, brain, eyes • Gastrointestinal tract and gall bladder
Fungi	• *Candida* • *Cryptococcus* • Histoplasmosis	• Mouth, oesophagus, gastrointestinal tract, vagina, skin, nails • Meninges and lungs • Lungs
Cancer	• Kaposi's sarcoma • Lymphomas – non-Hodgkin's • Ano-genital (human papilloma virus) • Liver (associated with hepatitis B or C) • Multi-centre (Castleman's disease)	• Skin, gastrointestinal tract • Lymph nodes • Ano-genital area • Liver

- The cytomegalovirus (CMV), a common inhabitant of the human body, can cause severe opportunistic infections in immune-depressed individuals. In Aids patients CMV often causes *retinitis*, an inflammation of the retina of the eye, which in many cases leads to blindness. CMV is a common cause of severe and often lethal *pneumonia* and it also targets the *gastrointestinal tract*. CMV is often excreted in the urine, saliva, semen, cervical secretions, faeces or breast milk of immune-depressed patients. CMV infections usually occur in the late stages of Aids when the CD4 levels fall below 50 cells/mm^3.
- *Kaposi's sarcoma*, a rare form of skin cancer, TC characterised by a painless reddish-brown or bluish-purple swelling on the skin and mucous membranes (e.g. in the mouth). Kaposi's sarcoma can also occur in the gastrointestinal tract and lungs. Kaposi's sarcoma responds well to chemotherapy and to alpha-interferon, but it can develop into invasive open lesions and cause death if not promptly treated. Kaposi's sarcoma is less common in black Africans.
- *Lymphoma* or cancer of the lymph nodes may present with enlargement of lymph nodes, the spleen or liver.
- Various other cancers such as ano-genital cancer (caused by the human papilloma virus) and liver cancer (associated with hepatitis B or C) may attack the body.
- *Tuberculosis* (TB), often extrapulmonary (outside the lungs), is a very serious opportunistic infection in people with Aids. According to a UNAIDS Report (2004), up to 70% of tuberculosis patients in sub-Saharan Africa are also infected with HIV. TB is such a critical health problem in Africa that it will be dealt with in more detail in section 3.5 on page 47.
- Other sexually transmitted infections are discussed in more detail in section 3.6 on page 53.

Table 3.1 on page 44 gives a summary of the common opportunistic infections, causing agents and cancers associated with Aids (based on Evian, 2003:33).

Enrichment

The importance of regular pap smears

Because HIV infection may increase the risk of cervical cancer, it is important to do a pap smear of the cervix on all HIV-positive women every one to two years. Encourage women to come back for the results of their pap smear, and refer them for gynaecological evaluation if their results are abnormal (Evian, 2000).

3.3 SYMPTOMS OF HIV INFECTION IN CHILDREN

Children with HIV infection often present with non-specific conditions that are common in childhood. The symptoms and conditions most often associated with HIV infection and Aids in children are:

- failure to thrive and weight loss (due to the direct effect of the virus on the gastrointestinal tract, secondary opportunistic infections or poor nutritional intake);
- prolonged fever;
- recurrent oral thrush (candidiasis);
- chronic diarrhoea and gastroenteritis;
- tuberculosis (pulmonary or extrapulmonary);
- recurrent bacterial infections (infections of the upper respiratory tract, otitis media or ear infections, pneumonia, tonsillitis, septicaemia, cellulitis, urinary tract infections, skin infections, osteomyelitis and meningitis);
- lymphoid interstitial pneumonitis, an otherwise rare lung disease found in HIV-positive children and characterised by a continuous cough and mild wheezing (usually has a good prognosis);
- anaemia, pallor, nose bleeds;
- PGL (swelling of the lymph nodes in the neck, armpit and groin);
- hepatomegaly (enlargement of the liver);
- splenomegaly (enlargement of the spleen);
- skin conditions such as severe nappy rash and allergic skin eruptions; extensive seborrhoeic dermatitis (an inflammation of the skin characterised by a yellowish, greasy scaling);
- herpes infections such as herpes zoster, herpes simplex;
- enlargement of the parotid gland and parotitis (inflammation of the parotid gland);

- delays in reaching developmental milestones or the loss of those already attained;
- neurological abnormalities such as seizures and reduced head growth;
- severe herpes simplex infection;
- complicated chickenpox or measles;
- *Pneumocystis carinii* pneumonia (PCP): occurs most commonly in children aged under one and is usually associated with a very poor prognosis;
- any other Aids-defining condition such as Kaposi's sarcoma, toxoplasmosis, or cytomegalovirus infections.

(Sources: Evian, 2000, 2003; Paediatric HIV Working Group, 1997; WHO, 2000a)

Symptoms such as diarrhoea, recurrent fever and dermatitis, common to many treatable conditions in children, tend to be more persistent and severe in HIV-positive children. HIV-positive children also do not respond to treatment as well as non-infected children and are more likely to suffer life-threatening complications.

Infections in children should be recognised and treated as early as possible. Parents and caregivers should therefore be encouraged to seek medical help as soon as they can if the child develops any unusual signs or symptoms. Hospitalisation should be avoided as far as possible, since the hospital environment exposes the immune-deficient HIV-positive child to many harmful pathogens or germs.

The clinical course of HIV infection in children differs significantly from that in adults. The time lapse between infection and the onset of Aids is usually much shorter in children than it is in adults, and most infected infants develop the disease during the first year of life. We estimate that 75% of all HIV-positive children will have died before their fifth birthday unless given antiretroviral therapy.

HIV viral activity in children is different from that in adults. In adults, high viral levels occur in the first weeks after infection and levels reach a steady state 4–6 months after the primary infection (see Figure 3.1 on page 39). In babies infected at birth there is a very rapid increase in the HIV viral level in the first weeks of life, and the level remains very high for a year or two, after which it gradually declines, reaching a steady state by the age of 5 or 6 (Evian, 2003:159).

Children who acquire HIV infection during pregnancy, birth or breastfeeding can be divided into two main groups: *rapid progressors* and *slow progressors*. Rapid progressors usually develop symptoms of HIV/Aids between 6 and 12 months of age. They are usually sickly from birth, have constant diarrhoea, never thrive and usually die within the first 2 years of life. About 40–60% of children with HIV infection are rapid progressors, and they usually have high viral loads and low CD4 cell counts. Children who are slow progressors usually develop mild symptoms some time after the first year of life. They often survive to older childhood and even into the early teenage years.

The progress of Aids in children may be accelerated by poor nutrition and illnesses such as gastroenteritis, TB, respiratory infections, malaria and measles.

It is often difficult to diagnose HIV infection in a child under 18 months of age because an HIV antibody test may react to the antibodies transferred from the mother to the child during pregnancy (see 'When a baby can be tested for HIV infection' on page 68). A p24 or HIV PCR test should be done in children younger than 18 months.

Activity

- Make a sketch of the adult human body. Label the different parts of the body: the head, eyes, mouth, throat, lymph nodes, lungs, abdomen (stomach), skin, genital and anal area, and feet. Use each of these body parts as a heading. Also make one heading for 'general problems'. Arrange all the symptoms and conditions usually associated with advanced HIV disease or Aids under these labels. The symptoms and diseases usually associated with Aids should be clear after one glance at your sketch of the human body.
- Make a sketch of a young child and indicate the symptoms usually associated with Aids in children (as you did in the activity above, but adapted for children).

3.4 THE PREVENTION OF OPPORTUNISTIC INFECTIONS

There are a number of opportunistic diseases (see the enrichment box 'A definition of opportunistic diseases' on page 43) that are common in HIV-positive people with depleted immune systems. It therefore makes sense to prevent these infections from occurring by initiating treatment for them before they can develop. Prophylactic (or preventive) treatment for opportunistic diseases is generally based on CD4 cell counts. A low CD4 count (< 200) is usually a sign of immune deficiency as well as a certain indication that the patient will develop opportunistic infections. If CD4 lymphocyte tests are not available, conditions such as oral thrush, skin infections, herpes simplex (cold sores) or herpes zoster (shingles) may be signs of immune deficiency, and a good sign that prophylactic treatment should be started. The following opportunistic infections can be prevented with timely treatment:

- TB is the commonest opportunistic infection in Africa, and TB prophylaxis (preventive treatment against the disease) should routinely be given to patients whose CD4 cell counts drop below 350 cells/mm^3 (this prevents the reactivation of latent TB bacilli). If CD4 cell counts are not available, TB prophylaxis should be considered in a patient who shows signs of immune deficiency. To avoid drug resistance, it is important to make sure that the patient does not have active TB, and that he or she will be able to take the medication as prescribed. (See 'Tuberculosis and HIV: the curse of Africa'.)
- Prophylaxis for PCP should be started when the CD4 cell count drops to lower than 200 cells/mm^3 (PCP is usually treated with co-trimoxazole, e.g. Bactrim or Septran).
- Oral, oesophageal and vaginal candidiasis commonly starts to appear when the CD4 count drops below 350 cells/mm^3 and can be prevented by using a locally applied agent or fluconazole.
- Toxoplasmosis can be prevented (with co-trimoxazole) when the CD4 count drops below 200 cells/mm^3.
- If herpes infections are recurrent, severe and very debilitating, prophylaxis should be considered if affordable by using aciclovir or valaciclovir.
- Patients can also be offered immunisation against various diseases such as influenza and hepatitis B.

It is important to prevent opportunistic infections in children with HIV infection. Prophylactic treatment should be considered for infections such as TB, PCP, candidiasis and recurrent bacterial infections. It is recommended that prophylaxis against TB and PCP in children should start as soon as the child shows clinical signs of HIV infection or as soon the HIV PCR test is positive (Paediatric HIV Working Group, 1997).

Pregnant HIV-positive women may receive prophylactic treatment (e.g. co-trimoxazole) from the second trimester onwards if necessary, but should not receive any vaccinations.

3.5 TUBERCULOSIS AND HIV: THE CURSE OF AFRICA

TB is the most serious and most common opportunistic infection that attacks HIV-positive people, especially in Africa. It is estimated that 50% or more of the HIV-positive people in Africa are co-infected with TB (Coker & Miller, 1997; UNAIDS, 2000c). The greatest impact of HIV on tuberculosis has been in sub-Saharan Africa, where up to 70% of TB patients are also infected with HIV (UNAIDS, 2004). TB is the most common cause of death in Aids patients because it is reactivated as the immune system fails. TB accelerates HIV disease and is responsible for 32% of all HIV-related deaths in Africa.

Researchers are deeply concerned about the high incidence of TB in HIV-positive people in South Africa. In 1996 the World Health Organization declared the TB epidemic in South Africa to be the worst in the world. In Hlabisa, a community of 205 000 people in KwaZulu-Natal, the percentage of adults with TB increased from 8.7% in 1991 to 70% in 1997. Most of these TB patients are co-infected with HIV ('True terror', 1997).

But why is this dual infection with TB and HIV so dangerous?

The dangers of the TB-HIV combination

The combination of TB and HIV is a disastrous combination for the following reasons (Evian, 2000, 2003; South African TB Control Programme, 2000; Van Dyk, 1999; WHO, 2000a):

- An HIV-positive patient with a deficient immune system has a ten times greater risk of developing TB or of having his or her old infection reactivated.
- HIV shortens the time between exposure to the TB bacillus (the agent that causes TB) and the development of active TB.
- The mortality (death) rate from TB is as much as four times higher in people who are infected with HIV.
- TB can shorten the time it takes for HIV to become final-phase Aids, and it can also worsen the condition of someone suffering from Aids.
- HIV-positive people have a much greater chance of developing extrapulmonary TB (i.e. TB *outside* the lungs). These forms of TB include TB of the lymph glands, brain, bone, spine, joints, heart, kidneys, liver, genital tract, and so on.
- Miliary TB is more common in patients with HIV infection. Miliary TB results from widespread blood-borne dissemination of TB bacilli and is often an under-diagnosed cause of end-stage wasting in HIV-positive individuals.
- TB can diminish the number of CD4 cells in the body while correspondingly increasing the HI viral load.
- The presence of HIV reduces the accuracy of the methods used to detect TB infection. HIV-positive people with a low CD4 cell count may not be able to mount an immune response to a tuberculin (Mantoux) skin test, so the skin test will give a false negative result. Sputum smears may also be negative, and even chest X-rays can be unreliable. Such false results lead to non-diagnosis, giving TB the chance to spread even more widely in the community.
- There is a higher chance of TB treatment failure.
- The recurrence of TB is more common in HIV-positive individuals.
- Adverse or unwanted reactions to the drugs used to treat TB may be more likely in HIV-positive patients. These reactions to the TB drugs may also be confused with HIV/Aids-related conditions such as peripheral neuropathy (nerve problems in the feet and hands), visual disturbances, skin reactions and diarrhoea.
- The diagnosis of TB can be confused with the diagnosis of other HIV-related lung conditions such as PCP and other forms of pneumonia. This could delay treatment of these conditions.
- Unusual forms of TB such as MAI (*Mycobacterium avium-intracellulare*) are more common, especially in the advanced Aids stage.
- The development of multiple drug resistance in HIV-positive people is grounds for great concern. HIV-positive patients with TB may find it particularly difficult to comply conscientiously with the treatment regimen, because the side effects they experience from taking TB medicines may be far more severe than in people who are HIV negative. They may therefore be tempted to skip doses or stop taking the medication altogether. Such interruptions of treatment facilitate the development of TB bacilli that are increasingly resistant to medication.
- Interactions may occur between some TB drugs (such as rifampicin) and some HIV-related drugs (such as some protease inhibitors).

Because HIV and TB frequently occur together in Africa, it is vitally important for health care professionals to be well informed about TB and to recognise its symptoms when they see them.

The cause of TB

TB is an infectious disease caused by a microorganism, the bacillus *Mycobacterium tuberculosis*, which usually enters the body by inhalation. *Mycobacterium tuberculosis* usually affects the lungs, but it may also spread from the lungs to almost any part of the body via the bloodstream, the lymphatic system, or the airways.

Pulmonary TB (in the lungs) is the infectious and common form of the disease, occurring in over 80% of cases. Extrapulmonary TB results from the spread of the disease to other organs, most commonly the pleura, lymph nodes, meninges (of the brain), spine, joints, genito-urinary tract, intestines and pericardium (of the heart), kidneys, bones or abdomen. TB may affect any part of the body. While TB in these sites may cause serious illness, the infected person is not likely to transmit the disease unless they *also* have TB of the lungs.

TB develops in two stages in the human body.

- The first stage occurs when an individual breathes in the TB bacilli and becomes infected. The immune system usually brings this original infection under control, but (in contrast with most other infectious agents) the TB bacillus usually remains dormant in the body for a number of years. The TB-infected person shows no symptoms of TB during this dormant phase of infection. Among those who do become infected, most (90%) will never become ill with TB.
- If, during this dormant period, the immunity of the host is suddenly weakened or compromised (as happens when a person suffers from continuous malnutrition, or when the immune system is suppressed, for example by HIV, stress, cancer or diabetes), the TB bacilli immediately begin to multiply. This multiplication leads to the second stage of the disease, which includes any one of the several TB diseases. If the patient's body can recover from this illness, the TB bacilli once again revert to dormancy.

About a third of the world's population (including most South Africans) carry latent tuberculosis infection (where *Mycobacterium tuberculosis* bacilli lie dormant in the body without causing disease). In the absence of HIV only about 5% of people with latent TB bacilli will *ever* progress to the active disease. However, infection with HIV dramatically increases the probability that someone already harbouring latent tuberculosis will develop active TB (up to 5–10% *annually*) (UNAIDS, 2004).

The spread of TB

The infectiousness of a person with TB is determined by the concentration of TB bacilli in the lungs, and their spread into the air surrounding that person (SA TB Control Programme, 2000). When a person with active pulmonary TB coughs, spits or sneezes, he or she produces small droplets that contain TB bacilli. If a susceptible person inhales these droplets, he or she may become infected and may later develop active TB.

The most infectious cases are those with a positive smear by microscopy (smear-positive cases). Patients in whom micro-organisms cannot be seen directly under the microscope (smear-negative cases) are far less infectious. As stated earlier, patients with extrapulmonary TB are almost never infectious, unless they have pulmonary TB as well.

Health care professionals should protect themselves by wearing tightly fitting masks and by teaching patients with active TB to cover their mouths and noses when coughing or sneezing.

Enrichment

TB – a risk for all

The growing wave of TB is not only a menace for those infected with HIV. TB can spread through the air to HIV-negative people. It is the only major Aids-related opportunistic infection that threatens HIV-negative people in this way (UNAIDS, 1997).

The symptoms of TB

The symptoms of pulmonary (lung) TB are:

- persistent cough for 3 weeks or more;
- blood-stained sputum (coughing blood);
- shortness of breath and chest pain;
- loss of appetite;
- loss of weight and sunken cheek bones;
- night sweats and fever;
- a general feeling of illness (malaise);
- tiredness, loss of motivation and loss of strength; and
- anaemia.

Health care professionals working with HIV-positive people should always be alert to the possibility of TB, especially in patients who present with persistent coughs, night sweats and weight loss. Voluntary HIV counselling and testing (VCT) clinics should use TB checklists and refer patients with symptoms to their nearest TB treatment clinic. TB clinics likewise should look out for symptoms of HIV and refer the patient for counselling, testing and treatment.

The diagnosis of TB

TB can be diagnosed in the following ways:

- sputum for acid-fast bacilli;
- chest X-rays;
- TB sputum culture;
- other tissue cultures for extrapulmonary TB; and
- tuberculin (Mantoux) skin test (not very helpful in communities where TB is common, as in South Africa).

1. *Sputum (phlegm) for acid-fast bacilli (AFB).* A sputum examination for AFB is the most important test for diagnosing TB. A sputum specimen is spread on a slide, stained by the Ziehl-Neelsen method and examined microscopically. If AFB are detected by this method, the patient is said to have smear-positive TB. A smear-positive result indicates active TB with large numbers of TB bacilli in the lungs. Such a person is likely to spread TB to other people.

   Although sputum tests are the most important tests for diagnosing TB, they sometimes show false negative results in HIV-positive patients, and chest X-rays should therefore be done in HIV-positive cases where TB is strongly suspected.
2. *Chest X-rays.* Although chest X-rays are convenient and quick, reliance on chest X-rays as the primary means of confirming a diagnosis of TB is often questionable. Many diseases (such as PCP and viral and fungal diseases) mimic TB on chest X-rays, and this may lead to incorrect diagnosis. X-rays may also show lung fibrosis or destruction due to old TB, leading to over-diagnosis and erroneous treatment of pulmonary TB. Chest X-rays are, however, important in cases where the sputum results are negative but TB is nevertheless suspected. Sputum-negative TB is more common in HIV-positive patients than in HIV-negative patients (Evian, 2003; SA TB Control Programme, 2000).
3. *TB sputum culture.* TB sputum culture is an expensive diagnostic technique, and is seldom used to diagnose TB. It is also not necessary to do this test if the sputum is definitely positive for TB (i.e. AFB are present). However, sputum cultures may be needed for diagnosis when smear microscopy is negative but TB is suspected. The use of sputum culture is also suggested for the diagnosis of drug-resistant TB in patients who do not respond to treatment or whose clinical condition is deteriorating in spite of treatment. TB cultures are also helpful in the diagnosis of some of the unusual forms of TB.
4. *Other tissue cultures.* Blood cultures are sometimes used for diagnosing extrapulmonary TB; stool or urine may be used for the diagnosis of gastrointestinal tract or urinary TB; and tissue biopsy may be done to diagnose extrapulmonary disease such as TB in the lymph nodes, liver or bone marrow.
5. *Tuberculin skin test.* The tuberculin skin test (Mantoux test) is not a good diagnostic indicator of TB in adults from communities where TB is common. Tuberculin skin tests should, for example, not be used in South Africa (and other African countries) to diagnose TB, because most South Africans have been exposed to TB and will therefore test positive on tuberculin skin tests. In the South African mines, for instance, 97% of mineworkers test positive on tuberculin skin tests because of previous exposure to TB bacilli. (Note that a positive Mantoux test indicates that a person was *in contact* with a TB patient and is therefore *infected* with TB, but it does not necessarily mean that the person has *active* TB disease. The bacilli can be dormant and the person healthy.)

? What does a positive tuberculin skin test mean in a child under 5 years old?

A strongly positive tuberculin skin test in a child under 5 years old indicates recent infection, which is a risk factor for progression to disease. If other factors are present, such as contact with a TB patient, signs and symptoms of TB and X-ray changes, the child should be treated with TB medications for 3 months (SA TB Control Programme, 2000). A negative tuberculin skin test, however, does not exclude the possibility of TB in children. Various conditions may suppress the tuberculin test and give a false negative result. Such conditions could be HIV infection, malnutrition, severe viral infections (e.g. measles, chickenpox), cancer, immunosuppressive drugs (e.g. steroids) or severe disseminated TB. If a child has a negative skin test but a chest X-ray raises the suspicion of TB, TB can be diagnosed.

The treatment of TB

TB can be completely cured in almost every case of infection if the patient completes a course of antibiotic treatment. Active TB is usually treated with the simultaneous administration of a combination of drugs that destroy the infective organisms. The following drugs are used in different combinations to kill the TB bacilli and to cure TB. (Fixed-dose combination tablets are also available.)

- Isoniazid (INH)
- Rifampicin
- Pyrazinamide
- Streptomycin
- Ethambutol

> Because treatment regimens change from time to time, the specific combinations, dosages and durations of anti-TB medications are not given here. Consult the following booklet on TB treatment regimens as used by the South African Department of Health: *South African Tuberculosis Control Programme – Practical guidelines.* This brochure is regularly updated and is available free of charge from:
>
> Director General, Department of Health, Private Bag X828, Pretoria, 0001

The principles of managing TB patients who are co-infected with HIV

HIV-positive people are treated for TB in exactly the same way as HIV-negative people. The following are the principles of managing TB patients (Evian, 2003:251):

- Pulmonary and extrapulmonary TB are treated with the same anti-TB drugs.
- The treatment regimen for first-time TB patients differs from that of second-time patients or those in whom treatment has failed.
- A combination of drugs is always used. For example, patients may be given a combination that includes rifampicin, INH, pyrazinamide and ethambutol, with streptomycin added for second-time users. Specific combinations and dosages depend on whether the patient is a first- or second-time user.
- First-time users receive therapy for at least 6 months (2 months of intensive treatment and 4 months of continuation or maintenance treatment).
- Second-time users (recurrent TB, failed or interrupted treatment) receive therapy for at least 8 months.
- Treatment is usually given for 5 days a week, Monday to Friday, as a daily dose.
- Compliance (taking the drugs as prescribed) is absolutely essential to avoid the development of multi-drug-resistant TB bacilli (MDR TB). Directly observed treatment short course (DOTS) is indicated for individuals who find it difficult to take every dose of medication (see enrichment box 'DOTS to enhance compliance with TB treatment' on page 52).
- TB treatment should not begin before there is a definite diagnosis of TB (sputum or culture).
- Multi-drug resistance should always be considered if treatment fails in spite of patient compliance.
- Weight loss should stabilise and cough and night sweat symptoms should show definite signs of alleviation within 4 to 6 weeks of commencing treatment.
- Sputum samples should be negative after 3 to 5 months.
- Health care professionals should pay close attention to any side effects that arise from taking TB medication. Possible side effects are peripheral neuropathy (numbness, tingling or pins and needles in the feet or hands), hepatitis, fever and rash, renal failure, visual disturbances, hearing loss, bleeding tendency and shock. If these serious side effects occur, the drug(s) responsible should be stopped temporarily or permanently. However, it is

important to note that some of these symptoms may be confused with symptoms of HIV-related disease.

- TB medications such as rifampicin may interact with some antiretroviral medications, and this may result in a reduction in the levels of the antiretroviral medication. TB should therefore always be managed by public-sector TB clinics where they are aware of these drug interactions. If the patient is already on ART, the ART regimen is usually changed to be compatible with rifampicin (see 'Interactions between antiretrovirals and other medications' on page 78).

Enrichment

DOTS to enhance compliance with TB treatment

Compliance with TB treatment can be enhanced by implementing the DOTS (or directly observed treatment short course) strategy in communities. The DOTS strategy uses 'patient observers' to watch TB patients swallow each dose of medicine for the complete treatment period of 6 to 8 months. Trained health care workers, responsible members of the community (such as traditional and religious leaders, teachers and employers) and other volunteers (such as shopkeepers, family members, friends and former TB patients) are appointed in the community to ensure that patients stick to their daily regimen and take their medication as often as they need to for the prescribed time.

The principles of managing children with TB

- Combinations and dosages are different for the treatment of children under 8 years of age (see SA TB Control Programme – Practical guidelines).
- Children receive treatment for 6 months (a 2-month initial phase of treatment 5 times a week, and a 4-month continuation phase).
- All children with severe forms of TB (meningitis, spine, peritonitis, miliary, bones) should be referred to a hospital for management.

Prevention of TB in patients with HIV/Aids

It is possible to reduce the incidence of TB in HIV-positive patients by treating them prophy-

Enrichment

BCG

BCG is a vaccine routinely given to babies to provide them with TB antibodies. BCG immunisation gives up to 80% protection against the progression of TB infection to active TB disease. However, the main benefit of BCG is protection against the development of serious extrapulmonary forms of TB such as TB meningitis or miliary TB in children.

lactically with INH for 9 months. INH prophylaxis works mainly by preventing reactivation of latent or dormant TB bacilli in the lungs. (A combination of rifampicin and pyrazinamide given for 2 months can be used as an alternative to INH prophylaxis.)

INH prophylaxis should be offered to all HIV-positive individuals with a CD4 cell count of under 350 cells/mm^3 provided that (1) they make a commitment to adhere to therapy, and (2) they show no signs of active TB. If patients are not reliable and do not take every single dose of the medication for the full prescribed period, INH drug resistance may develop. The development of drug resistance is also the reason why INH prophylaxis should never be given to patients who already show symptoms of active TB infection (such as weight loss, cough, chest pain or abnormal chest X-ray). Patients with active TB are never treated with only one drug (e.g. INH), but always with a combination of drugs. To treat a patient with active TB with only one drug (such as INH) will encourage the TB bacilli to become resistant to the effects of the drug. This same drug will then have no effect on the TB bacilli when used in the future.

The difference between TB *prophylaxis* and TB *treatment* can be illustrated with the following examples:

- Joan is HIV positive with a CD4 cell count of 300. She does not have any symptoms of active TB. To prevent Joan from developing TB, she should take isoniazid (INH) prophylactically for 9 months.
- Peter is HIV positive with a CD4 cell count of 300. He has had a persistent cough for the past month, he is always tired, he has lost a lot of weight, and he complains of night sweats and

fever. Peter has active TB and if he is a first-time patient he should be properly treated with a *combination* of TB drugs, such as rifampicin plus INH plus pyrazinamide plus ethambutol for the first 2-month initial phase, and then a combination of rifampicin plus INH for a further 4 months. If Peter is treated prophylactically with INH only, the treatment will be inadequate to cure his TB, and this will lead to INH-resistant TB bacilli.

Multi-drug-resistant TB

The emergence of MDR TB is the most serious aspect of the TB epidemic. Multi-drug-resistant bacilli are resistant to at least INH and rifampicin. Multi-drug resistance develops when treatment for TB is inadequate, or when patients do not comply with treatment. Multi-drug resistance is a very serious situation because the patient is at a much higher risk of developing progressive life-threatening TB; it is very expensive to treat MDR TB; and these drug-resistant bacilli could spread to others, including health care personnel, with serious results. MDR TB is very difficult to treat, and the cure rate is currently less than 50% (SA TB Control Programme, 2000). According to Evian (2003:257), 1% of new patients and 4% of those needing retreatment in South Africa are multi-drug resistant.

MDR TB is present if:

- a patient does not respond to treatment with a drug regimen containing INH and rifampicin; and
- there is clinical and laboratory evidence of resistance to these drugs.

MDR patients should be referred to a TB specialist centre for correct management and therapy. Treatment of MDR TB should continue for at least 12 months after the sputum converts to negative. This means that full treatment for MDR TB should last 18–24 months.

3.6 SEXUALLY TRANSMITTED INFECTIONS AND HIV: A DEADLY COMBINATION

Sexually transmitted infections (STIs) constitute a major public health problem in southern Africa. It has been estimated that more than 1 million people a year seek treatment for STIs at municipal clinics and in private practice. Many more are seen at hospitals and primary health care clinics. However, it is believed that most STI cases in Africa do not attend health facilities, but are treated by traditional healers (Green, 1994).

For the following reasons, patients who have STIs are particularly prone to HIV infection:

- Patients with genital ulcers (sores) are especially susceptible to HIV infection because the sores create openings in the mucous membranes – openings through which the HI virus can easily move.
- Statistical evidence suggests that STIs that do not cause ulcers can also facilitate the transmission of HIV (Green, 1994). Genital inflammation causes the migration of millions of lymphocytes to the site of the infection (in and around the genital tract). As we noted earlier, these cells have special receptors on their surfaces, receptors to which HI viruses attach themselves in preparation for easy entry into the body (Evian, 2000). STIs (especially genital ulcers) thus make it five to ten times easier for the HI virus to enter the body.
- The concentration (number) of HI viruses is very high in genital discharges and secretions, which are increased in STIs. An HIV-positive person who also suffers from an STI is therefore extremely infectious.
- People with STIs are also more vulnerable to HIV because they are likely to have sex with a number of partners, increasing their risk of coming into contact with other STIs and HIV.
- Because an HIV infection may delay the healing and cure of STIs, HIV infection often makes STIs more severe and difficult to treat.

Special attention should therefore be paid to patients who frequently visit STI clinics, and health care professionals should always be on the lookout for HIV infection. Most non-viral STIs are curable and preventable. It is therefore of the utmost importance for health care professionals to identify people with STIs as soon as possible, to treat them, and to refer them for HIV testing after pre-test counselling. *Many Aids researchers in Africa believe that the control of STIs may be the key to combating HIV.* In South African mines, for example, one of the strategies of health care professionals in the attempt to combat Aids is the prevention and treatment of STIs.

 Enrichment

Condoms and sexually transmitted infections

Latex condoms, when used consistently and correctly, are highly effective in preventing the transmission of HIV. In addition, their correct and consistent use can reduce the risk of transmission of gonorrhoea, chlamydia, and trichomoniasis. Latex condoms can also reduce the risk of transmission of genital herpes, syphilis, chancroid and HPV (human papilloma virus), but *only* when the infected areas are covered or protected by the condom. The use of latex condoms has also been associated with a reduction in risk of HPV-associated diseases, such as cervical cancer (CDC prevention messages, 2002).

Diagnostic versus syndromic management of sexually transmitted infections

The ideal approach in the management of STIs is to establish a definitive diagnosis of the STI by identifying the causing organism, and to treat the infection with absolute precision. However, this *diagnostic approach* is very difficult to follow in southern Africa because of its dependence on laboratory support. Laboratories with sophisticated techniques and facilities are often not available in remote or rural areas. Waiting for laboratory results to confirm a diagnosis delays the test results. Because it is often not possible for patients to return for test results at a later stage, the STI goes untreated and the danger of infecting sex partners remains.

A more practical alternative for the management of STIs in Africa is the *syndromic approach*. Syndromic management of STIs involves recognising clinical signs and patient symptoms (or a syndrome) and prescribing treatment for the major causes of that syndrome. A syndrome can be defined as a combination of symptoms or complaints. The syndromic approach enables health care workers who lack specialised skills and access to sophisticated laboratory tests to treat most symptomatic infections effectively during a patient's first clinic visit. A study of community-based syndromic management of sexually transmitted infections in Mwanza, Tanzania, showed that the number of new HIV infections in the study population was cut by 42% (UNAIDS report, 2002:90).

The following are the most important STI-related syndromes (Ballard et al., 2000:54):

- urethral discharge in men;
- scrotal swelling;
- vaginal discharge;
- lower abdominal pain;
- genital ulcers in men and women;
- inguinal bubo (swelling) without ulcer; and
- balanitis/balanoposthitis in men.

Syndromic case management offers several advantages: it is easy to use; it is inexpensive; it does not require highly trained STI specialists; it does not require laboratory support; and it allows treatment of the infection at the time of the first visit with no delays or need for a return visit. The treatment recommended covers the whole range of infections known to cause the syndrome, and the success rates are high. For example, if a certain syndrome is known to be caused by either *gonorrhoea* or *chlamydia*, the syndromic approach requires medications that will treat both conditions. One of the disadvantages of the syndromic approach is over-treatment of patients, who may receive more drugs than are actually necessary. This approach also does not address the problem of people with asymptomatic infection who do not come for treatment.

Syndromic flowcharts

The WHO has recognised flowcharts as essential tools in syndromic case management. A flowchart shows a series of consecutive decisions and actions that need to be made, starting from a given problem, in this case the identification of an STI syndrome. The flowcharts designed for use in southern Africa to treat and manage STIs (Protocols for the management of a person with an STI according to the Essential Drug List) can be ordered free of charge from:

Gauteng Directorate for Aids and Communicable Diseases, Private Bag X 085, Marshalltown, 2107

The discussion that follows will not deal in depth with treatment regimens, because these are changed from time to time. Only general guidelines will be given – the government protocol should be consulted for more details. (See page 314 for home-based care of STIs.)

Syndrome I: Urethral discharge/burning on urination in men

The common causes of urethral discharge (or discharge from the penis) are *gonorrhoea* and *chlamydia* (or non-gonococcal urethritis). The discharge is usually an abnormal white, yellow or greenish colour and it is often profuse and purulent (containing pus). Rectal gonococcal infection is common in homosexual men and it may present with rectal discharge and a burning pain in the rectum. Gonococcal pharyngitis (throat infection) often occurs in both sexes after oral-genital contact (oral sex).

Although *candidiasis* usually occurs in women, it is also found in men, especially among uncircumcised men. It often occurs in men with Aids. The symptoms are that the foreskin and the area underneath it become very sore and red. There may be a yellow discharge under the foreskin. The skin of the penis, scrotum and around the anus sometimes also becomes red, sore and itchy.

Urethral discharge is treated with the following two antibiotics: *ciprofloxacin* (to treat gonorrhoea) plus *doxycycline* (to treat non-gonococcal urethritis). (Alternative medication is also available.)

Syndrome II: Scrotal swelling

Men with STIs often complain of severe pain in the testes accompanied by scrotal swelling and tenderness (epididymo-orchitis). This is usually caused by *gonorrhoea* and *chlamydia* (or non-gonococcal urethritis). Scrotal swelling is treated with the following two antibiotics: *ciprofloxacin* (to treat gonorrhoea) *plus doxycycline* (to treat non-gonococcal urethritis). Scrotal support and pain relief should also be offered if necessary.

Syndrome III: Discharge from the vagina

Abnormal vaginal discharge is usually caused by STIs such as *gonorrhoea, chlamydia, trichomoniasis, genital candidiasis,* and *bacterial vaginosis.*

Trichomoniasis in women produces vaginitis and to a lesser extent cystitis (bladder infection). If the infection is mild, only a slight discharge may be noticed. If it is extremely severe or acute, patients may complain of a copious, thin, offensive-smelling white, yellow or yellow-green discharge which may be frothy in appearance. On examination, acute inflammation of the vulva and inner thighs is often visible. The vaginal walls and cervix may be covered in a thin discharge. The mucous surfaces may be observed to be extremely red after the discharge has been removed.

Genital candidiasis (thrush) usually occurs in women and manifests as infections of the vagina and vulva. Genital candidiasis is often found in association with HIV infection. The symptoms in women are irritation of the vulva and vaginal discharge, but many women may be symptom-free. The discharge is usually scant and watery, but it can be profuse, thick and white (like cottage cheese) in severe cases. The vulva may be red and swollen and fissures (cracks) may be present.

Bacterial vaginosis, or non-specific vaginitis, is one of the most important causes of vaginal discharge. It is characterised by a grey, homogeneous, adherent vaginal discharge which is usually malodorous (bad-smelling). Bacterial vaginosis, unlike other causes of vaginal discharge, is not associated with pruritus (itchiness), dysuria (painful urination) or dyspareunia (painful sexual intercourse). The main complaint is the discharge itself, which may be profuse and is usually described as having a fishy odour.

Women with discharge from the vagina sometimes also show symptoms of pelvic inflammatory disease or PID (see syndrome category IV).

Abnormal vaginal discharge is treated by administering *ciprofloxacin* (treatment for gonorrhoea) plus *doxycycline* (treatment for chlamydia) plus *metronidazole* (treatment for trichomoniasis and bacterial vaginosis). *Clotrima-*

zole (topical treatment for candidiasis) is added if the patient also complains of vulval itching and/or curd- or cheese-like discharge.

Syndrome IV: Lower abdominal pain (pelvic inflammatory disease)

Pelvic inflammatory disease (PID) is caused by the spread of micro-organisms from the vagina and cervix to the uterus, fallopian tubes and pelvic organs. PID is often caused by gonorrhoea, chlamydia or anaerobes. It is characterised by severe lower abdominal pain and a typical PID gait, which includes slow walking and grasping of the lower abdomen. A vaginal discharge which often smells bad is frequently noted, and the patient has a high temperature (fever). PID is usually treated with *ciprofloxacin* (treatment for gonorrhoea) plus *doxycycline* (treatment for chlamydia) plus *metronidazole* (treatment for anaerobes). If vaginal discharge is also present, refer to the treatment protocol for syndrome category III (discharge from the vagina).

Syndrome V: Genital ulceration

A thorough and proper understanding of genital ulcer disease is vital for our fight against HIV infection because (as we noted earlier) open lesions (cuts) and ulcers contribute to the spread of HIV infection by facilitating the transmission of the virus across non-intact and inflamed mucosal and skin surfaces. Most genital ulcers or sores are caused by *syphilis*, *genital herpes* and *chancroid*. Open lesions and ulcers are most commonly found on the glans penis and penile shaft in men, and on the labia, vulva, vaginal walls or cervix in women. Anal and rectal syphilis ulcers are also frequently seen in homosexual men.

Genital ulcers are usually associated with enlarged lymph nodes in the groin area. These enlarged nodes can become very painful and precipitate pustule formation in some cases of chancroid. Chancroid (followed by syphilis) is the most common cause of genital ulceration in Africa. Chancroid has also been found to be a major co-factor in the heterosexual transmission of HIV in developing countries. It is therefore extremely important to be able to diagnose and treat chancroid as accurately and as quickly as possible.

Genital ulcers are usually treated with *benzathine penicillin* (treatment for early syphilis) plus *erythromycin* (treatment for chancroid, lymphogranuloma and secondarily infected herpes lesions). Individuals often present with STIs that cause genital ulcerations or sores *as well as* genital discharge. Such cases should be treated with a *combination* of medication. Thus one might prescribe *benzathine penicillin* (for example) to cure the ulcers *together with ciprofloxacin* (for example) to cure the discharge.

Genital herpes

Herpes simplex (genital herpes) is very common, especially in individuals with HIV infection. Herpes is caused by the *herpes simplex* virus. The infection is life-long, it is recurrent, and ulcers will reappear periodically throughout an infected person's life. It recurs most frequently when a person is ill or is suffering from stress, or around the time of menstruation. Herpes simplex presents with small blister-like sores that often blend to form larger sores. Genital herpes is very painful, but it usually settles after about 2 weeks. In patients with HIV infection, herpes may occur more frequently, be more severe and painful, and remain active for longer (Evian, 2000). While herpes simplex (which is caused by a virus) unfortunately cannot be treated with antibiotics, genital ulcers can be suppressed with *aciclovir* or *valaciclovir* in severe cases. Because these medications are very expensive, their widespread use in poor countries is not possible. Secondarily infected herpes lesions should be treated with erythromycin.

Several studies have indicated that it is very likely that the *herpes simplex virus-2* (HSV-2) makes people more susceptible to HIV. A study in South Africa has found that HSV-2 was the most significant factor associated with HIV among both men and women, and that men infected with HSV-2 were seven times more likely to be HIV-positive as those without it. The occurrence of HSV-2 in combination with HIV indicates that HSV-2 control (both prevention and treatment) may be a valuable part of HIV prevention (UNAIDS Report, 2002:90).

Herpes management should include counselling on the nature of the disease with emphasis on the recurrence of the infection. Lesions should be kept clean and dry, using talcum powder, and pain relief should be offered if necessary.

Syndrome VI: Inguinal bubo (without ulcer)

Inguinal bubo is a tender, enlarged lymph node in the groin area, resulting from absorption of infective material. It is caused by early syphilis or lymphogranuloma venereum and the patient usually complains of swollen lymph glands which can be very painful. Inguinal bubo is treated with *benzathine penicillin* (treatment for early syphilis) plus *doxycycline* (treatment for lymphogranuloma venereum). Glands should be aspirated when necessary. If the patient also has genital ulceration, see 'Syndrome V: Genital ulceration' on page 56 for treatment.

Syndrome VII: Balanitis/balanoposthitis (without ulcer)

Balanitis is an infection of the glans penis characterised by thrush on the foreskin and head of the penis. It is caused by candidiasis. If a patient complains of itching of the glans and/or foreskin of the penis (without an ulcer or urethral discharge), the condition should be managed by washing the area with soap and water and painting it with an aqueous solution of gentian violet, or by applying nystatin ointment. If ulceration or urethral discharge are present, the appropriate treatment should be added.

Table 3.2 on page 59 gives a summary of all the major sexually transmitted infections.

General points in managing sexually transmitted infections

Apart from treating patients with STIs using a syndromic approach, health care professionals should also do the following:

- Make services accessible and user friendly. Integrate STI services with other primary care and HIV services, and try to provide clinic services at convenient times, for example during weekends and in the evenings.
- Avoid stigma, blame and negative attitudes towards patients. Treat the patient with respect and consideration for his or her dignity.
- Always be on the lookout for other STIs, and treat if present.
- Encourage the patient to go for voluntary HIV counselling and testing.
- Counsel the patient on compliance and risk reduction.
- Counsel the patient on safer sex practices and promote and provide condoms. Condoms should be used until the infection is fully healed, and thereafter to prevent re-infection.
- Sex partners should be notified and treated.

Enrichment

Preventing HIV infection by eliminating STIs

HIV/Aids forces us to think holistically. Health care professionals can no longer afford to focus on only one aspect of illness: somehow the possibility of HIV/Aids will always be hovering somewhere in the background. When clients present with an STI, treatment of the STI should be only one part of the total health care package delivered. The client should also be counselled about safer sex practices and HIV testing. Condoms should be provided and partners should be referred for treatment. Holistic and comprehensive care and counselling is unfortunately not always delivered. Analysis of data from Carletonville miners in South Africa in 2000 shows just how great the impact of prevention might have been on clients with STIs – had it been offered. The Carletonville studies found that fewer than 25% of miners presenting at the clinic for the first time with an STI were infected with HIV. Among those who had further bouts of STIs and came back for treatment a second, third or fourth time, the rate of HIV infection rose to over 40%. By the time the same men had been treated for their tenth episode or more, 80% of them were HIV positive. (These figures tell their own story.) Most of the men who were interviewed said that they never used condoms in their primary relationships. This means that many of these infections were acquired from or passed on through sex with a spouse or regular partner. If effective preventive measures had been directed at these men when they presented with their first episode of STI, many would have been able to avoid being infected with HIV (UNAIDS, 2000c:72–73).

- Take blood for RPR and VDRL (syphilis tests).
- Encourage the patient to return for a follow-up visit, especially if treatment does not cure the infection.
- If the syndromic treatment fails, refer the patient to a skilled STI (sexual health) practitioner or clinic for further investigation (e.g. serological tests or swabs).

Activity

A colleague of yours doesn't feel well and you think she looks feverish. She complains of painful urination, itchiness and a yellow, smelly discharge. Her husband works on a mine and she usually sees him only at weekends. What advice will you offer her?

Failure of syndromic treatment

If syndromic treatment fails, the following should be considered (Evian, 2003:269):

- The medication may not have been taken properly and completely.
- The sexual partner may not have been treated, and the patient is being reinfected.
- The STI may be resistant to the medication the patient is taking.
- The patient may be immune-depressed due to HIV infection, and therefore may need prolonged or more aggressive STI treatment.
- Herpes infection may have an unusual appearance, especially in the presence of HIV, or it may be secondarily infected. Also, remember that herpes does not respond to the usual syndromic protocols (because herpes is caused by a virus).

3.7 CONCLUSION

HIV/Aids is an immune system disease. As the HIV-positive person's immune system becomes weaker, many different diseases and symptoms may present themselves. HIV infection can be managed by keeping the immune system as healthy as possible – mainly by ensuring that the CD4 count stays as high and the viral load as low as possible. To manage HIV infection properly, it is imperative to diagnose it as soon as possible. The diagnosis of HIV infection and Aids will be discussed in more detail in the next chapter.

Table 3.2
Sexually transmitted infections

Infection	How do you get it?	Causing agent	How long before the disease manifests itself?	What are the symptoms?	How is it treated?	What are the effects of no treatment?
Candida (thrush, yeast)	*Men:* Sexual contact *Women:* Frequently acquired infection from the bowel, where *Candida albicans* naturally occurs	Fungal infection caused by *C. albicans*		*Women:* Thick, white discharge, swelling of vulva, painful and frequent urination, itching around the genitals *Men:* Swelling, redness, itching of the penis. Can cause balinitis in men and, rarely, urethritis	Vaginal cream or pessaries	Extreme discomfort; babies may develop oral or genital thrush
Chancroid	Sexual contact	*Haemophilus ducreyi*	Less than 1 week	Multiple painful ulcerations erupting from intradermal abscesses Ulcers bleed easily Ulcers often confused with other STI ulcers	Antibiotics	Abscess formation of the lymph nodes Inguinal ulceration
Chlamydia	Sexual contact	*Chlamydia trachomatis*	1–3 weeks	*Women:* Pelvic pain, vaginal discharge, painful and frequent urination, bleeding after sexual intercourse (Sometimes no symptoms at all) *Men:* Discharge from penis, painful urination, scrotal swelling (Sometimes no symptoms at all)	Antibiotics	Severe infection of reproductive organs *Men:* Sterility *Women:* PID; tube pregnancy and infertility Infection can be passed on to babies
Genital warts	Sexual contact and skin-to-skin contact with genital warts	Human papilloma virus (HPV)	1–6 months	Small, painless bumps grow on the genitalia, with slight itching or burning. They may be on the vulva, vaginal walls and cervix in women and on the urethra in men Peri-anal and rectal warts often seen There may be no outward signs. Determined with pap smear	Patient-applied therapy for external warts; can also be removed by burning, freezing and minor surgery	Grow large and spread Lead to cervical cancer Infection can be passed on to babies
Gonorrhoea (drip, clap, dose)	Sexual contact	*Neisseria gonorrhoeae*	1–10 days	*Women:* Most women have pelvic pain, painful urination, vaginal discharge or fever *Men:* Painful urination, discharge or drip from penis or no symptoms at all	Antibiotics	Vaginal infection Severe damage to reproductive organs may lead to infertility in women and sterility in men Heart trouble; skin disease Infection can be passed on to babies

Table 3.2 (continued)
Sexually transmitted infections

Infection	How do you get it?	Causing agent	How long before the disease manifests itself?	What are the symptoms?	How is it treated?	What are the effects of no treatment?
Hepatitis B	Sexual contact, body fluids, e.g. blood, semen, vaginal fluid and saliva	Hepatitis B virus	2–5 months (average 3 months)	*Stage 1:* Flu, fatigue, weight loss, painful joints *Stage 2:* Jaundice, skin and whites of eyes are yellow *Stage 3:* Gradual recovery Fatality rate varies: 1–10%	Adequate fluids, rest, nutrition; a vaccine can be given to prevent hepatitis B	Associated with liver cancer Can lead to death Infection can be passed on to babies
Genital herpes (blisters)	Sexual contact, direct contact with sore (oro-genital or purely genital)	Herpes simplex virus	2–20 days (usually 1 week)	*Onset:* Itching or burning; fever, malaise, and painful lymph nodes with primary infections Painful blisters break into open sores Sores can be found on the mouth or sex organs.	Once infected, the virus stays in body – no cure Aciclovir may provide relief	Sores will go away without treatment, but often reappear when the person is ill or stressed Infection can be passed on to babies
Non-gonococcal urethritis (NGU)	Sexual contact	Number of causative organisms (usually no specific causative agent)	1–3 weeks	*Women:* Frequent painful urination and a discharge *Men:* Painful and frequent drip or discharge from penis, painful urination. Often symptom free in men	Antibiotics	Infertility
Non-specific urethritis (NSU)	Sexual contact and can be caused by chlamydia	Depend on cause of NSU		*Men:* Burning while urinating; discharge from the penis *Women:* Few symptoms	Antibiotics	Severe infection of organs, infertility
Pelvic inflammatory disease (PID)	Sexual contact, can be caused by gonorrhoea or chlamydia	Caused by ascending spread of micro-organisms from vagina to pelvic organs. Mainly *N. gonorrhoeae*		Fever, nausea, vomiting, low abdominal pain, pain during intercourse, pain during menstruation, profuse vaginal discharge, typical PID gait (slow walking, grasping of lower abdomen).	Antibiotics	Sterility, abscesses on tubes
Pubic lice (crabs)	Sexual contact, close physical contact Using the same clothing or bed	Infestation by the crab louse (*Phthirus pubis*)	Immediately	Infestation mostly confined to pubic and peri-anal areas, but might spread to thighs, chest, axillae, eyelashes and eyebrows. Never the scalp. Lice feed on blood. Chief symptom is itching due to bites. Crawling lice and small eggs (nits) on hair or clothing	Special shampoos or lotions. All clothing and bedding must be washed in hot, soapy water. Dead lice and nits are removed with fine-toothed comb	Skin irritation and secondary infections due to scratching

Table 3.2 (continued)
Sexually transmitted infections

Infection	How do you get it?	Causing agent	How long before the disease manifests itself?	What are the symptoms?	How is it treated?	What are the effects of no treatment?
Scabies (itch)	Sexual contact, close physical non-sexual contact (families, schools, overcrowded conditions)	Parasitic mite *Sarcoptes scabiei* Poverty and poor standards of hygiene contribute to spread	4–6 weeks symptom free after infection, but infectious to others	Itching at night. Red lines in the skin as the female mites burrow. Ulcers develop after scratching. Sites commonly affected are the genital area, lower abdomen, buttocks, inner thighs, finger webs, axillae, but rarely the head and neck	Special cream and preparations that should be applied to whole body, except head and neck. All clothing and bedding to be washed before applying. Repeat after 3 days	Spread all over body. Secondary infections as a result of scratching. Extremely severe manifestations of the disease may be seen in patients co-infected with HIV
Syphilis (the pox)	Sexual contact	*Treponema pallidum*	*Stage 1*: 9-90 days *Stage 2*: 3-6 months *Stage 3*: over 2 years after acquiring disease	*Stage 1*: a painless sore called a chancre *Stage 2*: Fever, headache, malaise, general rash, general lymphadenopathy *Stage 3*: Very ill. The cause is not easy to find. Late syphilis phase not infectious	Antibiotics (superficial lesions of early syphilis (stages 1 and 2) are infectious; those of late syphilis are non-infectious)	Severe infection, infertility, skin diseases, arthritis, baby can be born blind or dead, heart, blood vessel and brain damage
Trichomoniasis (trich)	Sexual contact	*Trichomonas vaginalis*, which is a flagellate protozoan	1 week	*Women:* Copious, thin, offensive white, yellow or greenish frothy discharge. Acute inflammation of vulva, perineum, inner thighs and itching around genitals. Sometimes cystitis. In many cases symptom free *Men:* Urethritis and balanitis, but mostly symptom free	Flagyl	Fever and infection of organs. Pass infection on to baby. Can cause prostatitis and very rarely, epididymitis

chapter

4 Diagnosing HIV Infection and Aids

Definite signs of Raka's presence
The men saw the signs of his strength in the bush:
it must have been the work of his hands,
the carcass of a buffalo lying in a footpath,
with its knees buckled beneath its dead body.

HIV infection can be diagnosed by assessing the clinical history; by identifying risk factors; by clinical assessment of signs and symptoms; and by testing for HIV antibodies or for viral antigens. The diagnosis of HIV infection is usually based on clinical assessment as well as subsequent confirmation by means of an HIV antibody or viral test. However, testing is sometimes not possible, for example in remote rural areas where rapid tests are not always available, and not all tests can be used on babies under 18 months of age. Many health care professionals therefore have to rely on clinical diagnosis of HIV infection.

4.1 CLINICAL DIAGNOSIS OF HIV INFECTION: SIGNS AND SYMPTOMS

In order to make a clinical diagnosis of HIV infection, the first important step is to take a detailed case history. Ask the patient how long he or she has been ill and enquire about any other symptoms experienced in the past such as tuberculosis or sexually transmitted infections. Ask about sexual practices and about the health of sexual partner/s and children.

A physical examination should include a thorough of the skin, the oropharynx (mouth and throat) and the lymph nodes. Dermatological (skin) conditions are among the most common early manifestations of HIV infection, as are infections of the mucous membranes and generalised lymph node enlargement.

The World Health Organization (WHO) has developed criteria for the diagnosis of HIV infection where access to HIV antibody tests is limited. These criteria are based on the recognition of certain major and minor features. (These symptoms and diseases are discussed in detail in chapter 3.)

Clinical criteria for diagnosing HIV infection in adults

The following clinical criteria (Table 4.1) for diagnosing symptomatic HIV infection in adults were developed by the WHO for health care professionals who do not have access to HIV antibody tests.

In Africa the WHO criteria should be adapted to the local illness pattern. Researchers in Botswana found that the most common symptoms in individuals who tested HIV positive on the ELISA (enzyme-linked immunosorbent assay) test were weight loss (47%), persistent cough (30%), prolonged fever (23%), chronic diarrhoea (21%), TB (16%), herpes zoster (13%) and oral candidiasis (11%). Bacterial pneumonia was evident in only 8% of cases; failure to thrive was evident in 7%; and the least common symptom was generalised lymphadenopathy (6%) (Edhonu-Elyetu, 1997).

Table 4.1
Criteria for diagnosing HIV in adults
(Source: Friesen et al., 1997:102)

The presence of opportunistic conditions such as Kaposi's sarcoma or cryptococcal meningitis is sufficient for the diagnosis of Aids. HIV infection (or Aids) is also diagnosed if at least two major criteria and one minor criterion are present in the absence of other known causes of immune suppression such as malnutrition.

Major criteria (x2)	Minor criteria (x1)
• Fever that has lasted for more than one month • Weight loss of more than 10% of the usual body weight • Chronic diarrhoea for more than one month • In Africa: – Herpes zoster (shingles) – Non-healing genital ulcers	• Cough that has lasted for more than one month (often associated with TB in Africa) • Generalised pruritic dermatitis • Oral candidiasis or thrush • Chronic or aggressive ulcerative herpes simplex • Herpes zoster (or shingles) • Persistent generalised lymph node enlargement

It was also noted that chronic diarrhoea, weight loss, herpes zoster (or shingles) and non-healing genital ulcers, *if found together*, predicted a positive ELISA result in 95.5% of cases. It is therefore recommended that, in the absence of an ELISA test, these symptoms can be used to diagnose HIV infection for intervention purposes. It is also suggested that shingles should be given the status of a *major* diagnostic symptom in the WHO clinical case definition for HIV/Aids – at least for use in Africa in areas that cannot afford HIV antibody tests. Note that the occurrence of shingles in young people in Africa is *almost always* associated with HIV infection.

Clinical criteria for diagnosing HIV infection in children

Table 4.2 lists clinical criteria for diagnosing HIV infection in children. These criteria were developed by the WHO to help health care professionals make symptom-based diagnoses when HIV antibody tests are not available.

Table 4.2
Criteria for diagnosing HIV in children
(Source: Evian, 2000:161)

A child is considered to have Aids if *two major* and *two minor* criteria are present in the absence of any other known cause of immune deficiency.

Major criteria (x2)	Minor criteria (x2)
• Weight loss, abnormally slow growth or failure to thrive • Prolonged fever that has lasted for more than one month • Chronic diarrhoea for more than one month	• Chronic cough that has lasted for more than one month • Generalised lymph node enlargement • Recurrent common infections (such as those of the ear and throat) • Chronic dermatitis (skin infections or rash) • Fungal infections of the mouth and/or throat (oral candidiasis or thrush) • The mother has been proved to be HIV positive

4.2 HIV TESTING AS DIAGNOSTIC TOOL

After Montagnier discovered HIV in 1983, and Gallo demonstrated its propagation in cell culture in 1984, one of the greatest struggles in medical history began: to develop a test to diagnose HIV infection. This effort was especially driven by the blood banks, who urgently needed a test to screen blood (Schoub, 1999). Gallo's laboratory played a huge role in the development of HIV diagnostic tests, and the first kits for antibody testing became available in April 1985. Later that year commercially produced HIV diagnostic tests were licensed by the Food and Drug Administration of the United States.

These tests were designed on the ELISA (enzyme-linked immunosorbent assay) principle, which is the most widely used test for detecting viral antibodies in the blood. Although the earlier ELISA tests lacked specificity, which means that they frequently gave a positive result in individuals who were not infected, major advances in the design of these tests have now improved them to a level of very high sensitivity and specificity (Schoub, 1999:129). (See 'The sensitivity and specificity of tests' on page 65.) The tests we use to diagnose HIV infection are now very reliable.

There are three main reasons why HIV antibody testing is carried out:

- to screen donated blood;
- to research the transmission patterns and prevalence of the virus; and
- to diagnose HIV infection in individuals.

HIV testing was previously used mainly to confirm or diagnose suspected HIV infection in patients who experienced certain symptoms or diseases. People are now encouraged to make use of voluntary counselling and testing (VCT) services to find out their HIV status (see 'Voluntary HIV counselling and testing as HIV prevention strategy' on page 103). It is hoped that people who know their HIV status and are seronegative will be motivated to use preventive measures to prevent future infection, and that if they know they are seropositive they will learn to live positively; use care and support services at an earlier stage; learn to prevent transmission to sexual partners; and plan for their own and their families' futures (WHO, 2000a:1–4).

Pre- and post-HIV-test counselling must always be done before and after testing a client for HIV infection. The reason for testing, the nature of the test, the implications of a positive or a negative result, and the client's prospects (in either case) should be discussed with every client before testing. Informed consent and confidentiality are mandatory. Pre- and post-HIV-test counselling are discussed in chapter 11. Legal and ethical aspects of HIV testing are discussed in chapter 19.

The diagnosis of HIV infection is based mainly on the testing of blood samples. There are two broad classes of tests:

- *HIV antibody tests,* which react to *antibodies* that have formed in reaction to the virus; and
- tests that detect the *actual virus* (HIV) or viral elements in the blood.

A combination test is also available (the HIV Ag/Ab Combo) which is based on the detection of HIV antibodies as well as viral proteins.

4.3 HIV ANTIBODY TESTS

HIV antibody tests are usually done on blood (serum). However, HIV antibodies can also be detected in other body fluids such as saliva and urine. Two of the best-known HIV antibody tests are the ELISA and the Western Blot tests. These tests cannot trace the virus in the blood, but they react to the HIV *antibodies* that are formed when the immune system tries to protect the body against the virus. These antibodies can usually be detected in the blood 3–6 weeks after infection, depending on the test being used. While first generation ELISA tests took about 42 days to show positivity, the latest third generation ELISA tests can detect HIV antibodies after approximately 23 days. Note that an antibody test becomes positive only after the host (or patient) has mounted an immune response, and has seroconverted (see 'The primary HIV infection phase' on page 40). The latest ELISA antibody tests can detect antibodies to both HIV-1 and HIV-2, as well as antibodies to the known variants of HIV-1. In some very rare cases it may take as long as 3–6 months to develop antibodies. In such cases, follow-up testing for 6 months is recommended to exclude infection after exposure.

The ELISA and Western Blot tests are usually done in a laboratory, but rapid HIV antibody tests are also available for use outside laboratories.

The ELISA antibody test

The ELISA HIV antibody test is the most popular and commonly used test. It is widely available and not expensive. The test is very sensitive and reliable, and produces very few false negative results. Because false positive results (test result positive, person actually HIV negative) can occasionally occur (usually less than 1%), an HIV-positive test result should *always* be confirmed by means of a second test. A positive ELISA test is usually confirmed by means of a second ELISA test.

In South Africa, with its high HIV prevalence, two positive HIV ELISA tests are considered adequate evidence of HIV infection (Evian, 2003). The second ELISA test is usually done on the same blood specimen, preferably with a different testing method or design. Rapid HIV antibody tests can also be used to confirm a positive ELISA test, especially in remote or rural areas where resources are limited. Rapid tests are as accurate as the ELISA test, and many doctors believe that the use of rapid tests in conjunction with the ELISA is as reliable as (or even more reliable than) the combination of the ELISA and Western Blot tests (Schoub, 1997b).

It is not necessary to confirm a positive HIV antibody test result if there are clear indications of HIV infection such as obvious signs and symptoms of immune deficiency or Aids (see Tables 4.1 on page 63 and 4.2 on page 63), HIV-related opportunistic infections, and/or laboratory evidence of immune deficiency such as a low CD4 cell count (Evian, 2003:43).

Enrichment

The sensitivity and specificity of tests

The two factors that determine the accuracy of a serological (blood) test are sensitivity and specificity.

- The *sensitivity* of a test is its ability to pick up very low levels of antibodies (its ability to detect HIV positivity and not give false negative results).
- The *specificity* of a test is its ability to ignore the presence of antibodies that are not specific, or in other words, to distinguish specific HIV antibodies from other cross-reacting non-specific antibodies (i.e. its ability to demonstrate HIV negativity and not give false positive results) (Evian, 2000; Schoub, 1999). The most common cause of false positive tests is vaccination. In such cases the test should be repeated after about 30 days, or an HIV viral test should be used to diagnose HIV infection.

Specificity and sensitivity are usually expressed as percentages – the *sensitivity* of a test is that percentage of infected individuals who are detected by the test, while the *specificity* of a test is that percentage of non-infected individuals who have a negative test result. The ELISA test has a sensitivity of 99.6% and a specificy of 99.4% (Schoub, 1999:129).

Rapid HIV antibody tests

The ELISA tests are also available as rapid tests. Rapid HIV antibody tests can be performed outside a laboratory (in places such as clinics, consulting rooms or even at the patient's bedside), and the results are usually available within 10-30 minutes. Rapid HIV tests are relatively easy to use (they involve a prick of the finger with a lancet), not expensive, and reliable if used correctly. Rapid tests are very useful for the diagnosis of HIV infection in areas far from diagnostic laboratories where clients often cannot afford to come back for test results. The tests can be performed and read by non-laboratory personnel such as nurses if they have had adequate training and experience.

All positive rapid HIV test results should preferably be confirmed with a laboratory-based ELISA antibody test. In rural areas where this may be a problem (for the reasons mentioned above), confirmation of the first rapid test should automatically be carried out by conducting a second but *different* rapid test (Evian, 2000). A standard ELISA should then be done only in the case of an indeterminate result (where it is not clear if the test result is positive or negative). However, a second confirmatory test will not be necessary if the person tested shows clear symptoms of immune depression or Aids (see Tables 4.1 and 4.2).

Rapid HIV diagnostic home-kit tests are available, but should be used with extreme care.

It is not advisable to do the home test without proper pre- and post-test counselling because of the potentially serious consequences for individuals who discover their HIV status without support. Also, the results can be incorrect if the testing instructions are not followed exactly; if the test kit was not stored at the required temperature; if the kit is older than the expiry date shown; or if a poor-quality test kit is used. A positive result on a home test should *always* be confirmed by a subsequent laboratory test.

Saliva HIV antibody tests

Saliva tests (such as Orasure) detect the presence of HIV antibodies in saliva. Saliva testing has a number of advantages over blood testing: it is less intrusive; it is painless; it avoids the potential hazard of a needle-stick injury to the person doing the test; and it can be used where blood is difficult to take, for example in children and intravenous drug users whose veins are often difficult to access.

Saliva tests are very easy to use. The saliva is usually collected by placing an absorbent pad under the tongue. The sensitivity of saliva tests is good, but positive results must be confirmed by conventional ELISA testing on blood before a patient can be diagnosed as HIV positive (Schoub, 1999). The saliva test is often used in unlinked, anonymous surveillance studies, and it also offers opportunities for home testing. Saliva tests are not recommended for home use without proper pre- and post-test counselling.

? If a saliva test can diagnose HIV infection, does it also mean that saliva can spread HIV?

This question can best be answered by making a clear distinction between *antibodies* in saliva and the actual *HI virus* in saliva. HIV antibodies are abundant in saliva, but the concentration of the actual virus is extremely low. The saliva (or oral) test is based on detecting the antibodies in the saliva, not the virus. The viral concentration in saliva is so low that transmission through kissing, for example, is highly unlikely. (Blood in saliva may of course change the situation.)

If the health care professional has the slightest suspicion that the test results are falsely negative (for instance, one positive and one negative ELISA, for a person who is known to practise high-risk behaviour), he or she should advise that person to be tested again after 3 weeks. If the person concerned is in the 'window period', complete seroconversion should have taken place after 3 weeks. The test will then produce more accurate results.

In very rare cases, patients may lose detectable antibodies late in the disease because of overwhelming immune depression. An antibody test will therefore be negative, but it will nevertheless be very clear from the person's clinical condition that he or she has Aids. The viral load in the person's blood will be very high.

The Western Blot antibody test

The Western Blot test is an antibody test that relies on the development of antibodies to give an HIV-positive result. The Western Blot test is more expensive and less widely available than the ELISA. It is never used as a screening test (to diagnose HIV infection), but only as a confirmatory test under special circumstances, for example to confirm a positive result in a newborn baby, or in the case of an indeterminate ELISA test. The Western Blot should not be used routinely as a confirmatory test.

The window period

The window period is the time between HIV infection and the appearance of detectable antibodies to the virus (when antibody tests will give positive results). In the case of the most sensitive HIV antibody tests currently available, the window period is about 3–4 weeks. For less sensitive tests, the period can be longer (approximately 6 weeks). In some cases the window period can be as long as 12 weeks or (in rare cases) as long as 6 months, and any HIV antibody tests conducted during this window period may give false negative results. This means that, although the virus is present in the person's blood, antibodies cannot yet be detected. The tests will indicate, incorrectly, that the person is not infected. Remember that an antibody test will become positive only after the host has mounted the initial immune response – namely to develop antibodies.

The window period is usually much shorter for tests that detect the presence of the virus itself. Such tests do not have to wait for the immune system to form antibodies, but respond to the presence of the actual virus particles.

During the window period the individual is already infectious and may unknowingly infect other people. People who are exposed to or who practise high-risk behaviour are well advised to arrange for a repeat test after 3–6 months, and to practise safer sex (for example by using condoms) while waiting for their results.

4.4 HI VIRUS TESTS

HI virus tests detect the *actual HI virus* in the blood, and do not rely on the development of *antibodies*. Diagnosis of HIV infection using viral tests is based on the following:

- detection of *viral antigens* such as p24 (a core protein of the virus);
- detection of *viral nucleic acid* (the genome of the virus either in its RNA or DNA form); and
- isolation of the virus in lymphocyte cell culture. (This process is cumbersome and seldom used for diagnostic purposes.)

Two of the best-known HIV viral tests are the p24 antigen and HIV PCR tests. Because these tests detect the actual HI virus (HIV antigens or viral nucleic acid) in the blood, they yield a positive result much sooner after infection (usually within 11–16 days) than do the ELISA, Western Blot or rapid tests. Although the window period is much shorter for viral tests than for HIV antibody tests, the test is more reliable a month after infection. It is therefore recommended that 30 days be allowed after possible infection before testing. A negative test result in the first 2 weeks after infection may be false negative and the test should be repeated. Unfortunately HIV antigen tests are very expensive and not always available in remote areas.

The HIV p24 antigen test

The HIV p24 antigen test detects the predominant HIV antigen (p24). The p24 antigen is the main protein of the core of the virus (see Figure 1.3 on page 11), and can usually be detected in the blood shortly (16 days) after initial HIV infection (pre-seroconversion period) and again in the late stages of infection. The p24 test is especially useful when there is a high viral load in the blood, as occurs in the very early phase of HIV infection and again in the final phase of Aids. It is not very useful after the initial phase of infection, because the immune response reduces the number of p24 antigens, so there are fewer p24 proteins to be detected. The p24 antigen test is useful in certain clinical situations where early detection is important (e.g. for newborn babies or for blood and tissue banks to screen donations during the window period).

The PCR technique

The most valuable diagnostic test for directly detecting the presence of the HI virus is the PCR (polymerase chain reaction) technique. The main function of the HIV PCR technique is to detect the nucleic acid (in its RNA or DNA form) of HIV (see Figure 1.3). The test is so sensitive that it can detect as little as one fragment of the nucleic acid of HIV in 100 000 host cells (Schoub, 1999:141). The HIV PCR technique can be used for diagnostic as well as post-diagnostic purposes.

A *qualitative* PCR test is used for diagnosing an individual as HIV positive or HIV negative by detecting the presence of HIV genome. The qualitative PCR test is especially useful when early diagnosis is required (e.g. for post-exposure prophylaxis); for diagnosing babies born to HIV-positive mothers (see enrichment box 'When a baby can be tested for HIV infection' on page 68); for use as a post-rape test before beginning antiretroviral therapy; and when antibody tests are indeterminate. The estimated window period for an RNA PCR test is 11 days, while the estimated window period for a DNA PCR test is 16 days.

A *quantitative* PCR test is used mainly *after diagnosis*, during treatment (see 'The viral load' on page 72). The quantitative PCR test makes it possible to measure the amount of virus in a particular body fluid by determining the number of copies of the viral RNA. This test is also called the

Enrichment

When a baby can be tested for HIV infection

HIV antibody tests such as ELISA, Western Blot or rapid tests are often used to test whether babies born to HIV-positive mothers are infected with HIV. However, these tests cannot be used until babies are 15–18 months old because in younger babies it is not certain whether antibodies in the baby's blood were produced by the baby or by the mother.

During pregnancy antibodies pass across the placenta from an HIV-infected mother to the fetus. These maternal antibodies can stay in the baby for as long as 18 months and will show up on an HIV ELISA antibody test. This means that, up to the age of about 18 months, a baby who got the antibodies but not the virus from the mother can test HIV antibody positive without actually being infected.

It is possible to test the HIV status of the baby 11–16 days after birth with the HIV p24 antigen and HIV PCR tests, although it is preferable to wait until 30 days after birth as earlier results can be false negative. These tests detect the HI virus itself in the blood and do not depend on the existence of antibodies. The p24 antigen and the PCR tests are too expensive and sophisticated for general use, but they are often used for abandoned children who are up for adoption, or for children requiring major surgery. (See 'The rights of children' on page 364.)

Activity

- A young HIV-positive mother in your community is very worried about the HIV status of her baby, who is three months old. She says to you: 'They refuse to test my baby at the clinic. They keep saying that my baby is too young to be tested. What do they mean, too young?' How would you go about counselling this young mother?
- The same young woman has another question for you. She asks: 'The clinic also tested my husband, but he is HIV negative. They told him to come back for another test in three months' time. They said something about a "window". What did they mean? Is he infected or not?' What would you tell her?

Write a brief summary of your answers with all your main points clearly indicated. Use metaphors to explain the concepts.

HIV viral load test. The viral load is usually a reliable indicator of the infected individual's prognosis (outlook), and it is also used to measure an individual's response to antiretroviral therapy.

4.5 THE ANTIBODY/VIRUS COMBINATION TEST

There is also a diagnostic test available that detects both *antibodies* to the HI virus and the *p24 antigen* (the HIV Ag/Ab Combo test). Because the p24 antigen can be detected in serum or plasma soon after infection (even before seroconversion), it was hoped that the combination test would shorten the window period dramatically, improving early detection of HIV infection. Although the combination antibody/antigen test detects infection about 1–3 days earlier than the ELISA antibody test, it does not reduce the window period as much as a p24 antigen test does on its own. A positive HIV Ag/Ab Combo test should always be confirmed with a second test.

What is meant by a positive (or reactive) HIV antibody test?

A *positive HIV antibody test* means that the individual has been infected with HIV and is able to spread the HI virus during sex, through his or her blood, or during pregnancy, childbirth and breastfeeding. A positive HIV antibody test does *not* reveal for how long the person has been infected. The test also gives no indication of the stage of infection, or how long it may take to develop Aids. It is important to keep in mind that a positive HIV antibody test does not necessarily mean that the person has already developed Aids (the last stage of HIV infection).

What is meant by a negative (non-reactive) HIV antibody test?

A *negative HIV antibody test* means that no antibodies against HIV were found in the blood. This means either that the person has not been infected with HIV, or that he or she may have been infected but antibodies have not yet formed (because of the window period).

The test may be falsely negative if done within the first 6 weeks after HIV infection, so tests done within this period should be repeated 12 weeks after the possible exposure to HIV. A very small percentage of HIV-positive people (usually in the last stage of infection) have no HIV antibodies in the blood, and their tests will repeatedly produce false negative results. This happens when the immune system is so depressed it can no longer form antibodies.

What is an indeterminate test result?

An *indeterminate test* means that the result is not clear either way and it is therefore not possible to tell if the person is HIV-antibody positive or negative. The test should be repeated after a few weeks or an HIV antigen test (p24) or PCR test should be done.

Are people immune to Aids when they have HIV antibodies in the blood?

No. The antibodies formed against HIV do *not* protect the individual from the devastating effects of the virus. These antibodies, unlike the antibodies in other infections, do not provide immunity against HIV or Aids. They are formed as the body *unsuccessfully* attempts to defend itself against the virus.

When should a person who has an HIV negative test result be retested?

Retesting for HIV should be done on people and their sexual partners who have been at risk for acquiring HIV in the 6–12 weeks before the test. Ask the client and his or her sexual partner for a history of any risky sexual behaviour in the past 3 months; of any sexually transmitted infection; of any sharing of needles and syringes; and of blood transfusions. Rape and needle-stick injuries during the past three months will also fall into this category (Evian, 2003).

HIV testing is only a tool. That tool is blunted to the degree that it is used to harm other people (Coates, 1990:1).

4.6 CONCLUSION

The early diagnosis of HIV infection is important because in many cases the onset of Aids can be drastically delayed if the HIV infection is managed by medication, by boosting the immune system and by changing to a healthier lifestyle.

The advantages of voluntary HIV counselling and testing will be discussed in chapter 6.

chapter

5 Managing HIV Infection and Antiretroviral Therapy

Delaying Raka

Behind him he heard the angry grunt of the beast . . .
He swung around.
In its tracks the big thing came to a halt.
With a grin, it retreated a few steps,
angered, but afraid, half ashamed of itself.

There are no hard-and-fast rules about caring for people with HIV/Aids, and there is no single specific management protocol. The management of HIV infection should always focus on the specific needs of the patient at the time. The care and treatment offered will therefore depend on many and varied factors such as the following:

- How far has the patient's disease progressed?
- What are the patient's symptoms now?
- What opportunistic infections are attacking the patient?
- What kind of medical care (hospital, clinic, home-based or hospice) is available to the patient?
- In the case of antiretroviral therapy (ART), how committed is the patient to adhering to treatment?

The clinical assessment of the patient's health, as well as the use and function of antiretroviral drugs, will be discussed in this chapter. The management and care of specific symptoms and HIV-related conditions in the hospital and clinic and in home-based care will be discussed in chapter 17.

5.1 CLINICAL ASSESSMENT

Once a patient has been diagnosed HIV positive, it is important to do a full clinical assessment of his or her health. Regular check-ups (at least every 4–6 months if the person is healthy, but more frequently if he or she has symptoms) should be done to monitor changes in the person's health. Regular check-ups can help health care professionals to identify and treat physical as well as psychological problems at an early stage and to promote the general health of the patient. Clinical assessment also helps the health care professional to make decisions on when to start prophylaxis (treatment to prevent opportunistic diseases) and when to start antiretroviral treatment. Always be on the lookout for any clinical features that may indicate early opportunistic infections, cancers or other HIV-related conditions.

Regular medical and growth checks (at least once every 2–3 months) are important for monitoring the health of HIV-positive children. Clinical aspects that should be monitored in adults and children with HIV infection, at the first visit and also at each follow-up visit, are listed in Table 5.1.

5.2 ASSESSING IMMUNE STATUS AND VIRAL LOAD

In order to manage HIV infection, opportunistic infections and Aids, it is important to monitor the individual's CD4 lymphocyte count as well as the viral load in the blood on an ongoing basis. CD4 cell counts are important to:

- evaluate the status of the immune system;
- indicate when to start to prevent or treat opportunistic infections and diseases; and
- indicate when to start antiretroviral treatment.

A viral load test is important to:

- assess the severity of the HIV infection (or the prognosis) by telling us how far the immune system has been eroded;
- prescribe relevant antiretroviral medication; and
- measure the patient's response to antiretroviral therapy.

Immune status and the CD4 cells

The single most important test for determining an individual's immune status is the CD4 lymphocyte count. The CD4 count tells us to what extent the immune system is compromised. It also gives an indication of what phase of infection the patient has reached. CD4 cell counts are further the best predictors of the risk of opportunistic infections in HIV-positive people. CD4 values

Table 5.1

Clinical assessment of adults and children with HIV infection

	Adults	Children
General assessment	• Weight • Examination of skin, mouth, teeth, eyes, lymph nodes and genitals • Examination of respiratory system (e.g. for signs of TB) and abdomen (for signs of an enlarged liver or spleen) • Neurological assessment (e.g. memory, general mental state, pupil reaction, sensation, power, reflexes and gait)	• Weight • Developmental progress • Growth • Head size • Immunisation status • Nourishment and feeding • Any symptoms that may indicate opportunistic diseases
Laboratory tests	• Full blood count (especially lymphocyte and neutrophil count, haemoglobin level and platelet count) • Syphilis serology • Liver enzymes (if antiretroviral therapy is considered) • CD4 cell count and percentage (or total lymphocyte count if CD4 count is not available) • HIV RNA viral load test	• Full blood count and platelet count • Total lymphocyte count • CD4 cell count and percentage • HIV PCR viral load test
Tests as needed	• Chest X-rays, sputum test (if TB is suspected) • Hepatitis B and C • Pap smear in women • Renal and liver function • Toxoplasmosis • CMV	• Chest X-rays in cases of respiratory problems or TB • Throat swabs • Urine, stool or blood cultures in cases of fever or infection

below 350–400 cells/mm³ usually indicate immune suppression and vulnerability to opportunistic infections. Preventive treatment against specific infections such as TB and *Pneumocystis carinii* pneumonia should be based on CD4 cell counts. This is preferable to waiting for symptoms to occur and *then* treating these very serious conditions (see 'The prevention of opportunistic infections' on page 47). The CD4 cell count is also the best indicator of the best time to start antiretroviral treatment.

What is a normal CD4 cell count?

A normal CD4 cell count is approximately 1 000 cells/mm³, but it varies, and some healthy (HIV-negative) people may have CD4 cell counts as low as 600 cells/mm³ or as high as 2 000 cells/mm³. It is very important to take a baseline CD4 cell count as soon as possible after infection. This initial CD4 count can then be used as the baseline against which any changes can be measured.

Unfortunately it is not always possible to do CD4 cell counts – they are expensive, and sophisticated laboratory facilities are not available everywhere. Health care professionals in such situations have to rely on their observation of the general clinical condition of the patient and symptoms of opportunistic diseases in particular.

The viral load

The HIV RNA viral load test (measured with a quantitative PCR technique) measures the number of viral particles (virus copies) per ml of blood. It is important to know the actual number of HI viruses in the blood in order to manage HIV infection effectively. An increasing viral load is usually an indication of active HIV disease and the rapid development of immune deficiency. It therefore predicts a poor health prognosis (or future) for the patient.

Knowing the viral load is also very useful for assessing the effect of antiretroviral therapy (ART) as well as for the ongoing monitoring of ART. *A rising viral load in a person on ART is an indication that the treatment is not working.*

Enrichment

Other useful measures of immune status

The percentage of CD4 cells of the total lymphocyte (white blood cell) count is a useful measure of immune status. CD4 cells normally make up more than 30% of the total lymphocyte count. Levels below 30% generally indicate immune deficiency, and the lower the percentage, the more severe the deficiency (Evian, 2003:74).

The CD4/CD8 ratio is another measure of immune status. In healthy individuals there are four times as many CD4 lymphocytes as CD8 (or suppressor T) lymphocytes. With the depletion of the CD4 lymphocytes this ratio drops, and eventually reverses as the number of CD8 lymphocytes overtakes that of CD4 lymphocytes (Schoub, 1999:150).

The viral load is also monitored to detect antiretroviral drug resistance.

Viral levels in patients with HIV infection may range from *undetectable levels* (in a patient on ART) to *very high levels* such as 3–5 million copies/ml. An undetectable HIV RNA viral load means that the viral level is too low for the test to detect – it does not necessarily mean that the virus is truly absent. Undetectable levels are < 50 or < 400 copies/ml, depending on the laboratory doing the test (Evian, 2003:74). An increasing viral load is usually accompanied by a decreasing CD4 cell count (see Figure 3.1 on page 39).

CD4 cell counts and viral loads may vary from time to time. The CD4 count can increase or decrease in response to factors such as infection, stress, smoking, exercise, the menstrual cycle, positive living and relaxing.

It is therefore important to monitor the trend of the CD4 cell count over time and not to rely on a single reading. If the patient has an infection such as flu or herpes it is also best to delay taking a CD4 count until they feel better.

Viral load measurements can also vary significantly. If a person has an infection or has recently received a vaccination, he or she may have a temporary increase in viral load. It is therefore best to avoid having a viral load test for at least a month after the vaccination or illness.

5.3 ANTIRETROVIRAL THERAPY

The first antiretroviral drug, AZT (zidovudine), was approved for use in 1987. In 1994 ART was used for the first time to prevent mother-to-child transmission of HIV. In 1995 the use of triple-drug therapy or HAART (highly active antiretroviral therapy) was introduced. The knowledge that the opportunity to save lives has been available to us for more than a decade, makes the following statement so much more tragic:

> The magnitude of HIV infection in southern Africa and the number of impoverished people who desperately need antiretroviral therapy (ART) but who will never receive this, is overwhelming, and unparalleled in the history of infectious diseases.
>
> (SA HIV Clinicians Society, 2002a)

Although treatment and care, including access to antiretroviral drugs, are recognised by all the world's governments as an essential element of the response to the global HIV/Aids epidemic, the cost associated with ART and the lack of political will to roll out national treatment programmes remain the most important obstacles to adequate management of HIV infection in many countries. There are, however, many success stories (e.g. in Botswana) where the right of all HIV-positive adults and children to receive an optimal standard of care (including free access to antiretroviral drugs) is respected.

Goals of antiretroviral therapy

Antiretroviral therapy has the following four primary goals:

1. *Virological goal:* to reduce the HIV viral load as much as possible – preferably to undetectable levels – for as long as possible.
2. *Immunological goal:* to restore and/or preserve immunological function so as to improve immune functioning, reduce opportunistic infections and delay the onset of Aids.
3. *Therapeutic goal:* to improve the quality of the HIV-positive person's life.
4. *Epidemiological goal:* to reduce HIV-related sickness and death, and to reduce the impact of HIV transmission in the community.

The four goals of ART are achieved by suppressing viral replication as intensely as possible for as long as possible by using tolerable and sustainable treatment for an indefinite period of time. By doing so, the impact of HIV on the immune system may be minimised and the morbidity and mortality associated with HIV infection can be improved (SA HIV Clinicians Society, 2002a). Effective therapy has been shown to reduce the number of new cells infected by HIV and to interfere with the ability of the virus to evolve drug resistance.

Antiretroviral therapy (ART) is used mainly:

1. to *treat* established HIV infection (long-term treatment) as discussed in section 5.3; and
2. to try to *prevent* HIV infection (short-term treatment), including:
   - the prevention of mother-to-child transmission of HIV (see section 5.4 on page 82);
   - the prevention of HIV infection after occupational exposure (see section 5.5 on page 83); and
   - the prevention of HIV infection after rape or sexual assault (see section 5.6 on page 84)

The effect of antiretroviral drugs on the HI virus

The HI virus uses *enzymes* to replicate itself inside CD4 cells (see 'The effect of HIV on the immune system' on page 17). Two of the most important enzymes used by the virus are:

- *reverse transcriptase* enzymes, which are essential for completion of the early stages of HIV replication by transforming viral RNA into proviral DNA; and
- *protease* enzymes, which are required for the assembly of new viral RNA and viral proteins, and for the maturation of fully infectious new viruses that bud from the CD4 cells.

Antiretroviral drugs act by blocking the action of these enzymes. There are three main classes of antiretroviral drugs that interfere with the enzymes:

- *nucleoside reverse transcriptase inhibitors* (NRTIs);
- *non-nucleoside reverse transcriptase inhibitors* (NNRTIs); and
- *protease inhibitors* (PIs).

Figure 5.1 illustrates the effect of these three classes of antiretroviral drugs on the HI virus.

The *reverse transcriptase inhibitors* disturb the life cycle of the HI virus by interfering with the reverse transcriptase enzyme in the early replication of the virus (see Figure 5.1, A). Interference with this enzyme prevents the virus from changing its RNA into proviral DNA. The *protease inhibitors* interfere with the formation of new viruses by 'paralysing' the protease enzyme and so preventing the assembly and release of newly replicated HI viruses from the infected cells (see Figure 5.1, B).

The war against HIV is fierce. New drugs and new categories of drugs are constantly being developed and tested. Two of the most promising new classes of drugs (not yet on the market at the time of publication) are *fusion (T20) inhibitors* and *integrase inhibitors*. Fusion (T20) inhibitors prevent HIV from entering the host cell by affecting the interaction between the virus and the cell (they stop the viral proteins gp120 and gp41 from

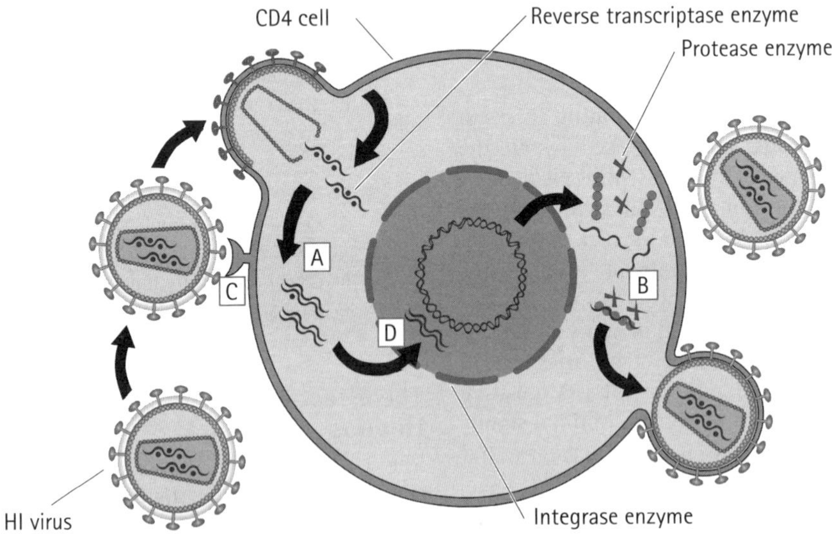

A **Drugs that work here:**
- Non-nucleoside reverse transcriptase inhibitors (NNRTIs)
- Nucleoside reverse transcriptase inhibitors (NRTIs)

(Drugs interfere with the reverse transcriptase enzyme and prevent the transformation of viral RNA into proviral DNA.)

B **Drugs that work here:**
- Protease inhibitors (PIs)

(Drugs interfere with the protease enzyme and prevent the formation of new viruses.)

C **New development:**
- Fusion (T20) inhibitors

(Drugs block binding, fusion and entry of HIV into the cell.)

D **New development:**
- Integrase inhibitors

(Drugs interfere with the integrase enzyme and prevent integration of viral DNA into the cell's core.)

Figure 5.1
The effect of antiretroviral drugs on the HI virus

forming a stable interaction with the CD4 molecule). In this way, binding, fusion and entry of the host cell is blocked (see Figure 5.1, C).

Integrase inhibitors interfere with the integrase enzyme and prevent the process by which HIV integrates into the host genome, or core of the CD4 cell. The virus is therefore unable to replicate because it cannot be integrated into the host cell's DNA (see Figure 5.1, D). Health care professionals should stay informed about the latest developments in antiretroviral medications by reading about them in medical journals, on the Internet and in other sources.

Classes of antiretroviral drugs

There are currently three main classes of antiretroviral drugs. Table 5.2 gives a summary of the classes and their mechanisms of action as well as a list of the antiretroviral drugs currently available in South Africa (based on SA HIV Clinicians Society Clinical Guidelines, 2002a).

As new treatments regularly become available for clinical use, health care professionals are advised to contact the Southern African HIV Clinicians Society for the most current version of treatment guidelines (e-mail: sahivsoc@sahivsoc.org; website: http://www.sahivcliniciansociety.org).

Health care professionals can also obtain the South African Government's *National Antiretroviral Treatment Guidelines*, published in 2004, from the South African Department of Health (HIV/Aids and STI Directorate) in Pretoria (tel: 012 312-0121). The guidelines are available free of charge.

Activity

If you are a teacher, make (or ask the children in your class to make) a model from different coloured clays or plasticine to demonstrate the interaction between the HI virus and a CD4 cell. Use the model to explain to the children what antiretroviral drugs do to the virus.

Table 5.2
Classes of antiretroviral drugs and their mechanisms of action

	Classification of antiretroviral agent		
	Nucleoside reverse transcriptase inhibitor	Non-nucleoside reverse transcriptase inhibitor	Protease inhibitor
Abbreviation	• NRTIs	• NNRTIs	• PIs
Enzyme inhibited	• Reverse transcriptase	• Reverse transcriptase	• Protease
Specific action	• Mimics the normal building blocks of HIV DNA	• Directly inhibits reverse transcriptase	• Inhibits late stages of HIV replication
Antiretroviral agents available in South Africa	• zidovudine (AZT) (Retrovir®)* • didanosine (ddI) (Videx®)* • zalcitabine (ddC) (Hivid®) • lamivudine (3TC) (Epivir®)* • stavudine (d4T) (Zerit®)* • abacavir (ABC) (Ziagen®)* • tenofovir	• nevirapine (NVP) (Viramune®)* • efavirenz (EFV) (Stocrin®) • delaviridine	• indinavir (IDV) (Crixivan®) • saquinavir (SQV) (hard gel formulation) (Invi-rase®) • saquinavir (SQV) (soft gel formulation) (Forto-vase®) • nelfinavir (NFV) (Vira-cept®)* • ritonavir (RTV) (Norvir®)* • amprenavir (Preclir®)* • lopinavir/ritonavir (Kaletra®) • atazanavir

*Antiretroviral agents available in paediatric formulations

Guidelines for the use of antiretroviral therapy

The South African HIV Clinicians Society (2002a) recommends that maximally suppressive antiretroviral regimens should be used whenever possible in order to obtain the best clinical results and to prevent resistance. HAART (or highly active antiretroviral therapy) is therefore recommended for optimal results.

- *Single-drug regimens (or monotherapy)* should not be used in the *treatment* of HIV infection. Monotherapy (one drug only) produces a temporary reduction in viral load, and will almost always lead to rapid development of drug resistance (see 'The development of drug-resistant viruses' below). Single-drug regimens do, however, continue to play a very important role in the prevention of mother-to-child transmission (e.g. nevirapine as a short-term limited-course treatment).
- *Dual-drug regimens (treatment with two antiretroviral agents)* are moderately effective, but are unlikely to produce long-term durable benefits in most patients. Although it is not the standard of care (or best available care), treatment with two drugs is considerably better than no therapy at all, and should be considered in patients who cannot afford triple combinations (or HAART). Dual-drug regimens should be given only to patients who have already developed Aids. If dual-drug therapy is prescribed to patients without symptoms, development of resistance is a major problem. Dual therapy (prescribing two drugs) is more effective than monotherapy (one drug) and leads to a greater reduction in viral load.
- *Triple combinations (the combination of three antiretroviral agents that work together)* are recommended as the standard of care. A combination of three different antiretroviral drugs (or HAART) has been shown to produce the best effects in terms of both viral suppression and reducing the development of drug-resistant viruses. Effective combination therapy attacks the virus at all the different levels (sites A and B shown in Figure 5.1). Substantial reductions in medication prices continue to make triple-therapy regimens more affordable.

The development of drug-resistant viruses

There are two main factors influencing the development of drug resistance in HIV:

- the high genetic variability of HIV; and
- the relative 'fitness' of these variations in the presence of antiretroviral drugs.

HIV replicates extremely fast, and 1–10 billion copies are produced daily. HIV also has the ability to mutate or change very fast, owing to its proneness to make mistakes in the reproduction cycle (see 'Variability and subtypes of HIV' on page 19). Many spontaneous genetic mutations of HIV therefore arise every day – including changes in the enzymes that are targeted by the antiretroviral drugs. In *untreated* HIV-positive individuals, one genetic variant usually dominates and reproduces more rapidly, and we call this dominant variant a 'wild-type' virus. The mutations usually persist at very low levels in the plasma (or blood).

The introduction of antiretroviral drugs changes the ecology of the virus population in the body dramatically. If, for example, a single-drug regimen is used (e.g. only AZT), it will only repress the reproduction of the wild-type viruses, giving the drug-resistant viral mutations the chance to become the dominant viruses in the population and remain so as long as the drug is administered. The aim of treatment with combination drugs (HAART or triple therapy) is to suppress viral replication completely. When virus replication is suppressed, mutations do not occur and resistance does not develop.

A resistant virus compromises future therapy of the patient and poses a significant public health challenge, because these resistant viruses are spread into the community.

Drug resistance also occurs when patients do not take their drugs regularly. It is important to have enough drugs in the bloodstream 24 hours a day to keep the virus depressed. Each time a dose is missed, the concentration of drugs in the blood falls too low for several hours, and the virus gets a chance to break through and develop ways to resist the drugs. The patient's viral load will rise again, and the drug to which the virus has become resistant can also no longer be used for this or any other patient infected with this drug-resistant virus. Also, resistance to one drug may result in resistance to other drugs in the same class. This is known as cross-resistance (Brouard et al., 2004; Maartens, 2003; Project Inform, 2002).

Choice of drug regimen

Internationally there is no agreement as to which antiretroviral drug regimen is best. The choice of regimen depends on many factors, including (Evian, 2003:84):

- what is affordable?
- what is the clinical history of the patient?
- at what stage is the disease? The more advanced the stage of disease, the greater the need for more potent drug regimens;
- what dosage will be convenient? For example, is it easier for the patient to take drugs once a day rather than three times a day?
- what antiretroviral drugs has the patient used in the past?

The SA HIV Clinicians Society provides the following guidelines for treating adults with antiretroviral drugs (Table 5.3). These guidelines are based on WHO and UNAIDS recommendations.

As can be seen in Table 5.3, the three classes of antiretroviral drugs (NRTI, NNRTI and PI) can be subdivided into 5 categories for treatment purposes. These categories can be combined as follows:

NRTI and NNRTI combinations are usually recommended for starting therapy: two NRTIs (one drug from Category I and one from Category II) and one NNRTI (one drug from Category IV) are usually prescribed.

The PIs (Category V) are usually added when NNRTI (Category IV) treatment fails. There is broad cross-resistance against the currently available NNRTIs, and resistance to one NNRTI precludes the use of any other NNRTI. Most clinicians prefer to keep the PIs for later use in patients who develop resistance to the NRTI and NNRTI regimens, and for patients who cannot tolerate NRTIs or NNRTIs due to toxicity or side effects, or develop treatment failure on these regimens. The reason for avoiding PIs in the initial regimen is their greater toxicity.

Individuals in whom an NNRTI-containing regimen does not succeed may be given a triple NRTI regimen by adding abacavir (Category III) to the other two NRTIs, but this combination of NRTIs may only be used if the viral load is less than 55 000. In all other cases, the use of triple NRTIs should be avoided.

It is an ongoing research challenge to find new drugs, new categories of drugs and the most suitable combination of drugs for various groups of patients with their distinct needs. It is a further challenge to eliminate treatment failure and determine how to assess the likelihood that a patient will develop resistance to antiretroviral drugs.

Table 5.3

Antiretroviral regimens for use in South Africa for the previously untreated adult patient

Category	Drugs
• Category I:NRTI	• Stavudine (d4T)* • Zidovudine (AZT)
• Category II: NRTI	• Didanosine (ddI)* • Zalcitabine (ddC) • Lamivudine (3TC)
• Category III: NRTI	• Abacavir (ABC)
• Category IV: NNRTI	• Nevirapine (NVP) • Efavirenz (EFV)†
• Category V: PI	• Nelfinavir (NFV) • Indinavir (IDV) • Ritonavir (RTV) • Saquinavir soft gel formulation (SQV) • Lopinavir/ritonavir combination

*Stavudine (d4T) and didanosine (ddI) should not be used during pregnancy and lactaction.

†Efavirenz is teratogenic (harmful to the fetus) and should be avoided in women of childbearing age unless effective contraceptives are used, and then only where no other antiretrovirals are available.

Side effects of antiretroviral therapy

One of the important factors in the success of treatment is how well the patient tolerates the antiretroviral drugs. Some of the milder side effects, usually occurring in the first few weeks of antiretroviral therapy, are indigestion, change in bowel movements, diarrhoea, nausea, skin rashes, headaches and dizziness, weakness, tiredness and lethargy. More serious side effects and complications of antiretroviral agents are:

- myelosuppression (bone marrow suppression), which results in bleeding and anaemia) (NRTIs, especially AZT);
- gastrointestinal intolerance, nausea, vomiting and abdominal pain (NRTIs, NNRTIs and PIs);
- pancreatitis (NRTIs);
- peripheral neuropathy (NRTIs);
- allergic reactions (NNRTIs, rarely NRTIs and PIs);
- lipo-atrophy (wasting of the fatty tissue of the body) (NRTIs);
- liver diseases (NRTIs);
- lactic acidosis (NRTIs);
- lipodystrophy (disturbance of fat metabolism) (NRTIs, PIs);
- raised cholesterol and triglycerides (NNRTIs, especially efavirenz, and PIs);
- insulin resistance in diabetics (PIs);
- reduced bone density (PIs);
- neuropsychiatric problems (NNRTIs, especially efavirenz);
- skin rashes, which may be very severe or may present with large red blisters as in Stevens-Johnson syndrome (nevirapine). Stevens-Johnson syndrome is often characterised by ulceration in the oesophagus;
- renal calculi (kidney stones) (indinavir);
- hepatitis (nevirapine).

Carry out routine laboratory monitoring to pick up side effects of some drugs, e.g. liver function for nevirapine; full blood count for AZT; and lipid profile for PIs.

Interactions between antiretrovirals and other medications

Many antiretroviral drugs may react with other commonly used medications. For example, some antiretroviral drugs may interact with TB medications such as rifampicin, which may reduce the levels of antiretrovirals in the blood. If the patient is already on ART, the regimen is usually changed to be compatible with rifampicin. The SA HIV Clinicians Society (2002a) recommends that if a patient's CD4 cell count is above 200, ART should commence only after completing TB medication. If the CD4 count is below 200, ART should be delayed until after the intensive phase of TB therapy (2 months) unless the patient has another serious HIV-related illness or a very low CD4 count, in which case ART should be introduced only once the patient is stabilised on TB therapy.

Clinicians should always consult the drug information inserts before prescribing any drugs.

Antiretroviral therapy for children

Most antiretroviral drugs used for adults are also available in paediatric formulations (see Table 5.2). An experienced paediatrician should be consulted for the treatment of children, because dosages need to be adjusted to suit the age or weight of the child. Antiretroviral therapy in children preserves or restores immune function (CD4 cell count); provides sustained suppression of the viral load; promotes or restores normal growth and development; improves the quality of life; prevents complicating infections and cancers; and prolongs the child's life.

ART in children should be considered when there is an early diagnosis of HIV infection (in a baby younger than 3 months old whose mother is HIV positive and who tested positive on an HIV PCR test) or when a baby or child is diagnosed late because an HIV-related symptomatic disease develops. Good adherence to drug therapy is critical to achieve a satisfactory viral and immunological outcome. The following factors may have an impact on adherence (SA HIV Clinicians Society, 2002b):

- Affordability of ART. Before initiating ART, the clinician should make sure the parents or caregivers of the child can afford a proposed treatment regimen over a prolonged period of time.
- Motivation and commitment of the caregiver or parent to the child's lifelong therapy. Care-

givers should understand that adherence involves giving every dose of medication, one to three times daily, every day of every year. Caregivers or parents need to anticipate and plan for weekends away, schooling and other activities that could mean that doses are missed.

- Parental or caregiver understanding that poor adherence is the single most important factor associated with drug failure and resistance. Parents should understand that resistance implies loss of future treatment options for the child. Good adherence should be emphasised at each visit.

Parents or caregivers often understand adherence better if ART is compared to treatment of diabetes or hypertension, both of which may require lifelong therapy and where poor adherence is associated with disease progression. Clinicians should keep in mind that the doses of ART are likely to need modification at each visit as the child gains weight and grows. The SA HIV Clinicians Society also suggest that clinicians dispense the ART themselves, or have them delivered to their rooms if possible, in order to keep track of those patients who are not collecting their medications on time. This could alert the clinician to a potential adherence problem.

When to start antiretroviral therapy

Antiretroviral therapy should be delayed until patients are prepared to commit themselves to long-term treatment and to maintaining good adherence to the therapy. It is becoming more common to delay the start of antiretroviral therapy until immune deficiency becomes measurable and the probability that diseases will develop has become high (WHO, 2000b). Current guidelines suggest that therapy should be initiated as follows (SA HIV Clinicians Society, 2002a):

- All patients with *symptomatic* HIV infection, or with current or previous HIV-associated diseases (such as unexplained weight loss of more than 10% of body weight; unexplained diarrhoea lasting for more than a month; oral candidiasis or oral hairy leukoplakia; recurrent herpes infections or shingles; and uncontrolled skin disorders) should be treated with antiretroviral drugs, regardless of CD4 counts and viral load.
- Asymptomatic patients with CD4 cell counts below 200 cells/mm^3 should be treated with antiretroviral drugs. A CD4 count between 200 and 350 should be monitored, and treatment should start if the annual decline is more than the expected 20–80 cells/year. When the CD4 cell count is over 350, treatment is deferred. ART is, however, less effective when started in patients with advanced disease. In Uganda it was found that patients who started ART at an advanced stage of disease (CD4 count less than 50 cells/mm^3) were three times more likely to die than those who started above this level. Note that the criteria for commencement of ART differ from country to country. In some cases ART is initiated when the CD4 cell count reaches a threshold of 250 cells/mm^3, while others start when it reaches 350 cells/mm^3.

The effectiveness of antiretroviral therapy should be monitored with HI viral load, CD4 cell counts and other supportive laboratory tests to monitor toxicity. These tests should be done every 2–3 months until stable, and then every 4–6 months. If the medication is effective, the viral load should eventually stabilise at acceptably low levels. An increase in the viral load indicates that the treatment is not working. The patient's drug therapy then needs to be re-evaluated and changed (see enrichment box 'Health care professionals in ART programmes' on page 82).

Issues in deciding to take ART

Antiretroviral therapy will cause irreversible changes in a patient's life, and the health care professional should consider every advantage and disadvantage treatment is likely to bring before recommending or prescribing it to any patient. When considering antiretroviral therapy, each of the following factors should be taken into account (based on Evian, 2000:80):

- Patients who want to take antiretroviral therapy must be committed, well informed, and able to keep to a strict medication regimen. This means that they should be able to take 2–3 tablets two to three times a day (taking some doses with food and some on an empty stomach). They will have to live by the clock to make sure that they take the right medicines at exactly the right times.

- Some patients may experience side effects such as nausea, vomiting, abdominal discomfort, diarrhoea, skin rashes, fatigue, headache, anaemia, liver toxicity, fever, peripheral neuropathy (see page 44) and kidney stones (see 'Side effects of antiretroviral therapy' on page 78). Patients should be made aware of possible side effects and they should be advised to report side effects immediately.
- Patients should be warned about harmful interactions with some other drugs (e.g. St John's Wort, which should not be used with some antiretroviral drugs).
- Current treatments are permanent and lifelong and it is absolutely essential for the patient to keep strictly to the regimen prescribed. Patients often stop treatment because of side effects, and this may lead to the development of viral resistance to the drugs.
- Drug therapy should be monitored regularly by checking the viral load as well as the CD4 count. This monitoring indicates whether the viruses are being successfully suppressed and whether ART is effective. Patients on ART therefore need to be able to visit their doctors or clinics regularly for check-ups.
- Because antiretroviral therapy is expensive, it is beyond the reach of many people who are HIV positive. They may not be able to afford optimal drug regimens.

When to change treatment

Antiretroviral medication should be changed under the following circumstances:

- when the patient shows intolerance of the medication, despite adequate and appropriate treatment;
- when significant side effects appear;
- when virological failure occurs, e.g. when the viral load increases or shows an insignificant decline despite treatment.

When a patient shows *intolerance* towards a specific medication, the drug can simply be replaced with another drug. When *virological failure* occurs, it is essential to change at least two of the drugs in the regimen.

Can HIV be eliminated completely?

Unfortunately HIV cannot be completely eliminated from the body. The virus remains latent or dormant throughout the body and it can easily become reactivated in the right conditions. When the virus is reactivated, it continues attacking the infected person's immune system (see Figure 3.1). The function of antiretroviral therapy is to slow down disease development by lowering the viral load in the blood. When the viral load becomes undetectable, it simply means that the viral load is too low to be detected by the blood tests. *It does not mean that there are no more viruses in the body.* Research has also shown that once antiretroviral therapy is discontinued, viral replication usually resumes and viral loads begin to rise again (Evian, 2000).

Can the antiretroviral medication cure Aids?

Although HIV infection can be treated so that the viral load is kept low and the immune system is kept as healthy as possible, *there is still no cure for Aids or HIV infection.* The current emphasis in treating HIV is to keep the viral count as low as possible and strengthen the immune system to keep the individual as healthy as possible for as long as possible, and to treat opportunistic infections (see chapter 17).

Adherence to antiretroviral therapy

Strict adherence to antiretroviral therapy is extremely important to achieve viral suppression and avoid the risk of mutation, the development of resistant strains, and drug failure. Drug resistance can develop very rapidly with missed or inadequate doses of medication. Missing even a few doses in a week may lead to the development of drug resistance. A study in San Francisco found that 65% of patients who adhered 100% to their drug regimens had undetectable viral loads, but of those whose adherence was down to 80%, only 36% had undetectable viral loads (Gray & McIntyre, 2002). Adherence of 95% or more is critical to achieve viral suppression and to slow the time to treatment failure and subsequent development of resistance (Paterson et al., 2000).

It is very important to develop strategies to help patients take responsibility for their own care, adhere to antiretroviral therapy, and maximise the chances of successful treatment. It is therefore important to understand the factors that may affect adherence. Gray and McIntyre (2002) propose that adherence is a complex issue determined by factors related to:

- the patient;
- the disease process and stage;
- the treatment regimen itself;
- the interaction between patient and health worker; and
- the environment in which the patient lives.

The following questions should be asked in order to find out whether the patient will adhere to ART:

- *The patient.* Is the patient motivated to take ART? Does he or she have a social support system? What does he or she know and believe about sickness and health in general? What was the patient's previous level of adherence to medications such as TB medication or other antibiotics? Does he or she have proper coping skills? What is the level of cognitive ability of the patient? Will he or she be able to follow a strict treatment regimen?
- *The treatment regimen or disease factors.* How many pills will the patient have to take, and how often? What is the size of the pills, what do they taste like, and how easy is it to take them? How must the pills be taken (for example with water, with fatty foods, on an empty stomach)? What are the side effects, and how severe are they? Will there be interactions with other drugs? Does the patient suffer from any other associated conditions, and if so, for how long?
- *Relationship between the patient and the health care worker.* Is there a relationship of trust between the patient and the health care worker? Is the health care service consistent? Does the health care worker offer support and reassurance? Does he or she give clear explanations, and explain the possibility and symptoms of side effects?
- *Environment.* Are health care services easily accessible to the patient? Does he or she have access to a broad scope of services? Does he or she have transport to clinics? Will the patient have enough tablets at all times? Does the person have enough food if the ART has to be taken with food?

Strategies to improve adherence to antiretroviral therapy and the development of effective but patient-friendly regimens are needed. In the developed world many resources are available to Aids carers and their clients. These include printed materials, electronic media, websites, SMS messages, training courses, support groups, electronic pill counters, and alarm beepers. Such resources are not readily available everywhere in Africa, and we will have to find our own unique ways to help clients adhere to antiretroviral therapy. When developing adherence programmes, health care professionals should take into account factors specific to Africa. These include cultural perceptions of what causes disease, attitudes to health and sickness, a culture of non-disclosure and therefore no community support, stigmatisation, illiteracy, differing concepts of time, practical problems such as distance to clinics, difficulties in communication, and lack of time in medical facilities to discuss treatment issues (Gray & McIntyre, 2002).

Studies on adherence promotion in some African countries found that adherence to antiretroviral programmes could be improved by patient empowerment, information provision, social networking and support, educational activities such as photonovels, and other innovative patient-centred approaches. The TB Control Programme (DOTS) may also prove helpful for ART adherence, but there are special challenges involved in HIV/Aids that may make such a programme problematic, such as the significant differences in infectiousness, legal controls, issues of confidentiality, disclosure, duration of therapy, and the non-availability of a once-a-day treatment regimen in the form of one pill.

Some strategies for improving adherence in Africa are suggested below (based on Gray & McIntyre, 2002).

Enrichment

Health care professionals in ART programmes

Health care professionals will have a very important role to play in the government's plan to roll out a comprehensive care plan, including an antiretroviral treatment programme. One of their major functions will be to educate the general public on the protocol of ART, and the following points will have to be explained:

- Not all HIV-positive people can now be treated with ART. ART can be started only when the CD4 cell count goes down to 200 cells/mm^3 or when there is a significant deterioration of the immune system, with clear Aids-related symptoms.
- Only patients who are absolutely committed to adhering to the strict medication regimen for the rest of their lives, can be considered for ART.
- Possible side effects should be explained and patients should be encouraged to report any signs and symptoms of side effects immediately.
- Regular follow-up visits to establish viral load and CD4 cell count are mandatory for people on ART to see if ART is depressing the viral load in the patient's blood sufficiently.

Strategies for improving adherence to antiretroviral therapy

Establish whether patient is ready to take medication regularly

- Take a history of the patient's pill-taking commitment in the past (e.g. STI or TB treatment).
- Do a trial run with something like peppermints or jelly tots to measure commitment.

Patient education

- Use pamphlets and visual aids (in the patient's language) that describe how to take the medications.
- Use teaching techniques, e.g. ask the patient to repeat information; encourage questions; and concentrate on skills development.
- Encourage frequent follow-ups, such as clinic visits and telephone calls.
- Offer peer education and support.

Reminder strategies

- Identify routine activities to which taking the medication can be linked (e.g. taking a tablet when brushing the teeth in the mornings and evenings).
- Medication boxes.
- Electronic reminders (e.g. preprogrammed SMSs).

Management of side effects

- Instruct patients on the side effects they may experience.
- Monitor and manage side effects pro-actively.

Reduce complexity of regimens

- Simplify regimens where possible (e.g. reduce number of pills or the frequency at which they have to be taken).
- Avoid unnecessary medication.
- Pay attention to food requirements where relevant.

Enhance patient-provider communication

- Express personal interest in the patient. Establish respect and unconditional acceptance.
- Use positive reinforcement (e.g. praise adherence, share results of viral loads and CD4 cell counts).
- Develop shared goals.

Enlist a support system

- Enlist the help of partners, family, friends, peers, support groups in the community, the church and allied health care professionals to reinforce adherence to treatment.

Optimise psychosocial functioning system

- Provide counselling services.
- Provide substance abuse treatment if needed.
- Provide financial support and ensure availability of antiretroviral drugs.
- Help the patient to plan ahead, e.g. to have extra medication for holidays.
- Minimise barriers to care (e.g. access, transportation, child care).

5.4 USING ANTIRETROVIRAL THERAPY TO PREVENT MOTHER-TO-CHILD TRANSMISSION OF HIV

The use of ART has been shown to be the most important strategy in preventing mother-to-child transmission of HIV. ART prophylaxis (e.g. AZT) can reduce mother-to-child transmission by 68% if started early in pregnancy (at 14–34 weeks), and by 30–50% if started later in pregnancy (after 34 weeks). ART should therefore be considered for HIV-positive pregnant women and their babies, as well as for HIV-positive mothers who are breastfeeding.

There is no single preferred treatment regimen, and current treatment protocols should be followed. AZT (which has the best-known safety profile in pregnancy) and nevirapine (NVP) are often used (Evian, 2003). Health care professionals should stay informed about new developments in antiretroviral therapy for HIV-positive pregnant mothers in their regions/countries.

The South African recommendation for best practice in women who are found to be HIV-positive at the time of labour, and who have had no prior treatment with antiretrovirals, is as follows (Gray et al., 2001):

- single-dose nevirapine (NVP) (200 mg orally) at onset of labour and a single dose of NVP (2 mg/kg orally) to the baby at 48–72 hours; or
- oral AZT/3TC during labour and then one week of therapy with AZT/3TC for the baby; or
- AZT injected intravenously or administered orally during delivery, followed by AZT orally to the infant for 6 weeks.

Nevirapine is usually given at the time of the rupture of the membranes. It should be noted that the nevirapine dose should not be repeated. If the woman took nevirapine and it turns out that she was in false labour, she should not receive nevirapine again when she goes into labour at a later stage. The reason for this is to prevent drug resistance. Women should be warned to be on the lookout for possible side-effects of nevirapine, such as fever, rash and a sore throat, which may indicate Stevens-Johnson syndrome.

How does nevirapine work to prevent mother-to-child transmission?

As an antiretroviral drug, the main function of nevirapine is to lower the HI viral concentration in the blood of the mother. The baby's chance of becoming infected during the birth process is much lower if the viral load in the mother's blood is lower. If the mother takes antiretroviral drugs while she breastfeeds her baby, the effect is the same: ART reduces the viral load (or concentration of viruses) in the milk, so there is less chance that the baby will become infected.

What are the chances of developing drug resistance due to a single dose of nevirapine?

The development of drug resistance due to the administration of a single dose of nevirapine to HIV-positive women in labour poses a real risk, and cases of nevirapine-resistant viruses have been reported. According to the World Health Organization (International Aids Conference in Bangkok, 2004), the use of nevirapine to prevent mother-to-child transmission is currently the best option we have – despite the possibility that resistance may develop. To minimise the risk of resistance, only a single dose of nevirapine should be given to the woman in labour, and it should not be repeated.

Women who are already on ART should generally continue during pregnancy. However, the safety of ART in the first 14 weeks of pregnancy is not fully established, and it is therefore safest to stop taking the medication during the first trimester. The ART can then be restarted from about 12–14 weeks of pregnancy. Any antiretroviral drug that may harm the fetus should be discontinued and substituted with another safer drug.

5.5 USING ANTIRETROVIRAL THERAPY TO MANAGE OCCUPATIONAL EXPOSURE

Although the risk of contracting HIV after occupational exposure to the virus is very low (0.3%), everything possible should be done to protect health care professionals against HIV infection. Research has shown that antiretroviral drugs such as AZT, 3TC and protease inhibitors can significantly reduce the risk of HIV infection after percutaneous (through the skin) exposure to HIV-infected blood. Post-exposure prophylaxis (PEP) with antiretroviral therapy must start as soon as possible (within the first hour or two after the injury, and no later than 72 hours) to reduce the chances of viral reproduction as much as possible.

Antiretroviral treatment after accidental exposure is recommended if the source patient is HIV positive. If the source patient's HIV status is unknown, PEP should be considered if the patient has one or more signs of HIV infection and/or if the needle-stick injury occurred in a community where HIV is prevalent.

A combination of AZT and 3TC is usually recommended for a 4-week treatment period. If viral resistance to AZT is a distinct possibility (e.g. if the source patient has been on AZT treatment for longer than 6 months), or in rare cases such as massive exposure following a blood transfusion with contaminated blood or an injection with a substantial volume of blood, a protease inhibitor (such as indinavir) should also be added to the prophylaxis regimen for 4 weeks. The use of nevirapine is not recommended for PEP, because it resulted in severe hepatitis in some health care workers.

Any fluid contaminated with blood or serous fluid, semen, vaginal fluid, cerebrospinal fluid (CSF) or pleural fluid should be considered to be potentially infectious. These body fluids pose the same risk of transmitting HIV as does infected blood. Non-infectious body fluids are urine and faeces (unless they are contaminated with blood). Post-exposure prophylaxis is not recommended if exposure has been to urine and faeces alone.

Post-exposure prophylaxis is unfortunately not always successful. Treatment may fail if (Evian, 2000):

- the health care professional has been exposed to an HIV viral strain that is resistant to the antiretroviral drugs that he or she takes for prophylactic purposes;
- the viral load in the source patient is very high; or
- the post-exposure prophylaxis is given too late or for too short a time.

Side effects of the antiretroviral medication may include symptoms such as fatigue, headache, nausea and vomiting and diarrhoea (in the case of PIs). Health care professionals on ART should also receive counselling to help them adhere to the medication and deal with the psychological turmoil and uncertainty after the injury.

NOTE: Post-exposure prophylaxis starter packs are often available for health care professionals who are exposed to HIV-infected blood. A starter pack contains enough antiretroviral drugs for only 3 days. The health care professional should be advised to start taking the drugs immediately, and to get a prescription for the rest of the medication. ART should be taken for 28 days to have an effect on the replication of the virus (also see enrichment box 'Starter packs for rape survivors' on page 85).

Activity

While working in a hospital as a volunteer counsellor, you notice that a nurse is pricked with a needle while working with a very confused Aids patient. What advice would you give to the nurse?

The hospital pharmacy gives the nurse a 'starter pack' of antiretroviral drugs, but no information on how to use it. What advice would you give her?

What do you think are the counselling needs of the nurse, and how would you counsel her?

Make a wall poster indicating all the steps that health care professionals should take after accidental exposure to HIV-infected blood in the health care situation. (See 'Management of accidental exposure to blood and other infectious body fluids' on page 347.)

5.6 USING ANTIRETROVIRAL THERAPY AFTER RAPE OR SEXUAL ASSAULT

Because of the high incidence of violent crime in South Africa, health care professionals are often called upon to treat the trauma that accompanies rape or sexual assault on adults and children. The risk of HIV infection after rape depends on factors such as the HIV status of the rapist, the viral load in the blood of the rapist, and the co-existence of STIs – especially ulcerations. The risk of HIV infection may also be higher in cases of violent rape and rape of children, because of the considerable physical trauma inflicted by the rapist. Incidents of male rape (e.g. forced anal sex) are often reported, and counsellors should not underestimate this problem. Oral sex can also put the rape survivor at risk of HIV.

It is very important to begin prophylactic treatment with antiretroviral therapy as soon as possible (within the first hour or two and no later than 72 hours) after the first act of penetration or attempted penetration. Children who are sexually assaulted or raped especially need to be treated with ART as soon as possible (within the first 2 hours) after the incident. A combination of AZT and 3TC is usually recommended for a period of 28 days. In high-risk situations such as when, for example, the assailant *is known* to be infected with HIV or where considerable trauma and bleeding are evident, a protease inhibitor, such as indinavir, is also administered for 4 weeks.

The rape survivor should be counselled and tested for HIV (preferably with a rapid HIV antibody test) before ART is started. The following protocol should be followed:

- If the rape survivor tests HIV positive on the rapid HIV antibody test, ART should not be given, because the person was not infected by the rape, but previously. Treating an already HIV-positive rape survivor (or health care worker after a needle-stick injury) with short-term antiretroviral drugs may lead to drug resistance, and compromise future treatment.
- If you have to wait for HIV test results, start treating the patient with ART. If the HIV test is negative, continue with treatment for 28 days. If the HIV test is positive, discontinue treatment and refer the client for proper counselling on positive living and keeping the immune system healthy.

Clients on ART should be counselled about the possible side effects that the drugs might have on them.

In South Africa, rape survivors are provided with free antiretroviral drugs at state hospitals and some clinics. If the drugs are not available, rape survivors should be advised to call the Aids Helpline (0800-012-322) to find out where they can get ART for free (see also 'Websites and Toll-free Helplines' on page 369). ART is also available at chemists, but a prescription will be needed and the medicines may be expensive. Rape survivors should be counselled to go back for HIV antibody testing at 6 weeks, 3 months and 6 months after the assault, and if they wish at one year, to determine whether HIV infection has occurred. An HIV PCR test can be done approximately 2–4 weeks after exposure. The rape survivor should practise safe sex for 6 months after sexual assault.

The rape survivor is at risk not only of HIV infection, but also of other sexually transmitted infections such as syphilis or hepatitis B. It is therefore important for rape survivors:

- to be tested and treated prophylactically for STIs; and
- to be vaccinated with hepatitis B vaccine.

There is also a 'morning-after' pill available to prevent women from becoming pregnant from the rape.

Enrichment

Starter packs for rape survivors

Rape often takes place 'after hours' or over weekends when it is difficult to get antiretroviral medication. 'Starter packs' consisting of a 3-day supply of antiretroviral drugs are available to rape survivors (or to health care professionals after accidental exposure to HIV-infected blood). Starter packs should be available at all health care services and some police stations for the immediate initiation of post-exposure prophylactic treatment. It should be noted that the starter pack is designed to provide medication for only the first 3 days because it is designed as an emergency measure. To suppress viral replication effectively, antiretroviral prophylaxis should be taken for a full 4 weeks after the assault or accident. The client should therefore be advised to visit a doctor or clinic to obtain follow-up medication.

Can children take antiretroviral drugs after sexual assault or rape?

Yes, children can take antiretroviral drugs (dosages are adjusted according to the weight of the child). It is important that children be treated with ART as soon as possible (within the first 2 hours) after sexual assault. Children older than 14 years do not need their parents' or guardians' permission to have an HI test, or to take antiretroviral medication. For children younger than 14 years the consent of one of the parents, the guardian or the hospital superintendent is needed for an HIV test and for taking ART. In emergency situations where a child younger than 14 years has been raped and needs urgent assistance, doctors should be guided by the best interests of their patients and their duty to give emergency medical treatment.

Prophylactic ART can also help to prevent HIV infection in situations where the condom slipped off or broke during sex with a partner who is known to be HIV positive, or in other situations when unwanted or risky sex has occurred. However, ART should be used with care, and it should not be used routinely or frequently in place of general safer sex practices.

How does ART work to prevent HIV infection after needle-stick injuries or rape?

If ART is given as soon as possible (within hours) after rape or a needle-stick injury there is a good possibility that the viruses that entered the body will be eradicated *before* they have a chance to attack CD4 cells, replicate and establish themselves in the body. Remember that ART interferes with the *replication mechanisms* of HIV (see Figure 5.1 on page 74) and prevents the virus from reproducing. Unfortunately ART does not always succeed in preventing HIV infection after needle-stick injury or rape, for example when the viral load of the rapist is very high and the rape was accompanied by violence and physical trauma, or if ART is started too long after the rape or injury.

5.7 IMMUNISING CHILDREN AND ADULTS WITH HIV INFECTION

Children with HIV infection should be fully immunised. Many children with Aids die of diseases that can be prevented by immunisation. No vaccines are contraindicated in HIV-positive children, with the exception of BCG (the TB vaccine) which should not be given to children with advanced HIV disease.

The following guidelines apply to BCG:

- BCG should be given to *all* HIV-positive babies who show *no symptoms* of HIV/Aids at birth.
- BCG should *not* be given to HIV-positive children who *show symptoms* of advanced HIV infection or Aids.
- BCG should also not be given to HIV-positive adults under any circumstances.

Because TB is so common in HIV-positive individuals, the siblings of HIV-positive children (or the children of HIV-positive parents) should all be immunised with BCG. Because recommendations for BCG in HIV-positive children may change, local protocols should be followed.

Why should BCG not be given to symptomatic HIV-positive children (or to adults)?

Some vaccines are prepared from a weak form of the infecting agent (the virus or micro-organism). BCG, for instance, is prepared from a weak form of the TB bacillus (*Mycobacterium tuberculosis*). If this weakened form of the TB bacillus is injected into a person with an already weakened immune system (as is the case with a patient who shows symptoms of advanced HIV infection or Aids), it may actually *cause* active TB in this patient. So, instead of BCG *preventing* TB, it can actually *cause* the disease in a patient with a depleted immune system. A patient with a depressed immune system due to Aids should rather be treated prophylactically with TB medications if the CD4 cell count is below 350 cells/mm^3, and if he or she shows no symptoms of active TB (see 'Prevention of TB in patients with HIV/Aids' on page 52).

The WHO recommends that babies and children with HIV infection (healthy as well as symptomatic children) should be immunised with the following vaccines:

- Oral polio (OPV) at birth, 6 weeks, 10 weeks, 14 weeks and again at between 4 and 5 years of age.
- Diphtheria, tetanus, pertussis (DTP) at 6 weeks, 10 weeks, 14 weeks and again at 18 months.
- Diphtheria and tetanus at 4–5 years.
- Mumps, measles, rubella (MMR) at 9 months and measles at 18 months.
- Hepatitis B (HBV) at 6 weeks, 10 weeks and again at 14 weeks.
- *Haemophilus influenzae* type B (Hib) at 6 weeks, 10 weeks and again at 14 weeks.

- Annual immunisation against influenza (flu) is strongly recommended. (In the southern hemisphere it should be given in March or April for protection in the coming winter.)
- A single dose of polyvalent pneumococcal vaccine should be given to HIV-positive children older than 2 years.

If a child is very ill, immunisation with live vaccines should be delayed until the child is better. Annual immunisation against influenza is also strongly recommended for HIV-positive adults. HIV-positive adults should also be vaccinated against hepatitis B if they are at risk or living in an area where hepatitis B is prevalent.

5.8 CONCLUSION

In Part 1 we were concerned largely with the physical aspects of HIV and Aids: how the virus is transmitted and what effect it has on the body. Although all this information is vitally important in the fight against HIV/Aids, *behaviour change* remains the most important means of preventing the spread of this disease while no real cure or effective vaccine is available. Part 2 will deal specifically with how to prevent HIV/Aids by changing behaviour that increases the risk of infection, and will explain how ordinary people may learn the life skills necessary to prevent infection.

part

2

Prevention and Empowerment in the HIV/Aids Context

INTRODUCTION TO PART 2

Because there is no cure for HIV infection or Aids, our best defence against infection is prevention. But prevention means much more than what to do and what to avoid. Effective prevention requires accurate knowledge of how people behave in different situations. It is important to know *when* or *under what conditions* people will be prepared to change their sexual behaviour. To be successful, HIV/Aids prevention programmes should take into account cultural differences, beliefs and customs. Because changing learned sexual behaviour is extremely difficult, our best hope for success in preventing the spread of HIV infection lies in empowering our children with the knowledge, attitudes, values and life skills needed both to prevent them becoming infected themselves and to help them care for those who are less fortunate.

The building blocks of a successful HIV/Aids education and prevention programme are discussed in *Chapter 6*. This chapter reviews various theories that describe the conditions needed for people to change their behaviour. The chapter also discusses the basic principles of adult education, the methods and strategies that promote learning, and the facilitation skills we need to help people learn new skills and attitudes. Voluntary HIV counselling and testing (VCT) as an HIV prevention strategy is also discussed in this chapter.

HIV/Aids prevention programmes will never succeed in Africa if we do not take the traditional African world-view into account. *Chapter 7* gives an overview of traditional African

Learning outcomes

After completing Part 2 you should be able to:

- develop an HIV/AIDS education and prevention programme for the workplace that is based on sound theoretical principles of behaviour change and appropriate methods of learning
- explain the traditional African perceptions of illness, sexuality, condom use and community life, and develop an education and prevention programme that incorporates these beliefs
- demonstrate the correct use of the male and of the female condom
- develop an HIV/AIDS education and life-skills training programme for schoolchildren that takes the age and the developmental characteristics of the children concerned into account

perceptions of illness, sexuality, children, community life and condom use. The chapter examines the implications of traditional African beliefs and customs for HIV/Aids prevention programmes in Africa.

Chapter 8 gives practical advice on how to prevent HIV infection. *Safe*, *safer* and *unsafe* sexual practices are all discussed, and numerous ideas and tips are given on how to practise safer sex. The prevention of HIV in injecting drug users is also addressed in this chapter.

HIV/Aids education and life-skills training for children are discussed in *Chapter 9*. Children's developmental characteristics, their perceptions of illness in general, and their understanding of HIV and Aids in their different developmental phases are all discussed. This chapter provides guidelines for educators about the kind of content they can include in HIV/Aids education and life-skills programmes for children in both the primary and the secondary phase of schooling.

chapter

6 Principles and Strategies for Prevention

How Raka can be kept at bay

This swift beast must die,
or he will reign over us
and he will bring a great and prolonged pain with him.

Aids differs from any other epidemic disease that has ever plagued the world. It is not only incurable; it is like the beast Raka from N.P. van Wyk Louw's epic poem because it challenges our deepest secrets and taboos about sex and death – whether as individuals or as a community. People vainly try to defend themselves against this *Raka* of destruction and fear by building defensive walls of myth, stigma, prejudice and blame around themselves. Although we can understand the feelings that make people want to distance themselves from anything to do with HIV and Aids, their denial makes us all more vulnerable to the effects of the disease.

Health care professionals are therefore faced with the tremendous task of trying to break down the walls of prejudice and lack of knowledge so that they can convince every member of the community that HIV/Aids touches the core of every person's life and that we should all work together to prevent the great and prolonged pain that this disease brings with it.

In 1990 Osborne said that 'the Achilles heel of HIV is its dependence on behaviour that is voluntary. Our best attack is that which enlists the community in his or her own defence' (p. 3). To enlist and train a whole community in its own defence is no small task. In this chapter we will examine the most important components of any successful HIV/Aids prevention programme.

6.1 THEORETICAL PRINCIPLES: WHEN WILL PEOPLE CHANGE THEIR BEHAVIOUR?

The initial reaction of the public health authorities in many countries as they tried to cope with the Aids epidemic was to try to persuade individuals and targeted groups to change their behaviour by providing them with relevant information about HIV/Aids. We now know that if we hope to change behaviour we need to do more than supply correct information to vulnerable groups. According to Fishbein and Middlestadt (1989:109):

> There are certain types of information that are necessary for developing effective educational communications or other types of interventions. The Aids epidemic is much too serious to allow interventions to be based upon some educator's untested and all too often incorrect intuitions about the factors that will influence the performance or nonperformance of a given behaviour in a given population.

If health care professionals want to be successful in changing people's sexual behaviour, they must have an understanding of the theories about how behaviour can be changed. We will not discuss the various theories in detail, but review the most important principles of behaviour change that form the basis of all these theories. These principles are based on:

- the theory of reasoned action (Fishbein & Ajzen, 1975)
- the theory of planned behaviour (Ajzen, 1991)
- the health belief model (Becker & Maiman, 1975; Rosenstock, 1974)
- the Aids risk reduction model (ARRM) of Catania et al. (1990)
- the social-cognitive learning theory of Bandura (1977)
- the learning theory of Rotter (1966).

According to the theories of *reasoned action* and *planned behaviour*, people are defined as *reasonable* beings who systematically process and use all information available to them when they *plan* their *behaviour* (Ajzen, 1991; Fishbein & Ajzen, 1975). To change people's behaviour, it is therefore necessary (in terms of this theory) to understand and change the cognitive structures that govern specific behaviour. Health care professionals can, for example, not begin to understand and change a person's behaviour if they do not have an appreciation or understanding of that individual's intentions, beliefs, attitudes, subjective norms and self-efficacy. Figure 6.1 gives an overview of the cognitive, emotional and social components that should be included in any programme designed to bring about sexual behaviour change.

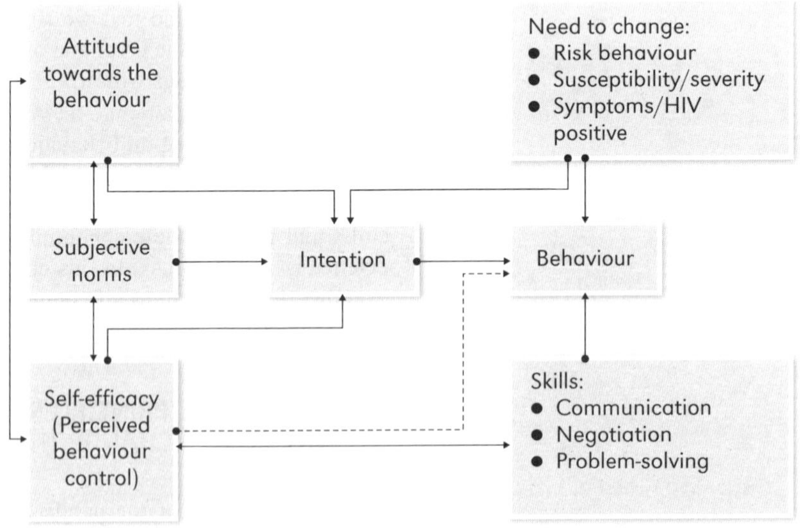

Figure 6.1
Cognitive, emotional and social factors influencing behaviour change
(Source: Adapted from Ajzen, 1991:182)

Recognition of the need to change

Before people can change any particular behaviour, they first need to recognise the *need* to change that behaviour. The factors that often contribute to the realisation that high-risk sexual behaviour should change are (Becker & Maiman, 1975; Fishbein & Middlestadt, 1989):

- the individual's self-description of being at risk;
- the perception of an individual's own susceptibility or vulnerability to HIV infection;
- the perception that the disease will have serious consequences and that it will affect the person's whole life;
- the belief that performing a specific behaviour will reduce susceptibility to (or the severity of) the illness;
- a concern about good health in general;
- experiencing the symptoms of illness;
- personal contact with somebody who is HIV positive or who has Aids; and
- an HIV-positive diagnosis.

Be specific about the behaviour you want to change

The health care professional should be absolutely specific about the behaviour that needs to be changed. Talking to people about 'safer sex practices' in general will rarely have any effect on their behaviour because the concept 'safer sex practices' is vague and refers to a whole category of behaviours instead of to one specific behaviour.

If we want to change a specific behaviour in an individual, we must identify that behaviour in cooperation with that person. For example, we might, together with the client, construct the following definite statements: 'I must always use a condom'; 'I should have only one sex partner'; or 'I must always use sterile needles for injecting drugs'. (See 'The male condom' on page 131 and 'The female condom' on page 134 on how to be specific about condom use.)

Every behaviour consists of four components: action, target, context and time. In order to change behaviour, it is important to identify the *action*, *target*, *context* and *time* of the behaviour that you want to change. For example, we should recognise the vital conceptual differences between *buying* and *using* a condom (*action*); *latex* versus *non-latex* condoms (*target*); a *primary long-term relationship* and *casual sex* (*context*); and casual sex *once a week* or casual sex *once a year* (*time*). Prevention strategies will vary according to the particular aspect of behaviour that we are considering. It is also important to remember that a prevention programme developed to *change* sexual behaviour (e.g. a strategy to increase or to decrease a specific type of behaviour) will not necessarily be effective for *maintaining* sexual behaviour (e.g. a strategy for continuing to use a condom every time the person has sexual intercourse). Cognitive factors associated with the *initiation* of specific behaviour may be totally different from the factors that are associated with the *increase*, *decrease* or *maintenance* of that same behaviour (Fishbein & Middlestadt, 1989).

If we want to have success in developing sexual behaviour change programmes, we must focus on behaviour that is under the *control* of the individual, rather than behaviour that depends on external factors. If a (disempowered) woman has no power to negotiate the use of male condoms with her unwilling partner, a counsellor should rather concentrate on convincing her to use the female condom, because this might be the only area of behaviour that she can control.

Intentions to perform a specific behaviour

If individuals want to change their behaviour, they must develop the *intention* of changing that behaviour. According to *the theory of reasoned action*, we can predict someone's behaviour if we can determine whether he or she has an *intention* to carry out that specific behaviour. Intentions reflect all the motivational factors that influence specific behaviour. Intentions are indications of how hard people are willing to try, or of how much effort they are planning to put into performing a behaviour (Ajzen, 1991:181). Generally, the stronger the intention or the commitment to do something, the greater the probability that it will be done.

Aids educators should therefore also concentrate on people's behavioural intentions in their HIV prevention programmes. The same principles that apply to behaviour change (in terms of specificity, action, target, context, and time) should also be taken into account in trying to change or reinforce intentions. In order to change behaviour, it is necessary to reinforce the intention that directly corresponds to that specific behaviour. If the desired behaviour is 'to use a latex condom every time I have sexual intercourse', the intention to be reinforced will be the intention 'to use a latex condom every time I have sexual intercourse' and not the intention 'to practise safer sex' or merely 'to use a condom' (both of which are too vague to be of any use).

However, intentions do not always predict behaviour. When people do not have control over their own behaviour (as in the case of disempowered women who cannot negotiate condom use with their sex partners), the best intentions in the world may not necessarily translate into behaviour. Good intentions are also often hampered by the *unavailability* of opportunities and resources such as time, money, condoms and the necessary skills.

Attitudes towards the specific behaviour

The intention to change sexual behaviour (by using condoms, for instance) depends on a person's *attitudes* towards that particular behaviour (e.g. condom use). If people truly believe that condom use will have a positive outcome for them, the probability that they will actually use condoms will be much greater. However, if they feel negative about using condoms (or find the use of condoms problematic, for whatever reason), a great deal of explanation, negotiation and persuasion may be required before they will actually use condoms (the desired behaviour). It is therefore very important for the counsellor to establish a person's attitude towards *the specific behaviour* that needs to be changed before the change can be expected to occur (Fishbein & Ajzen, 1975).

The strong predictors of behaviour are strongly positive attitudes, attitudes based on a lot of thinking, attitudes with great personal relevance, and attitudes based on direct personal experience – not vague, generalised attitudes based on impersonal second-hand and indirect information (Petty, 1995). Behaviour change can be predicted more accurately by considering attitudes to alternative courses of action. For example, you can predict more accurately whether or not a person will use condoms if you measure his or her attitude to using condoms as well to *not* using condoms (Petty, 1995). For predictions based on attitudes to be accurate, we must also know what a person's attitude is to all alternative forms of behaviour.

The influence of subjective norms on behaviour

The intention to change behaviour depends also on the *subjective norms* of the individual. Subjective norms are influenced by:

- the beliefs of important reference groups or individuals in a person's life; and
- the desire to please these reference groups or individuals.

If condom use is *not* acceptable to friends or lovers, and if it is important for the person to impress his or her friends, it will be very difficult for that person to change his or her behaviour and start using condoms. In such cases it may be necessary to counsel peer groups or partners before individuals will consent to use condoms (Fishbein & Ajzen, 1975).

Before a person's behaviour can be changed, it is important to establish whether this specific behaviour is under *attitudinal* or *normative* control. If a teenage boy's decision not to use condoms is under attitudinal control (i.e. he has a negative attitude towards condom use because it decreases his sexual pleasure), the counsellor's attempt to change his behaviour by using normative or peer pressure will fail, because his behaviour (in this case) does not depend on what his friends think (normative control). On the other hand, if a young woman who has no personal objections to condom use does not use them because her friends think that condoms are not 'cool' to use, the counsellor should concentrate his or her efforts on changing the group norm.

Self-efficacy or perceived behaviour control as a predictor of behaviour change

To have an intention to change behaviour is not enough: people should also *believe* that they have the *ability* to perform the desired behaviour. Bandura (1977) refers to a person's *belief* in his or her *ability* to control behaviour, or to carry out specific behaviour successfully, as *self-efficacy*. According to Bandura (1991:257), self-efficacy is central to any person's ability to function:

> People's beliefs in their efficacy influence the choices they make, their aspirations, how much effort they mobilise in a given activity, how long they persevere in the face of difficulties and setbacks, whether their thought patterns are self-hindering or self-aiding, the amount of stress they experience in coping with difficult environmental demands, and their vulnerability to depression.

Ajzen (1991) uses the term 'perceived behaviour control' to refer to people's perception of the ease or difficulty of performing a specific task. People with high self-efficacy (or a high perception of behaviour control) are better motivated to master new situations and behaviour, and more persistent in their attempts to reach specific goals, than people with low self-efficacy.

Low self-efficacy has been identified by many researchers as an obstacle to sexual behaviour change. Low self-efficacy has been found to correlate positively with high-risk sexual practices, with an unwillingness to change behaviour, and with relapses from low- to high-risk behaviour (recidivism) (Montgomery et al., 1989). On the other hand, subjects who were categorised as being in the lowest category of risk for HIV infection generated the highest self-efficacy scores.

Aids educators must not underestimate the importance of self-efficacy in their programmes. They should increase or reinforce people's self-efficacy by making sure that people possess the required communication, negotiation and problem-solving skills to carry out the desired actions, and that they know exactly how to apply their newly acquired behaviour (e.g. how to use a condom). The person's belief in his or her ability to use a condom and to discuss condom use with partners should also be reinforced. Researchers found that the intention to change behaviour, along with the perception that the behaviour can be controlled (high self-efficacy), significantly increased the probability that behaviour could be changed for the better.

The chances that a person will change his or her behaviour (e.g. by using condoms) are much better if that person:

- forms a strong intention (in this case, to use condoms);
- demonstrates a favourable attitude (in this case, towards condom use);
- has positive subjective norms; and
- also has a high level of self-efficacy and a perception that he or she *can* control that behaviour.

However, intentions, attitudes, subjective norms and perception of behaviour control may all be undermined if a person becomes discouraged and disheartened by perceived obstacles or difficulties that seem to block progress towards behaviour change.

Obstacles and rewards that impede or encourage behaviour change

People will change their behaviour only if they perceive the new behaviour as potentially effective, beneficial and feasible in practice (Rosenstock, 1966). The probability of a person changing his or her behaviour therefore depends on that person's perceptions of the *benefits* or *rewards* that will be gained from the new behaviour, as well as perceptions of the *disadvantages* or *obstacles* that will result. Researchers have found that people are prepared to change their sexual behaviour in various ways if they believe that this behaviour is beneficial (in terms of decreasing their risk of infection), and if they know that they have social support (i.e. support from friends and the community) (Montgomery et al., 1989).

One of the main reasons why people do not change their behaviour is that they perceive the existence of obstacles that (in their *perception*) hinder and obstruct the possibility of behaviour change (Janz & Becker, 1984). Research into the prevention of HIV infection identified the following factors as obstacles that hindered sexual behaviour change (Montgomery et al., 1989; Schurink & Schurink, 1990; Van Dyk, 1991):

- People abandon all attempts to use condoms if they find it *stressful* to initiate or to maintain the behaviour.
- *Society's intolerance* towards certain sex practices and safer sex makes it more difficult for people to change their behaviour.
- *Unsupportive sex partners and peers* lead to abandonment of all attempts at safer sex. Research found that people often do not use condoms because they do not want to offend their sex partners; because sex partners don't 'like' condoms; or because they are afraid that the partner will leave them. Partners often refuse to use condoms because it 'feels different' and because of the stigma attached to the use of condoms (in some circles). Condoms are often associated with syphilis, filth, uncleanliness, unfaithfulness and family planning.
- The lack of *communication skills* is one of the greatest obstacles in the way of behaviour change. People find it difficult to ask partners to use condoms, especially if they do not know the partner well. They are also often afraid that the partner may think that they have Aids. Women, in many cases, do not have the power to negotiate condom use with their husbands or partners.
- People find it difficult to handle a partner's *refusal* to use condoms.
- It is very difficult for people to change their sexual behaviour if they are not offered *alternative sex practices* that can replace risky behaviour. (See 'General safer sex rules' on page 136 for examples of alternative sex practices.)
- A *fatalistic attitude to life* hinders sexual behaviour change. Many young South Africans, for example, currently believe that they are at much greater risk from the possibility of violence than from the possibility of infection by HIV. As one student puts it: 'With Aids I still have a chance to live for many years. My neighbourhood is so dangerous, I am not sure that I will still be alive tomorrow morning.'
- In a Zimbabwean study, students listed the following obstacles to condom use: the necessity for advance planning, inaccessibility (i.e. difficulties in obtaining condoms), a lack of privacy (problems with storing condoms or being found with condoms in one's possession), and an inability to *communicate* with their partners (Sherman & Bassett, 1999).
- The use of *alcohol* and *recreational drugs* diminishes the power of individuals to make responsible decisions. Even subjects who had a firm intention always to use condoms and who had often used condoms in the past reported that they often had sex without condoms when they were under the influence of alcohol or drugs (their responsibility threshold was drastically lowered).
- Condoms are often not *available* and *accessible*. People, especially young people, do not use condoms if they are not readily available. They are either ashamed to ask for condoms over the counter, or they don't have the money to buy them.
- *Cultural norms* and *religious beliefs* are often not conducive to condom use (see 'Perceptions of condoms' on page 122).

It is up to health care professionals to try to identify the obstacles that stand in the way of safer sex practices and to help people to surmount these obstacles. People are more likely to change their behaviour if the rewards that come with changed behaviour (rewards such as peace of mind) are made obvious. Encourage individuals to make lists of rewards as well as obstacles. This will enable you to discuss each individual's concerns and (if at all possible) find suitable solutions. Some solutions are quite easy to put into practice. Many people are simply unaware of their existence.

Perception of health control: Internal versus external locus of control

It is important for the prevention of illness and for the promotion of health to know to what extent people believe that they have control over their own health status. According to the health locus of control theory, people who believe that they have no control over their own health (external locus of control) will be less inclined to get involved in preventive and promotive behaviour than people who believe that they can do something to improve their health (internal locus of control) (Rotter, 1966; Wallston et al., 1978).

People with an internal locus of control believe that they can influence and control their own health through personal behaviour. People with an external locus of control believe that they don't have much control over their own health because their health depends on external factors such as luck, chance, fate, other people, or uncontrolled forces outside themselves. People with an external locus of control will therefore not do much to prevent illness or to improve their health.

Research on locus of control and sexual behaviour change has generally found that people with an internal locus of control will be more inclined to change high-risk sexual behaviour than people with an external locus of control. The implications of these findings for educational programmes to change high-risk sexual behaviour are complex. Simply to say that 'educators should change people's locus of control from external to internal' is a demonstration of arrogance and ignorance.

Locus of control is not only a personal issue, it is also a cultural issue. Many cultures (including many indigenous African cultures) have a collectivistic world-view (i.e. a world-view that emphasises the dominance of group over personal interests). People from such cultures are acculturated to operate on the assumption of an external locus of control. According to Mbiti (1969:106) the identity of the traditional African is totally embedded in his or her collective existence, and all decisions (including decisions about health) are taken with the group's knowledge and approval (external locus of control). It is obvious that it would be almost impossible (as well as impractical) to imagine that health care workers would be able to change the underlying cultural and philosophical framework of an entire group of people.

Health care professionals who work in Africa should therefore accept that many Africans have an external locus of control, and learn to work *with it* rather than against it when they devise means to change high-risk sexual behaviour. In collectivist cultural contexts of this kind, the family, the community and peer counsellors should be involved in prevention programmes, because they have the authority and prestige to dictate sexual mores and customs (see 'Community involvement in Aids education, prevention and counselling' on page 124).

Skills for converting intentions into actions

Intention or a strong commitment to change behaviour can be translated into action only if people have the skills and help to do so. It may require complex negotiations with sexual partners who may not have the commitment to change. Verbal communication skills, negotiation skills and problem-solving skills are all needed before one can successfully get one's partner to commit to safer sex behaviour (such as, for example, condom use). Health care professionals should help people practise their communication and negotiation skills through experiential, 'hands-on' activities such as modelling and role play.

Theories of behaviour change: a summary

The theories of behaviour change provide a tremendous amount of information that is extremely useful for understanding behaviour and for implementing interventions that will be effective in changing behaviour (Ajzen, 1991: 206). These theoretical principles underlying behaviour change should be kept in mind by health care professionals when they develop programmes to prevent HIV infection in the community. Aids educators should ask themselves what role the social, cultural and economic context plays in inhibiting or promoting behaviour change, and what social changes are required to bring about individual change. Table 6.1 on page 98 summarises the principles that underlie behaviour change.

Table 6.1
A summary of the theoretical principles of behaviour change

People will be more likely to change their sexual behaviour if they:

- realise the need for behaviour change (e.g. feel vulnerable to HIV infection during unprotected sex with multiple sex partners);
- know exactly what specific behaviour needs changing and how to change it (e.g. that a new condom should be used for every act of intercourse);
- have the intention or commitment to perform the behaviour (e.g. the intention to use a condom every time they have sex);
- have positive attitudes to the behaviour (e.g. believe that condom use will prevent HIV infection, and that condoms are quite comfortable to use);
- have the support of friends in changing the behaviour (e.g. the peer group totally accepts and approves of condom use);
- have a strong belief (high self-efficacy) in their ability to perform the specific required behaviour (e.g. know exactly how to use condoms effectively and easily, and be able to insist – without fear of retribution – that condoms be used every time they have sex);
- know exactly how to perform the behaviour effectively (e.g. how to use the condom so that it will not break or leak);
- perceive that the benefits and rewards from the new behaviour (e.g. condom use) will outweigh obstacles; and
- have the necessary skills to perform and maintain the behaviour (e.g. the communication, negotiation and problem-solving skills to make condom use an acceptable behaviour).

Activity

Read the enrichment box 'The stages of behaviour change' and consider the following questions:

Why do you think it is important to be able to identify the exact stage of behaviour change in which a person currently finds himself or herself? How would it influence your HIV/Aids prevention message if you knew that a person was in the precontemplation phase? Or if you knew that a person was in the action phase?

Enrichment

The stages of behaviour change

According to Prochaska and DiClemente (1984:24–29), behaviour change involves movement through four different stages of change.

- In the first stage of *precontemplation*, people are unaware of having any problem at all, and so they can logically have no intention of changing their behaviour (e.g. they will not even be considering the use of condoms).
- The second stage of change is *contemplation*. This is the stage in which people become aware that a personal problem exists (e.g. they are aware of the dangers of unsafe sex and they are seriously thinking about using condoms, but they have not yet made a commitment to change).
- The third stage, *action*, is the stage in which people change their overt behaviour and the environmental conditions that affect their behaviour. In this stage people are acting on their beliefs in personal self-efficacy (e.g. people start using condoms and they believe in their ability to maintain this behaviour).
- The last stage of behaviour change is the stage of *maintenance*. In this stage people work to maintain their newly acquired behaviour and to prevent relapses to the kind of behaviour from which they made the change. Maintenance is not an absence of change; it is a continuance of change (e.g. people use condoms, but they still have to work very hard to maintain the behaviour and to prevent relapses into unsafe sex practices). Cessation of a problem occurs only when people no longer experience any temptation to return to the problem behaviour, and if they no longer have to make any effort to prevent themselves from relapsing.

6.2 PRACTICAL ASPECTS OF PREVENTION PROGRAMMES

The purpose of HIV/Aids education is not only to disseminate information, but also to change attitudes and behaviour, to equip people with the necessary life skills, to empower them to prevent the spread of HIV infection and to help them care for people who are already infected. The following practical aspects should be kept in mind when developing HIV/Aids prevention programmes (based on UNAIDS, 2000c, 2002; Van Dyk, 1999; WHO, 2000a):

National support

HIV/Aids prevention programmes can be successful only if they are backed by political will and leadership. No prevention programme can be successful without the support, commitment and high-profile advocacy of a country's leaders. A single, comprehensive, powerful national Aids plan involving a wide range of role players ranging from government to the private sector is necessary. Successful programmes should impart knowledge, counter stigma and discrimination, create social consensus on safer behaviour, and boost HIV prevention and care skills. These can be cost-effectively accomplished through mass media campaigns, through peer or outreach education, through life-skills programmes in schools and workplaces, and by ensuring that voluntary counselling and HIV testing are available.

Partnerships

Partnerships are essential for effective prevention programmes. Because multiple programmes in multiple populations are needed, it is crucial to create partnerships between different role players and stakeholders, including people with HIV/Aids.

Peer support

Behaviour change is most likely if peers educate and support each other. Youth programmes run by the youth, or programmes run by groups that comprise street children, injecting drug users or refugees, are all extremely effective in promoting practices and behaviour leading to reduction of HIV transmission. Sexual practices, drug-taking and other risk behaviours are much more likely to be openly discussed, explored and understood within such safe group environments.

Peer education programmes both empower and educate people. According to Harrison et al. (2000:287), a successful peer education programme transfers the control of knowledge from the hands of experts to lay members of the community, thereby making the educational process more accessible and less intimidating. Peer education also allows group debate and the negotiation of messages and behaviours that lead to the development of new collective norms of behaviour rather than attempts to convince individuals to change their own behaviour on a basis of rational decision making.

All over the world there have been powerful examples of the success of peer involvement in prevention strategies. Peer counselling has, for example, been very successfully applied by the South African mining companies. Willing and enthusiastic people should be identified and then trained to work as peer counsellors in their own communities. Health care professionals, teachers and religious leaders can play an important role in facilitating the formation of these groups and providing expert knowledge where necessary.

Involving people living with HIV/Aids

People living with HIV/Aids are often the best advocates and activists for social and behaviour change, and they should be included in the developmental and implementation stages of HIV/Aids prevention programmes. The personal story of someone living with HIV presents a powerful message. These messages can mobilise people and resources and so initiate successful prevention programmes. Involving people living with HIV/Aids in prevention programmes in their own communities helps to ensure that the programmes are relevant and meaningful to the community or population group in question.

Cultural, religious and social sensitivity

There is no standard programme that will be meaningful, relevant and effective for *all* people in *all* times and places. Prevention programmes must be contextualised so that they are sensitive to local customs, cultural practices and religious beliefs and values, as well as to other traditional norms and practices. Traditional African beliefs and customs that should be taken into account when developing HIV prevention programmes in Africa are discussed in chapter 7.

Facilitating empowerment

Empowerment can be facilitated by involving and encouraging individuals, groups and communities to address their own health concerns and to find solutions to their own problems. People who are empowered to come up with their own plans and solutions are more likely to implement effective HIV prevention programmes.

Individuals (especially women in disadvantaged positions, and young people) should be empowered by being taught communication skills, negotiation skills, assertiveness, decision-making strategies, self-esteem, self-efficacy, life skills, and the basics of competent sexual behaviour, problem solving and conflict resolution.

Although the personal and social disempowerment of women in Africa is often emphasised (and is indeed sometimes a serious problem), the inherent strength and autonomy of African women, especially in women's groups (where such qualities are more than evident), should not be overlooked by health care professionals working in Africa. Ulin (1992) commented that rural African women have always been able to mobilise and organise themselves informally to meet the needs of their communities by making the best use of the advantages and opportunities for solidarity inherent in family ties, neighbours and other informal networks. Ulin believes that the solidarity of women in rural African communities may be their greatest source of strength for coping with the Aids epidemic.

Condom distribution

Condom distribution should be an important component of any HIV prevention programme. Condoms should be easily accessible to men and to women. They should be available and distributed in places where people will feel a maximum sense of privacy and a minimum of embarrassment – through self-service (i.e. where people can simply help themselves to however many they need) in clinics, hospitals, factories, mines and bars and on campuses. Condoms should also be distributed free of charge if possible. Health care professionals need to know where free condoms are available and they should keep a supply themselves, if possible.

A holistic approach

Counselling, education, support and care services and resources should be combined to provide a holistic continuum of HIV prevention and care. A comprehensive prevention programme that addresses the various aspects of HIV/Aids in different contexts (churches, schools, hospitals and tertiary institutions) will prevent the stigma and discrimination often associated with HIV specific programmes.

6.3 CHANGING NEGATIVE ATTITUDES

Aids-related stigma and discrimination remain the greatest obstacles to people living with HIV infection or Aids. Stigma and discrimination increase people's vulnerability, isolate them, deprive them of their basic human rights, care and support, and worsen the impact of infection. Stigma and concerns about discrimination are the main reasons why people do not come forward to have an HIV test, to access antiretroviral drugs, to adopt safe feeding methods for their babies, or to change high-risk sexual behaviour.

But stigma and discrimination do not arise in a vacuum. They emerge from and reinforce other stereotypes, prejudices and social inequalities relating to gender, nationality, ethnicity and sexuality. They also feed into activities that are criminalised such as sex work, drug use or sex between men. 'Stigma, discrimination and human rights violations form a vicious circle, legitimising and spurring each other' (UNAIDS, 2002:67).

The following efforts should be implemented worldwide to fight stigma and discrimination (UNAIDS, 2002:67):

- Leaders at all levels and in all walks of life should be encouraged to visibly challenge and act against the many forms of HIV-related discrimination and to spearhead public action.
- People living with HIV/Aids should be actively involved in the response to the epidemic.
- Violations of human rights should be monitored, people should be able to challenge discrimination, and institutions should be designed to safeguard human rights.
- Governments should take urgent action to protect women's property and inheritance rights, and to protect children against sexual exploitation.

- A legal environment able to support the fight against discrimination should be created.
- Prevention and treatment, care and support services should be accessible to all.

Combating stigma, isolation, stereotypes and discrimination

By showing their own support and responsibility to care for all people, regardless of their health or social status, health care professionals can act as role models for others in helping to combat stigma, discrimination and the isolation of people living with HIV/Aids. Prevention strategies will become far more successful if and when HIV is treated like any other disease, and when people feel safe to be open about their HIV status. However, health care professionals can become advocates for acceptance and care only if they look inward and first examine their own beliefs, values, assumptions and attitudes towards HIV/Aids. This can be done individually or in groups by asking and reflecting on the following questions (WHO, 2000a:6-5):

- What fears or misunderstandings do I have?
- How might these fears or misunderstandings affect my work?
- Where do these fears or misunderstandings come from?
- How can I overcome these fears or misunderstandings in order to provide care, support, counselling, education, and advice in the prevention and care of HIV/Aids?
- What influence do I have on others who care for people infected and affected by HIV/Aids?
- What is my role in providing and promoting safe, moral and ethical care to people living with HIV and their loved ones, caregivers and communities?

Health care professionals should also think about and listen to the 'language' they use when they speak: prejudiced language may alienate them from their target group. While saying 'He caught Aids' and 'He has Aids' may mean the same thing, the first sentence is loaded with negative meanings that betray the implicit attitudes of the speaker. (Such a negative meaning may be that Aids is something over which we the, innocent, have no control, something that we 'catch' from 'them' – the contaminated 'others'). People often say 'He is HIV' instead of 'He is HIV positive'. A sentence constructed like this implies an identity with the virus, i.e. the person *is* the virus, instead of the person *has* the virus.

Aids educators should also be careful not to use sexist language. Always to refer to *he* and *him* in the context of HIV/Aids may imply that men are always the 'guilty' party. Victimising language should also be avoided. Instead of saying 'She suffers from Aids' one should rather say 'She lives with Aids' or 'She is HIV positive'. Rather than referring to 'rape victims', use positive language and refer instead to 'rape survivors'. Be careful not to fall into the trap of using prejudiced or discriminatory language. If you refer to people with HIV infection as 'those people', you are clearly dividing the world into two groups: the innocent, healthy *us*, and the guilty, diseased *them*.

While we all sometimes think in terms of stereotypes, we should make every effort to be aware of our own stereotypes so that we can root them out and thus avoid offending others and hurting feelings. If we interact with members of a stereotyped group, we will quickly learn to recognise our own prejudices and eliminate them.

The irrational and often exaggerated fears associated with HIV/Aids can be directly addressed through educational programmes based on sound medical, social and psychological knowledge. To be successful, such programmes must be sustained and supported over time. Prevention strategies will continue to be compromised if fear, ignorance, intolerance and discrimination against HIV-positive people persist. Health care professionals have a responsibility to help 'normalise' HIV in the communities where they work so that modes of transmission and prevention can be addressed without the emotional and attitudinal values that are currently getting in the way of open dialogue.

Counsellors and other health care professionals should not only 'advocate for Universal Precautions, but also for universal tolerance and knowledge about HIV/Aids' (WHO, 2000a:6-4).

Enrichment

Stereotypes, prejudice and discrimination

- *Stereotypes* are frames of reference or patterns of expectations that strongly influence the processing of incoming social information. A stereotype is usually an oversimplified, one-sided and relatively fixed generalisation or rigid view of a group, an individual or certain activities or roles. An example of a stereotype is the belief that all members of certain groups share traits or characteristics.
- *Prejudice* is a negative attitude to members of a group, based solely on their membership of that group.
- *Discrimination* refers to negative behaviour or actions based on prejudice – it is prejudice in action.

(Baron & Byrne, 1994:218–219).

Countering harmful gender norms

Programmes should seek to counter harmful gender norms that lead to the sexual coercion and exploitation of women and girls. Through the use of media, public information campaigns, the arts, schools and community discussion groups, such programmes should (UNAIDS, 2002:84):

- encourage discussion of how boys and girls are brought up and expected to behave;
- challenge concepts of masculinity and femininity that are based on inequality and aggressive and passive stereotypes;
- encourage men and boys to talk with each other and their partners about sex, violence, drug use and Aids;
- teach female assertiveness and negotiation skills in relationships, sex and reproduction;
- teach and encourage male sexual and reproductive responsibility;
- teach and promote respect for, and responsibility towards, women and children;
- teach and promote equality in relationships and in the domestic and public spheres;
- support actions to reduce male violence, including domestic and sexual violence; and
- encourage men to be providers of care and support in the family and community.

Long-term strategies to change harmful gender norms should be directed at underlying cultural and social structures, and their aim should be to promote mutual respect between men and women and equal access to all types of resources. The goals of long-term strategies include (Brouard et al., 2004):

- changing ideas and social norms that keep women in an inferior social position;
- achieving shared decision-making power between men and women at all levels: in relationships, community affairs and political and economic bodies;
- creating structural changes to give women equal access to education, training and income-earning opportunities; and
- reallocating work responsibilities so that men and women share them fairly.

A greater understanding and acceptance of men who have sex with men should also be encouraged. This population accounts for 5–10% of all HIV cases worldwide (UNAIDS, 2004). Men who have sex with men typically do not see themselves as gay, homosexual or bisexual, and many of them may also have unprotected sex with women. Typical situations in which there may be sexual expression among men who are not gay-identified are prison or military service. Prevention programmes must take into account that this group is highly stigmatised, and they are often 'driven underground' and out of reach of most prevention efforts. Peer-based interventions that target social networks of men who have sex with men can be very effective in promoting risk reduction.

Respecting human rights and improving social structures

HIV/Aids is also a developmental challenge. Society as a whole would become less vulnerable to HIV and the stigma surrouning it in the long run if governments were to make a serious attempt to grapple with social problems such as poverty, unemployment, migratory labour, the subordinate status of women, and child abuse. Social goals such as education, the empowerment of women and human rights should therefore be promoted.

Activity

Devise an exercise to make people aware of their stereotypes, negative attitudes or prejudices. Or use the following riddle in a group:

> A man and his son were involved in a serious car accident. Emergency vehicles sped to the gruesome scene. On arrival, paramedics applied CPR to both victims. Once stabilised, the patients were rushed by ambulance to the hospital. However, the man's injuries were fatal, and he died during transit. The boy was rushed to the emergency theatre, where medical personnel were waiting. But, just before starting the operation, the surgeon cried out: 'I can't operate. This is my son!'
>
> Who is the surgeon?

Ask the participants to write the answer down, and to raise their hands if they believe they have the answer. Do you know the answer? The surgeon, of course, is the boy's mother. If you could not figure the riddle out, is it because you are strongly imprinted with the stereotype that only men can be surgeons?

6.4 VOLUNTARY HIV COUNSELLING AND TESTING AS HIV PREVENTION STRATEGY

Voluntary HIV counselling and testing (VCT) has emerged as a major strategy for the prevention of HIV infection and Aids in Africa. Voluntary HIV counselling and testing should therefore be a key component of any prevention and care programme offered to communities. VCT is a process whereby an individual undergoes counselling to enable him or her to make an informed decision about being tested for HIV antibodies. Many studies show that knowing one's HIV status, whether it is positive or negative, is instrumental in effecting behaviour change and the adoption of safer sex practices (Mkaya-Mwamburi et al., 2000; Serima & Manyenna, 2000). Depending on the results of VCT, people usually take steps to avoid becoming infected or infecting others.

Within care programmes, HIV test results and follow-up counselling mean people can be directed towards relevant care and support services (e.g. treatment for sexually transmitted infections, tuberculosis and other opportunistic diseases, access to antiretrovirals, counselling about family planning and prevention of mother-to-child transmission, and support for adherence to medications). Wider access to VCT may also lead to greater openness about HIV/Aids, raised awareness and less stigma and discrimination (UNAIDS, 2002:122).

Availability of accessible and affordable VCT services is a problem in many countries, and this should be addressed by governments. The use of rapid HIV antibody tests is preferred because distances from the clinic and lack of transport often make it difficult for people to come back to the clinic for test results. Rapid HIV antibody tests can be carried out by staff with no formal laboratory training. If VCT services do exist, the community should be well informed about such services. They should be widely advertised and health care professionals and community workers should be sensitised to and trained in pre- and post-HIV-test counselling.

Figure 6.2 on page 104 illustrates VCT as the main entry point for prevention, care and support services. With plans for expanded antiretroviral drug access (both for treatment and prevention of mother-to-child transmission) in many countries, there will be an increasing need for hospitals and community care programmes to provide VCT. This stems from the simple fact that antiretrovirals are of little use unless people know their serostatus. In addition, ongoing counselling will be necessary to ensure that people taking antiretroviral therapy are supported, adhere to regimens and cope with possible adverse affects. Family and couple counselling will be particularly beneficial in the context of mother-to-child transmission, both for adherence and support. It is, therefore, all the more important to ensure that testing is supported by effective counselling with adequately trained counsellors, in user-friendly venues, and with guaranteed confidentiality (UNAIDS, 2002:124).

A South African VCT study: 'What is the point of knowing?'

In a South African study on the psychosocial barriers to voluntary HIV counselling and testing, conducted in 2002, the 1 422 participants expressed their needs, attitudes and beliefs about VCT as follows (Van Dyk & Van Dyk, 2003a,b):

Beliefs about HIV testing in general

Although the participants generally believed that everyone should know his or her HIV status, only 51% had been tested for HIV. Seventeen per cent of black and 5% of white participants who had not been tested for HIV before, said that they would definitely not go for VCT. They gave the following reasons:

- they felt that they had no treatment options;
- they feared prejudice and rejection by loved ones, health care workers and the community;
- they believed that knowledge of their HIV status would lead to depression, despair and an early death.

Of those subjects who were prepared to go for VCT, 19% of white and 40% of black participants said that they would go only to a clinic, hospital or doctor where absolutely nobody knew them – the main reasons being:

- lack of trust in the health care system;
- fear that confidentiality will not be observed; and
- fear of prejudice and rejection by health care professionals and by loved ones.

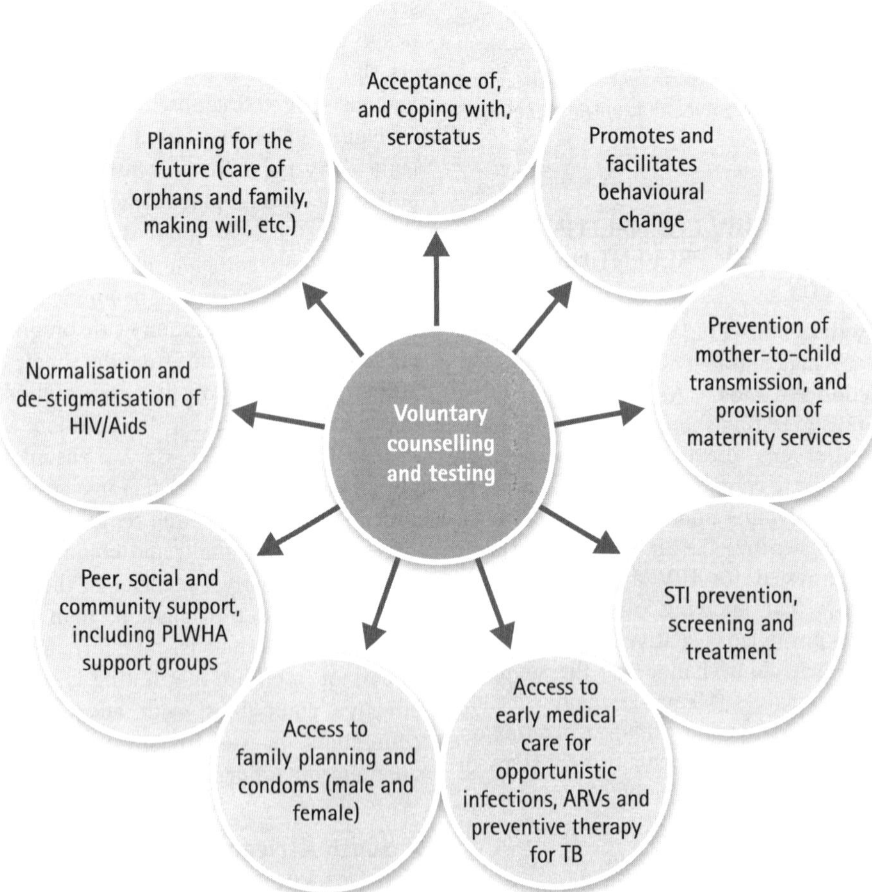

Figure 6.2
Voluntary counselling and testing as an entry point for HIV prevention and care
(Source: UNAIDS, 2002:123)

Most of the participants (85%) preferred rapid HIV antibody testing, mainly because they found the waiting period stressful, and because they often did not have the money or transport to return for their test results later. However, 15% said that they did not want their test results immediately, because they needed time to adjust to the possibility of being HIV positive and because they were not sure that they wanted to know the results.

Attitudes to disclosure

Eighty-four per cent of the participants said that they would disclose their HIV-positive status (but not necessarily to sex partners); 16% said that they would keep their results secret (this group consisted mainly of subjects who were younger, male, rural, and with fewer years of education); and 13% of married participants, mainly men, indicated that they would keep their results secret. It is interesting to note that fear of rejection was the main reason both men and women gave for not being prepared to inform sex partners, but the *source* of the fear was different for men and women. While women's fears were based in powerlessness, loss of security and the possibility of violence, men most feared the loss of their sexuality and sex appeal to women. Men also feared that nobody would take care of them when they were sick.

Behaviour change

Although most participants said that they would change their sexual behaviour if they tested HIV positive, 14% said that they would definitely not change their sexual behaviour and 9% were not sure. A fatalistic or 'why bother' attitude and a lack of in-depth knowledge of HIV/Aids were evident in some of the reasons participants gave for not changing their sexual (or health) behaviour if they tested HIV positive. Some subjects who practised high-risk sexual behaviour said that they would not change their behaviour if they tested HIV negative because 'it is obviously not necessary' and 'maybe I am immune like those prostitutes in KZN'. Subjects who knew someone who had died of Aids were significantly more prepared to change their own sexual behaviour if they tested HIV negative. They saw it as a 'new lease on life' or a 'second chance'.

Counselling experiences and needs

The counselling experiences of subjects who had received VCT before were mostly favourable. Counselling was described as being professional, compassionate, supportive and informative. Unfavourable experiences included the following:

- too few counsellors and long lines;
- lack of privacy;
- the use of group counselling;
- long waiting periods for results when rapid testing was not available;
- impersonal contact, like 'reading and signing a form' as pre-test counselling;
- presentation of the formal laboratory results so that the client 'can see for himself' without any proper counselling or explanation;
- lack of counsellor knowledge, experience, skills and sensitivity;
- cultural insensitivity of counsellors (in terms of language, age, sex, eye contact, or the remarks they make);
- too much emphasis on risk assessment.

Participants expressed the following needs:

- advice on how to live a positive life after diagnosis;
- how to change sexual behaviour;
- more advanced information on new developments in the HIV/Aids field;
- counselling or help to disclose their serostatus to sex partners (subjects felt totally disempowered in this regard, and because they don't know how to disclose, they often stay silent);
- a strong need was expressed for follow-up counselling and support, spiritual counselling and a comprehensive referral system – not only for themselves but also for their families. Generally, the feeling was: 'Why bother if there are no incentives?'

It is clear from this study that a comprehensive VCT service in South Africa faces various challenges, such as: appointing sufficient counsellors; establishing trust in the counselling services; setting up adquate testing sites; and making rapid testing generally available. A comprehensive VCT service further needs to emphasise confidentiality, positive incentives for testing, disclosure support and follow-up services or referral.

6.5 TEACHING AND LEARNING ABOUT HIV/AIDS

Health care professionals are increasingly required to act as HIV/Aids educators in various contexts.

Basic principles of *how* to teach HIV/Aids prevention, care and counselling will be discussed in this section. *What* we teach (content) will depend on the needs of the target group. The information given in this section is based on the WHO Fact Sheets on HIV/Aids (WHO, 2000a: 9-2 to 9-6).

Basic principles of adult education

Before commencing any educational programme it is important to assess the learning needs of the group and to be familiar with the cultural environment from which the participants have come. Use a questionnaire to establish the group's needs. Find out what they already know, what they don't know, and what misconceptions they have. Ask the participants what their needs and expectations are and what they expect to gain or learn from the course. This information will make it possible for you to plan relevant educational sessions and materials and deliver information that is meaningful and useful to the participants.

Evaluation of the educational strategies used and the learning outcomes of the participants is also critically important. Most adults learn best if they are actively involved in the learning process. It is important to realise that different people learn through the medium of different educational strategies. If we remember this, we will be careful not to use just one single learning method in all situations. For example, it might be important on one occasion to provide an opportunity for learners to practise a particular technique, but on another occasion it might be more appropriate to lecture, to review a textbook or to utilise another kind of document. Learners also need time to reflect on their learning and to revisit what they have learned through the use of techniques such as practice, discussion, critical questioning, research, or active participation in teaching others.

Educational sessions should be conducted in such a way that learners feel safe about admitting their ignorance when they do not understand something. Educational sessions should also empower learners actively to seek additional teaching/learning and support. The facilitator should create an atmosphere in which no student will feel too embarrassed to ask for information about any kind of behaviour and practices whatsoever – for example, the meaning of specific sexual practices such as fellatio, cunnilingus, fisting or rimming. A workshop facilitator who does not create the right atmosphere for free, frank and full discussion and enquiry should not be working in the field of HIV/Aids education or counselling.

Timing is important in the teaching/learning process. Learners learn best when they feel that they have a need to know. It is the responsibility of the teacher to foster this need to know. The retention of learning should be assessed periodically and supported over time (WHO, 2000a).

Aids education involves raising sensitive issues such as sexuality, different sexual practices, drug use, and other risk behaviours. Traditionally, health care professionals have not been educated to feel comfortable with openly discussing sensitive, embarrassing, or 'offensive' practices. Practice in discussing these subjects should begin in a safe learning environment. Finally, it is important to teach risk analysis and risk-avoidance strategies.

Preparing educational sessions

When you are engaged in preparing an HIV/Aids educational session, you should ask yourself the following questions:

- Who are the people in the audience? Are they male, female, young or older, educated or less well educated? What do they know about the subject? It is important to have a very clear idea of who your participants are before you choose or produce educational materials.
- What do you hope to achieve? What outcome do you expect the educational session to pro-

duce? What is your main message? Do your expected outcomes match the learning needs of the group?

- How will you access the information you need to conduct the session?
- How long will the educational session take? Will the participants be able and willing to stay for the entire session?
- How much will the educational session cost? Is enough money available to finance the course?
- Have you made provision for tea and lunch breaks?
- What equipment will you need? Is the equipment available, or can you adapt your session so that you will be able to use whatever is available?
- Is existing material available to you? If material is available, use this (and adapt it if necessary) rather than starting from scratch. Contact the Department of Health and Aids centres to get posters, pamphlets, etc.
- Is the language appropriate? Are you presenting the information at the educational level of the learner? Is your language too complex or too simple for the participants? What is the literacy level of the group?
- Are the illustrations appropriate and culturally sensitive? Are they clear enough for the participants to understand? Do the illustrations reflect issues and images with which the participants are familiar?
- Is video material appropriate for your specific group? Although it is important to be specific about sex practices and preferences, participants may be offended if they perceive the material to be pornographic.
- Do the educational materials look good and attract people's attention? Are the designs and colours attractive? Are they culturally sensitive? Can the participants identify with the materials?
- Does the educational material avoid discrimination? Does the material use examples of people who are similar in racial origin, age, and sexual orientation to the target group? Do the illustrations foster stigma or fear? Showing a person dying of Aids might, for example, lead some people to believe that *all* people living with HIV are about to die.
- Does the educational material generate feelings of fear? Messages such as 'Aids Kills' might scare people away. Such scare tactics rarely help to promote effective behaviour change. Positive messages, on the other hand, often promote changes in attitudes and behaviour. However, even some 'negative illustrations' can be effective in raising awareness if they catch people's attention. The key to success is to know the target group well and choose your messages accordingly.
- Does the educational material avoid moralising and preaching? People resist listening to someone telling them what they *should* and *should not* do. Such practices often make learners resistant to opening themselves to the message, and therefore far less likely to engage in open and productive discussions. For example, once young people have been told in a session that they should 'never engage in sexual intercourse before marriage', they will probably make no contribution at all to any subsequent discussion about safer sexual practices. The best materials provide information in a clear and respectful way and they empower people to make their *own* decisions.
- Are your educational strategies built on skills that have already been acquired and do they promote confidence? It is important to build on the expertise of the group. What do they already feel confident about doing? How can that confidence be carried over to other circumstances?
- Does the educational material help to build a supportive environment? People learn best when they feel cared for and supported. If people work together towards the same ends, much can be achieved. Does the learning session provide participants with opportunities for supporting one another? Can your group be supported in promoting effective change in other people, in changing health care practices, and even changing legislation?
- What educational materials work best for the participants? Consider using attractive posters, local radio, TV or newspaper announce-

ments, leaflets, fact sheets, case studies and training aids such as flip charts or flash cards. Open discussions, interviews with people living with HIV/Aids and their families, listening to stories from other care providers or patients, and advertisements, all deliver powerful educational messages. It is also important for participants to visit people living with HIV/Aids in hospital and in the community.

- How will you distribute educational material? Sadly, excellent educational materials are often not used simply because they are not distributed properly.
- Do the learners leave with any materials (handouts) that will reinforce their learning? Learning takes place over a period of time and needs repeated reinforcement. What methods of reinforcing learning have you considered? Do you have fact sheets ready for distribution? Will the posters you select reinforce learning? Do you provide additional educational sessions? Do you test the learners at a later date? Do you require supervised practice after a teaching/learning session? Is a library and a list of recommended reading available? What other strategies have you considered to reinforce learning?
- Have you considered pre-testing the educational material before it is printed or published? Pre-testing educational material can be a very important step towards ensuring that the message is understood, is well received and has the potential to motivate behaviour change and promote best practice.
- What methods of evaluating the educational sessions have you considered? Evaluation of student learning can be done by using questionnaires before and after the programme. Observation of practice and observation or anecdotal reports of behaviour change are other forms of evidence. Did the participants also evaluate the facilitator and the educational sessions? Has behaviour change been observed over time (i.e. has there been retention of learning)? What other forms of evaluation have you considered? What will you do with the evaluation information? Will you make changes to your educational material and teaching/learning processes if necessary?

It is a good idea to ask the participants to evaluate the educational sessions at the end of each day so that you can adapt the next day's sessions if necessary.

Activity

Visit your nearest health department or Aids training, information and counselling centre and collect all the pamphlets, posters, fact sheets and other training material you can get. These are usually distributed free of charge. Evaluate the material by using the relevant criteria for the development of effective educational material discussed above. List the strengths and weaknesses of the pamphlets or the other material that you have collected.

Methods of teaching/learning

Many teaching methods or strategies can promote learning. Your choice should take the needs of the learners into account. A combination of methods is likely to be most effective.

Lectures and mini-lectures

Certain factual information (e.g. technical or medical information) can best be explained by lectures or mini-lectures. The facilitator should make the lecture as interesting as possible by using visual aids such as power-point presentations, pictures and drawings. Densely formatted text-only material will soon have your learners nodding off.

Group participation

Evidence shows that people learn best when they participate rather than merely observing passively. In the past, students were placed in rows and then lectured to by the teacher of the group. Although this method is sometimes useful for communicating a body of knowledge quickly, reinforced learning leading to behaviour change is best accomplished through active participation of the learners. It is often extremely effective to *reverse* the lecture/group participation process by:

- asking the participants to brainstorm a specific problem (e.g. the basic principles of HIV/Aids counselling);

- letting them present feedback to the group; and then
- wrapping up the session with a mini-lecture on 'the basic principles of HIV/Aids counselling'.

Enrichment

Ice breakers

When people do not know each other well or when they come from varying backgrounds and are expected to participate in group discussions, it may be a good idea for a facilitator to introduce an 'ice breaker' at the beginning of the session. An ice breaker is an exercise that helps people to get to know each other and feel comfortable with each other. It also helps to break down some of the barriers that often exist between people (Nel, 2000).

Some ideas for ice breakers:

- Ask participants to devise their own imaginary T-shirts with their personal motto on the front, a picture of themselves (how they see themselves) under the motto, their likes on the one sleeve, their dislikes on the other sleeve, their achievements and their dreams on the back, and so on.
- Ask each participant to choose an animal that represents him or her, and then ask each person to explain to the group why he or she chose that particular animal.
- Ask participants to name three things (not people) that they would like to take with them if they had to leave this planet.

Can you think of a few original ice breakers of your own?

Group discussion

Group discussions are useful if group members feel comfortable with one another and if individuals are not reluctant to speak. Feelings of group safety can take time to develop and are not always achieved. However, the group facilitator (the educator) can use his or her skills to facilitate group discussions and provide encouragement. Group discussions expose members to the beliefs, values and practices of others, and usually lead to peer support. Topics can be discussed in one big group, or the participants can split up into smaller 'buzz' groups which then report back to the big group.

One of the best ways to encourage group discussion is through problem posing and problem solving. These problems can either be developed by the facilitator or from the experiences of the participants. For example, if the facilitator poses a problem like the one described in the following paragraph, a lively debate is guaranteed:

> You are an Aids counsellor working in a voluntary counselling and testing centre. One of your clients, Peter, is HIV positive. He refuses to tell his wife of his HIV status and he strictly forbids you to inform his wife. However, he does not want to start using condoms, because his wife might get suspicious. What do you do? Do you tell his wife?

(See chapter 19 for ethical and legal implications.)

Role play and simulation

Learners often find it beneficial to practise new learning by acting in, or observing, a role-play or simulated exercise. This kind of practice makes learners more confident and skilful in expressing in the 'real world' what they have learned through role play. The 'fish bowl' technique is a very effective learning tool: the role players sit in the middle of a circle formed by the rest of the group who observe the interactions in the role play (e.g. a health care professional counselling the family of an HIV-positive individual). After the role play has ended, the group can discuss and analyse the processes that they have observed. Debriefing should always be done after a role-play session so that the participants can be reminded that their role playing was only a make-believe situation. People can become very emotionally involved in role play, and they often leave the session with feelings of depression and sadness if proper debriefing is not undertaken.

Building on successes of learners

Find out what your learners have been successful in achieving and use these experiences of success to teach other learners. This strategy provides learners with a sense of confidence and empowerment. Ask the learners to bring ice breakers, exercises and examples that work for them in the communities where they work. Your aim as a facilitator should not only be to teach, but also to learn from your learners.

Group activities

People seem to learn best when they are actively engaged in their learning. Often the group develops its own teaching/learning sessions. Young people usually learn best from their peers and when they are actively engaged in the development of peer group learning. They enjoy group activities such as games, making collages and jigsaw puzzles.

Group excursions

If there is time (as in, for example, a ten-day course), it is always a good idea to organise excursions to facilities that care for people with HIV/Aids, such as hospices and hospitals. Visits to Aids training, information and counselling centres, voluntary HIV counselling and testing sites and community projects providing home-based care or Aids-orphan care are also very valuable experiences for students.

Visual and learning aids

Posters, photographs, pictures, overhead projections, slide presentations, videos and works of art can all be powerful educational tools. Discussion can follow the use of such visual aids. For example, the group can be asked what the visual aid meant to them, what they liked or disliked about it, what was unclear, disturbing, or helpful. Another interesting technique is to ask learners to make their own collages (from magazines, for example) showing their feelings about issues discussed in the class. One can then ask learners to explain to the rest of the group what their collages mean. Discussions provoked by newspaper clippings can also be informative and thought-provoking.

Flip charts, fact sheets, a white board, flash cards, wall charts, drawings done by the group or others, diagrams, tables, and graphs also provide clear and easy access to information. These visual aids can be used to promote group discussion: 'What does this graph tell you?' 'What is missing from this information?' 'How could you go about getting this information?' 'What does this drawing tell you?' 'How would you have drawn this picture differently?' Models of anatomy can be used to help learners understand how HIV and other sexually transmitted infections are passed from one person to another. Models (e.g. dildos) are also suitable for practising correct condom use. Because models (e.g dolls) can be used to demonstrate many basic nursing care procedures, they can be helpful for training caregivers who will provide home-based care.

Enrichment

Learning aids don't have to be expensive

Nthabiseng Seepamore (2000), a social worker and Aids educator, uses a bottle, two glasses, water, red food colourant, and a condom to illustrate to her learners why a condom prevents transmission of the virus from one person to another.

She fills the water bottle and the glasses with tap water. She then adds the red food colourant to the water in the bottle and explains to the learners that the red colour represents the HI virus in the body. The water in the bottle is now red, while the water in the glasses is still clear, representing two people without HIV infection. Then she slowly pours red water from the bottle into one of the glasses. The clear water in the glass turns red, showing how the HI virus spreads from the infected to the uninfected person. Now she puts a condom over the neck of the bottle and tips it over the second glass of clear water as if she was going to pour red water into that glass. But the red water is kept in place by the condom, and the water in the second glass stays clear. She explains to her learners that this is exactly what happens in the body: the HI virus is trapped in the condom and therefore cannot infect the sex partner.

Case studies

Ask the learners to draw on their own work experience as Aids educators to prepare and present a case study. Discuss the case study in the group. Many new and alternative views on handling problems usually come up, and they can be a valuable learning experience for all. Keep confidentiality issues in mind constantly and encourage everyone to use fictional names and places in order to protect the identity of HIV-positive people. (See 'The Caregiver's Bookshelf' on page 367 for references to books with case studies that can be used in workshops.)

Interviews with HIV-positive people

If you can arrange an open interview with an HIV-positive person, it will be a very powerful learning experience for most learners. Not only do they get first-hand information; the experience also challenges their stereotypes and prejudices. Afterwards learners will often say things like 'But I thought HIV-positive people look different' or 'She can't be HIV positive because she's not thin and skinny!' or 'He is a person just like me.'

Guest speakers

Learners usually enjoy listening to guest speakers who are experts in their fields. It also breaks the boredom of always listening to the same presenter.

Story-telling and sharing one's experiences

Story-telling and sharing personal experiences can often promote effective learning. People like to hear about the experiences of others, and they often find that it is easier to relate to these experiences than to grasp facts that seem to have little relevance to themselves. Fictional stories are also helpful for sharing important messages. Even though a story is about a fictional character, a listener will be able to relate to and understand the message.

The World Health Organization's *Aids Home Care Handbook* (1993) uses an example to illustrate how a story can be a very effective means of explaining sometimes difficult issues to people in such a way that they can really relate to the people in the story. The story tells how HIV came into Yulia and Musaka's family and what happened to them and their children over several years. Pictures showing events in their lives (such as their wedding, Musaka's loneliness and casual sex in the city, Yulia's pregnancy, the funeral of their baby, and so on) are used to bring the characters in the story to life. By changing the names, the setting (rural or city), and the background, this story can be adapted to suit any audience.

Participating in drama

Staging a play can be a powerful way of conveying important information. Not only do the participants in the play learn from this method, but the audience can also be brought into the drama. Young people are particularly open to this form of learning.

Learning through games and play

Board games, making models out of clay or dough, and puppets can all be used to present important messages. Puppets often help to make the subject matter more playful and less intimidating. Puppets can be made by the students and they can also collaborate in the creation of the story that the puppets will present.

Singing, dancing, drumming and drama

Teaching in the African context should include traditional healing and learning methods to tell the story of Aids. The African tradition of social sharing, rituals, story-telling, dramatisation, singing, clapping, dancing and drumming should be explored and creatively used by Aids educators to get the HIV/Aids message across. Dance, for instance, is and has long been a medium of education in Africa for teaching important cultural values (Pasteur & Toldson, 1982). Metaphors, song and dance are especially useful when there is a language barrier between the Aids educator and the learners, and they can be used very successfully to integrate the message of Aids with the traditional African concept of sickness. People often best express what they have learned by writing songs and poetry. Many black Aids

> Health care professionals often work in contexts and cultures unfamiliar to them. Be open-minded and remember that you are there to help. Be yourself and be honest. If you do not feel comfortable with the customs of a specific community, then don't participate in those customs. If you do something you don't believe in, you will be insincere and it is likely to show. Nevertheless, it is important for you to show respect for the community and for their beliefs and customs. If you show yourself to be consistent and honest, people will listen to your message.

counsellors include spiritual aspects, prayer or ancestor consultation in their presentations.

Social marketing and use of the media

Social marketing and use of the media can be powerful methods of sharing information. Posters can be displayed at places where people live, work and play. Leaflets and written information can be left for people at health care centres, shopping centres, parks, shebeens, sports stadiums, gyms and other recreational facilities. The media can be involved in getting educational messages across to the larger community. Students can be encouraged to participate in media presentations. Cartoons and comic strips can reach wide audiences and be useful methods for peer support and education.

Community fairs or meetings

Places where communities come together, such as fairs or meetings, can be used to present important information. Such community gatherings can increase public awareness of the issues and challenges of HIV/Aids and encourage the wider community to become actively involved in the care and prevention of HIV.

6.6 FACILITATION SKILLS

To facilitate means to help people discover how much they already know; to enable them to explore their own potential; to build upon their experience; and to generate their own further learning. Facilitation involves creating an environment that is conducive to learning, experimentation, exploration and growth (Rooth, 1995:9). The role of the facilitator is to guide a process that will help participants reach their stated goals and objectives within the time allotted. A successful facilitator needs special skills. A facilitator should always bear the following points in mind (Nel, 2000; Van Dyk, 1999; www.dfid.gov.uk/foi/tools/annex_02_frame.htm):

- One of your main roles as facilitator is to set the initial mood or climate of the group.
- Establish a set of agreed-upon ground rules for the group as soon as possible (these ground rules may, for example, include agreed rules about confidentiality, equal participation, honesty, feedback, time management, comfort breaks, use of cell phones, leaving the group, taboo subjects, mutual respect and language issues).
- Encourage everyone to participate but remember that individuals participate in different ways. Encourage silent participants without shaming them and without discouraging those who have a lot to say.
- Remember that people have the right to differ and disagree.
- Keep the group focused on task and process but try to keep the discussion on track without controlling the process too much.
- As facilitator you may share opinions with the group, once the appropriate climate has been established, but do so in ways that do not demand or impose, but represent simply a personal sharing that group members may take or leave.
- Remain as objective as possible.
- Be alert to signs of confusion (puzzled or frustrated looks, people asking neighbours questions, resistance, etc.).
- Do not force your ideas on the group. Allow learners the freedom to explore, regardless of what you as the facilitator believe is the solution.
- Remember to pose open-ended questions. When you ask a question, allow group members time to think before answering. Allowing participants time to think is essential if you want thoughtful answers.
- Listen more than you talk.
- Adapt to various learning styles.
- As an informed guide, it is your role to help the group to chart its course and accomplish its goals.
- Don't do the group's work. Learning is more effective and lasting if individuals and small groups discover on their own.
- Circulate, but don't become a permanent part of any one group because you may too easily influence the group.
- Spend sufficient time with each group during small-group work to be certain that they have grasped the tasks and concepts supporting it.

- Review portions of the small-group tasks that are causing confusion if several individuals or groups are having difficulty.
- Ask frequently whether there are questions.
- Encourage reflection. Give participants the time and space to reflect on activities and to absorb, consolidate and transform their experiences into lasting and meaningful learning.
- Ensure that most participants agree with the conclusions reached, or at least that they have had the chance to express their views.
- Be flexible. Assess the group's needs and expectations. Be respectful of their prior knowledge, and try to engage them on the level on which they habitually function. Changing the programme as you go along doesn't mean poor planning; it probably means that you are listening, watching, and adjusting your plans to fit the situation.
- Remember that a successful facilitator guides, listens, advises, assists, affirms, manages and probes. A successful facilitator allows people to empower themselves in a safe environment.
- Be sensitive to group dynamics, communication and behaviour dynamics.
- Throughout the group experience, remain alert to expressions that indicate deep or strong feelings. Use debriefing whenever necessary by allowing the group to share their feelings with each other.
- Protect members of the group from attack by others.
- Observe confidentiality at all times.
- Energise the group or slow it down, as needed.
- Recap what has happened in the workshop occasionally and help the group to make connections between the sessions.
- Be sensitive to gender and cultural issues. In a traditional African setting it is, for instance, not advisable to mix sexes and different age groups, especially when a sensitive and often 'taboo' subject such as sex is discussed. Out of respect for the men (or elders) in the group, women and young people will often not respond or take part in the discussions. Since wisdom is often associated with old age in some black cultures, adults may be reluctant to pay attention to a younger facilitator. Men are also often not willing to listen to women, who traditionally are regarded as minors. The nurse's uniform may, however, in some cases invest a woman with authority. Drawing on the expertise of the older people in the group and learning from them will make sessions more effective. The use of peer educators is probably the most effective means of educating traditional African people in sexual matters.
- Speak the 'language' of the group. Slang words and the use of subgroup terminology may cause a total communication breakdown between facilitators and their learners. It is therefore important for facilitators to become acquainted with the terminology used by the group. Don't refer to sexual behaviour and body parts in unfamiliar medical terms. Use the words that are familiar to the group.
- Be aware of the different meanings of certain concepts in different subgroups, and make sure that you are understood correctly. The concept of 'high-risk sexual behaviour' may, for example, mean different things to different people. Within the teenager subgroup, two sexual relationships per year may sometimes be defined as 'safer' sex – as opposed to frequent casual sex. Words such as 'promiscuity' and 'prostitution' also have different connotations in diverse cultures. If it is customary, for example, for a married man to have more than one sex partner, he will not perceive himself as being promiscuous. Women classified by men from a particular culture as prostitutes (sex workers) may simply be considered to be lady friends by men from a different culture. Even when such women are rewarded with presents, these gifts are not necessarily regarded as payment for prostitution (Zazayokwe, 1989). Aids counselling programmes that warn against prostitution without explaining the concept might therefore easily fail in communities where men define prostitution differently.
- In your functioning as a facilitator of learning, recognise and accept your own limitations.
- If you don't know something, say so. If a participant asks you a question to which you

don't know the answer, just say, 'I don't know but I will find out for you.' Don't give wrong or vague information to save face. Make sure that you do find an answer and tell the person as soon as possible. In this way you will show respect for the person's question, and he or she will not lose confidence in you or respect for you.
- Don't feel that you must be an expert in everything. Remind yourself and the group that you are a facilitator. Remind them of their own expertise and experience. Ask other participants for their ideas on a question, and don't feel that you should always answer everything.
- Take at least two breaks of 15–20 minutes each – one in the morning and one in the afternoon. Suggest short comfort or stretch breaks as needed.
- Remember that the four cornerstones of being a good facilitator are empathy, respect, genuineness and concreteness ('concreteness' means presenting all material in a structured way and using clear, unambiguous terms and concrete explanations).

6.7 CONCLUSION

Aids educators should be creative in exploring and using different methods and materials and transferring information effectively. They should be sensitive to their group's needs and should keep the theories of behaviour change in mind when they devise their programmes.

chapter

7 Prevention in Traditional Africa

Raka sniffs around the kraal
And then Raka came up from his sleeping place
and peered at the red streaks and glow of the fire,
falling through the wooden pole fence of the kraal.
Then they heard his cry, like that of an animal
And when the coals of the fire were white and
cold –
they heard him sniffing loudly at the thin spars of
the kraal.

In the beginning it was called 'Juliana's disease'. It was first noticed in the village of Lukunya, on the Ugandan border, in early 1983. A handsome Ugandan trader had come through selling cloth for women's kangas patterned with the name Juliana. A village girl with no money traded sex for a kanga, as did several other women who coveted the beautiful Juliana cloth. Some months later the first girl became sick: she had no appetite, could hold down no food, and had constant diarrhoea, which filled her with shame. In a few weeks she wasted away, grew weak, and had to be carried everywhere. Before she died, two other women, also adorned in Juliana's cloth, came down with the strange disease. The people of Lukunya decided that the Ugandan was a witch, and that Juliana's cloth had evil powers. To conquer Juliana's disease, traditional healers toiled to lift the stranger's curse. But the curse was too powerful and the death toll continued to rise. Within a year the curse had spread to the neighbouring villages. Rumours of widespread witchcraft spread throughout the Kagera region, and traditional healers felt compelled to solve the Juliana mystery (Garrett, 1995:334–335).

If education and prevention programmes are to be successful in Africa, it is important for us to understand and appreciate the traditional African world-view.* The story about 'Juliana's disease' and the causes of Aids illustrates how people can experience the world in a unique and very spe-

*The people of sub-Saharan Africa differ widely in terms of culture, geography, language, religion and ways of life, but a dominant socio-religious philosophy is shared by many, and we refer to these similarities, rather than the differences, when we talk of a common African perspective or world-view (Gyeke, 1987; Okwu, 1978; Sow, 1980). Because of a constant process of westernisation, many Africans internalise traditional African as well as Western beliefs.

cific way that is different from the way in which Westerners experience it. This unique world-view has for far too long been ignored by the Western world. HIV/Aids education and prevention programmes have mostly been based on Western principles, and no attempt has been made to understand or integrate the diverse cultural and belief systems of Africa into such programmes. Might this not be one of the reasons why HIV/Aids prevention programmes have tended to fail so dismally in Africa? It is important for health care professionals who work in Africa to understand what health, sickness and sexuality mean in the traditional African context, and to incorporate these beliefs into their HIV/Aids prevention programmes. It is also important to appreciate the importance of community life in African societies (Van Dyk, 2001a).

7.1 PERCEPTIONS OF ILLNESS

When bad things happen, traditional thought does not simply attribute it to bad luck, chance or fate. Instead, there is a belief that every illness is directed by an intention and a specific cause. In order to fight the illness, it is therefore necessary to identify, uproot, punish, eliminate and neutralise the cause, the intention behind the cause, and the *agent* of the cause and intention. In an attempt to understand illness, traditional Africans will always ask the questions 'Why?' and 'Who?' (Sow, 1980). There are beliefs that mental as well as physical illness can be caused by disharmony between a person and the ancestors, by a god or spirits, by witches and sorcerers, by natural causes, or by a breakdown in human relationships.

The ancestors and God as causal agents of illness

Some traditional religious systems in Africa see God as a supreme being or creator who has withdrawn himself from people, and is distant and remote. Although these religious systems believe in and honour God, God is deemed too important to bother with everyday problems. The living spirits of the deceased ancestors are the 'mediators' between the people and God (Mbiti, 1969; McCall, 1995; Sow, 1980).

Ancestors form a very important and intrinsic part of the daily lives of many traditional Africans. Ancestors are seen as benevolent spirits who preserve the honour and traditions of a tribe, and they usually protect their people against evil and destructive forces. Ancestors can, however, punish their people by sending illness and misfortune if people do not listen to their wise counsel, if certain social norms and taboos are violated, and if culturally prescribed practices and rites are neglected or incorrectly performed.

In some cases it is believed that ancestors do not actually send illness themselves but merely allow it to happen by withdrawing their protection. When ancestors express their anger or displeasure by withdrawing their protection, their descendants are left exposed to attacks by witches and sorcerers. The illnesses caused by the ancestors are seldom serious or fatal, and the relationship with the ancestors can be restored through offerings and sacrifices (Beuster, 1997; Bodibe, 1992; Hammond-Tooke, 1989; Mbiti, 1969).

God, the ancestors and Aids

There is no indication in the literature that *traditional* Africans attribute Aids to the anger of ancestors or to God's punishment. The influence of Christianity can, however, be seen in the beliefs of some African Christians who believe that Aids is God's punishment for immorality and sins (Van Dyk, 1991).

Witches and sorcerers as causal agents of illness

Traditionally, the fate of people is seen as being regulated and controlled by the complex relations between humans and the invisible but powerful beings and creatures who inhabit an intermediate other-worldly zone of existence. This zone is the territory of evil spirits, witches and sorcerers. Nearly all forms of illness, suffering, misfortune, conflict, accidents and death are ascribed to beings who operate from this zone (Sow, 1980).

Both an *immediate cause* and an *ultimate cause* for disease or misfortune are recognised. A person with Aids may, for instance, fully understand that the *immediate cause* of her illness is a virus, but she will nevertheless still ask: 'Why me and not my neighbour? While I sleep only with my husband, my neighbour is running around with many men.' The only answer that will really satisfy this woman is that *someone*, by means of magical manipulation, has 'caused' or 'sent' the virus to make her, rather than her neighbour, ill (this is the *personal or ultimate cause* of the illness) (Van Dyk, 2001b).

Many people therefore consult traditional healers as well as Western health care professionals for the same condition: the traditional healer is consulted to diagnose the *personal cause* of the condition (e.g. bewitchment) or to *prevent* a recurrence of the illness (e.g. by performing a ritual); the Western doctor is consulted for medication to *treat* the condition *symptomatically* (Hammond-Tooke, 1989; Herselman, 1997; Mbiti, 1969). If health care professionals do not understand this belief in immediate and ultimate causes of illness, they may feel threatened by the erroneous idea that black people do not 'trust white medicine'.

Witches or sorcerers are often blamed for illness and misfortune in traditional societies (Felhaber, 1997). People who believe that the services of witches and sorcerers can be sought to send illness, misfortune, bad luck and suffering to enemies, also believe that whatever bad luck or illness befalls them is sent by witches or sorcerers. Hammond-Tooke (1989) compared the perceived causes of illness in a conservative Ciskeian rural area in South Africa with those in an urban area, and found a strong belief in witchcraft in *both* the rural and the urban areas. Table 7.1 reflects the causes of illness and misfortune as divined by traditional healers in Ciskei.

Table 7.1
Perceptions of the causes of illness in an African context
(Source: Hammond-Tooke, 1989:123)

Perceived cause	Rural	Urban
Ancestors	8%	7%
Witchcraft or sorcery	72%	45%
Non-mystical (accidents and alcohol)	17%	48%

Enrichment

The difference between witches and sorcerers

Witches are thought to have supernatural abilities, commit evil deeds and cast spells with the help of mythical animals and supernatural creatures (or 'familiars'). One of the most widely known mythical monsters used by witches is the uthikoloshe or tokoloshe. Witches also use small animals such as wildcats, owls, snakes or skunks to do their evil bidding.

Sorcerers, on the other hand, do not have mystical powers, but they act anti-socially to cause harm to people. Sorcerers usually misuse their natural ability or knowledge of medicine or herbs for nonhealing purposes. They put poison in food or place objects charged with malevolent force on a path or in a place where they will be 'picked up' or accidentally touched by the passer-by (the targeted victim). Sorcerers can also use the victim's urine, hair or nails to harm him or her. Some people will refuse to use bedpans or urine bottles in hospitals because they are afraid that the contents may fall into the hands of sorcerers (Hammond-Tooke, 1989).

Witchcraft and HIV/Aids

Witchcraft is believed by some to be the causal agent in HIV transmission, Aids and death in many African countries, especially among the rural poor or people with the least education (Boahene, 1996; Bond, 1993; Yamba, 1997). More than 25% of Zambian subjects in Yamba's study ascribed STIs to witchcraft. 'Why else,' they argued, 'will one man become infected and the other remain uninfected when *both* men have had sexual contact with the same woman?'

The psychological function of witchcraft beliefs

Accusations of witchcraft and sorcery are usually levelled against others when the harmony of a group is threatened or disturbed because conflict, jealousy, tension and unhealthy competition have become too prominent and are threatening to overwhelm the stability of relationships in community life (Beuster, 1997; Hammond-Tooke, 1989). The harmony of Africa has been disastrously disrupted by the advent of Aids because it has caused the untimely death of innumerable young people and has led to an unprecedented lowering of life expectancy among all groups and classes of people. In African societies, death is accepted as natural only when old people die. In most other cases (where 'the queue of dying is jumped'), death is seen as a punishment or as the work of evil spirits and witches (Okwu, 1978; Yamba, 1997). The psychological rationale of blaming witchcraft for the breakdown of African societies is therefore understandable. A belief in malevolent witchcraft helps in making sense of the horrors and disruptions caused by HIV/Aids (Yamba, 1997). If external factors such as witches and sorcerers are blamed for Aids, this projection of responsibility consoles the family, victims and society as a whole. It also explains HIV/Aids in a way that can be understood in terms of a traditional world-view, and so helps to alleviate feelings of guilt and anxiety.

The belief in witches helps people give meaning to the things that happen to them. Such beliefs provide answers that science cannot provide – such as an explanation of the personal or the ultimate causes of illness. According to Seeley et al. (1991), witchcraft beliefs are both an expression and a resolution of a community's need to explain why some people who are 'at risk' do not contract Aids and why some people die much more quickly than others.

Attributing HIV infection to witchcraft may also help the bereaved family to avoid feeling stigmatised by their community (Campbell & Kelly, 1995). Ironically, Boahene (1996) found that people who believe that Aids is caused by witches are more likely to be supportive of HIV/Aids patients because their understanding is that the patients have became infected with the virus through the agency of sources that are 'beyond their control'.

Witchcraft beliefs nevertheless also have very negative implications for Aids counselling and education in Africa. The belief that *everything* that happens to a person can be attributed to external, supernatural beings or powers (an external locus of control) implies that individuals cannot be held responsible or accountable for their own behaviour. This outlook tends to prevent people from trying to solve their problems themselves (Viljoen, 1997). Boahene (1996) found that many people in Africa do not consider their own behaviour as a possible reason for HIV infection. Because of this misconception, they cannot appreciate the need for using HIV-preventive methods.

Witch-blaming may be a 'healthy' psychological move for the victim, but the personal cost for perceived witches in African society can be very high indeed, because it may result in their death. Witches are still hunted down and killed in some places. It is often feared that accusations of witchcraft may follow the disclosure of a positive HIV test result if confidentiality is broken (Seeley et al., 1991).

Enrichment

Witchcraft in Western Europe

The motives behind the witch myth lie deep in the human psyche and are not confined to traditional Africa. The last English witch was burnt in 1722. Witchcraft in Western Europe can also be explained in terms of social tensions and antagonism. Waves of witch hysteria coincided with the rise of Protestantism and the breakdown of the feudal system in Europe (Hammond-Tooke, 1989:49). Scapegoating, stereotyping, prejudice and discrimination can clearly be seen in beliefs about witches when the routine tensions of social life are projected onto a marginalised person or group of people.

Implications of the belief in witches for HIV/Aids education

Experience has taught Aids educators working in Africa that ignoring and ridiculing traditional witchcraft beliefs has adverse effects on their HIV/Aids prevention programmes. These beliefs should rather be taken into account and integrated into HIV/Aids prevention programmes. Programmes should, for example, recognise the belief that the *personal* or *ultimate cause* of an illness may be witchcraft, but it should be stressed that the *immediate cause* is a 'germ' which is sexually transmitted. In her counselling of traditional Africans in South Africa, Zazayokwe (1989) dealt successfully with the problem of causality by telling people that *they* may know where the HIV infection originated, but *she* knows what the disease does inside the body and how they can avoid contracting it. In their research in Uganda, Seeley et al. (1991) found that, as Aids has become more widespread, an explanation that combines scientific fact and witchcraft theory is more frequently used and is more accessible to people. Among the Rakai people of Uganda, for example, people are aware that HIV is sexually transmitted, but many attribute the chance of being infected through a sexual act to the power of witchcraft.

Some people believe that witches or sorcerers use sexual intercourse as the contact point for their medicine or spells to infect people with STIs and HIV (Green et al., 1993). And throughout the ages there have been forms of prophylaxis against witches and sorcerers. To protect themselves against diseases, misfortune and death, people wear charms or amulets which they believe have preventive and protective powers (Hammond-Tooke, 1989; Okwu, 1978). (Nurses are familiar with babies in hospital wearing protective strings around their necks or waists.) One may therefore ask why – in cases of casual sex – the condom cannot be introduced as a preventive charm to block the sexual contact point against the evil spells of witches. The services of traditional healers should be sought to 'fortify' the condoms with protective power before they are distributed among the community *as protective charms*. This will encourage traditional people to take responsibility for the *immediate cause* of HIV infection by obstructing the entry point of evil in the form of HIV. The following African proverb applies in these situations: 'If you know there is a snake in your house, you don't ask where it comes from: you kill it.'

'Pollution' as cause of illness

There is a belief that people sometimes get sick because they neglect to purify themselves from pollution by failing to carry out the age-old prescribed rituals for everyday life. The crucial difference between this set of beliefs (pollution) and the others (ancestors and witchery) is that illness caused by not performing rituals is not actually *sent* by a person or spirit, but is the consequence of neglect. Illness of this kind is regarded as originating from an *impersonal causation* (Hammond-Tooke, 1989).

Enrichment

Are Christianity and traditional African beliefs compatible?

In her book, *A change of tongue*, Antjie Krog (2003:308–309) relates the following story: 'In my home town lives this retired professor, Gabriel Setiloane, and he wanted to understand why African ancestral ritual plays such a significant role in how black people practise Christianity. As a fourth-generation Methodist, his mother, for example, would dish out food for the ancestors at night after evening prayers. After going to church they would also visit a sangoma. He was curious why neither he nor his parents, devout Christians that they were, experienced any contradiction or betrayal. When Gabriel Setiloane became a minister, his white colleagues pressured him to purify himself of these heathen practices. It was then that he realised, that in his mind and heart the two religions did not exist separately from each other. For him, Christianity formed a compartment inside the traditional African religion, and not the other way around. The religion of his ancestors was so spacious that Christ fitted comfortably into it as a main Ancestor.'

Ritual impurities are usually associated with sexual intercourse (in particular sex with a prohibited person); with the activities of the reproductive system; or with situations in which a person comes into contact with corpses and death. The violation of sexual prohibitions in particular can give rise to a variety of health problems. If a man, for example, has sexual intercourse with a woman during menstruation, it is believed that 'bad blood' rushes to his head and causes delirium. In some cultures widows, women who have had an abortion or miscarriage, and people who have handled corpses or twins, are considered to be ritually impure or polluted. In order to cleanse himself or herself from ritual impurity, a person has to perform extensive cleansing rituals that involve washing, vomiting and purging (Beuster, 1997; Bodibe, 1992; Felhaber, 1997; Green, 1994; Hammond-Tooke, 1989).

Pollution and Aids

Although Aids is not ascribed to states of pollution or ritual impurity, some of the sexual prohibitions may be helpful in HIV prevention programmes. Prohibitions such as the prohibition against sexual intercourse with a woman during menstruation; with a widow before she is cleansed (her husband might have died of Aids); or with a woman who has had an abortion or miscarriage, should be encouraged because they can prevent HIV infection.

Germs as a cause of illness: the STI–Aids connection

Traditional beliefs do not ascribe all illness to evildoing. Some diseases (such as colds, influenza, diarrhoea in children, STIs and malaria) are seen as caused by natural causes such as 'germs' (Felhaber, 1997). Although witches may sometimes *use* germs and sexual intercourse to cause illness, it is accepted that the *immediate* cause of STIs is germ-related; that they are transmitted through sexual intercourse; and that they can be prevented by behaviour change (Green, 1994).

Unfortunately, the connection between STIs, Aids and sexual behaviour change is often not made in Africa. People often cannot understand why they have to change their sexual practices to prevent HIV infection, because HIV attacks everything except their sexual organs. They believe that the place where a germ or disease *enters* the body is the body part that becomes ill (the genitalia are usually affected in the case of syphilis, but not in the case of HIV infection).

The Aids message should therefore be strongly linked to STI prevention in Africa. The knowledge and help of traditional healers should be actively used in the control and prevention of Aids (Green et al., 1993). Many patients consult traditional healers for STI treatment, and these healers are particularly competent in handling STIs. They often give sound biomedical advice to their STI patients, advice that is also conducive to Aids prevention. Among other things, they advise patients to abstain from sex while undergoing STI treatment; to choose healthy sex partners who are unlikely to have STIs; not to have sex with sex workers (prostitutes) and soldiers; and to locate and advise all recent sex partners to be treated (Green, 1994).

Green (1994) believes that the spread of HIV in Africa can be curtailed only if STIs are more effectively treated and prevented. He feels that more financial and other resources should be devoted to STI control programmes instead of being allocated only to condom promotion and distribution.

Enrichment

Identify and correct misconceptions

Aids educators should be very sensitive to cultural beliefs. They should accommodate them where possible, and also identify misconceptions that may have adverse implications for responses to Aids. For example, some of the Shona people in south-eastern Zimbabwe believe that a man who has sex with another man's wife will get a fatal disease called runyoka. A married man places this permanent curse on his wife so that he can punish any other man who has an illicit sexual relationship with her. This disease will only strike the guilty man who has sex with the wife and not the wife or her husband. Scott and Mercer (1994) found that 22% of the Zimbabwean respondents in their study (25% in rural areas) believed that Aids and runyoka are the same disease.

The implication of such a misconception is obvious. Men may think that they are safe from HIV if they do not have sex with married women or if they adhere to sexual taboos (runyoka is also believed to strike a man who breaks sexual taboos by having sex with a woman who is menstruating or has miscarried). Once such misconceptions are identified, Aids educators can make adjustments such as, for example, teaching people how Aids differs from runyoka and emphasising that all kinds of unprotected sexual practices expose one to the danger of HIV infection.

7.2 PERCEPTIONS OF SEXUALITY

Sex not only serves a biological function in African societies. Traditionally sex also conquers death and symbolises immortality.

Personal immortality through children

Many traditional people consider it as extremely important to acquire personal immortality through their children. In traditional African thought, according to Mbiti (1969), history does not move forward into the future, but backwards in time toward the *Zamani* – the Swahili word for the past. As a person grows older, he or she moves gradually from the *Sasa* (the now-period that represents a person's present experiences) to the *Zamani*. After physical death, people continue to exist in the *Sasa* period as the 'living-dead' for as long as they are personally remembered by name by relatives and the friends who knew them during their life and who have survived them. So long as they are alive in the memories of those who knew them, they are in a state of *personal immortality*. Mbiti explains this in the following way:

> Unless a person has close relatives to remember him when he has physically died, then he is nobody and simply vanishes out of human existence like a flame when it is extinguished. Therefore it is a duty, religious and ontological, for everyone to get married; and if a man has no children or only daughters, he finds another wife so that through her, children (or sons) may be born who would survive him and keep him (with the other living-dead of the family) in personal immortality.
>
> (Mbiti, 1969:26–27)

To be forgotten after one's death and to be cast out of the *Sasa* period into the spirit world of the *Zamani* is the worst possible punishment.

Procreation is therefore one way of ensuring that a person's personal immortality is not destroyed. According to Mbiti (1969:26) a traditional woman might consider the failure to bear children a worse fate than committing genocide. She has not only become a dead end for the family's genealogical line: she has also failed to perpetuate her own self through her children. When she dies, nobody of her own immediate blood will be there to 'remember' her, to keep her in the state of personal immortality: she will simply be 'forgotten'. Some people from the Shona ethnic group in rural Zimbabwe believe that those who die childless cannot be accepted into the spirit world of the ancestors and they are doomed to wander the earth as evil, aggrieved or haunted spirits (Mutambirwa in Scott & Mercer, 1994:86).

The importance of having children for day-to-day functioning

Traditionally, children are not only valued for ensuring immortality, but are also very important in day-to-day existence because people can prosper on the land of their ancestors only if they have many wives and children to help them work their land. There are many duties, such as looking after the cattle, babysitting, working in the fields, and fetching firewood and water, that cannot be performed adequately if the family is too small. A man's wealth depends upon the growth of his tribe.

Implications for Aids education

Once Western health care professionals understand the importance of personal immortality and the value of children, they can appreciate why polygamy (the practice or custom by which one man has more than one wife, or one woman has more than one husband, at the same time) is practised in many African cultures. They can then also understand why convincing people to use condoms is so difficult, and why women often insist on having children, even if they are found to be HIV positive.

Polygamy

Western health care professionals often frown upon polygamy in African societies, but polygamy often helps to prevent or reduce unfaithfulness, prostitution, STIs and HIV. In Mbiti's (1969) opinion polygamy is particularly valuable in modern times when men are often forced to seek work in the cities and towns. If a husband has several wives, he can afford to take one at a time to live with him in the town, while the other wife or wives remain behind to care for the children and family property. Polygamy can provide a healthy alternative or solution to problems inherent in certain cultural customs. In some African societies, for example, sexual intercourse between a husband and his wife is prohibited while she is pregnant and this abstinence is observed until after childbirth or in some cases even until after the child is weaned. In such situations, polygamy prevents husbands from turning to casual sex.

In societies where polygamy is practised, Aids educators are wasting their time when they try to advocate monogamy. Much more will be achieved by emphasising loyalty and fidelity between a husband and all his wives and by discouraging sex outside that group. Polygamy is, of course, only safe if all the partners in the relationship are HIV negative.

Protection while planning to have children

Population control remains a sensitive issue in Africa because it has a negative impact on the growth of a tribe; it deprives parents of needed labour; and it undermines traditional beliefs and values (Hickson & Mokhobo, 1992). Instead of telling people in Africa to use condoms (and thereby inevitably to prevent pregnancy), it is better to tell them how to protect themselves from STIs and HIV while sometimes allowing 'unprotected' sex to make children. They should be advised not to use condoms until the wife conceives, and to start using condoms again while she is pregnant and nursing the baby. Although this solution is imperfect, it is more realistic than advising people to abstain from procreation, and it would at least *reduce* the risk of partner infection and perinatal transmission in stable relationships (Schoepf, 1992). The importance of voluntary HIV counselling and testing (VCT), measures to prevent mother-to-child transmission, and the possible use of antiretroviral medications should be discussed with the parents.

Although having many children is still important to many Africans, women in Africa are increasingly accepting the idea of birth spacing and maternal protection.

The devastating effect of HIV on babies

The fact that HIV (and other STIs) can infect newborn infants is of great concern to traditional healers in Africa because they realise that Aids may jeopardise future generations, and indirectly also the immortality of their tribe. The devastating effect of HIV on unborn babies should therefore be emphasised in Aids education programmes as an incentive for change (Green, 1994; Schoepf, 1992). Schoepf found that many young women in the Democratic Republic of the Congo (DRC) who are aware of this fact have sought a return to their ancestral traditions which placed a high premium on premarital virginity. Some married women have urged their husbands to join religious groups to support their resolve to remain faithful. Schoepf also found that although many women in the DRC were not in a position to negotiate the conditions of their sexual practices or condom use for their own safety, they had taken steps to change their children's behaviour. Many of the mothers had in fact broken the taboo against discussing sex with unmarried children in order to help them understand the need for condom protection. Although it may now be too late for many mothers, there is still hope for the children of Africa.

7.3 PERCEPTIONS OF CONDOMS

Condoms have not been popular everywhere in Africa. Green (1994) found that although Aids awareness was reasonably high in Uganda in 1993, and although millions of condoms had been distributed, only about 3% of Ugandan men were regularly using condoms. Taylor (1990) similarly found that although the people of Rwanda were well informed about Aids and had modified their sexual behaviour on the basis of their perceptions, none of the people in his study were using condoms. Young people are using condoms increasingly, but in 2005 condom use remains a serious problem in Africa.

Many Western authors incorrectly ascribe the lack of condom use in Africa to promiscuity, permissiveness and a lack of moral and religious values (Caldwell et al., 1989). This is clearly due to a lack of understanding of the African philosophy behind sexuality and a disrespect for African cultural beliefs. Apart from social and political problems, there are deep-rooted cultural beliefs against the use of condoms in some parts of Africa. The challenge is not to condemn Africa, but to make the hidden cultural logic behind the resistance to condoms known and thereafter to find ways to work with or around it (Scott & Mercer, 1994). Some of the cultural reasons for not using condoms, and their implications for Aids education, will now be discussed.

Condoms block the 'gift of self'

Taylor (1990) found that the resistance to condom use in Rwanda had nothing to do with ignorance, but with a very specific social and cultural dimension of Rwandan sexuality. Many Rwandans believe that the flow of fluids involved in sexual intercourse and reproduction represents the exchange of 'gifts of self' which they regard as being of the utmost importance in a relationship. The use of condoms is thought to block this vital flow between two partners, and such a blockage is seen as preventing fertility and also causing all sorts of illnesses. Many Rwandan women fear that the condom might remain in the vagina after intercourse and that they therefore risk becoming 'blocked beings'. In a culture where health and pathology are conceptualised in terms of 'flow' and 'blockage', it is understandable that women cannot imagine how a 'blocking' device could also be a healthy device.

Zazayokwe's (1989) research found that some women in South Africa expressed similar fears: they were afraid to use condoms because they believed that the condom might remain behind in the vagina and eventually suffocate them by moving through the body to the throat. Zazayokwe ascribed this misconception to a lack of basic anatomical knowledge and corrected it by explaining the reproduction system to the women with the aid of models. Determining the *reasons* behind certain beliefs is vitally important for Aids educators because they cannot attempt to rectify what they don't properly understand.

Implications for Aids education

Because of their cultural beliefs, many Rwandans will not easily be persuaded to use condoms. Aids educators should therefore rather expend their energy in looking for other ways to prevent the spread of HIV. Existing cultural forms of sexual intercourse should be investigated and encouraged if they seem to be safe – even though Western educators may find them strange. For example, Taylor (1990) described a safe but exotic form of sexual intercourse practised by Rwandans – called *kunyaza* – where the focus is on heightening both partners' sexual pleasure while keeping penetration to a minimum. Safer behaviour like this should be identified and encouraged.

Condoms prevent the 'ripening of the fetus'

There is a widespread belief in many parts of Africa (East Africa, the DRC and among the Zulus in South Africa) that repeated contributions of semen are needed to form or 'ripen' the growing fetus in the womb (Heald, 1995; Ngubane, 1977; Schoepf, 1992). One of the objections often raised against condoms is that condoms are 'not natural' – not only because they inhibit pleasure, but also because they interfere in the process of natural fetal development. It is also believed that semen contains important nutrients necessary for the continued physical and mental health, beauty and future fertility of women.

Implications for Aids education

In correcting the 'ripening of the fetus' belief, Schoepf (1992) found an ally in the traditional healers of Kinshasa (DRC) who were able and willing to reinterpret traditional beliefs in ways that facilitate condom use. Traditional healers realised that while their ancestors were correct in stressing the health value of frequent sexual intercourse, they were not confronted by an Aids epidemic which makes infected semen dangerous. The traditional healers of Kinshasa were therefore prepared to tell their clients that semen should be seen as a *metaphor* for repeated intercourse.

Repeated intercourse is necessary to nourish the mutual love and understanding between the parents, which is essential for providing a nurturing environment for fetal growth. A nurse explained this as follows to a group of mothers: 'When the mother knows she is pregnant, the baby is already on its way to growing. The ancient ones meant that the husband should take an interest in his wife and not run around with other women while she awaits the child' (Schoepf, 1992:231). Clients are assured that the actual semen is not needed to 'ripen' the fetus and that condoms can therefore be used after conception to reduce risks of HIV infection to partners.

Although current practices relating to the prevention of HIV/Aids are sometimes alien to traditional thinking, many traditional healers are prepared to introduce new ideas and practices into their healing repertoire. They even have specific rituals for asking for the approval of the ancestral spirits before introducing unfamiliar objects or practices among their people. Green et al. (1995) found that traditional healers in South Africa were prepared to use lifelike dildos to demonstrate the use of condoms to their clients, but that they first sought the approval of their ancestor spirits by ritually presenting the dildos and condoms to their ancestors and explaining their beneficial use. After the ancestors had signified their approval, the healers were prepared to incorporate the dildos and condoms as a useful part of their standard healing instruments.

7.4 THE IMPORTANCE OF COMMUNITY LIFE

The community plays a very important role in traditional life in Africa. Traditional beliefs are based on principles such as the value of the *collective interest* of the group; the *survival of the community* or tribe; and the *union with nature*. One cannot exist *alone*: personal identity is totally embedded in the collective existence (Sow, 1980). Mbiti (1969:108) explains the importance of the community to the individual in the following way:

> When he suffers, he does not suffer alone but with the corporate group; when he rejoices, he rejoices not alone but with his kinsmen, his neighbour and his relatives whether dead or living. Whatever happens to the individual happens to the whole group, and whatever happens to the whole group happens to the individual. The individual can only say: I am, because we are; and since we are therefore I am.

The collective existence gives rise to values such as communality, group orientation, cooperation, interdependence and collective responsibility (Viljoen, 1997).

Community involvement in Aids education, prevention and counselling

The collective existence and the unity of the person with the community should be kept in mind by Aids educators working in Africa. Education and healing always take place in a social setting. For example, a sick person is usually accompanied by family members who understand, support and accept the patient (Bodibe, 1992; Chipfakacha, 1997). It is therefore strongly recommended that healing ceremonies involving relatives and incorporating the guidance and cooperation of the 'living-dead' kin should be included in the education and treatment of Aids patients (see enrichment box 'Confidentiality: a controversial issue' on page 125).

Dancing, singing, rituals and ceremonies should be encouraged, because these forms of dramatisation enable people to express their emotions, to overcome anxiety, and to accept and integrate into their personal reality what may seem like very threatening parts of themselves. Incorporating the family and community has the additional benefit that their fears and emotions can also be attended to.

Aids educators should be creative and imaginative in incorporating traditional beliefs and healing methods into Aids education programmes. The tradition of social sharing, of rituals, of story telling, of drama, of singing, drumming and dancing should be used to convey the threat of HIV infection to traditional people. The story of Aids is already told very successfully in many African countries by using these media, and they should be cultivated further.

Community involvement in the planning, implementation and evaluation of Aids education programmes is also important for the success of such programmes. A community's essential norms and values, cultural images and language can only be appropriately understood and incorporated with the help of the target community (Airhihenbuwa, 1989; Boahene, 1996; Campbell & Kelly, 1995; Scott & Mercer, 1994; Walters et al., 1994).

The influence of the traditional community and significant others should never be underestimated by Aids educators working in Africa. A 1991 South African study found that black South Africans' health and sexual behaviour and decisions were determined by 'other people' (external health locus of control) rather than by themselves (internal health locus of control) or by fate or chance (Van Dyk, 1991). Community resources that are already established, such as elders, traditional healers, community leaders and peer counsellors, should therefore be trained and co-opted in the fight against HIV transmission.

Enrichment

Confidentiality: a controversial issue

Health care professionals working in Africa should be very sensitive to the issue of confidentiality in the areas in which they work. Because community and collectivity are so important, Westerners often think that the notions of privacy and individualism are alien to Africans, and that they usually share all their experiences with one another. However, there are norms that regulate the kinds of information that can be shared, and the people with whom one may share it. In Tanzania, for example, sharing of information may be regulated in terms of categories such as gender, age groups, specified relationships among relatives, extended family networks, elders, traditional midwives and healers (Lie & Biswalo, 1994).

Many traditional people are especially concerned about secrecy and confidentiality where Aids is concerned, because they fear rejection by the community if their HIV status becomes general knowledge. In Lie and Biswalo's study, 98% of the subjects indicated that secrecy and confidentiality are very important to them. They pointed out that they would prefer to talk to somebody 'who can keep a secret' about their HIV status. Such people (who can keep secrets) are usually trusted relatives, medical personnel, religious leaders and traditional healers. One of the subjects in this study communicated his trust in his traditional healer as follows: 'He is a wise man with much life-experience. He will help me and show me respect. I trust him. He is used to secrets. He knows more secrets than anyone. He knows our history – our forefathers' (p. 144).

The plea for secrecy is understandable in the light of real events. In December 1998 the brutal killing of an HIV-positive woman from KwaMashu (in KwaZulu-Natal) shook the country: Gugu Dlamini, an HIV/Aids activist, was beaten to death by her neighbours for disclosing that she was HIV positive ('Brave Gugu', 1999). The critical issue, according to Lie and Biswalo (1994), is who should be informed and how. This should be done in such a way as to minimise the risk of rejection and to maximise the mobilisation of social support and existing coping resources. It is therefore a major challenge to the HIV/Aids counsellor to identify, in cooperation with the HIV-positive person, which significant others should be informed, in what sequence and by whom.

Traditional healers as vehicles of change

No Aids prevention programme can succeed in Africa without the help of traditional healers. Traditional healers are effective agents of change because they have authority in their communities. They function as psychologists, marriage and family counsellors, physicians, priests, tribal historians and legal and political advisers. They are the guardians of traditional codes of morality and values; they are legitimate interpreters of customary rules of conduct; and they have the authority to change or invent new rules and to influence their people in matters relating to sex. Traditional healers have greater credibility in their communities than village health workers, especially with regard to social and spiritual matters (Green et al., 1993; Holdstock, 1979; Schoepf, 1992; UNAIDS, 2000b).

About 80% of people in Africa rely on traditional medicine for many of their health care needs. Traditional healers are well known in the communities where they work for their expertise in treating STIs, and since the early 1990s the World Health Organization has advocated the inclusion of traditional healers in national Aids programmes (UNAIDS, 2000b). Collaborative health programmes involving traditional healers are under way in many African countries, and indications are that traditional healers can effectively be involved in HIV/STI prevention programmes.

The aims of these programmes are to convince traditional healers to promote the use of condoms and safer sex practices and to counsel their clients on the prevention of STIs and HIV. Traditional healers are also encouraged to sterilise their instruments whenever they come into contact with bodily fluids so as not to put themselves at risk of HIV infection. They are encouraged to refer Aids patients to hospitals. Condoms are often deemed acceptable by traditional healers, especially if they fit into their belief systems. Research has also shown that traditional healers abstain from dangerous practices when they are educated about the risks. Thus, for example, traditional healers often ask their clients to bring their own sterile razor blades for invasive procedures (Green, 1988, 1994; Green et al., 1993, 1995; UNAIDS, 2000b).

The South African government hired a traditional healer who has many years of experience to train fellow healers. She immediately suggested that traditional healers need to be involved in a *participatory* approach to training and that they need to be shown the utmost respect. Her advice was: 'Let them burn their incense in training.' This means that if their customs are respected, the training will be successful. She also emphasised the importance of using fellow-healers to train others because healers are far more receptive to hearing new things from their peers (UNAIDS, 2000b).

According to a UNAIDS report on collaboration with traditional healers in HIV/Aids prevention and care in sub-Saharan Africa (2000b), most healers had little difficulty in understanding and accepting information about Aids symptoms, HIV transmission and prevention, condom use, and condom promotion and distribution. The areas in which they experienced problems were home care, death and dying, mother-to-child transmission, and condom use in countries where the people had a strong desire to have more children.

Training of traditional healers should therefore also concentrate on home-based care and the care of orphans and other children made vulnerable by HIV/Aids. Traditional healers will in future have a very important role to play in the care and support of Aids patients, their families and the Aids orphans who remain behind after their parents have died. Because national health systems will not be able to cope with the high Aids toll in Africa, it will in many cases be the responsibility of traditional healers to advise people about proper home care, to treat opportunistic infections, to counsel young people about HIV prevention and to give psychological and spiritual support to those living and dying with Aids (Green et al., 1993).

7.5 USING TRADITIONAL BELIEFS IN AIDS EDUCATION

Health care professionals who work in Africa should resist the temptation to stigmatise beliefs and practices that are different from their own as ridiculous, superstitious and harmful. They should rather focus on those beliefs that can promote Aids education and prevention. Airhihenbuwa (1989) proposed a strategy or model (the PEN model), in terms of which traditional cultural health beliefs and behaviour can be categorised as positive (P), exotic (E) or negative (N) – thereby providing a basis for health care professionals to understand and cope with traditional cultural health beliefs and behaviour with which they are not familiar.

Encouraging and reinforcing positive cultural behaviour

According to the PEN model, positive cultural beliefs and behaviours are values and behaviours known to be beneficial. These should be encouraged and reinforced. Examples of positive values and behaviour are those that discourage or forbid sexual intercourse before marriage, immediately after birth, during menstruation, with widows (the husband might have died of Aids), and with women who have aborted or miscarried. Other helpful beliefs are the belief that intercourse with a person with an STI is dangerous and the belief that encourages traditional 'thigh sex' or other forms of non-penetrative intercourse sometimes practised by young and unmarried people, or by a husband when his wife is menstruating (Airhihenbuwa, 1989; Green et al., 1993, 1995).

Accepting and respecting exotic cultural behaviour

'Exotic' behaviours are customs and behaviours unfamiliar and strange to anyone from outside a particular community, but not harmful to health. These 'exotic' behaviours, such as polygamous marriages (provided that all partners are uninfected and faithful to each other), cultural rituals, ceremonies and herbal remedies, need not be changed and should be respected.

Health care professionals should appreciate the importance of rituals for the corporate existence of people. If they find that a ritual (such as male circumcision or tribal markings) is harmful to people's health, they should not attempt to *change or put a stop to the ritual* but rather suggest *ways to make it safer* (by, for example, encouraging the use of clean instruments so that

HIV will not be transmitted). In many societies, a child can only become fully integrated into his or her society after going through extensive rites of incorporation (initiation). To prohibit or discourage these rituals would be to make an outcast of the child in those circumstances where rituals are regarded as important (Mbiti, 1969).

Rites, rituals, incisions and tribal marks signify identification, incorporation, membership and the enjoyment of full rights and privileges in the community. They unite the individual with the community, both the living and the dead, and they should be respected by outsiders.

Some people are even currently pleading for Africans to look into their own past and to bring back some of the long-lost customs that advocated 'safe sex'. Many of these customs were denounced by Western colonialists and missionaries as pagan or evil, without any attempt to understand the reasons or logic for them and without the provision of any healthy alternative (see enrichment box 'A plea for Africa: "Bring back your long-lost customs!"').

Changing negative cultural behaviour

Although Aids educators should take care not to interfere in cultural beliefs and behaviour, some traditional behaviours are indeed harmful to people's health, and attempts should be made to change these. Examples include:

- having multiple sexual partners;
- cleansing rituals such as those in Zambia and Botswana whereby a widow has to have sexual intercourse with a close relative of her deceased husband to cleanse her of her husband's spirit (Hickson & Mokhobo, 1992);
- the custom of inheriting the wife of a deceased brother (who might have died of Aids);
- the impregnation of an impotent or sterile brother's wife;
- the use of sex to express hospitality where the host offers his wife or sister to a visiting guest (Mbiti, 1969);
- female genital mutilation (or female circumcision); and
- the practice of 'dry sex' to heighten sexual sensation for men, or (more traditionally) to

Enrichment

A plea for Africa: 'Bring back your long-lost customs!'

Ahlberg (1994) described the very strict sexual customs and mores among the Kikuyu people of East Africa before Christianisation. The Kikuyu people were fairly open about sexuality and there were many occasions when public discourses about sexual activity were held. During initiation and ritual ceremonies related to marriage and childbirth, the community openly addressed sexual matters through songs and dances. Sexual activity was never indiscriminate or casual, and penetration was strictly prohibited among newly initiated adolescents. It was obligatory for members of the tribe to practise strict sexual discipline, and the rules of sexual conduct were strictly observed. But because European missionaries found these ritual ceremonies, songs and dances and the collective public discourses offensive, they prohibited such valuable practices and traditional disciplines. This had the tragic consequence that customs such as circumcision were simply performed in secret, but the associated discipline of morality was lost and forgotten.

According to Ahlberg (p. 233), 'sexuality was dramatically transformed from a context where it was open but kept within well defined social control and regulating mechanisms, to being an individual, private matter surrounded largely by silence. The link between community moral values and sexual behaviour was broken.' The Kikuyu people of East Africa should have been encouraged to practise and preserve their sexual rituals, songs and dances because, although they might have seemed 'exotic' to outsiders, they were incredibly valuable for regulating and maintaining balanced and healthy sexual and personal relationships within the community. It is one of the great tragedies of African colonialisation and Westernisation that such valuable knowledge and practices have now largely been lost. Ahlberg believes that if Aids educators expect any success in combating Aids in Africa, they should begin to encourage and facilitate a discourse from a point in the 'idealised past'. The Kikuyu people should be reminded that they once had an open sexual model which protected adolescents from engaging in sexual activity outside marriage, and they should be urged to re-establish their old traditional ways rather than merely order adolescents to desist from their current permissive sexual behaviour.

'clean the temple for creation' from undesirable vaginal secretions (Moses & Plummer, 1994; Runganga & Kasule, 1995). (See enrichment box 'The dangerous practice of "dry sex"' on page 138.)

The traditional practice of virginity testing might also be dangerous if it is not properly done. (See 'Virginity testing: a women's rights issue' on page 363.) Ways should also be devised to make the practices involved in the preparation and cleansing of bodies for burial safer. In Sudan, for example, some cultures remove undigested food and excreta from corpses by hand – a procedure that was implicated in the 1976 and 1979 Ebola outbreaks in the DRC and Sudan (Garrett, 1995).

It is absolutely essential to obtain the cooperation of community leaders and traditional healers before even attempting to change dangerous cultural behaviour or practices. Success stories do exist. A positive and global community response was seen in Côte d'Ivoire where people living with HIV/Aids (in cooperation with women selling food) held a conference for 400 young women to reduce their vulnerability to HIV in the face of risky cultural practices. Follow-up sessions a year after the conference have shown that many families have abandoned female genital mutilation; that condom use among adolescents has increased; and that wife inheritance by another male member of the family has diminished (Sidje et al., 2000).

Activity

Set out to make one friend from a culture other than your own this year. Share your own customs and beliefs with this person and take the time and trouble to learn whatever you can about his or her culture.

7.6 CONCLUSION

It is necessary to impress vividly upon health care professionals and other Aids educators who work in Africa that they should not merely criticise and condemn beliefs with which they are not familiar, but rather try to understand the philosophical or cultural and historical reasons that underlie the world-view, and show the utmost respect for ancient beliefs and practices. Aids education and prevention programmes in Africa will succeed only if traditional cultural beliefs and customs are recognised and taken into account. Counselling in a traditional African context is discussed in chapter 10, page 195.

chapter

8 Changing Unsafe Behaviour and Practices

Koki prepares to fight Raka
. . . and then she named the dark creature,
who concealed himself in the cover of the night
and sheltered in the green slime of the ponds.
And she sang about Koki's courage –
the play of his weapons and the boldness of his feet
as he danced out into the darkness of the forest
to fight against something beastly and strong.

There is only one weapon against HIV infection and Aids and that is *behaviour change*. It is unfortunately the most difficult and complex weapon to use, because people find it extremely difficult to change their sexual behaviour. Connor and Kingman (1988:1) wrote:

> The disease that spreads with the help of sex is a formidable foe, because it is transmitted during the most intimate and compulsive of human activities – sex.

One of the main educational functions of health care professionals is to encourage changes in unsafe sexual behaviour. This is very difficult because sex comprises deeply pleasurable and meaningful acts that touch the very core of what it means to be a human being. In addition, sex is also laden with symbolic and other meanings and resonances for human beings. Health care professionals should therefore set themselves realistic goals: although people will never stop having sex, they can be taught to practise safer sex. In this chapter, safer sex practices and the prevention of HIV transmission in injecting drug users will be discussed. The importance of life skills for the implementation and maintenance of safer sex practices (or abstinence) will also be discussed.

8.1 LESSONS FROM THE PAST

Evidence from around the world confirms that well-designed and skilfully executed prevention programmes can reduce the incidence of HIV. Studies from all over the world have shown that behaviour interventions (including information, education and communication programmes, condom promotion programmes and other behaviour change initiatives) can bring about changes in high-risk sexual behaviour. Programmes encouraging abstinence from sex and freely accepted postponement of the onset of sexual activity by young people (sexual initiation) have also been successful (Harrison et al., 2000; UNAIDS, 2000c).

The San Francisco gay community demonstrated to the world in the nineties that people *can* be persuaded to employ safer sex. Education about safer sex practices and the dangers of unsafe practices such as unprotected anal intercourse caused the rate of infection among gay men in that city to drop from 8 000 infections a year in 1982 and 1983 to 1 000 a year by 1993, and to less than 400 a year by 1998 (Coates & Collins, 1998). Unfortunately it now seems that, because of the availability of antiretroviral therapy, many have once again become indifferent to the risk of HIV infection. The incidence of unprotected anal sex and rectal gonorrhoea is on the increase in some of the world's major cities because of this 'new (but false) sense of security' (UNAIDS, 2000c).

Success stories are not limited to the developed world. As a result of rigorous prevention efforts, a similar trend may be observed even in resource-poor settings. In Rwanda, for example, condom use in 'discordant' heterosexual couples (those in which only one partner is HIV positive) increased from 3% to 57% after counselling programmes had communicated the dangers of unprotected sex to sexually active couples. In the Congo, the use of condoms in similar circumstances has increased from 5% to 77%. A mass-media campaign that advocated safer sex in the Congo caused condom sales to increase from 800 000 in 1988 to more than 18 million by 1991 (Coates & Collins, 1998). In Uganda the percentage of teenage girls who had sex with a partner using a condom trebled between 1994 and 1997. More teenage girls reported condom use than any other age group. This indicates that the acceptability of condoms is growing more rapidly among young people than among older people. Condom use among men having sex with younger women has also increased significantly (UNAIDS, 2000c, 2004).

Unfortunately, in many parts of Africa our prevention efforts are not yet adequate. A study in western Kenya found that 63% of unmarried men and women who had sex in the past year did not use condoms. The rate of condom use among married people having sex with partners outside their marriages was even lower. Four out of five married women (80%) reported that condoms were *never* used when they had sex with men who were not their husbands (UNAIDS, 2000c).

8.2 PREVENTION OF SEXUALLY TRANSMITTED HIV

The most common means of transmission of HIV (as well as STIs) is via sexual intercourse or contact with infected blood, semen, or cervical and vaginal fluids. HIV can be transmitted from an infected person to his/her sexual partner through man-to-woman, man-to-man, woman-to-man, or, to a lesser extent, woman-to-woman sexual intercourse. HIV transmission through sexual contact can occur vaginally, anally or orally. Man-to-woman transmission is now the most common form of HIV sexual transmission in Africa. Women (and of course men) who remain faithful to their partners (and who therefore do not feel that it is necessary to use condoms) run a very high risk of contracting HIV when their partner has had sexual contact with an HIV-positive person outside (or before) their relationship (WHO, 2000a). People who assume that their partners are faithful may in some cases be putting themselves at risk of HIV infection.

The only 100% effective way to protect oneself against sexual transmission of HIV is *total abstinence* from sex (i.e. not having sex at all). Young people in particular should therefore be encouraged to abstain from sex or at least to delay their commencement of sexual relationships for as long as possible.

However, in some instances abstinence is not realistic, and in a close and loving relationship it is certainly not desirable! A *mutually faithful relationship* with an uninfected partner is therefore the ideal. Sex with one loyal, uninfected partner cannot lead to HIV infection (as long as both partners *are* absolutely faithful and reliable). In cultures where a man has more than one wife (or vice versa), he and each of his wives should be uninfected and remain faithful.

Any additional sex partners will increase the risk of contracting HIV. It is therefore wise (if possible) to limit the number of sex partners; to ask searching questions about the sexual history of current and future sex partners; and always to practise *safer sex*. Note that we say 'safer sex', not 'safe sex', because the safety of sex cannot be guaranteed in the presence of the HI virus.

Safer sex that will give protection against HIV means sexual activities that do not allow semen, fluid from the vagina, or blood to come into contact with the mouth, anus, penis or vagina of the partner. Barrier methods (such as latex or polyurethane condoms) that prevent semen and other bodily fluids from passing from one partner to another are the most effective preventive methods to use if people are having sex with more than one sex partner. Barrier methods also reduce the risk of contracting other STIs.

The male condom

The male condom is a barrier method of contraception that is placed over the glans and shaft of the penis. Male condoms are available in latex, lambskin (not recommended), and polyurethane. The *consistent* and *correct* use of latex condoms is one of the most effective ways of combating the spread of HIV. Laboratory tests have shown that the virus cannot pass through latex condoms. This means that the virus stays inside the condom after ejaculation and cannot enter the partner's body. Various researchers have reported a significantly lower incidence of HIV and other sexually transmitted infections among people who insist on using condoms. Note, however, that condoms are never 100% safe because they can leak or tear. Condoms tear easily if they are used incorrectly.

Some people are allergic to latex and cannot use latex condoms. Male condoms made of polyurethane (a type of plastic also used to make female condoms) are available for use by people who are allergic to latex. Condoms made from polyurethane are thinner and stronger than latex condoms, provide a less constricting fit, are more resistant to deterioration, and may enhance sensitivity. Condoms made of polyurethane can be used with oil-based lubricants, unlike latex condoms, which must be used with water-based lubricants. Unfortunately male polyurethane condoms are not readily available. Individuals who are allergic to latex can also use the femidom (female condom).

Condoms made of other substances such as natural membranes (e.g. lambskin – made from the intestinal lining of lambs) should not be used. While lambskin condoms prevent pregnancy because they do not allow sperm to pass through, HIV and other viruses (like the hepatitis B virus and the herpes simplex virus) are so small that they can easily pass through the pores of natural-skin (non-latex) condoms. Note that HIV *cannot* pass through intact latex (or polyurethane) condoms, because the pores (holes) in these condoms are so infinitesimally small.

How to use a male condom

Not all people know how to use condoms. It is therefore important for health care professionals to feel comfortable in demonstrating their use. Show how to put a condom on a dildo (an artificial erect penis, usually made of rubber) and give clients the opportunity to practise. Videos and pamphlets are useful in illustrating the correct use of condoms. If dildos on which to demonstrate or practise are not available, the World Health Organization (2000a) recommends that objects such as bananas or cucumbers be used. If you have to use these, make sure that your clients understand that a condom should go onto an erect penis. (See page 170 for educational wooden condom demonstrators.) Present the following specific instructions on how to use a condom (Figure 8.1 on page 132 illustrates the use of a male condom):

- Use a new, unused condom for each act of sexual intercourse.
- Check the expiry date on the condom package and make sure that the condom is not brittle, sticky or broken.
- Open the package carefully – fingernails or teeth can tear condoms.
- Always use a condom from start to finish during any type of sex (vaginal, anal or oral).
- Always put the condom on the penis before intercourse begins.
- Put the condom on only after the penis is erect.
- Make sure the condom is the right way round. First unroll it a little bit to ascertain the

direction in which it unrolls. It should roll down easily when you are doing it correctly.

- If the male is not circumcised, pull the foreskin of the penis back (gently) before putting on the condom.
- In putting on the condom, squeeze the reservoir tip or empty space at the end of the condom to remove the air. Do not put the condom tightly against the tip of the penis; leave the small empty space at the end of the condom to hold the semen (if this isn't done correctly, the condom might break).
- Unroll the condom all the way to the base of the penis, to a point as close as possible to the testicles.
- Use only water-based lubrication. Do not use oil-based lubricants such as cooking or vegetable oil, Vaseline, baby oil or hand lotion as these will cause the condom to deteriorate and break.
- If the condom tears during sex, withdraw the penis immediately and put on a new condom before resuming intercourse.
- After ejaculation, withdraw the penis while it is still erect. Hold the rim of the condom as you withdraw so that the condom does not slip off and spill seminal fluid on your partner.
- Remove the condom carefully before the penis loses its erection so that seminal fluid does not spill out.
- Knot the used condom and wrap it in paper (such as a tissue, toilet paper or newspaper) until you can dispose of it in a safe place such as a toilet, pit latrine or closed rubbish bag, or until you can bury or burn it.

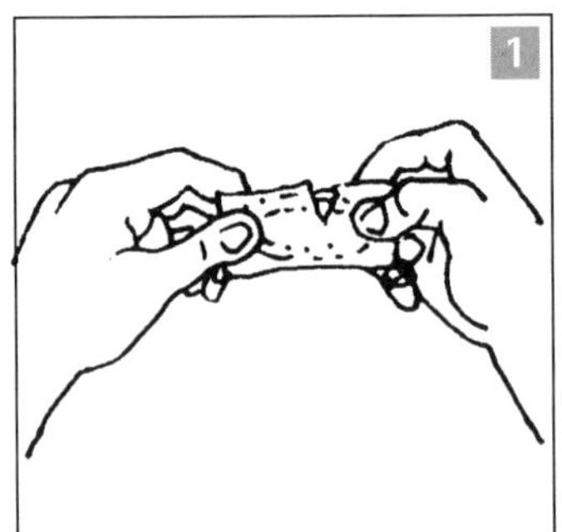

Open the package carefully, after checking the expiry date.

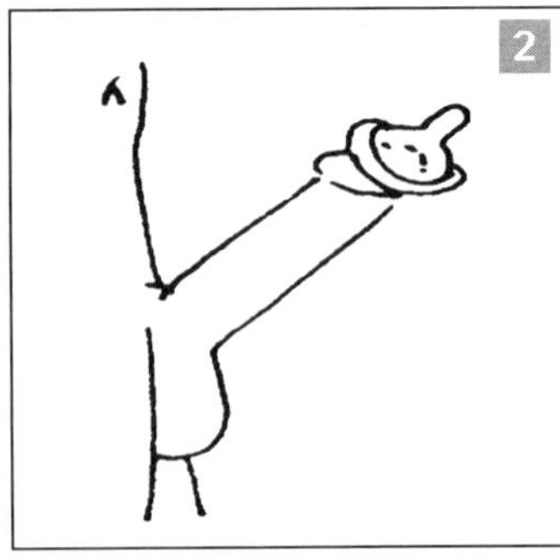

Put the condom on the tip of the erect penis.

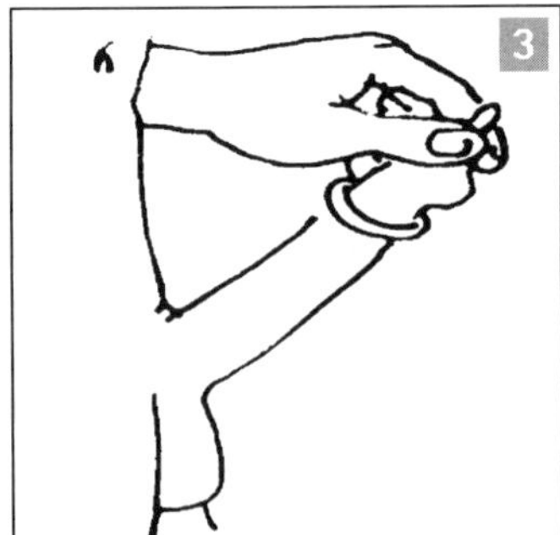

Pinch the tip of the condom to remove any air from the tip.

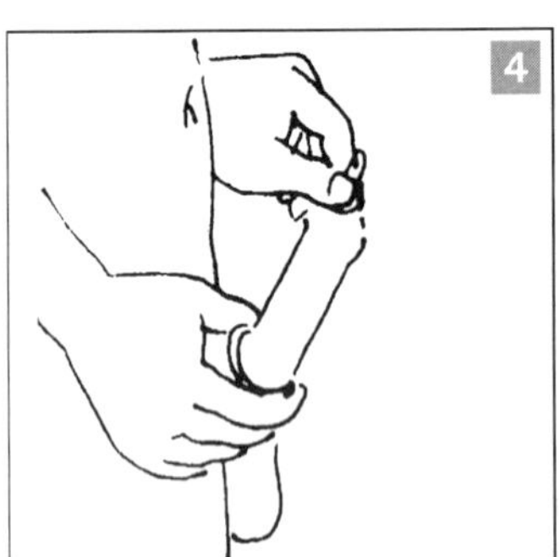

Unroll the condom all the way to the base of the penis.

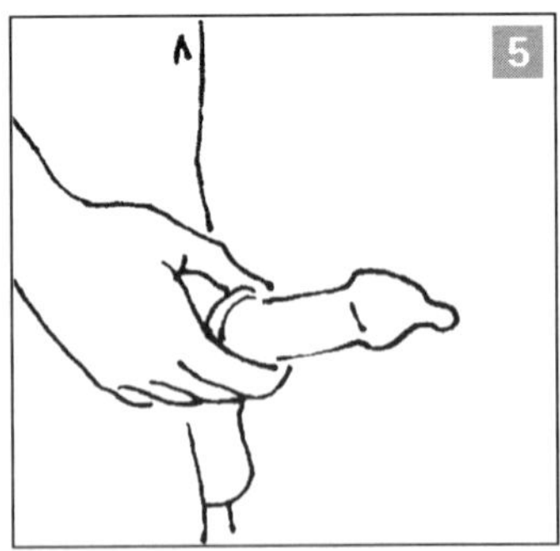

After ejaculating, hold the base of the condom and withdraw from your partner.

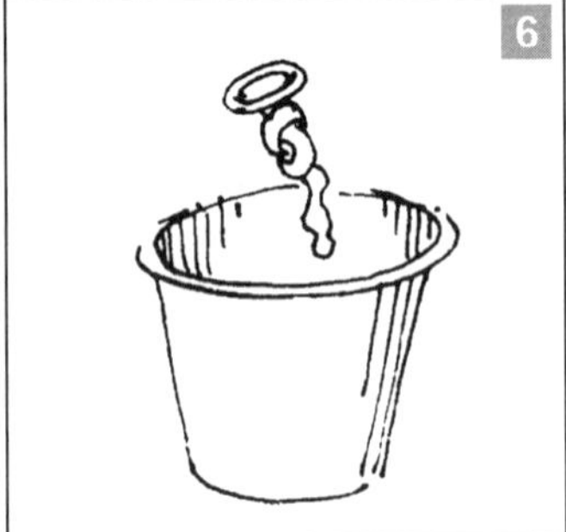

Knot the used condom and dispose of it in a safe container.

Figure 8.1
How to use a male condom

Activity

Ask a friend or colleague to play the role of a shy young man who visits your HIV/Aids prevention clinic. He has recently started his first sexual relationship with a woman and he is concerned about Aids. Talk to him about HIV and Aids (he is very uninformed) and show him how to use a condom. Prepare your role play on paper by jotting down the main points of your discussion with the young man.

Enrichment

Man-to-man sexual transmission

Unprotected penetrative anal sex creates a very high risk of HIV transmission – especially in the receptive partner. The risk is several times higher than in vaginal intercourse because the lining of the rectum is thin and because it tears easily – even small lesions can allow the virus easy access into the partner's bloodstream. According to a WHO report (2000a), a large percentage of men who have sex with men are either married or are also having sex with women. Most of these men will not identify themselves as homosexual or gay, and because sex with other men is often stigmatised and criminalised in many countries, it is very difficult to reach these men with health promotion and prevention programmes.

Enrichment

How are condoms tested?

For quality control, reputable condom manufacturers take a sample from each lot of finished, packaged condoms and examine them for holes by using a *water leak test*. International standards specify that fewer than 1 in 400 condoms may fail the water leak test. Condoms that pass the water leak test are essentially impermeable to particles the size of STI pathogens. Manufacturers also test condoms for physical properties using the *air burst test* and the *tensile* (strength) test. The U.S. Food and Drug Administration developed a test to determine a condom's ability to prevent the passage of viruses. In a laboratory they created 'viruses' the same size as STI pathogens, and they used high concentrations of these 'viruses' to test the permeability of condoms. The tests showed that condoms are highly effective barriers to virus passage, and that the chance of leakage is very small (Siecus Fact Sheet, 2002).

Lubrication

Ensure adequate lubrication during intercourse to avoid discomfort and friction. Condoms are generally well pre-lubricated, but if extra lubrication is needed with latex condoms, use only lubricants with a *water base* such as K-Y Gel, glycerine or lubricants specially made for use with condoms. Some women use plain, white yoghurt as lubricant. Lubricants with an *oil base* should *never* be used because they weaken, dissolve and break latex condoms. *Never* use Vaseline or petroleum jelly, baby oil, massage oil, body lotions with an oil base, cooking or vegetable oil, butter or fats as lubricants with latex condoms. Saliva should also not be used because it is not very effective as a lubricant. K-Y Gel or other water-based lubricants can be bought at any pharmacy and at some supermarkets.

Activity

Carry out the following exercise in a group as part of a safer sex workshop. It is great fun, and participants will never forget how important it is not to use oil-based lubricants with latex condoms. Give every person in your group a condom and ask them to inflate it like a balloon. Supply them with all kinds of water-based as well as oil-based lubricants such as K-Y Gel, Vaseline, cooking oil, massage oil and baby oil. Ask the participants to add their own hand lotions if they have any with them. Ask them to choose any of these lubricants, apply it to the inflated condom and rub it in. Set your stop watch to see how long it takes for the condom rubbed with Vaseline to burst!

Tips to prevent condoms from breaking or leaking

The following tips are helpful for preventing condoms from breaking or leaking:

- Choose prelubricated condoms specially packed in square wrappers that keep light out.
- Use a brand of condom that shows that it has been tested for reliability. Always check the information on the packet before buying condoms.
- Store condoms away from excessive heat, light, and moisture, as these cause them to deteriorate and perhaps break. Store condoms

in a cool, dark, dry place if possible. Don't store condoms in a wallet, where they can easily be damaged, or in the glove compartment of a car, where they can deteriorate due to heat.

- Check the expiry date on the condom wrapper. Don't use condoms after the expiry date or more than 5 years after the manufacturing date, because they may break.
- Do not use condoms that are sticky, brittle, discoloured or otherwise damaged.
- Open the wrapper carefully so that the condom does not tear. Be careful not to tear condoms with long nails, teeth, other sharp objects or jewellery.
- Make sure that the type of condom you use is strong enough for the type of sexual practice you engage in. Use extra strong condoms (e.g. Durex Extra Strong) for anal penetration. Ordinary condoms are generally made for vaginal intercourse, and the increased friction and strain placed on the latex by the narrow, less flexible anus may cause them to break.
- Don't ever use two condoms (i.e. one pulled over the other) as the friction will tear the condoms.

Enrichment

Heterosexual anal intercourse

People often assume that only homosexual men have anal intercourse. But research has shown that this is not the case and that 20–35% of men and women have heterosexual anal intercourse. Halperin (2000) sees anal intercourse as a neglected risk factor for heterosexual HIV infection: 'We tend to concentrate on classic risk factors (such as condom use, STIs, and multiple partners) in our prevention programmes, while we neglect practices such as heterosexual anal intercourse, "dry sex", and male circumcision.' Various European and US studies indicated that the chance of becoming infected with HIV after one act of unprotected receptive anal sex is approximately 20 times greater than after one act of unprotected vaginal sex. These studies also indicate that anal intercourse may account for up to half of heterosexual transmissions in some countries. Anal intercourse is often practised as a means of avoiding pregnancy, of maintaining 'virginity', or as a preferred pleasure. Young girls in traditional communities who fear the humiliation of failing a virginity test often practise anal sex as an alternative to vaginal sex. It is also practised by commercial sex workers and by men who prefer anal intercourse with women for reasons similar to the reasons they prefer 'dry sex' (Garcia et al., 2000; Halperin, 2000; Pando et al., 2000). 'Dry sex' is discussed later in this chapter, on page 138.

The female condom

The female condom (or femidom) is a strong, soft sheath made of polyurethane plastic that is inserted into the vagina before sexual intercourse. It is pouch-shaped and about the same length as the male condom, but wider. The female condom has two flexible plastic rings: a loose ring at the closed end that helps in inserting the condom and keeps it in place during sex, and a larger ring at the open end, which remains outside the vagina and spreads over the woman's external genitalia.

Because the female condom is made of polyurethane plastic (not latex), it requires no special storage. It can be inserted a few hours before having sex, it does not require immediate withdrawal after ejaculation, and it can be used with both oil-based and water-based lubricants. Because the external ring is usually visible during sex, a woman cannot easily use a female condom without her partner knowing about it, but women do have more control over use of this method than they do over the use of a male condom. Because it can be inserted hours before sexual intercourse, it can provide protection in situations where consumption of alcohol or drugs may reduce the chances that a male condom will be used. The female condom also provides protection during menstruation.

The female condom provides extra protection to men and women because it covers both the entrance to the vagina and the base of the penis, both of which are areas where STI sores make it easy for HIV to enter. Although research on the re-use of the female condom (after it has been thoroughly washed) is under way, the current recommendation by the World Health Organization is that it be used only once before it is discarded. Female condoms are much more expensive than male condoms and they are not as acceptable or easily accessible (UNAIDS, 2000c).

Activity

If you do not know what a female condom looks like, try to get one from a clinic or pharmacy. Unfortunately they are expensive compared with male condoms and not generally available. The female condom is manufactured by the Female Health Company (http://www.femalehealth.com)

How to use the female condom

Figure 8.2 illustrates how the female condom should be inserted. The following instructions should be presented:

- Do not use damaged, discoloured, brittle or sticky condoms.
- Check the expiry date.
- Before using the female condom, rub it between your fingers in order to spread the lubrication around evenly.
- Hold the condom at the closed end. Twist the inner ring into a figure-8 shape and hold it between your fingers, or just squeeze the inner ring. With the other hand, separate the outer lips of the vagina.
- The vagina must be relaxed when you insert the condom. Squat or sit with your knees apart, or stand with one leg raised.
- Gently push the inner ring into your vagina with your fingers (use the same insertion method you use to insert a tampon), and be

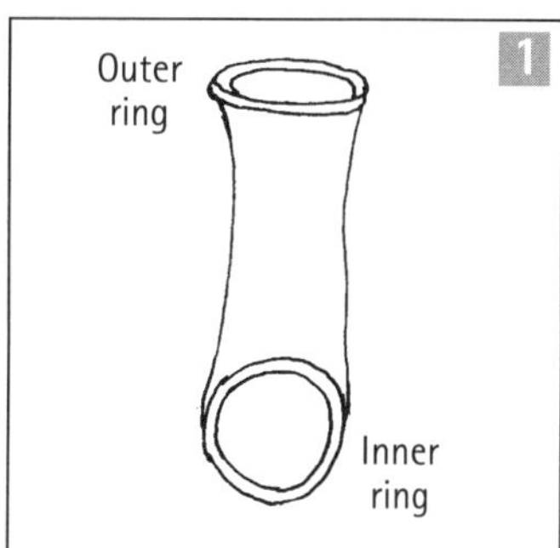

The open end covers the vagina, and the inner ring is used for insertion and to hold the condom in place.

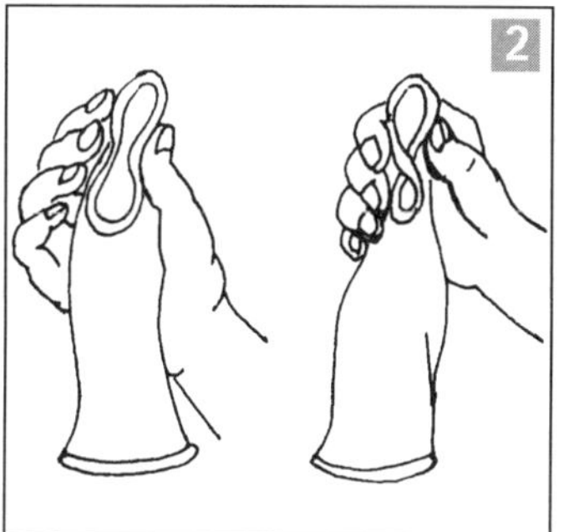

Hold the inner ring between your fingers and squeeze or twist the ring into a figure 8.

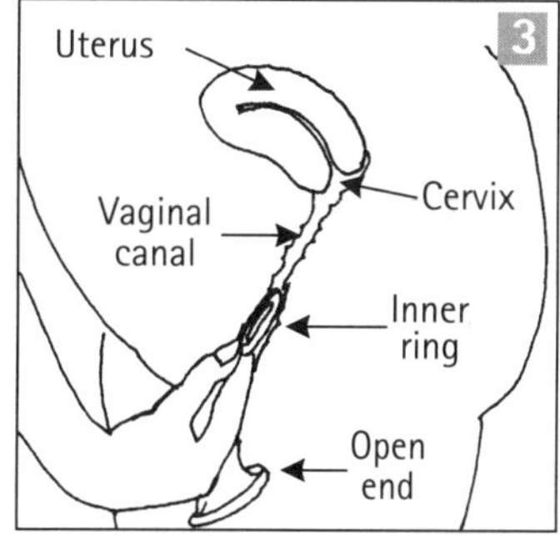

Push the inner ring into the vagina with your fingers (like you would a tampon).

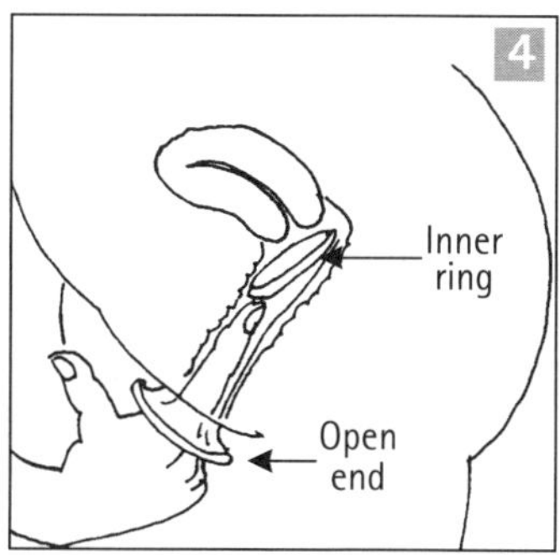

With your index finger, push the inner ring up as far as it can go.

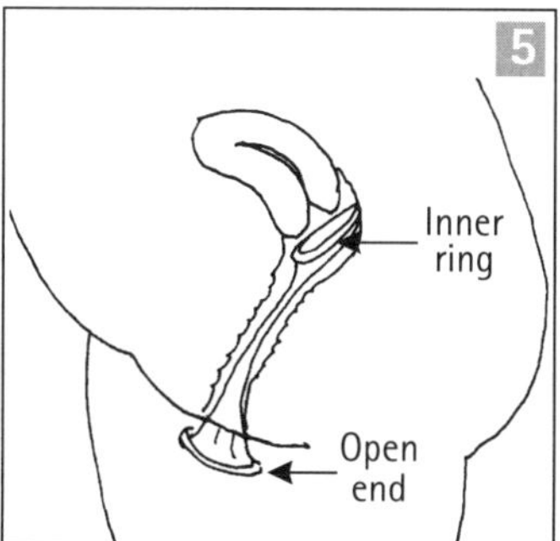

The female condom in place.

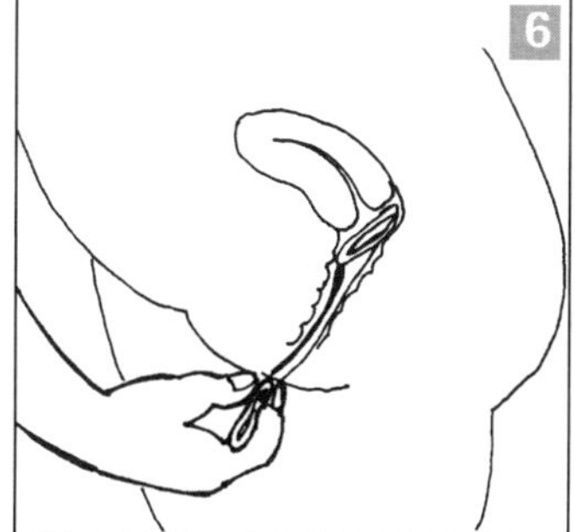

Remove the condom before standing up. Squeeze and twist the outer ring, pull gently, and dispose.

Figure 8.2
How to insert the female condom

careful to ensure that your fingernails or jewellery do not damage the polyurethane.

- Put your index finger in the condom and gently push the inner ring up into the vagina as far as it will go (similar to how a diaphragm would be inserted). The condom should fit snugly against the cervix (behind the pubic bone). If it is in the right place, you will not feel the ring.
- The outer ring should hang outside the vagina, and it should not be twisted.
- During intercourse it is necessary to guide the penis into the condom and to check that the penis has not entered the vagina *outside* the condom wall. Make sure that the condom is not pushed into the vagina by the penis.
- If there is a problem (e.g. if the condom rips or tears, if the outer ring is pushed inside or if the condom bundles up inside the vagina), remove the condom and insert a new one.
- Don't *ever* use a male condom at the same time as the female condom because the friction between them will move both condoms out of their proper positions.
- Remove the condom after male ejaculation by squeezing and twisting the outer ring and gently pulling the condom out of the vagina. Remove the condom before standing up.
- Wrap the condom in tissues or toilet paper and dispose of it in a rubbish bin and not in the toilet. Do not re-use it.

Add more lubrication (e.g. K-Y Gel) onto the penis and/or inside the female condom if the penis does not move freely in and out, if the outer ring is pushed inside, if sex is noisy, if you feel the condom when it is in place, and if it comes out of the vagina during sex. The female condom can also be used for anal sex (e.g. in case of allergies to latex), but the inner ring should be removed before use.

(See http://www.femalehealth.com/theproduct.html for pictures and information on the female condom.)

Although the female condom is not meant to replace the male condom, it increases the options available in the fight against HIV and other sexually transmitted infections. According to a Thai study among sex workers in brothels, the women experienced a 34% decrease in the number of new sexually transmitted infections in cases where a female condom was provided as an extra option to the male condom. The same study also found that sex workers who had access to both the female and the male condom were less likely to have unprotected sex than women who had access only to male condoms (UNAIDS, 2000c).

Research is currently under way to find effective microbicides in the form of a vaginal cream that can be controlled by women (see 'What is a vaginal microbicide?' on page 26).

General safer sex rules

- Avoid all high-risk sex practices such as vaginal, anal and oral sex without a condom. Avoid casual sex, sex with a commercial sex worker, sex with a partner who shares needles and syringes with other drug users, and sex with a person whose sexual history you do not know.
- Never allow semen, vaginal fluids, blood or menstrual blood to come into contact with or enter the vagina, anus, penis, mouth or broken skin. Wash your hands with soap and water if they have been in contact with semen or other body fluids. Rinse your mouth with cold (not hot) water if it has had contact with semen and *don't* brush your teeth immediately afterwards.
- Avoid deep, wet or 'French' kissing with an HIV-positive person if there is a possibility of trauma to the mouth, bleeding gums or sores that may result in an exchange of blood. Kissing is safe when there is no blood involved.
- Avoid sex when either partner has open sores on the genitals or any sexually transmitted infections.
- Avoid anal or rough vaginal intercourse. Do not do anything that could tear the skin or the moist lining of the genitals, anus or mouth and cause bleeding.
- Do not perform oral sex when you have a cold, a sore throat or open sores in your mouth or if you have brushed your teeth within the past few hours. Avoid oral sex if there are sores on your partner's genitals.

- It is a good rule not to share dildos, vibrators and other sex toys. But if you must share them, make sure that they are clean and that you use a new condom on the dildo or sex toy before sharing it.
- If you perform oral sex on a man (called fellatio) you should always use a condom. Although the risk of HIV transmission through oral sex is low, it appears that fellatio is the riskiest kind of *oral sex* if the partner performing the fellatio receives semen into his or her mouth. If the taste of latex puts you off, use the fruit- and mint-flavoured condoms available for oral sex. However, always make sure that they are of good quality before you buy them. (Durex make a variety of high-quality flavoured and coloured condoms.)
- If you want to perform oral sex on a woman (called cunnilingus), a dental dam (or latex sheath placed over the vagina) will make sure you do not get vaginal fluid or menstrual blood into your mouth. Non-porous plastic wraps, such as non-microwaveable plastic wrap (e.g. Glad Wrap), can also be placed over the vagina, or a condom can be cut open for this purpose. Added lubricants between the plastic wrap or sheath and the vagina will help to keep it in place. Although cunnilingus holds a low risk of HIV transmission (if the skin is intact and if the woman is not menstruating), other sexually transmitted infections can be transmitted in this way.
- The majority of sexually transmitted infections occur when infected mucous membranes come into contact with uninfected mucous membranes. When performing oral sex (both fellatio and cunnilingus), the herpes simplex virus and the bacteria that cause gonorrhoea and syphilis infections may be present on the lips or in the mouth or throat, and these can cause infections of the genitals, or vice versa.
- While oral-anal sex (called anilingus or 'rimming') does not appear to carry a high risk of HIV infection unless there is blood present, the possibility of contracting the hepatitis B virus, the herpes simplex virus, the cytomegalovirus and a number of different parasites from oral-anal sex is very high indeed. A latex sheath (dental dam), Glad Wrap or a spliced-open condom should be used to cover the anal area.
- If you have open wounds on your fingers, wear a condom over your finger before inserting it into the vagina or anus of your partner.
- If you practise vaginal and anal fisting (inserting the whole fist into the vagina or anus), you should use latex gloves during the process. You should also take care of your nails because sharp edges can tear gloves and condoms.
- Avoid alcohol and illicit drugs because they can impair your immune system as well as your judgement. If you use drugs, don't share needles, syringes and drug-preparation equipment such as cookers.
- Adopt alternative sexual practices that are less likely to result in infection by HIV, other viruses or infection-causing agents. Safe practices that are still enjoyable include the following:hugging, cuddling and body-to-body rubbing
  - erotic massage
  - petting
  - kissing
  - bathing or showering together
  - masturbating alone
  - masturbating together
  - sexual fantasies
  - phone sex
  - using personal sex toys
  - thigh sex (a healthy skin provides a protective barrier against the virus). Thigh sex is a practice where the penis is rubbed between the thighs of the woman, who crosses her legs. Note that no penetration occurs during thigh sex.

  (It is not possible to get HIV from direct contact with semen *on* the body – as long as it is not *in* the body.)

Is oral sex safe?

No, oral sex is not considered safe sex. Numerous studies have shown that oral sex can result in the transmission of HIV and other STIs. However, the risk of HIV transmission from an infected partner through oral sex is much lower than the risk of HIV transmission from unprotected anal or vaginal sex. Measuring the exact risk of HIV transmission as a result of oral sex is very difficult because most sexually active individuals practise oral sex in addition to other forms of sex. Several co-factors can, however, increase the risk of HIV transmission through oral sex, including oral ulcers, bleeding gums, menstrual blood, genital sores and the presence of other STIs. A number of other STIs can also be transmitted through oral sex, such as herpes, syphilis, gonorrhoea, genital warts (HPV), intestinal parasites and hepatitis A.

The risk of HIV infection from oral sex can be lowered by using latex condoms for every act of fellatio (oral contact with the penis). For cunnilingus (oral-vaginal sex) or anilingus (oral-anal contact), plastic food wrap, a condom cut open, or a dental dam can serve as a physical barrier to prevent transmission of HIV or other STIs. Oral sex is commonly practised by sexually active male-female and same-gender couples of various ages, including adolescents. Apparently many adolescents who engage in oral sex do not consider it to be sex, and use oral sex as a means of experiencing sex while believing that they remain abstinent. Many adolescents consider oral sex to be safe or a no-risk sexual practice. In a national survey conducted for The Kaiser Foundation, 26% of sexually active teenagers aged 15–17 believed that one 'cannot become infected with HIV by having unprotected oral sex', and an additional 15% didn't know whether or not one could become infected in that way (McIntosh, 2004).

Enrichment

The dangerous practice of 'dry sex'

'Dry sex' is practised by many women in Africa. Because some men believe that a dry vagina is a sign of faithfulness, or to heighten their sexual pleasure, they insist on 'dry sex'. In order to obtain this dry condition, women use herbs, snuff, antiseptic solutions (such as Dettol, soap, salt solutions or Betadine), chemical and other substances (toothpaste, washing powder, methylated spirits, vinegar, human urine, baboon's faeces), cotton wool, cotton cloth or newspaper to 'dry out' the vagina (Runganga & Kasule, 1995). Apart from being painful for the woman, this practice is potentially very dangerous because it may promote lacerations (or breaks) in the vaginal walls – a condition that helps the spread of HIV. Proper education (of women and of men), the empowerment of women and assertiveness training for women may be the only way to put a stop to such dangerous practices.

What is a 'dental dam', and what is it used for?

A dental dam is a square sheet of latex rubber used as a protective barrier during dental work. Because they are made of latex, they can also provide a barrier in situations where the mouth comes into contact with body fluids that may contain HIV – especially during cunnilingus (oral-vaginal contact) and anilingus (oral-anal contact). Anilingus and cunnilingus are relatively low-risk sexual acts with regard to HIV transmission (in the absence of blood). The placing of a latex barrier between the mouth and the vagina or anus brings the chances of contracting HIV through these acts to almost zero.

Can lesbians get Aids?

Lesbians who have sex with men as well as with women can contract HIV infection if they have sex with infected men. The risk of infection is low for women who have sex only with women. One of the ways in which lesbian women can contract HIV infection is by *sharing* contaminated sex toys (dildos or vibrators, for instance) for vaginal or anal penetration. Because sex toys can cause bleeding or irritation of the vaginal or anal lining, they can give the HI virus a chance to enter the body if people use them or share them. When sex toys are used, they should be thoroughly cleaned and preferably not shared. Women should also be careful during menstruation. Lesbian women who are survivors of sexual assault or rape by men are at risk of contracting HIV, which they might then transmit to their lesbian sex partners.

Does the female diaphragm prevent HIV infection? And does the contraceptive pill prevent HIV infection?

In both cases, no. The female diaphragm prevents semen from entering the cervix, but it does *not* protect the vagina or external genitalia from exposure to HIV. Cervical barriers such as a diaphragm, cap or sponge (used to prevent pregnancy) can, however, provide extra protection if a condom is also *always* used during penetrative vaginal intercourse. Some people erroneously believe that the contraceptive pill can protect them against HIV infection. They should be told that, although the pill prevents pregnancy, it does not prevent contact with semen (which contains the virus) in the same way that a condom does. The pill therefore does *not* prevent HIV infection.

Is there still a risk of HIV infection if the penis is withdrawn from the vagina (or anus) before ejaculation?

Interrupting intercourse by withdrawing the penis from the vagina or (anus) before ejaculating will result in reduced exposure to fluids, but withdrawal will not necessarily prevent a person from getting or transmitting HIV. Vaginal fluids come into contact with the penis *during* intercourse – regardless of whether the penis is withdrawn before ejaculation or not. The fluids that come out of the tip of the penis before ejaculation (pre-seminal fluids) contain sufficient amounts of HIV to cause infection. While withdrawal before ejaculation may reduce the chances of infection, it cannot protect against HIV (Kalichman, 1996).

Does cleaning (washing) the vagina or anus after sex reduce the risk of HIV infection?

There is no evidence to support the belief that vaginal or anal cleansing (douching or flushing) after sex can prevent HIV infection and other sexually transmitted infections. In fact, cleansing of this kind is *not advised* because it may actually facilitate HIV infection by washing infected semen *deeper* into the vagina or anus (Kalichman, 1996). Substances (cleansing agents) used for washing may also cause irritations or abrasions in the vagina or anus, which may give the virus easier access into the body.

Are condoms really safe and effective?

Yes. Scientific evidence shows that latex condoms are highly effective in preventing the transmission of HIV and some other STIs when they are used *consistently* and *correctly*. The effectiveness of condoms can be reduced by manufacturer errors and by user errors. All high-quality condoms are tested by the manufacturers, and according to the Food and Drug Administration in the USA, condoms are 99.7% defect-free. The effectiveness of condoms was tested in a 2-year study of heterosexual 'discordant couples' (couples with one HIV-positive and one HIV-negative partner) in Europe. Among 124 couples who used condoms consistently and correctly, *none* of the uninfected partners became infected. In contrast, when condoms were used inconsistently for vaginal or anal intercourse, 10% of the uninfected partners became infected, and 15% of HIV-negative partners became infected when condoms were not used at all (Centers for Disease Control, 2000).

Enrichment

Problems associated with condom use in Africa

The use of condoms poses certain problems that are specific to Africa. These problems should be recognised by health care professionals working in Africa. Apart from cultural and other problems with condoms (see 'Perceptions of condoms' on page 122), Green (1994) observed that condoms as they are actually used in practice in Africa may only have a 50% effectiveness rate in reducing most sexually transmitted infections because of incorrect use and the poor quality of condoms. Condoms are also sometimes inadequately stored and transported under tropical conditions. The high temperatures caused by the African sun can damage the lubrication of condoms and make them brittle and therefore useless. Because of this, Green feels very strongly that Aids prevention programmes should not rely solely on the use of condoms, but that they should also concentrate on the prevention and treatment of STIs in general.

Breaking or slipping off of condoms is almost always caused by user errors such as not putting the condom on correctly, using a petroleum-based lubricant, using deteriorated or out-of-date condoms, or storing condoms at a high temperature for a long time in places such as a car glove compartment or a wallet. Only tested, high-quality condoms should ever be used. As people's knowledge about using condoms increases, breakage and slippage decreases. Health care professionals therefore have a big responsibility to make sure that people know how to use condoms correctly (Centers for Disease Control, 2000).

A study published in the *American Journal of Public Health* observed female sex workers in Nevada brothels, where condom use is required by law. It was found that, of 353 condoms used by the sex workers during the study, none broke or fell off during intercourse, and only two (0.6%) slipped off during withdrawal. Other studies reported breakage rates during vaginal intercourse ranging from 0% to 6.7%. Most studies report that condoms break less than 2% of the time during intercourse or withdrawal. Breakage rates during anal sex for gay men in four prospective studies ranged from 0.5% to 12%, with rates of less than 2% in three of the studies. In most of these cases, the breakage of condoms was due to human error and incorrect use of condoms (Siecus Fact Sheet, 2002:3).

Is it still necessary to use condoms if both partners are HIV positive?

Yes. It is important for HIV-positive individuals to protect themselves against re-infection with other strains of HIV. Any new infection can also cause an increase in the viral load in the blood. This may in turn lead to a further decrease in CD4 cells, and an accompanying further weakening of the immune system. In addition to re-infection with HIV, a person can also of course contract *other* sexually transmitted infections and these may damage his or her overall health and immune status.

Is it safe to use spermicidal creams that contain nonoxynol-9?

The use of spermicidal creams containing nonoxynol-9 (N9) as an ingredient was recommended in the past because the substance was believed to kill HIV. It now seems that nonoxynol-9 may not be as safe as was formerly believed, because of the allergies and infections it can cause (we noted earlier in the text that, because allergies, infections and skin irritations cause broken or inflamed mucous membranes, they facilitate transmission of the HI virus). The Centers for Disease Control therefore recommended in 2000 that the use of nonoxynol-9 should be discouraged and discontinued (Gayle, 2000). It was also found that nonoxynol-9, when used with condoms, did not protect women from the bacteria that cause gonorrhoea and chlamydial infection any better than condoms used alone (Roddy et al., 2002). (Note: A spermicidal cream is a cream used by women for contraception. It contains a substance that kills sperm.)

A continuum of sexual practices: from no risk to high risk

If we want to determine the extent of risk generated by each different sexual practice, we must first ascertain exactly what *body fluids* are involved in each specific practice. The highest concentration of the HI virus is found in blood (including menstrual blood), semen, pre-seminal fluids ('pre-cum'), and vaginal secretions. The concentration of the virus is very low in saliva, tears, urine and sweat. In the light of this

Activity

The owner of a singles bar for women is very concerned about the health of the women who visit her club. She asks you, an HIV/Aids consultant, to create a pamphlet to inform her customers about women's health issues. What information would you include in your pamphlet?

Refer back to and re-read the section about the safety of women who have sex with women (page 138). Keep in mind that some of the women who have sex with other women also have sex with men.

Table 8.1
Continuum of sexual behaviours: From no-risk to high-risk behaviours

No risk
• Abstinence • Erotic massage • Hugging and body rubbing • Petting • Kissing • Bathing or showering together • Masturbation • Mutual masturbation (if there is no contact between broken skin and semen/vaginal fluids) • Sexual fantasies • Thigh sex • Phone sex • Using personal sex toys
Low risk
• Oral sex on a man (fellatio) who is wearing a condom • Oral sex on a woman (cunnilingus) with a latex barrier • Anilingus (oral-anal sex) with a latex barrier • Contact with urine ('golden showers' or 'water sports' on unbroken skin)
Some risk
• Oral sex (on a man or woman without a condom or barrier) • Vaginal penetrative sex with a condom • Anal penetrative sex with a condom (it is safer to withdraw before ejaculation)
High risk
• Vaginal penetrative sex without a condom • Anal penetrative sex without a condom (*very high risk*) • Swallowing semen • Sharing uncovered sex toys • Vaginal or anal penetrative sex with a condom if using a petroleum-based lubricant • Unprotected oral-anal contact if blood is present • Unprotected manual-anal intercourse (fisting) without a latex glove • Unprotected manual-vaginal intercourse (fisting) without a latex glove • Contact with menstrual blood

information, we can rate sexual practices on a continuum that ranges from behaviours that carry no risk of infection to those that carry a high risk. Table 8.1 gives an indication of the behaviours on the continuum between *no risk* and *high risk*. The risk will, of course, increase with the number of partners who are involved in unprotected sexual activities.

8.3 TALKING TO CLIENTS ABOUT SEX: THE DO'S AND DON'TS

It is often very difficult for counsellors to talk to their clients about sex. It is even harder for clients to discuss their most intimate and private behaviour with counsellors. What follows are a few do's and don'ts to keep in mind when talking to clients about sex (credit to Dr Elna McIntosh from DISA Health Care).

DO:

- Be comfortable with your own sexuality.
- Raise the issues of sex and safer sex practices rather than wait for the client to ask.
- Be aware of your own attitudes and beliefs about sexuality.
- Be aware of your own body language and what it will convey to the client.
- Have information available about sexuality that the client can take away.
- Normalise the client's problems and let him or her know that he or she is not alone.
- Use the same terminology that the client does.
- Discuss sex in a frank, forthright and professional manner.
- Feel comfortable to illustrate condom use.
- Discuss sexual issues openly, clearly, comfortably and with empathy.
- Refer the client to a sexologist or sex therapist if necessary (especially in cases of sexual dysfunction).

DON'T:

- Assume that all clients are heterosexual. Some clients are gay, lesbian or bisexual and sometimes transsexual.
- Assume that everyone is the same. Everyone has his or her own unique experiences.

- Assume that a client of a different race or gender is completely comfortable with you just because you are a counsellor, nurse or doctor.
- Assume that if a client does not ask any questions, he or she has all the answers. The client may feel too embarrassed to ask questions.
- Ask only YES/NO questions. Also ask open questions that invite clients to share their experiences.
- Make light of or joke about the client's sexual complaints.
- Be impatient when the client takes a long time getting round to describing or discussing sexual problems. The client may feel anxious about sharing this intimate information with you.
- Share your own personal sexual attitude or experiences with the client. This is not the time to have your own personal therapy session!
- Be afraid not to know everything. It is acceptable to get back to the client once you have done some investigating.

8.4 PREVENTION OF HIV IN INJECTING DRUG USERS

Sharing needles to inject drugs ('shooting up') is a major factor in the Aids crisis. In many countries the Aids epidemic is fuelled by the sharing of dirty needles. It is important for governments to plan their actions and laws accordingly. Drug injection poses a threat to drug users as well as to their sexual partners. Many drug users sell sex to pay for their drugs, and this spreads the virus in the general population.

We are fortunate in Africa because we do not (yet) have as many injecting drug users as other parts of the world. We should use this window of opportunity to get appropriate preventive measures into place. Programmes should focus on the primary prevention of drug use, especially among young people; on the rehabilitation of drug users; and on the prevention of HIV among drug users who do not want to (or cannot) stop the habit.

Anti-drug campaigns and rehabilitation

Comprehensive anti-drug programmes are needed to prevent drug use, and campaigns that deter young people from using drugs should be actively implemented in schools, colleges and universities.

Easy access to rehabilitation programmes should be made available to individuals who want to stop taking drugs, and they should be supported as they complete the treatment. Relapse-prevention programmes should also be offered.

Guidelines on how injecting drug users can reduce the risk of HIV infection

HIV-prevention programmes, including Aids education, condom promotion and drug treatment, should all be implemented among injecting drug users who are not interested in rehabilitation programmes. Sustained attempts should, however, be made to involve drug users in rehabilitation programmes.

The Centers for Disease Control give the following guidelines for drug users who cannot or will not stop injecting drugs:

- Never re-use or share syringes, needles, water, or drug preparation equipment.
- Only use syringes and needles that you obtain from a reliable source (such as a pharmacy or a needle exchange programme in countries where this is available to registered drug users).
- Use a new, sterile syringe and needle to prepare and inject drugs.
- If possible, use sterile water to prepare drugs. If you cannot obtain sterile water, at least use clean water from a reliable source (such as fresh tap water).
- Use a new or disinfected container ('cooker') and a new filter ('cotton') to prepare drugs.
- Clean the injection site with a new alcohol swab prior to injection.
- Safely dispose of the syringe and needle after each (one) use.

Note: These guidelines should NOT be misconstrued as implying any condoning of drug use. Instead they should be regarded as a means of reducing the considerable personal risks faced by drug users, as well as the health (and other) risks that drug users pose to the community at large.

Needle exchange and bleach distribution programmes

Many major cities in Europe and in the USA allow drug users to swap used needles and syringes for sterile equipment. Although needle exchange programmes are successful in preventing the spread of HIV, these programmes are very controversial because many people regard them as condoning drug abuse. In contrast to this view, many research studies in the USA have found that needle exchange programmes (or greater needle availability) reduce HIV transmission *without* increasing the use of illegal drugs (Coates & Collins, 1998).

Some countries have instituted less controversial strategies such as distributing bleach and other supplies for cleaning needles and syringes. Drug users are advised to sterilise their injecting equipment by using a bleach-water solution (one part bleach to ten parts water). They are advised to draw the bleach solution up through the needle to fill the syringe, to flush the solution through the needle twice, to rinse it in clean water twice after cleaning, and not to share rinsing water.

People who continue to inject drugs should have themselves tested for HIV on a regular basis.

8.5 THE PROMOTION OF HEALTH AND THE ACQUISITION OF LIFE SKILLS

The aims of health education in HIV-prevention programmes should not only be the prevention of illness; they should also focus on the promotion of physical and mental health. HIV/Aids education should therefore be part of a broader strategy to empower people with the necessary life skills to make the right health choices and to improve the overall quality of their lives. Health care professionals must help their clients develop responsible and effective coping skills which will not only enable them to prevent HIV infection but also help them to enhance their lives on various levels. Health care professionals should facilitate the following life skills:

- assertiveness;
- self-efficacy (a strong belief in your ability to do something);
- a strong self-concept and self-awareness;
- a belief in the right to make your own choices;
- the ability to handle peer pressure;
- taking responsibility for yourself and for others in the community;
- problem-solving skills;
- conflict resolution;
- effective communication skills (condom promotion programmes often fail because people are advised to use condoms but are not given guidance on how to *communicate* with their partners on this issue); and
- negotiation skills, which are absolutely vital in persuading 'difficult' partners to practise safer sex and to use condoms.

Life skills enable young people who are not yet sexually active to learn safe habits from the start. Life skills also enable people who have *already* acquired risky sex patterns to begin to practise safer sex. Women especially should be taught to be more assertive and self-efficient in sexual matters. Women should believe in their ability and right to make their own choices, to insist on condom use, and to say no to sex when they don't want it.

Various strategies may be used to promote life skills. Role play can teach new skills which can then be practised, and social modelling helps individuals observe (e.g. on video) and understand how to deal with interpersonal situations (Bandura, 1989; Franzini et al., 1990). People must be taught the ability to exercise control over their lives and behaviour. Some need to be trained to communicate effectively with their sex partners if the partners are resistant, defensive or manipulative (Sy et al., 1989).

Activity

You will often find a lot of giggling, laughing and joking in your safer-sex workshops. What do you think is the psychological function of humour in stressful situations like these? How can humour be used as an educational tool? Are you personally comfortable with using humour? When should one be careful or cautious about using humour?

8.6 CONCLUSION

Although it is true that a disease that spreads with the help of sex is a formidable foe, *we are not helpless victims.* We have the power to emerge from the war as victors, but only if we are prepared to use the only weapon we have: sexual behaviour change. When promoting safer practices, Aids counsellors should be specific and not hesitate to give detailed (but sensitive) explanations and demonstrations that enable people to fight the war pro-actively.

chapter

9 HIV/Aids Education and Life-Skills Training

The children
At the edge of the riverbed
the children played in the warm clay.
But Koki, filled with fear, saw that
the game was different this morning.

Our future lies with our children. This saying has never been as true as it is now, at a time when HIV/Aids is destroying countless human lives, especially in sub-Saharan Africa. If we cannot stop the current progress of the disease, we can at least try to ensure an Aids-free future for our children. The role of schools and religious and civic organisations is extremely important in the fight against Aids. We should empower our children with education and life skills, not only so that they can prevent themselves from being infected, but also so that they can learn to become compassionate, caring members of a society that will be struggling with the aftermath of HIV/Aids for a long time to come.

9.1 LEARNERS, TEACHERS AND HIV/AIDS: A GRIM PICTURE

HIV/Aids has had a devastating effect on educational systems in many parts of the world, wreaking havoc among learners and teachers alike. In its report on the global HIV/Aids epidemic, UNAIDS (2000c:29–30) presents the following disturbing facts about the effect of HIV/Aids on educational systems.

The Central African Republic (where approximately one in every seven adults is infected with HIV) has a 33% shortage of primary school teachers. During 1996 and 1998, almost as many teachers were lost to death as to retirement, and of those who died, 85% were HIV positive (they died an average of 10 years before reaching the minimum retirement age of 52). Because of staff shortages in the Central African Republic, 107 schools have closed and only 66 have been able to remain open. It is estimated that more than 71 000 children between the ages of 6 and 11 will be deprived of a primary education by the year 2005. The impact of Aids in Côte d'Ivoire presents the same grim dimensions. In that country confirmed cases of HIV/Aids account for seven out of ten deaths among teachers. Zambia lost 1 300 teachers in the first ten months of 1998 – the equivalent of around 65% of all new teachers who are trained annually. According to the South African Democratic Teachers Union, nationwide Aids-related deaths among teachers rose by over 40% in 2000–2001, as calculated from claims to the union's funeral plan between June 2000 and May 2001 (UNAIDS, 2002). Illness or death of teachers is especially devastating in rural areas, where schools often depend heavily on one or two teachers. Moreover, skilled teachers are not easily replaced. Swaziland has estimated that it will have to train 13 000 teachers over the next 17 years just to keep services at the 1997 level – 7 000 more than it would have had to train if there were no Aids deaths. A study in Manicaland, Zimbabwe, found that 19% of male teachers and almost 29% of female teachers were infected with HIV in 2002.

This kind of devastation also applies to learners who are either infected or affected by HIV/Aids. The presence of Aids in the family often means that children have to drop out of school, temporarily (or permanently) interrupt their schooling because of a shortage of money, or work full time in the home to help sick parents and to care for younger siblings. Research in Zimbabwe showed that 48% of the orphans of primary school age who were interviewed had dropped out of school – usually when their parents became too ill to look after themselves or when their parents died. Not one orphan of secondary school age was still in school. In a study of orphans in Kenya, boys tended to cite economic reasons for dropping out of primary school (64% said they could not afford the school fees or that they needed to earn cash from fishing), while 28% of the girls said that they had become pregnant and 41% said that they had left to get married (UNAIDS, 2000c:29).

According to the UNAIDS (2004:53) the number of orphans and other children made vulnerable by Aids is still growing in high-prevalence countries. 'It is crucial that they have locally appropriate, affordable, non-stigmatising, innovative educational options, such as home-based learning and distance education.'

A decline in school enrolment is one of the most visible effects of the Aids epidemic (due to dropouts, a decline in birth rate as a result of Aids-related infertility, and children themselves being infected and not surviving their school-going years). According to research by the University of Natal in South Africa, the number of pupils enrolling in the first year of primary school in 2001 in parts of KwaZulu-Natal was 20% lower than in 1998. In the Central African Republic and Swaziland, school enrolment is reported to have fallen by 20–36% due to Aids and orphanhood, with girls most affected (UNAIDS, 2002:52).

Sexual initiation may occur at a very early age for some children, especially in marginalised communities where sexual abuse and rape are relatively common. A survey of 1 600 children and adolescents in four poor areas of the Zambian capital, Lusaka, found that more than 25% of children aged 10 said they had already had sex (this figure rose to 60% among 14-year-olds). In South Africa, 10% of respondents in a study in six provinces said that they had started having sex at age 11 or younger. The South African Department of Health used the results of this study as the basis for its recommendation that sex education should be introduced to children at around the age of 12 so that it can benefit them before many of them become sexually active (UNAIDS, 2000c). A survey among adolescents in KwaZulu-Natal reported that 76% of girls and 90% of boys are sexually experienced by the time they are 15 or 16 years old. In the Free State province of South Africa, teenagers reported that they were sexually active at around 12 years of age. Relatively few of the teenagers interviewed practised safer sex (Coombe, 2000).

Education and information are fundamental human rights, and children and young people must not be denied the basic information, education and skills that they need to protect themselves against HIV/Aids. We should not allow religious values, social mores or cultural preferences to prevent children and young people from being empowered in this way.

9.2 BASIC REQUIREMENTS FOR SUCCESSFUL HIV/AIDS EDUCATION

HIV/Aids education should comply with the following requirements and standards if it is to be successful in schools:

- HIV/Aids education should never be presented in isolation – that is to say, in a special 'Aids period'. If HIV/Aids education is presented in isolation, children may acquire an irrational fear of the disease. Such a distorted emphasis may interfere with the child's healthy sexual development because the child may become accustomed to equating sex with disease and death (Centers for Disease Control, 1988; Post, 1988).
- HIV/Aids education should preferably form part of a life-skills education programme that includes sexuality education as well as information on HIV and Aids.
- HIV/Aids information can also be integrated into the existing school curriculum, either as part of other health-related subjects, or within one or more subject areas such as biology, science, social science, mathematics and religious studies.
- HIV/Aids education should begin as early as the foundation phase (or grade 1). At this early age, children's behaviour patterns have not yet been established and they are very receptive to the principles that govern healthy behaviour.
- HIV/Aids education should be an ongoing process. A single lecture or video, or an 'HIV/Aids information week' in the senior phase, is not sufficient. The life skills required to prevent HIV infection must be learnt at a young age. These lessons should be reinforced continually as the child grows older.
- It is important to include parents, community leaders and spiritual leaders for active input at all stages of programme development. If HIV/Aids programmes are to be successful, they have to have the active support of all stakeholders in the community – and they must also reflect the whole spectrum of religious, cultural and moral values found in any particular community.
- The Centers for Disease Control (1988) recommends that the class teacher should handle the HIV/Aids education of children in the lower or primary grades, because the teacher is familiar to the children and probably best equipped to use those teaching strategies that are appropriate to the children's age group. In the more senior grades HIV/Aids education and life-skills training should be carried out by specially trained teachers (such as guidance counsellors). The educator should feel at ease with the content of the HIV/Aids curriculum and should be a role model with whom learners can easily identify.
- Information about HIV/Aids should never be presented in a way that frightens children. Research has shown that anxiety-orientated approaches in HIV/Aids education are counterproductive because anxiety escalates to a point where people are inclined to evade or deny the truth of the information (Wyatt, 1989).
- HIV/Aids education that focuses on problems while ignoring sexuality as a normal aspect of all human life may well retard the normal sexual development of the child. The positive and delightful aspects of sexuality should never be ignored. Children must be made aware that sexual feelings and impulses – which are present from birth – are both pleasant and normal. They must nevertheless be helped to understand that, although sexual feelings are normal, the active expression of sexuality is not appropriate behaviour for young children (Quackenbush & Villarreal, 1988).
- Sexuality and HIV/Aids education should always be tailored so that it is appropriate to a child or young person's particular developmental stage. It is therefore important for us to have a clear idea of the degree of cognitive, emotional, social, moral and sexual development in children in specific age groups so that the sexual education we offer to children will be exactly appropriate and suited to the developmental stage through which they are passing. Teachers should always remain sensitive to *individual* and *cultural* developmental needs and differences and adjust their education programmes accordingly.

- Programmes must take account of traditional beliefs and value systems, as well as the popular myths that circulate among young people and their wider communities.
- All education programmes should be based on protecting and promoting the rights of the child, including the rights to information, education, health and health care, freedom from rape and sexual coercion and cruel and inhuman treatment, and the right of girls to equality in education, employment, inheritance, marital law, and sexual and reproductive decision-making (UNAIDS, 2002:73).

9.3 THE BUILDING BLOCKS FOR SUCCESSFUL HIV/AIDS EDUCATION

HIV/Aids education should never concentrate on the dissemination of information on HIV and Aids alone. To make responsible decisions, a child must have *knowledge* that is firmly based on healthy *values, norms and attitudes*, and *skills* to implement these decisions. For an HIV/Aids education programme to be successful, there should be a balance between knowledge, life skills, values and attitudes (see Figure 9.1).

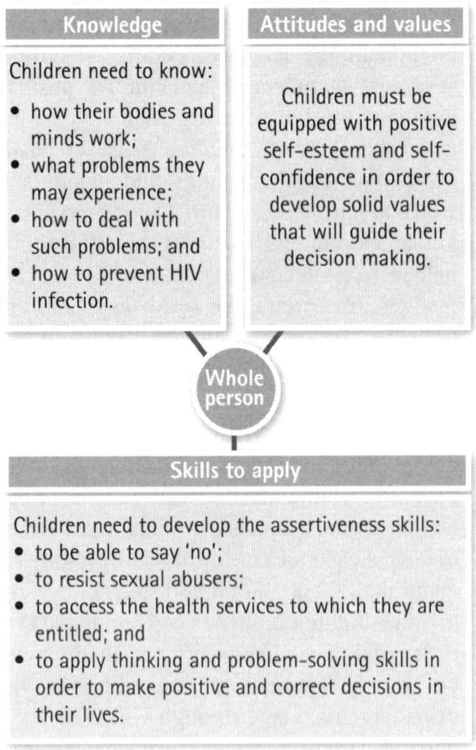

Knowledge

Children need to know:
- how their bodies and minds work;
- what problems they may experience;
- how to deal with such problems; and
- how to prevent HIV infection.

Attitudes and values

Children must be equipped with positive self-esteem and self-confidence in order to develop solid values that will guide their decision making.

Whole person

Skills to apply

Children need to develop the assertiveness skills:
- to be able to say 'no';
- to resist sexual abusers;
- to access the health services to which they are entitled; and
- to apply thinking and problem-solving skills in order to make positive and correct decisions in their lives.

Figure 9.1
The building blocks for successful HIV/Aids education
(Source: Adapted from Norton & Dawson, 2000:vi)

Basic knowledge, attitudes, values and skills (not exclusively HIV/Aids-related) should be established, promoted and reinforced in all the phases of a child's school career. The content, and the way in which this knowledge and these attitudes and skills are taught, should be adapted to the child's age and developmental phase (Edwards & Louw, 1998; Pilot Project on Life-skills, 1999).

Knowledge

An effective HIV/Aids education and life-skills programme should provide the following knowledge in a manner that is appropriate to the age of the child:

- How to conduct relationships with significant others, and with friends of the same and the opposite sex, and how to cope with strangers.
- How to deal effectively with peer-group pressure.
- What sexual abuse or molestation is, how it can be prevented, and where to find help in the case of actual or attempted sexual abuse or molestation (teach young children to distinguish between different kinds of touching).
- How to use leisure time creatively and in a way that brings satisfaction.
- How to keep the body safe and healthy and how to avoid harmful behaviour (such as sniffing glue, drinking alcohol or taking various kinds of drugs).
- Adequate knowledge about germs, viruses, HIV and Aids.
- The ability to identify health problems and seek appropriate help.
- Awareness of the universal precautions to be taken when handling blood.
- How to care for someone at home who is ill (e.g. how to make tea or run errands (a younger child) or how to feed a sick person (an older child)).
- How to cope with death in the family.

- Facts about sex, sexuality and gender and sexuality education that are appropriate to the age and developmental stage of the child.

Attitudes and values

The following attitudes and values, which are accepted by all cultures and religions as important for the survival of individuals and communities, should be included in HIV/Aids education and life-skills programmes:

- building a realistic, positive self-concept;
- respect for the self and others as unique and worthwhile beings;
- self-control;
- the right to privacy;
- the right to protect oneself;
- the right to say no to an older person or someone in authority;
- the right to chastity;
- loyalty and commitment in relationships;
- honesty;
- taking responsibility for one's actions;
- respect for life;
- non-discrimination towards and tolerance of anyone who is different from ourselves;
- forgiveness;
- loving and caring;
- social justice; and
- friendliness, kindness and sensitivity.

Life skills

We should help children develop the following life skills so that they can implement the knowledge, attitudes, values and decisions they make during the learning process:

- self-awareness;
- critical thinking;
- responsible decision making;
- problem solving;
- assertiveness;
- negotiation skills (e.g. negotiating abstinence, the postponement of sexual intercourse and safer sex practices such as using condoms);
- communication skills (including listening skills);
- refusal skills (also called 'how-to-say-no' skills);
- planning for the future: goal setting;
- conflict resolution;
- handling emotions (such as fear, uncertainty, anger, etc.);
- handling failure and coping with related feelings;
- tolerance towards others whose values, behaviour, manners or appearance may differ from our own; and
- a positive self-concept.

Enrichment

Sources for life-skills training in schools

Excellent outcome-based materials have been developed on sexuality education, HIV/Aids education and life-skills training for schools in South Africa. See 'The Caregiver's Bookshelf' on page 367 for the references.

For HIV/Aids education to be successful, it is important to know how children of different ages perceive *illness in general* and *HIV/Aids in particular.* We know that children's perception of illness depends on their developmental characteristics. In order to arrive at a clearer understanding of what we should include in HIV/Aids education and life-skills programmes, we will therefore review (in sections 9.4 and 9.7) the developmental characteristics of children between grades 1 and 12. (Only those developmental characteristics that are relevant to HIV/Aids education will be discussed.)

9.4 THE MIDDLE CHILDHOOD YEARS

The middle childhood years stretch from about 6 or 7 years to 12 years. What follows is a discussion of how children develop cognitively, emotionally, socially, morally, sexually and in terms of their self-concept during this phase of their lives.

Cognitive development

Cognition refers to how we acquire information about the world; how we represent and transform such information into knowledge; and how we store, retrieve and use that knowledge to direct our behaviour (Meyer, 1998:10). Egocentric thinking, concrete thinking and the ability to classify are especially relevant to HIV/Aids education in the middle childhood years.

Egocentric thinking

The young child in the middle childhood years (6–7) may still use egocentric and magical thinking. *Egocentrism* is the inability to see situations from any perspective other than one's own, and magical thinking is the belief that one's thoughts alone are powerful enough to effect events and changes in the world. (A typical example of magical thinking is when a young child wishes that his or her newborn sibling were dead. If that sibling then actually dies, the child will believe that it was his or her *wish* alone that caused the death.) In older children, this rigid, egocentric outlook is gradually replaced by thought processes that allow children to see things from the point of view of other people. Older children gradually become aware of a variety of points of view, and they become more sensitive to the fact that other people do not always perceive or view events exactly as they do. They also become able to postpone a particular action until they have evaluated alternative responses to situations, and their steady reduction in egocentricity begins to form the foundation on which they will construct an ability to think logically and develop and define concepts of morality as they grow older (Piaget, 1973; Wong et al., 1999:781).

Concrete thinking

Although the child in the middle childhood years is capable of operational thinking, such thinking is still concrete and not abstract. (According to Piaget, children in the middle childhood years are in the period of *concrete operations*.) *Concrete thinking* means that children cannot construct or manipulate abstract ideas or reason in terms of hypotheses or speculate about possibilities. They can reason only in terms of the observable reality or objects in front of them (Meyer & Van Ede, 1998; Piaget & Inhelder, 1969). During this phase (called the *concrete operational phase*) children gradually begin to understand the relationships between *things* and *ideas*. They progress from making judgements based on what they *see* (perceptual thinking) to making judgements based on the consequences of their *reasoning* (conceptual thinking). They are increasingly able to master symbols; to use their memory of past experiences to evaluate and interpret the present; and to classify or group objects together according to the characteristics that they share in common (Wong et al., 1999).

The ability to classify

The ability to classify develops through three stages:

- Young children (i.e. younger than 6 years old) classify objects in a very indiscriminate way. They do not have a specific characteristic or criterion in mind when classifying objects, and they often change criteria (for instance, from colour to shape) while classifying objects.
- Children from about 6 to 9 years old can classify objects on the basis of only one characteristic or criterion (such as, for example, colour).
- Only in the third stage of classification ability, which develops between the ages of 9 and 12 years, does the child begin to understand multiple and hierarchical classification. *Multiple classification* refers to the ability of a child to classify objects on the basis of more than one criterion simultaneously. *Hierarchical classification* implies class inclusion – which means that a person has the ability to understand that a subclass is always smaller than the more general overall class in which the subclass is included (subsumed).

Ability to classify may vary considerably from one child to another. According to Inhelder and Piaget (1964), who conducted their research on children in Europe, the ability to classify hierarchically usually develops in children between 7 and 11 years of age. Other studies, however, found that children often develop this ability only during mid-adolescence or beyond (Lowell, 1980). A South African study found that 9-year-old children could classify in terms of only one dimension, while older children (aged about 12 years) were more frequently able to classify objects in terms of two or three dimensions (Ramkisoon in Louw et al., 1998:327).

Emotional development

Children in the middle childhood years are relatively independent and self-sufficient and can express a variety of emotions. An emotion which is relevant to HIV/Aids education is the expression of fear.

Fear

Younger children (under 5) are afraid of specific things such as dogs, loud noises, the dark, unfamiliar objects, strangers, 'bad people' and being separated from their parents. Older children (6–8) experience an increase in fear of imaginary and abstract things such as supernatural creatures (witches and ghosts), monsters, darkness, thunder and lightning, burglars, physical injury, death, being alone at home, and media events (such as reports on Aids, war, violence and child-kidnapping). Older children (9–12) are often afraid of tests and examinations at school, school performance, physical injury, thunder and lightning, death and the dark (Botha et al., 1998:271). It has been generally observed by researchers that children's fears correspond to the times in which they live and the events with which they are familiar from the media and from listening to discussions. Today's children are generally afraid of Aids, pollution and nuclear war.

Social development

Social developmental abilities that are important for HIV/Aids education and life-skills programmes are a child's ability to socialise with friends and the ability to form prejudice.

Peer group

The peer group becomes increasingly important in the middle childhood years. The peer group plays a very important role in children's social development because it gives them experiences of comradeship (friendship) and relationships, opportunities for experimenting with new forms of behaviour, and opportunities to exercise limited forms of independence. Children also continue to learn to appreciate the numerous and varied points of view that are represented in their peer groups, and this experience helps diminish the rigidly egocentric outlook that was characteristic of an earlier developmental stage. The peer group also offers children opportunities for learning positive social skills such as negotiation, assertiveness and competitiveness. Excessive conformity and attachment to a peer group can lead to undesirable activities and behaviour such as experimentation with drugs or sex. Peer group pressure usually becomes a strong motivational factor for the 12-year-old child (Louw et al., 1998).

Prejudice

Prejudice (or negative attitudes towards other people) usually develops during the preschool years, but children continue to develop their capacity for prejudice during their middle childhood years because of the influence of reinforcement, modelling and imitation. Parents and teachers play a very important role in the development of attitudes in children – not only through the *information* that they convey to the child, but also through the *manner* in which they communicate this information. While some teachers may not, for example, express any *explicit* prejudice against homosexuality, their *implicit* prejudice may be revealed very clearly in their attitude and their facial expressions, body language and tone of voice when reacting to any kind of manifestation of homosexuality. The influences that cause children to become prejudiced are therefore often very subtle but powerful (Louw et al., 1998). The mass media also play a very influential role in reinforcing or dismantling the influence of stereotypes and prejudice.

Moral development

Moral development refers to the process by which children learn the principles that enable them to judge behaviour as good or bad and as right or wrong.

Rules and punishment

According to Piaget, children younger than about 5 years of age are *premoral*. This means that, because they do not understand rules, they are unable to judge whether or not a rule has been broken. Between the ages of 5 and 10 (in the phase of *moral realism*), children develop an enormous respect for rules, and they come to believe that rules must be obeyed at all times. They regard rules as absolute, unchangeable, 'holy', and an extension of the higher authority that they perceive to be invested in authority figures such as their parents, teachers or God. Although these children do not understand the reasoning behind rules, they regard rules as guidelines for acceptable behaviour and they believe that any violation of rules should be punished.

Children in this phase also believe in *immanent justice*. This means that they perceive sickness or hurt to be a *punishment* for the breaking of a rule. Children at this stage also believe that what *other* people (especially adults and authority figures) tell them to do is right, and what they themselves think is wrong. (This may become a problem if it leads children to accept criminal behaviour such as sexual molestation as right – or even as a punishment for something that *they* did wrong.) By about the age of 10, children reach the phase of *moral relativism*. In this stage they display greater moral flexibility. They realise that social rules are arbitrary, less absolute and authoritarian, and that rules can be legitimately questioned and even changed. Older children can judge an act by the *intentions* that prompted it rather than merely by its *consequences*. However, it is not until adolescence or beyond that children can understand morality as an abstract body of concepts constructed from sound reasoning and principled thinking. Older children in middle childhood are also able to understand and accept the concept of treating others as they would like to be treated themselves (Kohlberg, 1985; Louw et al., 1998; Piaget, 1932; Wong et al., 1999).

Sexual development

By the age of 5 to 7, the sex-role identities of children are usually formed and they know that their gender is fixed and that it cannot be changed. They can identify with their own bodies and they become increasingly inquisitive about body parts. Older children (grades 4 and 5) are often aware of their own sexual feelings and desires, and they often feel confused and conflicted about these feelings. They explore sex roles and they are usually quite comfortable about discussing human sexuality at this age (Davidson, 1988).

Curiosity about sex

Because they are curious about sex, children in the middle childhood years often engage in various forms of simple sex play. Sex play in middle childhood is usually experimental and it has nothing to do with love or sexual urges. Because children's attitudes towards sex are formed at an early age, the way in which parents and teachers handle sex play during childhood will have a decisive influence on a child's development. If parents react with anger or disgust to the sexual exploration in which children engage, this will communicate a powerful message (namely that sex is 'bad' and 'dirty'). It will also of course discourage children from ever asking any questions about sex. Such children will then look to others for the information they need to satisfy their curiosity. Their main source of information will usually be their peer group. Information gathered from a peer group often contains considerable misinformation and distortion, which can create anxiety in children. Negative reactions by parents to their children's questions may also give rise to adverse emotional reactions and guilt feelings in the children. The period of middle childhood should be used as an opportunity to teach children the correct terminology for sexual organs and sexual feelings so that they will be empowered to use the correct language when they are older (Wong et al., 1999).

Self-concept development

One of the most important resources that any child can have as he or she makes life choices is a positive self-concept. All the life skills necessary to implement knowledge, attitudes and values (life skills such as assertiveness, decision making, negotiation, communication, and refusal skills) are based on a healthy, positive self-concept.

Self-concept refers to the way in which a person views himself or herself. It is sometimes used interchangeably with 'self-esteem', which refers more specifically to the personal assessment of *value* or *worth* that we attach to ourselves (Gillis, 1994). In addition, the role that significant others play in a child's life is crucial for the development of a robust self-concept. The expectations and esteem that parents and teachers have for a child crucially influence the development of that child's self-concept. It is therefore essential for parents and teachers to make children feel that they are special, likable, worthwhile human beings who are valuable *in themselves* – quite apart from any capacity or ability they might have to make a contribution to the larger world in which they find themselves. Adults must help children to increase their self-confidence by being honest with them; by providing opportunities for creativity; by helping them to succeed in their activities; and by providing positive reinforcement (Wong et al., 1999). Teachers have an especially important role to play in the development of a sound self-concept in the child, because children with a poor self-concept are especially vulnerable to criticism and praise in the classroom (Gillis, 1994).

Studies show that a negative self-concept in children is produced by the following factors (Gillis, 1994; Wong et al., 1999):

- Insufficient appreciative attention or regard from parents or members of the family.
- The conviction that they are constantly ignored and not noticed (this makes children feel invisible and therefore worthless).
- Ridicule, excessive and irrational punishments and the insecurity that is caused by harsh and rigid (and inconsistently applied) rules, or (conversely) the insecurity caused by too few or no rules or parental guidelines.
- Physical violence and threatening or menacing behaviour; psychological neglect; sexual and emotional abuse; negative, cruel and humiliating labels (verbalised abuse) that make children feel worthless, useless and anxious.
- Inconsistency on the part of parents towards their children.
- Unrealistically high expectations or inconsistent standards applied to children by parents, teachers or significant others.
- Overprotective attitudes by parents towards their children (this makes children insecure about their own judgement and thus increases their levels of anxiety).
- Deprivation of basic necessities such as food, shelter and safety.
- Physical disability or a perceived physical disability.
- Unfavourable or humiliating comparisons based on racial characteristics.

Children with positive self-esteem were found to be more independent, creative, energetic, optimistic, self-reliant, sociable, assertive, self-confident, relaxed, extroverted and popular at school and less self-conscious than children with a low self-esteem (Coopersmith, 1967; Norton & Dawson, 2000). Self-concept is also influenced by a child's own achievements and by the degree to which he or she has the ability to regulate own behaviour. It is therefore vitally important for children to develop a high self-efficacy or faith in their ability to meet personal and social requirements.

General skills

According to Erikson (1968), children in the middle childhood years develop an interest in handling the 'tools' of their culture (whatever these may be) and become keen collaborators in any productive process (Meyer, 1997). Middle childhood is the phase in which children learn to read and write, and during which they also become ready and willing to learn and assume their share of household tasks. These tasks are usually related to the male and female roles that have been defined by their culture, and many children assume responsibilities for tasks inside and outside the home, such as baby-sitting, cleaning, and working in the yard (Wong et al., 1999). These skills are all the more relevant in our current HIV/Aids situation because many households have Aids patients who need to be cared for. Children can be involved in helping in small ways with such care. *However, it is very important not to overload a child with household or caring chores.* (See enrichment box 'Using children in home-based care – a warning!' on page 264.)

We can divide HIV/Aids education in the middle childhood years into two categories if we base it on the developmental characteristics discussed in section 9.4:

- The *foundation phase* for children in grade 1 to grade 3 (approximately 7 to 9 years old). HIV/Aids education in this phase is discussed in section 9.5.
- The *intermediate phase* for children in grade 4 to grade 6 (approximately 10 to 12 years old). HIV/Aids education in this phase is discussed in section 9.6.

9.5 HIV/AIDS EDUCATION AND LIFE-SKILLS TRAINING IN THE FOUNDATION PHASE

The grade 1–3 child (about 7–9 years old) is in the early stage of the *middle childhood* years. Although the child in the foundation phase may still show some of the characteristics of the preschool child, the middle childhood years are usually characterised by rapidly increasing levels of cognitive development.

Perceptions of illness, HIV and Aids in the foundation phase

Young children in the foundation phase do not really understand what illness is – mainly because they are unable to think operationally (Piaget, 1973; Piaget & Inhelder, 1969). Because the thought processes of young children are *concrete,* they tend to focus on external, observable, perceptual events, and they make no spontaneous references to internal, invisible ideas or concepts. Young children's perception of illness is therefore also concrete. They define illness in terms of the external, observable features that are associated with the disease, and they make no references to what might be happening inside the body or to the processes of illness. To young children, people merely 'look' ill, and they cannot understand the reality of what it means for people also to 'feel' ill and the fact that their internal organs are also affected by the illness (Walsh & Bibace, 1990).

Perception of cause, effect and prevention of disease

Children in the foundation phase have no concept of the causes, symptoms or consequences of illness. They cannot distinguish between 'cause' and 'effect' because of their limited ability to *classify* and to distinguish between different objects. Children in this phase tend to classify only in terms of one dimension. They therefore tend to group together different ideas or facts that have no logical connection with each other, and they group these ideas or facts into a confused (and confusing) class of their own. While children often group entirely disconnected and unrelated facts together on the grounds of their own subjective and 'egocentric' reasoning processes, they remain unable to *see* the correlation between facts that actually *are* connected (Piaget, 1970).

Because they are unable to conceptualise the *inside* of the body, young children do not understand how causes function and they therefore have no understanding of the meaning of prevention (Walsh & Bibace, 1990). Because of their *concrete thinking* processes, young children understand the consequences of HIV/Aids only in concrete terms, namely *immediate* death. They are unable to grasp the significance of intermediary factors such as time, medication or the process of dying.

Children in grades 1–3 are therefore not interested in the causes, symptoms, consequences or prevention of Aids or any other illness. If young children are asked what causes Aids, they usually give an answer based on one or other *observable* aspect of Aids that has nothing to do with its actual causes (as understood by adults). For example, when asked why he thinks people contract Aids, a young boy answered: 'Aids is throwing up a real lot' (Walsh & Bibace, 1990:257). While young children will often ascribe illness to germs, they don't usually know what a germ really is, what it looks like, and where it 'hides' (Quackenbush, 1988; Quackenbush & Villarreal, 1988). (They may have heard adults talk about 'germs'.)

While older children in the foundation phase often begin to distinguish between *illness* and *cause*, they can still not describe how the *cause* leads to the *illness*. Their explanations are often based on associations or *magical thinking* instead of on a description of the mechanisms of transmission (Walsh & Bibace, 1990). Children in the foundation phase who mention sex or drugs as causes of Aids usually do not really understand how such factors cause Aids. Their answers are generally based on what they have seen on TV or heard from adults.

Perceptions of people who have Aids

Egocentric perspectives and an inability to think logically dominate young children's perception of Aids. They associate Aids with people in their environment who (in their perception) seem likely 'Aids candidates'. Their perception of Aids as a 'fearful disease' also leads them to infer that all people who are seriously ill (such as cancer patients) have Aids. If someone in their immediate community actually *has* Aids, they often come to the conclusion that everyone who is similar to that person also has Aids. (They may therefore arrive at the ludicrous conclusion that, for example, 'All thin men with long hair have Aids'.)

Fear of Aids

In spite of their lack of understanding of what Aids really is, one of the main characteristics of the young child's perception of Aids is an overwhelming fear of the disease (Quackenbush & Villarreal, 1988; Walsh & Bibace, 1990). This fear of Aids may be ascribed to their emotional developmental characteristics. A child's fear of diseases is rather vague, supernatural and imaginative – and this in itself contributes to feelings of helplessness and being unable to exercise control over contracting diseases. These feelings of helplessness may lead to endless irrational fears and feelings of vulnerability in children. Exposure to television, pictures in magazines and frightening stories from parents and friends also serve to increase a child's fear of Aids.

Influence of friends and mass media on perceptions of Aids

Children in the foundation phase develop a sense of autonomy and independence from their parents, and friends play increasingly important roles in their lives. Children are also exposed to information about sex, violence and death by television programmes, videos, films and the Internet. The misconception often exists that young children are not aware of HIV and Aids. What in fact happens is that, as their social contacts broaden and as they are increasingly exposed to mass media, they hear more and more about Aids. Because of their limited cognitive abilities, children do not always understand what they see and hear, and they therefore often have many questions about HIV and Aids.

Perception of Aids as punishment for sin

Because the child in the foundation phase tends to evaluate behaviour only in terms of the consequences of that behaviour (reward or punishment), children often believe that people get Aids because they are 'bad' or as punishment for bad behaviour (Quackenbush & Villarreal, 1988). This view is related to a young child's fears and doubts about his or her own 'goodness' or 'badness' and the consequent fear of punishment. Misconceptions like these contribute to irrational fears about Aids and can also provide a powerful impetus to the development of prejudice in the minds of children.

Sexual transmission of HIV

Because children in grades 1–3 do not understand how sexual intercourse can be a means of transmission of the HI virus, it should not be discussed with children when they are this young. When teachers do present sexual information to children, they should treat sex as a normal part of development. (See enrichment box 'Children's questions about sex and Aids' on page 156.)

Summary

Children in the foundation phase do not really understand what HIV/Aids is and they have no cognitive understanding of or interest in the causes, symptoms, consequences or prevention of Aids. They are, however, afraid of Aids because it is something vague and menacing over which they have no control. Friends and the mass media and parents often contribute (unwittingly) to this fear. Children are also inclined to regard

Aids as a punishment for sin and they are often very afraid that *they* may contract the disease as a result of misbehaviour. In spite of the cognitive limitations that prevent them from understanding HIV/Aids, children often have many questions about the disease.

Implications for HIV/Aids education and life-skills training in the foundation phase

The main aim of HIV/Aids education in the foundation phase should be the reassurance of children and the eradication of irrational fears. In view of their cognitive limitations at this age, the HIV/Aids education of children should not include specific information such as causes, symptoms and prevention. They should instead be equipped with the necessary knowledge, attitudes and life skills to help them to avoid HIV infection *in the future* and to better understand those facts to which they will be exposed at a later stage in their education.

The following knowledge, attitudes, values and life skills should be included in HIV/Aids education and life-skills programmes for children in the foundation phase (Centers for Disease Control, 1988; Davidson, 1988; Pilot Project on Lifeskills, 1999; Walsh & Bibace, 1990):

- Children's fears of the epidemic and their anxiety about their own susceptibility to the disease must be addressed. Aids should simply be defined as a serious illness *which children of their age don't usually contract.* Adapt this information in a tactful way when there are children in the school, in the family or in the community who are in fact already infected with HIV.
- Assure children that it is not easy to contract HIV/Aids. Tell them that they need not fear playing with children who have Aids or children whose parents have Aids. Tell them that they will not contract the disease by sitting next to a child who has Aids or by sharing their lunch or cold-drink with such children, or by holding hands, or by giving someone with Aids a friendly kiss or a hug.
- We should make young children aware of the dangers of HIV infection in a very concrete manner – but without making them afraid. An excellent method that is very successful with young children is to teach them that germs have various 'homes' – and then to illustrate this concept visually by using pictures and

Enrichment

Children's questions about sex and Aids

Parents and teachers often find it difficult to answer young children's questions about sex and Aids. The following points should be borne in mind when answering a young child's questions (Wong et al., 1999:710–711):

- Answer the question honestly and matter-of-factly. This will encourage the child to continue to search for answers.
- Don't answer a question with a 'tall tale' or with anxiety. This will teach children to keep questions about sex to themselves, to create their own (sometimes harmful) fantasies and formulate their own (wrong) theories.
- First find out what the child knows and thinks. You may then be in a position to correct the child's (often wrong) explanation before you present the correct information. Using this method helps to prevent parents or teachers from giving answers to unasked questions.
- Be honest and use the correct anatomical words. Although the child may forget most of the information or words, your sincerity, openness and honesty will set the scene for further sexuality education at a later stage.
- Honesty certainly does not imply imparting to children every fact of life. When children ask one question, they are looking for one answer. They will ask the next question when they are ready.
- When children do not ask questions, take advantage of natural opportunities to discuss reproduction (e.g. a pregnant family member or a TV programme).
- Neither condone nor condemn the sexual curiosity that is expressed in sex play (e.g. playing 'doctor-doctor'). Rather express the view that if children have questions, they should preferably ask their parents or teachers for answers.
- If children ask questions about condoms, teachers can say that condoms are things grown-ups use to prevent infection with HIV. Children don't need them (because they do not make love like grown-ups do).

games. One can tell them that the cold or flu germ lives everywhere (on places such as tea-cups and glasses), and that this is why one catches a cold so easily. One could then go on to say that some dangerous germs (like HIV) live in the blood and one should be very careful to avoid those germs by never touching anyone else's blood with one's bare hands. Tell them that if a friend has a nose bleed or gets hurt on the playground, they should call a teacher or any other adult immediately and that they will put on gloves before they touch the blood. Universal precautions should be explained to young children in ways like this – ways that they will understand and be able to apply.

- Warn children never to play with syringes, injection needles or anything sharp that they may find on the playground, in the street or on rubbish dumps.
- Teach children how to keep their bodies safe and healthy and how to avoid anything that could harm the body. Educational material should focus on personal hygiene and health in general. Research has shown that people who care about their health in general are also less likely to become involved in high-risk sexual activity (Feldman, 1985; Van Dyk, 1991).
- Explain the dangers of drug abuse to children. Discuss drugs or behaviour in ways that can be comprehended by children who can only understand concrete experiences. For example, a warning not to take too much cough mixture or too many pain pills or to sniff glue makes far more of an impression on younger children than a general discussion of the evils of smoking dagga.
- Although formal sexuality education is not offered to children in the foundation phase, it is extremely important to equip children with the necessary life skills to cope with sex and HIV when necessary. From an early age, children should be encouraged to feel positive about their bodies and to know the body parts by the correct names. Sex and intimacy should never be presented in a negative light, and children should never be made to feel bad about themselves. If the question should arise, children must be assured that it is natural and healthy to feel curious about sex. Sexuality education for the younger child should focus on dispelling misinformation, on emphasising equality between the two sexes and on having respect for one's own and for everyone else's body.
- Teach children what sexual abuse is, how to try to prevent it and where to find help. Start by teaching young children that there are different types of physical touching – good and bad touches. A mother's caress or hug, or holding hands with a friend, are examples of good touches, while any kinds of touch (e.g. genitalia) that make the child feel uncomfortable are examples of bad touches. Teach children never to stay in situations where they feel uncomfortable. Teach them to shout for help, run away and ask an adult they trust for help. Let children practise this in school (shouting and running; saying 'No!' very clearly and assertively). Let them act out their reactions to different situations in role play.
- Although children are taught to respect older people, they should also be taught that such respect does not mean that they must do everything older people tell them to do – especially if it is wrong and makes the child feel uncomfortable.
- Teach children never to go to the home of a stranger, or walk in the street or fields with a stranger, or get into a stranger's car. They should also not do any of these things with someone they know (a family member, teacher or good family friend) if that person makes them feel uncomfortable or if the person is behaving strangely or abnormally.
- Teach children about the importance of family life.
- Teach children how to care for someone who is ill. They can be taught to do small things to make a sick friend feel better (e.g. make a card or take food) and to do simple things in the home, such as making tea.
- Help children to cope with death in the family. (See 'Children and bereavement' on page 247 for children's perceptions of death and how to help them to deal with bereavement.)

- The fear of Aids can be addressed by helping the young child to modify his or her absolute thinking about HIV/Aids. Explain, for example, that people do not die of Aids immediately, but that there is quite a lengthy period between the time they fall ill and the time of death. Because young children are unable to assimilate *reasons*, it is not necessary to provide explanations for these facts.
- Reassure children that the 'germ' that causes Aids 'does not know whether people are good or bad'. People with Aids are not bad people. Explain to them that contracting Aids is not a punishment for wrongdoing.
- Research indicates that people who have learned to be safety-conscious in general tend to be more careful in other areas of their lives as well (including their sex lives) (Baldwin & Baldwin, 1988; Williams, 1972). It is therefore to the child's advantage (in more than one way) to emphasise safety-consciousness. Children should, for example, be taught to be careful with electricity, fire and swimming pools and always to wear safety belts.
- One of the greatest gifts a parent or teacher can give a child is to help him or her develop a healthy, strong and positive self-concept. A positive self-concept and accompanying psychological strengths, such as self-efficacy and assertiveness, may help children to avoid child abuse, drugs, premature or unwanted sex and HIV infection.

Enrichment

Enhancing the self-concept of the child

Gillis (1994:80–81) suggests that parents and teachers can enhance a child's self-concept in the following ways:

- Establish a caring, personal relationship, and create an environment of acceptance and optimism. The child needs to feel worthy of your special attention, respect and appreciation.
- Emphasise whatever is worthy and good about the child, and boost morale by focusing on existing strengths rather than by trying to improve inadequacies or defects.
- Provide the child with opportunities for experiencing success and set goals that are relatively easy for the child to attain.
- Reward the child's achievements with approval. The child should perceive the approval to be genuine (and will experience it as genuine if it is sincerely given).
- Encourage children to change negative self-thinking attitudes (I can't) to positive self-thinking (I can).
- Use modelling, role play and assertiveness training to help the child reinforce feelings of confidence in his or her ability to perform a behaviour.
- Teach problem-solving skills.
- Encourage children to help other children in some activity (helping others is morale-building).
- When friends are present, arrange activities in which you already know that the child will succeed. Praise from friends (or praise given in front of peers) is very effective in enhancing self-concept.
- Initiate pride in mutual projects (e.g. with friends). It boosts the child's self-concept to be part of a team.
- Give the child responsibility at home or at school (e.g. allow him or her to care for a plant or a pet).

9.6 HIV/AIDS EDUCATION AND LIFE-SKILLS TRAINING IN THE INTERMEDIATE PHASE

Perceptions of illness, HIV and Aids in the intermediate phase

Although children in the intermediate phase (about 10–12 years old) are capable of operational thinking, their thinking is still mostly concrete and not abstract. In this stage they still find it difficult to think in terms of abstract hypotheses (Piaget & Inhelder, 1969). Their capacity for logical reasoning has, however, developed to some extent. This gives them the ability to consider different aspects of one issue simultaneously.

Perception of the causes, effect and prevention of disease

Children in the intermediate phase have developed the ability to distinguish between objects and to observe differences between things. They can distinguish between the physical and the psychological as well as between internal and external bodily experiences (Piaget, 1971). Children in this phase can distinguish between the causes and effects (or symptoms) of disease. They define illness in terms of specific symptoms experienced by the body. While they describe the symptoms of Aids as externally observable when they are younger, older children can realise that symptoms can also be internal (i.e. that they do also affect the 'inside' of the body) (Walsh & Bibace, 1990).

When they are younger, children ascribe the causes of illness to external factors such as concrete, superficial transmission (physical contact or touch). But as they grow older, they begin to realise that there are processes that permit the illness to get inside the body. Children will initially describe these processes in concrete and global terms (e.g. 'You swallow it' or 'It gets in your blood'). Children in this phase are also unable to think in terms of classes or categories of causes; they can only think in terms of discrete causes that do not necessarily have any connection with each other. When they are asked to explain what causes Aids, children in this age group will often offer a long list of causes from what they have heard in the media, from what other people have said, or from what they imagine to be the causes of Aids (Walsh & Bibace, 1990).

By the time they reach the intermediate phase, children can see a simple, linear relationship between cause and effect (symptoms). Although their understanding is still largely concrete and non-specific, children in this phase know that HIV can be transmitted through sex or blood, from mother to baby, and by 'using drugs' (Montauk & Scoggin, 1989). They are also able to make basic distinctions such as that 'not all kinds of sex' or 'not all drugs' lead to Aids (Walsh & Bibace, 1990).

Montauk and Scoggin (1989) found that the questions asked by children in grades 4–5 are dominated by their own everyday frame of reference. For example, when they asked about the safety of blood, their questions were about blood from their own or their friends' wounds. They also wanted to know whether HIV can be transmitted through 'blood-rituals' between friends, and by using pins as 'pea-shooters'. Children at this age also had a lot of questions about the 'French kiss' – not really because they were practising it, but because of curiosity.

Because their thinking processes are still concrete, children in the intermediate phase find it difficult to conceptualise prevention (Walsh & Bibace, 1990). In a study undertaken by Montauk and Scoggin (1989), only 4% of the questions asked by children dealt with the prevention of HIV/Aids; most of their questions were about condoms (no doubt out of curiosity).

The children in this study were, however, very interested in the clinical aspects of HIV/Aids. This is an indication of how preoccupied in general children of this age group are with the question: 'How does it work?' Most of the questions they asked concerned the difference between people having HIV and people having Aids, what the virus does to the body, and how the body works. Because their thinking processes are less absolute, the older child in the intermediate phase is also better able to understand that there is a time lapse between HIV infection, the final stage of Aids, and death.

In answering the questions of children in the intermediate phase, it is important to remember that their capacity for abstract thinking is still limited and that these children feel more comfortable with concrete answers to their questions and problems.

Acquisition of myths

Children between the ages of 10 and 12 years are very prone to the acquisition of myths. They get confused between fact and fantasy and between hypotheses and reality (Davidson, 1988). One of the reasons for this may be the fact that children at this age are not yet fully capable of hierarchical classification. They are therefore not able to classify things in subcategories of 'cause' and 'non-cause'. They are only able to form the overarching or super-class of 'causes' in which they combine real causes and myths.

Although older children often have a good general knowledge about HIV/Aids, they also nevertheless entertain many myths. Most of the questions asked by children in grades 5 and 6 in Montauk and Scoggin's (1989) study suggested the existence of myths. They asked questions about the transmission of HIV through toilet seats, swimming pools, food, coughing or playing with friends, and through animals, mosquitoes, rats and flies. Brown et al. (1990) found that 54% of the grade 5 children in their study believed that one can get HIV by using a friend's hair comb, yet 84% of them did know that HIV cannot be transmitted by touch. This finding illustrates children's inability to classify and their tendency to generalise. Because they learn in school that lice can be spread by using a friend's comb, they generalise from this correct information to the false hypothesis that HIV can also be spread through sharing a comb – although they know that HIV cannot be spread by touch (the super class). Concrete thinking is neatly illustrated by the following question from a young boy: 'If a man has Aids and gives it to a lady, does he still have it?' (Montauk & Scoggin, 1989:293).

It is extremely important to eradicate myths and misconceptions because they may lead to severe anxiety in children. People who believe in myths also tend to have more prejudices or negative attitudes towards people with HIV/Aids. For instance, Siegel et al. (1991) found that children with misconceptions about the transmission of HIV believed that children with HIV should not be allowed to attend school.

Perceptions of people who have HIV/Aids

A decrease in egocentrism in children in the intermediate phase can be seen in their description of people who have HIV/Aids. They describe people with Aids in more general terms and they do not see it in specific, personal terms (e.g. a specific person in their neighbourhood) as they might have done when they were younger. The older child usually associates HIV/Aids with *specific* groups of people such as 'drug users', 'adults' or 'naughty teenagers'. Children in this phase tend to dissociate themselves from groups that they identify as vulnerable to HIV/Aids. This is, of course, a defence mechanism because it helps them to cope with their own fear of HIV/Aids.

Because of their decreased egocentrism, children at this stage generally have the ability to see things from another person's point of view and to understand that the points of view of various people differ. They are also able to change their own understandings and adapt them if necessary (Piaget, 1932). They are often deeply moved by stories or by personal contact with people with HIV/Aids (especially children). This kind of contact helps them to acquire a greater understanding and compassion for people with HIV/Aids. Children are also more tolerant of uncertainties and ambiguities at this stage and they no longer insist on black-and-white solutions (Quackenbush & Villarreal, 1988).

Concrete fears about the transmission of HIV

The fears of children in the intermediate phase are more concrete. They are no longer afraid of vague, supernatural or imaginary things. Older children's fears about the potential transmission of HIV are therefore also more concrete. But because they have difficulty in distinguishing between myth and fact, causes and non-causes, children in this phase often entertain irrational fears about HIV/Aids.

The influence of friends on children's perceptions of Aids

Because the child in the intermediate phase is becoming less egocentric and more sensitive towards others, the peer group begins to play a bigger role in the child's social development. The child becomes increasingly sensitive to peer group pressure and wants to please friends (Davidson, 1988). Friends can influence the child in two ways in this stage: they are often the source of misinformation, myths and half-truths about sex, HIV and Aids; and they often coerce the child into experimentation with harmful behaviour.

The development of prejudices

Social development includes not only the formation of friendships, it also includes the development of prejudices and negative attitudes towards other people. Because prejudice usually develops in the preschool and primary school phases, special attention should be devoted to the eradication of prejudice. Children also tend to use a 'reversed' form of prejudice in the HIV/Aids context. This means that they will label other children who have characteristics that they don't like as having Aids. A child may therefore say something like: 'Susan is so fat, if you touch her you will get Aids' (Quackenbush & Villarreal,

1988:80). Children often tease and label others as having Aids in order to conceal their own fears and uncertainties about the disease. The unconscious belief is that if they ascribe Aids to other children with certain characteristics, they will magically 'protect' themselves from contracting the disease. 'I won't get Aids because I am not like that.'

Perception of rules about safety, health and HIV/Aids

Children in the intermediate phase can follow health rules, safety rules and rules to prevent HIV infection. Older children are also able to internalise rules and know what is right or wrong in terms of these rules. They no longer blindly follow rules to avoid punishment; they now follow rules because they perceive the rules to be rational and useful (Davidson, 1988; Piaget, 1932). If children in the intermediate phase are told not to touch blood with their bare hands, they will comply – not to avoid punishment, but because they know that touching blood might be dangerous if the blood is infected.

Perception of sexuality and the sexual transmission of HIV

Children in the intermediate phase are in different stages of pre-puberty and early puberty and they are very interested in learning about sexuality, gender roles and human relationships. They are aware of their own sexual feelings and needs, and they often feel very confused by them. Children in this phase can understand the sexual transmission of HIV.

Summary

Because the social world of children in the intermediate phase is in the process of expanding so rapidly, and because they can read well, they are very conscious of HIV/Aids and they usually have many questions about it. Although their thought processes are still concrete, they understand the concepts of cause, effect (symptoms) and transmission of illness (and HIV) well. However, children of this age cannot conceptualise *prevention*. Children in the intermediate phase are prone to the acquisition of myths and prejudice.

Implications for HIV/Aids education and life-skills training in the intermediate phase

The main purpose of HIV/Aids education in the intermediate phase is to help children identify concrete causes of HIV/Aids, to rectify myths and misconceptions about HIV/Aids and to prevent the formation of prejudice. The establishment and reinforcement of life skills are also important in this phase. The following factors should be taken into consideration in HIV/Aids education programmes in the intermediate phase:

- HIV/Aids education can begin by making an inventory of what children know, including what they have heard, what they have seen and what they think they know. The curriculum can then be adjusted so that it is relevant to a specific group of children, and so that it can prove, disprove or expand on what children already know.
- Affirm that people have natural sexual feelings. Provide basic information about human sexuality, and help children understand the changes occurring in their bodies.
- The transmission of HIV is one of the most important concepts to develop in the intermediate phase. Children in this phase are beginning to experience puberty and they are curious about sexuality and drugs. Information about the transmission of HIV must therefore be clear and straightforward. Give specific, concrete examples by using phrases and words such as: 'If you have sex with an infected person', or 'Using needles and syringes that have already been used by infected people', 'Blood transfusions with blood that has been infected'. Reassure children that all donated blood is tested and destroyed if it is found to be infected.
- Children at this stage are very interested in the functioning of the body. They find the functioning of the immune system and the effect of the HI virus on the body fascinating, and teachers should use this opportunity to explain both how a healthy immune system functions and how a deficient immune system (ravaged by HIV) functions. Make the explanations concrete by using metaphors, stories, video material, etc.

- One of the main problems with HIV/Aids education for young people is that they do not understand the long 'incubation' period of HIV infection. They do not understand how a person can be infected without also being sick. Use a metaphor to explain this important concept to children. (The story of the Trojan horse is an apt example because it explains how the enemy hid inside a wooden horse until night fell before coming out to slaughter the citizens of Troy.)
- Be sensitive when you discuss symptoms of HIV/Aids with younger children. Symptoms such as fever, cough, tiredness, night sweat and diarrhoea are so common that emphasising them may increase the child's anxiety. Most children (and their parents) often have symptoms like these, so they may begin to fear that they (or their parents) have Aids (Quackenbush & Villarreal, 1988). It is often more helpful to concentrate on the less general symptoms or HIV-related diseases such as *Pneumocystis carinii* pneumonia (PCP) or Kaposi's sarcoma when discussing symptoms with young children.
- The vocabulary of Aids should be increased extensively in the intermediate phase. How well children will understand Aids issues in the future will depend on the strength of their Aids vocabulary. Montauk and Scoggin (1989) found that children in grades 5 and 6 found it very difficult to ask questions about sex and HIV/Aids because their vocabulary did not include the necessary terminology. By the sixth grade a child should have come into contact with *most major terms* relating to HIV/Aids (Post, 1988).
- Explain the difference between HIV (the virus) and Aids (the final stage of the disease) in a simple way to children. Because the use of the different terms may be confusing to the younger child in this stage, it may be better to use the term 'Aids' to refer to *all* cases of HIV infection when discussing HIV/Aids with the younger child.
- Because children at this stage do not have a cognitive grasp of the principle of prevention, and because they are not really interested in prevention, teachers should concentrate only on those aspects of prevention that are relevant to the child of that age. A helpful way of introducing the concept of prevention to young children is by concentrating on general strategies to improve health (and therefore indirectly to prevent illness). Such an approach will focus on the principles and practice of hygiene and a healthy style of living. Note however that some children are sexually active *at a very early age*, and it is important for these children to know how to protect themselves by practising safer sex. Teachers must always have an open-door policy so that they can encourage children to talk to them when they have problems and questions of a sensitive nature. It may also be a good idea to display the telephone numbers of the Aids helpline, or the nearest HIV/Aids Training, Information and Counselling Centre, on the school's notice board for children to use in case they need private and confidential advice.
- Children must understand very clearly what is dangerous for them. One should establish a strong connection between dangerous behaviour that they should avoid and the everyday world of their own experience. Don't tell young children to avoid 'contact with body fluids'. Rather tell them not to share toothbrushes; not to shoot pins at other children; not to mix blood in 'blood-brother rituals'; not to play with needles; not to ask a friend to make holes in their ears for earrings; and not to touch the blood of a friend who has been injured. Children understand rules, and they will usually abide by these rules.
- To prevent the formation of myths, we must explain to children how they will *not* get Aids. Use examples from their everyday experience – examples that refer to matters that worry them. Don't ever tell children half-truths. Children should be reassured that they will not get HIV/Aids by sharing ice cream, water fountains, taps, toilet seats and toys, and that they will also not get HIV/Aids from the school nurse's (sterile) needles, or from travelling on a bus with other children. Reassurance on how they will not get HIV/Aids will help children feel less anxious about HIV, and

will create an atmosphere of greater tolerance towards people with HIV/Aids.

- Prevent the formation of prejudice. Language is a very powerful tool and it should be used wisely. Don't, for example, refer to 'risk groups'. Rather refer to 'risk behaviour'. Stress the fact that any person of any race or sex or occupation or status can get HIV/Aids. We don't only avoid prejudice in order to protect HIV-positive individuals; we also avoid it so that we can protect children. A child who is led to believe that 'only prostitutes and bad people' get Aids is lured into a false – and ultimately dangerous and self-defeating – sense of security. When Aids is ascribed only to certain groups, it is easy (and wrong) for a person to say 'I won't get it because I don't belong to that group'.
- When certain children in the school are teased about having Aids, it is important to act immediately. *Make a strict rule forbidding children to tease other children about Aids*, and find out what the children know about the disease, and why they are teasing a particular child. This cruel behaviour is often attributable to the child's own anxiety and unanswered questions about HIV/Aids.
- Concentrate on life-skills training such as general hygiene, positive self-concept, self-efficacy, assertiveness, handling of peer pressure, decision making and refusal skills. General safety rules such as avoidance of drugs and alcohol, and the prevention and handling of molestation should also be reinforced.
- Strengthen moral values and the love and security inherent in the family. Teach children to respect their own bodies as well as those of other people. Teach children that all behaviours have consequences, and that they should take responsibility for their own behaviour.
- Learners in grades 4–6 have a natural interest in 'how to fix things' and are often interested in what kind of treatment people with Aids are receiving. They want to reassure themselves that all problems have solutions. It is important to explain to children that there is no cure for HIV, but that HIV-positive people can prolong their lives by a healthy lifestyle and – in certain cases – by using antiretroviral medication.
- Teach children to have compassion for people with HIV/Aids.
- Teach children how to develop personal learning and research skills by looking for articles dealing with HIV/Aids in newspapers and periodicals. Teach them how to classify Aids-related issues into subcategories with headings such as politics, economics, human rights and statistics (Post, 1988).
- Teachers should be aware that information on HIV/Aids may upset some children – especially if somebody in their family (or they themselves) is infected with HIV; if they know people who are using drugs; or if they were sexually molested in the past. Children with special problems should be referred to an HIV/Aids centre or a psychologist for individualised help.

9.7 THE ADOLESCENT YEARS

The adolescent years range from about 12 or 13 to about 18 or 19. The developmental characteristics of the adolescent will be discussed below in terms of cognitive, emotional, moral, social, sexual, identity and self-concept development.

Cognitive development

Abstract thinking, decision-making abilities, scientific thinking, and adolescent egocentricity are all relevant to HIV/Aids education in adolescence.

Abstract thinking

Piaget (1972) described the shift from childhood to adolescence as a movement from concrete to formal operational thinking. Most adolescents develop *formal operational thinking* between the ages of 12 and 15. This means that adolescents can think in abstract terms and think about possibilities. They also have the capacity to think through and examine hypotheses. Adolescents also factor a future-time perspective into their thinking: they are not tied so much to the kind of here-and-now thinking that characterised their childhood. Hypothetical thinking enables adolescents to plan ahead and identify the possible future consequences of present actions. Health messages are often based on the ability *to think further than the here-and-now*. While health messages for younger children who primarily use concrete thinking should concentrate on the *immediate* risks or benefits of the behaviour, the emphasis of health messages for older adolescents should focus on possible future benefits. It should also demonstrate the very real connections between wrong choices and risky behaviour and the eventual manifestation of negative and undesirable consequences.

Decision-making abilities

As a young person's capacity for cognitive development increases during adolescence, so also does the capacity for decision making. Young people develop the ability to consider hypothetical risks and the possible benefits of various kinds of behaviour, as well as the potential consequences (whether desirable or undesirable) of such behaviour, and this ability helps them to make good decisions. However, the pressures of time, commitments, personal stress, unhappiness and peer pressure frequently compel young people to abandon their rational thought processes (Thom et al., 1998). Many adolescents are so overwhelmed by negative pressures of various kinds that they never find themselves in a position to make the kind of rational choices that would be in their own best interests. Such young people need special understanding, support and compassion. They should not be abandoned just because they never had the opportunity to make the kind of choices that would have made them happy.

Scientific thinking

Adolescents gradually develop the ability to think *scientifically*. This means that they can see the relationship between *theory* and *evidence*. They are increasingly able objectively to evaluate evidence presented to them and to change their theories in the light of new evidence. Scientific thinking often leads those who think in this way to eliminate stereotypes and myths. When theories that contradict stereotypes and myths are based on sound evidence, older adolescents are often able to change their beliefs. Scientific thinking also makes it possible for adolescents to consider all the aspects of a problem, and all possible solutions.

Adolescent egocentricity

Although adolescents are less egocentric than younger children, they often fail to differentiate between what is important to them and what is of interest to others. Adolescents are often very self-absorbed indeed. Elkind (1978) refers to this as *adolescent egocentricity* and explains it as the inability of some adolescents to decentre from their own focus. Adolescent egocentricity manifests in two ways that may have implications for their health-related beliefs and decisions:

- They are so self-conscious that they believe that they are the focus of everyone else's attention (*imaginary audience*).
- They believe that they are *unique* and that their personal experiences bear no resemblance to the personal experience of others (*personal fable*).

The influence of these two forms of adolescent egocentricity can be seen in adolescents who don't want to take their medication at school because 'everybody will notice' (imaginary audience), and in sexually active adolescents who refuse to use condoms because they truly believe that 'other people get HIV, but not me' (personal fable). Egocentrism usually diminishes as adolescents approach about 16 years of age. Despite adolescent egocentrism, adolescents can understand the points of view of other people and they can see how the thoughts or actions of one person can influence those of others. As their 'perspective-understanding skills' increase, adolescents develop the capacity to learn from others (Thom et al., 1998).

Emotional development

Adolescents experience certain emotional changes as a result of their physical, cognitive, personality and social development. They often experience negative emotions, mood swings and emotional outbursts. Their focus on themselves can contribute to feelings of anxiety, guilt, shame and embarrassment. On the other hand, because of their ability to think in an increasingly abstract and complex way, they are more likely to show insight into their own and other people's feelings.

Moral development

One of the most important developmental tasks of adolescents is to develop a personal value system or a clear view about what is right and what is wrong. In order to develop a personal value system, adolescents have to question existing values; decide which values are acceptable to them; and then incorporate these values into their personal value systems.

Once they can think in abstract terms and see that other people's perspectives and opinions may differ from their own, adolescents also develop the ability to approach moral issues in a more mature way. Although many adolescents are still at a *conventional level* of moral reasoning (a law-and-order approach), they begin to accept rules because they can identify with them and perceive them as essential for preserving the coherence of society (Kohlberg, 1978). Once adolescents develop some capacity for *principled moral reasoning*, they begin to see that absolutes and rules may be questioned because such rules may be based on someone else's subjective point of view – a point of view that is open to various interpretations and (therefore) disagreement. They will adhere only to rules that are useful, that support individual and social rights and that promote the common good.

Social development

Importance of the peer group

Because adolescents have an intense desire 'to belong', their social development is characterised by an increasing interest in and involvement with the peer group. The peer group plays an important role in the adolescent's psychosocial development. Interaction with friends satisfies the adolescent's emotional needs. The peer group serves as an important source of information and it also provides adolescents with opportunities for socialisation.

Enrichment

Moral development of adolescents

Thom et al. (1998:466–467) mention these factors as influencing an adolescent's moral development:

- *Cognition.* The adolescent's value system is influenced by the ability to formulate hypotheses, to investigate and test them, to make certain deductions, and to think in an abstract manner.
- *Parental attitudes and actions.* The relationship between the adolescent and his or her parents plays an important role in whether or not the adolescent will internalise moral values. Parents who are warm and loving, who are consistent models of commendable moral behaviour and who apply disciplinary techniques that promote calm discussion with their children of the effects of misbehaviour and the importance of upholding certain values, undoubtedly promote the development of moral maturity in their children.
- *Peer interaction.* Interaction among peers who confront one another with different viewpoints promotes moral development. Adolescents often advance to higher levels of moral development when they have opportunities to discuss moral issues with their friends.
- *Religion.* Some studies indicate that adolescents' attitudes to religion affect their moral development and behaviour. Hauser (1981) found that religious youths show greater moral responsibility than non-religious youths. They also identified more with their parents' attitudes, values and behaviour than youths who were not religious. Hauser also found less premarital sexual intercourse, alcohol abuse and drug abuse among religious adolescents.

Not everyone reaches moral maturity. Moral immaturity always has the following two characteristics:

- *Egocentrism.* This is an inability to see another person's point of view. In a moral dilemma, egocentric people consider only what is important to themselves. For example, sexually active adolescents who do not regard the use of condoms as a shared responsibility are reasoning in an egocentric moral fashion.
- *Heteronomous acceptance of others' value systems.* This means that the individual is under the authority of the values of others (such as, for example, his or her parents). Such an individual has not formed an independent and autonomous value system which they can truly call their own.

Conformity

A characteristic of adolescent peer-group relationships is an increase in conformity. *Conformity* refers to the tendency to give in to social pressure (in this case, peer pressure). Young adolescents tend to conform more than older adolescents because younger adolescents are very sensitive about the approval of the peer group and they conform so as to be accepted. They have not yet developed sufficient self-confidence and independence to make their own choices. Conforming to the peer group gives them the guidelines they need to make their choices. Conforming to the peer group might have some benefit, but excessive conformity can have a negative influence on the adolescent's identity development and on development of autonomy. Excessive conformity can also lead to high-risk behaviour such as early sexual activity, smoking, alcohol and drug abuse, and antisocial behaviour. Peer group pressure is, of course, not the only cause of such negative behaviour. One usually finds that the adolescent has been influenced by a complex interaction of personality characteristics, family pressures, cultural expectations, and educational and socio-economic factors.

Sexual development

Because of accelerated physical development during puberty, adolescents become increasingly aware of their sexuality, and their newly developed sexuality begins to play a large role in their interpersonal relationships. It is during this phase that adolescents also discover their sexual orientation (i.e. whether they have a sexual preference for people of their own sex, the opposite sex or both). They are often confused and worried if they experience homosexual feelings. Adolescents may also worry about the changes in their bodies. Although they may have many questions about sex, adolescents are often unwilling to ask these questions because they don't wish to be shamed by appearing to be uninformed (Davidson, 1988). The period during early adolescence may be the best time for conveying information about sex, for instilling values, and for encouraging critical thinking, because young adolescents don't feel the strong emotions (such as shame, fear and embarrassment) about sex and sexuality that many adults do (Pies, 1988). Even though older adolescents sometimes tend to think (or pretend) that they 'know it all', they often still remain open to information provided by trusted adults.

An important developmental task that adolescents face is to satisfy their sexual needs in a socially acceptable way so that their sexual experience will contribute positively to the development of their identities. There is widespread evidence that adolescents are sexually more and more active and at a younger and younger age. Perhaps these changes can be attributed to earlier sexual maturation, peer-group pressure, changed values and attitudes in society, and the powerful influence that mass media exert on young people. Although adolescents can understand that behaviour has consequences, they often do not believe that the consequences will affect them (personal fable).

Enrichment

Masturbation

Parents are often concerned about their children masturbating (the self-stimulation of the genitals). Masturbation occurs at any age and, if not excessive, it is normal and causes no physical harm. Masturbation is most common at the age of four and during adolescence. For preschoolers it forms a part of sexual curiosity and exploration. It may, however, be an expression of anxiety, boredom or unresolved conflicts if it is repeated too often and too openly (examples are a young boy who repeatedly touches his penis, and children who masturbate openly and publicly). Masturbation, like other forms of sex play, is a private act, and parents should emphasise this to children when teaching them socially acceptable behaviour (Wong et al., 1999:711). For adolescents, masturbation is seen as an opportunity to discover their own sexuality and to satisfy their sexual needs – especially if they are not ready for a sexual relationship. Masturbation nowadays is regarded as a safe sex practice and a way of satisfying one's sexual needs while avoiding HIV infection. Masturbation is regarded as a problem or as abnormal only when it replaces social and other activities to such an extent that it hinders the adolescent's development or social interactions (Thom et al., 1998).

They tend to be unconsciously under the spell of an illusion of personal immortality, and this dangerous illusion might well make them more willing to engage in unsafe practices.

Identity development and self-concept

According to Erikson (1968), one of the main psychosocial tasks of the adolescent years is identity formation – to ask and answer the questions: 'Who am I?' and 'What do I want from life?' Steinberg (in Wong et al., 1999:898) describes identity development during adolescence in the following way: 'Before adolescence the child's identity is like pieces of a puzzle scattered about the table. Both cognitive development and social situations encountered during adolescence push individuals to combine puzzle pieces – to reflect on their place in society, on the way others view them, and on their options for the future.' Social forces play an important role in the adolescent's sense of self. The people with whom the adolescent interacts serve as mirrors that reflect information back to the adolescent about who he or she is and who he or she ought to be.

As their identities develop, adolescents' views of themselves (self-concepts) also change. Adolescents' self-descriptions become less concrete and more abstract; they include less physical and more psychological components; they illustrate a greater awareness of themselves; and they include descriptions of themselves in terms of their social competencies (such as, for example, whether they are friendly, helpful or kind) (Thom et al., 1998).

We can divide HIV/Aids education during the adolescent years into two categories if we base it on the developmental characteristics mentioned in section 9.7:

- The *senior phase* for learners in grades 7–9 (approximately 13–15 years old). HIV/Aids education in this phase is discussed in section 9.8.
- The *further education and training* phase for learners in grades 10–12 (approximately 16–19 years old). HIV/Aids education in this phase is discussed in section 9.9.

9.8 HIV/AIDS EDUCATION AND LIFE-SKILLS TRAINING IN THE SENIOR PHASE

The young adolescent's perceptions of illness, HIV and Aids

The young adolescent in grades 7–9 (approximately 13–15 years old) has a much better understanding of illness in general and HIV and Aids in particular than the child in the middle childhood years.

Definition and causes of illness, HIV and Aids

The young adolescent can locate a specific disease in the context of a broader class of illnesses to which it belongs. They understand the concept of a *syndrome*, and do not see illness merely as a collection of symptoms without any causative link between them. They realise that an illness can result in external as well as internal symptoms. They can understand the causes of illness in more complex ways and can explain the interaction between multiple causes and the dysfunctions of internal body parts or processes.

While young adolescents understand that HIV/Aids can be caused by sex and drugs, they also appreciate that the causal factor (sex or drugs) does *not always* lead to HIV/Aids, but that infection will depend on the presence or absence of other important components (the most important being the presence of the HI virus). Younger children (in the middle childhood years) tend to think that sex, blood and drugs *on their own* cause Aids.

Young adolescents can also appreciate the *relative* susceptibility or vulnerability of all people. Although they still see some groups as being more susceptible than others, they realise that *anybody* can become infected under certain circumstances. They no longer restrict HIV/Aids to individuals or groups they perceive as different from themselves; they can distinguish similarities and differences between groups; and they can perceive themselves as members of these groups.

A complex understanding of the consequences of HIV/Aids

Apart from understanding the definition and causes of HIV/Aids, young adolescents also have a more complex understanding of the effect or consequences of HIV/Aids. Whereas the young child in the foundation phase sees death as *immediate* with no time lapse between the onset of infection and death, and the child in the intermediate phase sees only *time* as the variable factor between infection and death, the young adolescent in the senior phase can appreciate that there are *many variables* that are significant between the onset of infection and death. They understand that medication, care and a healthy lifestyle may prolong the life of the HIV-positive person. They know that HIV-positive people will eventually die of Aids, but that some will live longer than others.

Fear of HIV/Aids

Young adolescents have a more realistic fear of HIV/Aids than younger children do. Their understanding of the biological mechanisms underlying the causes and prevention of HIV/Aids makes them more realistic. They realise that, although anybody can become infected with HIV, certain forms of behaviour can prevent infection. In this way their fear is mitigated, because they know that they have control over the choices they will make. Although this knowledge unfortunately does not eliminate the irrational fear of Aids, it allows adolescents to cope more effectively with these fears, and to develop a more realistic and reasonable attitude to HIV/Aids. However, young adolescents' anxiety about being socially acceptable may put them at risk of being infected by HIV if they are pressurised into making wrong decisions. Some adolescents are afraid because they were already sexually active *before* they knew how to prevent HIV. Other adolescents are filled with anxiety because they have been the victims of sexual abuse or rape.

Prevention of HIV/Aids

The emphasis of HIV/Aids education programmes in the senior phase should be on *prevention strategies*. At this stage adolescents know how HIV is transmitted and how it is not transmitted. They also usually have a good grasp of the complex workings of the human body and of sexuality. The emphasis during this stage of education should be on the acquisition of life skills so that young adolescents will have the opportunity to acquire the skills to prevent infection with HIV.

Implications for HIV/Aids education and life-skills training in the senior phase

- Repeat the basic information given to the children in the intermediate phase about disease, sound health practices, basic human biology, attitudes, values and skills, but present this information with examples relevant to the *adolescent's* current world-view.
- Because young adolescents often experience confusion and stress (the result of their rapid emotional, physical and social development, and the constant onslaught of new experiences), it is very important to give them exercises to develop their self-concept in a positive way. A positive self-concept will instil self-awareness, self-confidence and personal pride.
- Because young adolescents are just *beginning* to develop the skills of abstract thinking, the facts and information they are given about HIV/Aids must be direct, specific, frank and concrete (Pies, 1988).
- What young adolescents need is a general and basic overview on HIV/Aids that includes a clear description of how HIV is transmitted, how HIV is not transmitted, and how they can protect themselves from the virus. It is vital to discuss all aspects of the disease, not only modes of transmission and prevention.
- Although young adolescents believe that nothing bad can happen to them, they do understand the concept of risk. The reduction of risk can be explained to the younger adolescent by using the metaphor of a seatbelt as protection in a car accident. It is important for adolescents to be able to identify the risk behaviours that they and their friends are involved in (not necessarily all sexual) and to

have a clear idea of how they can reduce the risks inherent in such behaviour.

- Young adolescents must have an absolutely clear understanding of what sexually risky behaviour is, and they should be equally clear about the risks of needle sharing. They should also be well informed about risk reduction techniques.
- Help adolescents to understand that it is perfectly acceptable to postpone sexual activity until they themselves really want to engage in it. They should be encouraged to understand that they do not need to engage in sexual activity because of peer pressure or the relentless pressure of modern media such as television, films, radio and magazines. Promote abstinence or advise adolescents at least to postpone engaging in forms of adult sexual expression such as intercourse. Stress the importance of having only one loyal sex partner in a stable relationship. Tell adolescents that if they are already sexually active (or using drugs), they *can* stop if they want to, they *can* seek help, and they *can* protect themselves effectively from infection.
- Be *specific* in your use of terminology. Make sure that adolescents know what you are talking about. If you use the phrase 'sexual behaviour', adolescents may think that it also includes kissing and hugging somebody. Rather use the phrase 'sexual intercourse' if that is what you are referring to.
- The importance of reinforcing life skills cannot be sufficiently emphasised. These include decision-making skills, communication skills, assertiveness, a positive self-concept, self-efficacy, self-confidence, handling peer pressure, and caring for oneself and others. Use role play so that adolescents can have opportunities to practise these skills in safe circumstances. (A good scenario for role play might be (for example): What would you say to a boy who says 'If you really love me, you will do it'?)
- Remember that the peer group is important for the social development of the adolescent and that participation in peer group activities should not be discouraged (unless such activities are harmful to the child). The teacher should rather use the peer group to influence the adolescent's behaviour. Peer education, where a member of the peer group provides the information, often works very well.
- Teach or reinforce the principle that men and women are equal and that they should respect each other. Emphasise that a man must always ask a woman's permission before having sex with her; that if a woman says no, a man should accept and respect her decision; and that any man who forces a woman to have sex with him when she has said no is a rapist (as indeed he is in South African law).
- Adolescents need to know how HIV/Aids affects their communities, their country and the world (Pies, 1988). Teach them to do research and to use the library, newspapers, journals and the Internet to get the latest statistics on HIV/Aids. They should also read about the financial and human cost of HIV/Aids.
- Adolescents should be given information on where to turn for advice, help and support if they should ever need it. Teach adolescents how to find resource and referral information in the phone book, on the Internet or from local community sources. Display the contact numbers for the Aids hotline, Aids training, information and counselling centres and local clinics in a place where adolescents can have access to them without having to ask for the information. The availability of confidential services is very important for adolescents – especially when they have concerns relating to sensitive issues such as sexual or substance-use behaviour. They will certainly be unwilling to seek help if they think that their parents may find out about the visit.

It is not enough to know *why* and *what* to teach young adolescents about HIV/Aids. It is also extremely important to know *how* to teach this information. Teachers should be trained to convey the information in a direct but non-threatening and sensitive way. They must have a very good knowledge about all aspects of HIV/Aids and the complex nature of the epidemic. They must also be given the opportunity to explore their own concerns about sexuality and drugs and to practise effective communication techniques.

Conveying safer sex messages is often a huge problem for teachers in the senior phase. Although some adolescents will be sexually active, others will be sexually 'naive', and teachers don't want to shock or offend them. This is a real dilemma because, while adolescents' rights 'not to have certain information' have to be taken into account, life-saving information that they will definitely need in future should not be withheld from them. One solution may be to give all the important 'theoretical' information in the first part of a session and to inform the students that you are going to demonstrate (for instance) condom use in the second part after the break. Inform the students that although you think it is important for them to have this information, they are welcome not to return to the class after the break if they feel uncomfortable with it. It is also preferable to separate boys and girls when demonstrating the use of condoms. Teenage girls often don't mind condom illustrations, but they frequently prefer the teacher not to use dildos (rubber penises) to demonstrate the use of condoms. In such cases, rather use an educational wooden condom demonstrator (available from Aids Education and Training, Johannesburg, tel: 011 726-1495) that does not resemble the penis too closely. Make sure that sexually active adolescents know where to go if they need information, condoms, etc.

> The value of promoting safer sex through education and communication campaigns risks being lost if young people do not have access to further information, advice, voluntary counselling and testing (VCT), reproductive health services, and treatment of sexually transmitted infections. Current best practice in youth-friendly health services shows that services should be affordable, cater to minors or unmarried adults, and offer free condoms in an atmosphere that guarantees confidentiality. Young people are especially concerned about lack of confidentiality and unresolved issues about parental consent. (In South Africa, a child of 14 years and older may, for example, request an HIV test, contraception or treatment for an STI without his or her parents' consent.) Flexible opening hours for young people who work or study will make a big difference to the number of people who use such services (UNAIDS, 2002:75).

9.9 HIV/AIDS EDUCATION AND LIFE-SKILLS TRAINING IN THE FURTHER EDUCATION PHASE

HIV/Aids education for adolescents in grades 10–12 (further education and training phase) does not really differ from adult education. However, it is important to remember that adolescents respond better to messages that emphasise their *rights* rather than their *responsibilities*. Assure adolescents that it is their right to have information, and it is also their right to protect themselves. The right to information and protection indirectly implies responsibility.

Davidson (1988:454–455) offers the following guidelines for HIV/Aids education in grades 10–12:

- Revise the information given in the senior phase, and make sure that the learners have correct information about the definition of Aids, the effect of the virus on the immune system, the transmission of HIV, the symptoms, the management of infection and testing.
- Reinforce the knowledge that adolescents can prevent HIV/Aids by abstaining from or postponing sex; by having sexual relations within the context of a mutually faithful relationship with an uninfected partner; by always using latex condoms (even in combination with other birth control methods); by not using drugs; and by never sharing needles or syringes.
- The needs of young people who are not heterosexual are often ignored or avoided, and they lack access to information about same-sex practices. Sexuality education must deal with the needs and questions of all young people, and if teachers feel uncomfortable about discussing safer sex with gay or lesbian adolescents, they should refer them to an organisation where they can access the appropriate information.

- While we should make HIV/Aids issues as real and vivid as possible, we should try not to frighten learners.
- Movies about HIV-positive people or classroom visits from people with HIV infection often help students to overcome their denial of the disease and give HIV/Aids a human face.
- The focus should be on *healthy behaviours* rather than on the medical aspects of the disease.
- Help adolescents to examine and affirm their own values.
- The ability to *plan ahead* is often a powerful deterrent to unsafe behaviour. Adolescents who have future plans (e.g. to study, to have a career, to have children) are often less inclined to engage in high-risk behaviour, especially young women when they know what devastating effects HIV can have on babies.
- Students should *rehearse* making responsible decisions about sex, and powerful and definite responses to risky situations.
- Students should know that they have a right to abstain from sexual intercourse or to postpone becoming sexually active. They should be helped to develop the skills they need to assert those rights.
- It must not be assumed that all students will choose abstinence.
- Information about HIV/Aids should be presented in the context of other sexually transmitted infections.
- It is important to be honest and to provide information in a straightforward manner. Be explicit. Use simple, clear words. Explain in detail. Use examples.
- Sexual vocabulary can be expanded to include the slang expressions or words used

Enrichment

Educational activities

Educational activities to build knowledge, attitudes, values and skills

Children and adolescents need a supportive environment in which to practise their decision-making and communication skills. It is not enough to teach young people to 'just say no' to drugs or sex. Young people should be given learning opportunities to practise effective and successful behaviour for living healthy lives (Pies, 1988). We can use various methods for instilling the necessary knowledge, attitudes, values, and skills. These include (Edwards & Louw, 1998):

- Graphic activities: the use of puzzles, games, collages, illustrations, cartoons, maps, charts, photographs, posters, transparencies and slides.
- Oral activities: panel discussions, short plays, role plays, dialogues, debates, reports, songs, talks and interviews.
- Written activities: essays, articles, letters, mock press releases, TV programmes, reviews, songs, plays, diary entries, poems, interviews and dialogues.
- Audio-visual activities: slides with commentary, stories on tape, pictures or photographs with commentary and videos.

Activity

- If you work with children (in a school, church, orphanage or any other capacity), identify the developmental stage in which the children are and then use the information in this chapter to develop an HIV/Aids education and life-skills training programme that will be appropriate for your group of children. Identify personal, social or cultural differences specific to the group, and devise ways to make provision for these differences in your programme.
- Many learners will become orphaned or lose close family members and will need emotional help and guidance from educators. Orphaned learners may face enormous financial hardship and have great difficulty in paying for school fees, uniforms and books. Others may be forced to remain at home so that they can look after their younger siblings and act as heads of their households. Some of these children may themselves be infected, or be caring for others who are infected and ill. If you are a teacher, develop a policy for your school to assist Aids orphans and children made vulnerable by HIV. If you are a minister of religion or a religious leader, develop a plan of action for your congregation or religious group to provide assistance to orphans.

by teenagers if that helps to get the message across more effectively.

- It is important to be non-threatening and to work in a way that alleviates (rather than creates) anxiety.
- Students should be given the opportunity to ask questions anonymously. They usually very much like the idea of a 'question basket'. (Put a basket somewhere in the class and invite them to put anonymous questions in this basket. Answer the questions in the group.)
- Discussion of dating relationships can provide opportunities and pretexts for teaching decision-making skills.
- Teaching about HIV/Aids can often be effectively enhanced by:
  - movies and other visual aids;
  - role plays and other participatory exercises;
  - same-sex groupings (to encourage more candid discussions) followed by sharing in a mixed-sex group (to increase comfort level in discussing sexual subjects with members of the opposite sex); and
  - involvement of students in planning and teaching – let young people (whenever possible) speak the message *to each other.*
- The importance of using adolescent models and peer educators should never be underestimated. Adolescents learn best when they learn from their peers.
- HIV/Aids education should include discussions of critical social issues raised by the HIV/Aids epidemic, such as protecting the public health without endangering individual rights, orphan care, the provision of antiretroviral treatment to all, etc.
- Teachers should have resources to help students find answers to detailed medical questions.
- Students should be taught the kind of research skills that will enable them to continue to evaluate the HIV/Aids crisis.
- Students should know where to go for help if they need it, and they should be taught how to access medical services if they need them.

9.10 CONCLUSION

The school has a very important role to play in empowering children with the necessary knowledge, attitudes, values and life skills to protect themselves against HIV infection and Aids. But the responsibility for protecting our children should not be left up to schools. Many children (school dropouts, orphans and others made vulnerable by HIV/Aids, and street children) cannot be reached by the formal education system. Churches, civic organisations, youth groups, NGOs and individual volunteers should all be involved in HIV/Aids prevention and life-skills training programmes so that children who do not go to school can also be reached.

The National Policy on HIV/Aids for Learners and Educators, and the establishment of a safe school environment are discussed in Chapter 19.

part 3

HIV/Aids Counselling

INTRODUCTION TO PART 3

There is a very great need for counselling and for skilled HIV/Aids counsellors. Professional psychologists, counsellors and psychiatrists often cannot cope with the demand, and many people don't have access to professional services. We must therefore train every helper in the HIV/Aids field to give basic counselling. Counsellors should also be trained to recognise serious problems and to refer clients if they don't know how to cope themselves.

The basic counselling principles and skills are discussed in *Chapter 10*. The values underlying the counselling process and the basic communication skills are explained, and practical guidelines for cross-cultural counselling are given.

The basic principles of pre- and post-HIV-test counselling are discussed in *Chapter 11*. Helpful guidelines and hints are given on questions to ask, information to provide, and how to handle the important issues of informed consent and confidentiality.

Specific issues in the lives of people living with HIV/Aids (such as disclosure, anxiety, depression and suicidal feelings) are discussed in *Chapter 12*. Particular attention is given to counselling children. Specific approaches to counselling, such as family counselling and couple counselling, are addressed.

Chapter 13 reviews the principles of bereavement and spiritual counselling.

Learning outcomes

After completing Part 3 you should be able to:

- apply basic communication skills to interviewing a client
- counsel a client who wants to be tested for HIV (pre-HIV test counselling)
- counsel a client who has tested HIV positive
- counsel a client who has tested HIV negative
- do basic counselling to help people living with HIV/Aids and their significant others to cope with the day-to-day demands of the illness
- do crisis counselling
- recognise serious problems such as severe depression and suicidal tendencies, and refer clients for professional help if necessary
- do bereavement and spiritual counselling

chapter

10 Basic Counselling Principles and Skills

Diving deep

And Koki swam through the black water
or he drifted silently with the sound of cool water in
his ears.
But sometimes he dived deep down
into the cold shadows of the pool.

HIV/Aids has forced us to think in terms of *caring* rather than *curing*. Because we have no *cure* for HIV/Aids, we must focus on *caring* for the physical and mental welfare of people living with HIV/Aids. After diagnosis HIV-positive people have to find ways of living psychologically healthy lives, and they need extensive counselling to be able to do this. This need will soon far exceed the capacity of all the trained counsellors in sub-Saharan Africa. The sad reality is that, except for pre- and post-HIV-test counselling, very few HIV-positive people in sub-Saharan Africa have access to trained counsellors. Everyone in the helping professions must therefore urgently acquire the skills of effective HIV/Aids counselling. According to Johnson (2000:2):

> The single most important requirement to be an HIV/Aids counsellor, is to have compassion for another person's struggle to *live* beyond the confines of a disease, and the willingness and commitment to walk the walk with this person and his or her significant others.

This chapter is based on the principles of the person-centred approach and the cognitive-behavioural approach. It will focus on the basic principles and procedures of the counselling process. It will also examine the values and skills that all counsellors need. Although the basic counselling principles, values and skills described in this chapter apply to *all* clients who seek help (irrespective of culture, age or presenting problem), the counsellor's approach may sometimes be adapted in line with individual or cultural differences.

10.1 DEFINING COUNSELLING

There are numerous definitions of counselling, but for the purpose of this book, the following definition will be used (based on Gillis, 1994:2; Sikkema & Bissett, 1997:14):

> Counselling is a facilitative process in which the counsellor, working within the framework of a special helping relationship, uses specific skills to assist clients to develop self knowledge, emotional acceptance, emotional growth, and personal resources.

The overall task of counselling is to give the client the opportunity to explore and discover ways of living more fully, satisfyingly and resourcefully. Counselling may be concerned with addressing and resolving specific problems, making decisions, coping with crisis, working through feelings and inner conflict, or improving relationships with others.

The counsellor's role is to facilitate the client's work in ways that respect the client's values, personal resources and capacity for self-determination. The intention of counselling is not to 'solve' everything by 'prescribing' treatment or giving advice, but to *help or assist* clients to review their problems and the options or choices they have for dealing with these problems (Egan, 1998).

10.2 THE AIMS OF COUNSELLING

Counselling must always be based on the *needs* of the client. Counselling has a dual purpose (Egan, 1998):

- to help clients manage their problems more effectively and develop unused or underused opportunities to cope more fully; and
- to help and empower clients to become more effective self-helpers in the future.

Helping is about *constructive change* and making a substantive *difference* to the life of the client. Constructive change can be measured by an increased self-understanding and self-control as well as by decreased emotional distress and progress toward self-identified goals.

The counsellor should have a specific focus: the client's response to being HIV-positive. This response can be affective (emotions or feelings), cognitive (understanding and thinking), behavioural (action and doing), or a combination of feelings, cognitions and behaviour. The counsellor cannot change the *adversity* inherent in the client's status or the events that caused it. The counsellor's sphere of influence is defined by the aftermath of the disclosure of the HIV-positive status – how the client reacts, how significant others react, and what impact these reactions might have on symptom development, the course of the disease and the quality of the client's life.

> The aim of counselling the HIV-positive individual is therefore to focus on life beyond infection and not to dwell unnecessarily on the constraints of the disease.
> (Johnson, 2000:3)

The counsellor's role is to help the client improve his or her quality of life by helping him or her to manage problems, make life-enhancing changes and cope with the kinds of problems that will arise in the future.

10.3 THE FOUR FUNDAMENTAL QUESTIONS OF THE COUNSELLING PROCESS

According to Egan (1998:24), all worthwhile helping models or processes that focus on problem management and change should help clients to ask and answer the following four fundamental questions for themselves:

- Current scenario
  What are the problems (issues, concerns, undeveloped opportunities) I should be working on?
  The answers to this question constitute the client's *current state of affairs* or *current scenario*. To elicit the *current scenario*, counsellors must help clients to tell their stories in such a way that the counsellor (as well as the client) will understand the problem situation. Counsellors must help clients break through 'blind spots' that prevent them from seeing themselves and their situations as they really are. Because clients often present with several problems and issues, it is up to the counsellors to help them identify and work on *those issues that will make a difference*.
- Preferred scenario
  What do I need or want instead of what I have?
  Answers to this question constitute the *preferred state of affairs*, or *preferred scenario*. The preferred scenario spells out possibilities for a better future, and it culminates in an

agenda for change. Counsellors must help clients to discover and commit themselves to what they need and want for a better future. Gelatt (1989:255) has said that 'the future does not exist and cannot be predicted. It must be imagined and invented.' Egan (1998:28) warns that counsellors should never move from 'What is wrong?' to 'What do I do about it?' without exploring the question 'What do I need and want?' Helping clients discover what they *really* want has a profound impact on the entire helping process.

- Strategies
  What must I do to get what I need or want?
  Answers to this question produce strategies for goal-accomplishing action. Clients now need to discover ways of bridging the gap between the current scenario (what they have) and the preferred scenario (what they need and want). They have to ask themselves what they have to do to get what they need or want. Counsellors must help clients to see that there are many different ways of achieving their goals. Counsellors should help clients organise their actions into coherent, simple, achievable *plans* that they will be able to carry out to accomplish their goals. A plan of action is a *map* the client uses to get to where he or she wants to go.
- Action
  How do I make all this happen?
  Answers to this question help clients to move from *planning mode* to *action, getting-it-done* or *accomplishment mode.* But action should not be the last stage of change. From the very beginning of the counselling process counsellors should encourage clients to act – even in small ways – to start the transition from the current to the preferred scenario. Helping is ultimately about getting the client to work towards constructive change. As Egan puts it: 'There is nothing magic about change; it is hard work. If clients do not act in their own behalf, nothing happens' (Egan, 1998:31).

To help the client answer fundamental questions about the current scenario, the preferred scenario, strategies and action, the counsellor should structure the counselling conversation so that the client, in telling his or her story, will be able to identify problems, set goals and bring about constructive changes. Dividing the counselling process into four phases provides a helpful framework to help the client answer the four fundamental questions.

10.4 PHASES IN THE COUNSELLING PROCESS

There is no recipe for good counselling, but dividing the counselling process into the following four phases might provide a useful framework:

- establishing a working relationship with the client;
- helping the client to tell his or her story;
- developing an increased understanding of the problem; and
- intervention or action.

These four phases are generic to most counselling or therapeutic models. They remain the same regardless of the counsellor's theoretical assumptions or model. The distinction between the phases is arbitrary (in practice the phases will overlap and interact), but they do provide a framework or map for the counselling process. This framework guides counsellors when they get stuck in the conversation; when they need to consider the requirements of the current phase (in which the counsellor and the client find themselves); and when they need guidelines before initiating new and unexplored therapeutic topics of conversation. Every interview or counselling session with clients consists of these four phases. A summary of the counselling model is given in Figure 10.1 on page 177.

The counselling phases, their goals, the counselling skills central to each phase, and how that phase helps the client are summarised under the four headings that follow (based on Brouard, 2002; Egan, 1998; Gillis, 1994; Johnson, 2000; Life Line, 1997; Pearce, 1997). Note that although the skills are *central* to specific phases, they are not *exclusively* relevant to those stages – the skills should be used throughout the counselling session when needed. The counselling skills will be discussed in more detail in Section 10.6 (page 185).

Phase 1: Relationship building

The *goal* of phase 1 (*relationship building*) is to establish an open and trusting relationship in which the client will feel safe enough to address personal issues and to disclose information to the counsellor.

The first step in relationship building is defining the relationship's objectives, process and parameters. This is crucial to effective and ethical counselling and is usually done in the first few minutes of counselling. The following points should be kept in mind:

- Provide a context that is unambiguously therapeutic. Establish a safe, confidential setting that clearly distinguishes the counselling relationship from social conversation.
- Provide a physical setting that is conducive to enhancing the therapeutic relationship.

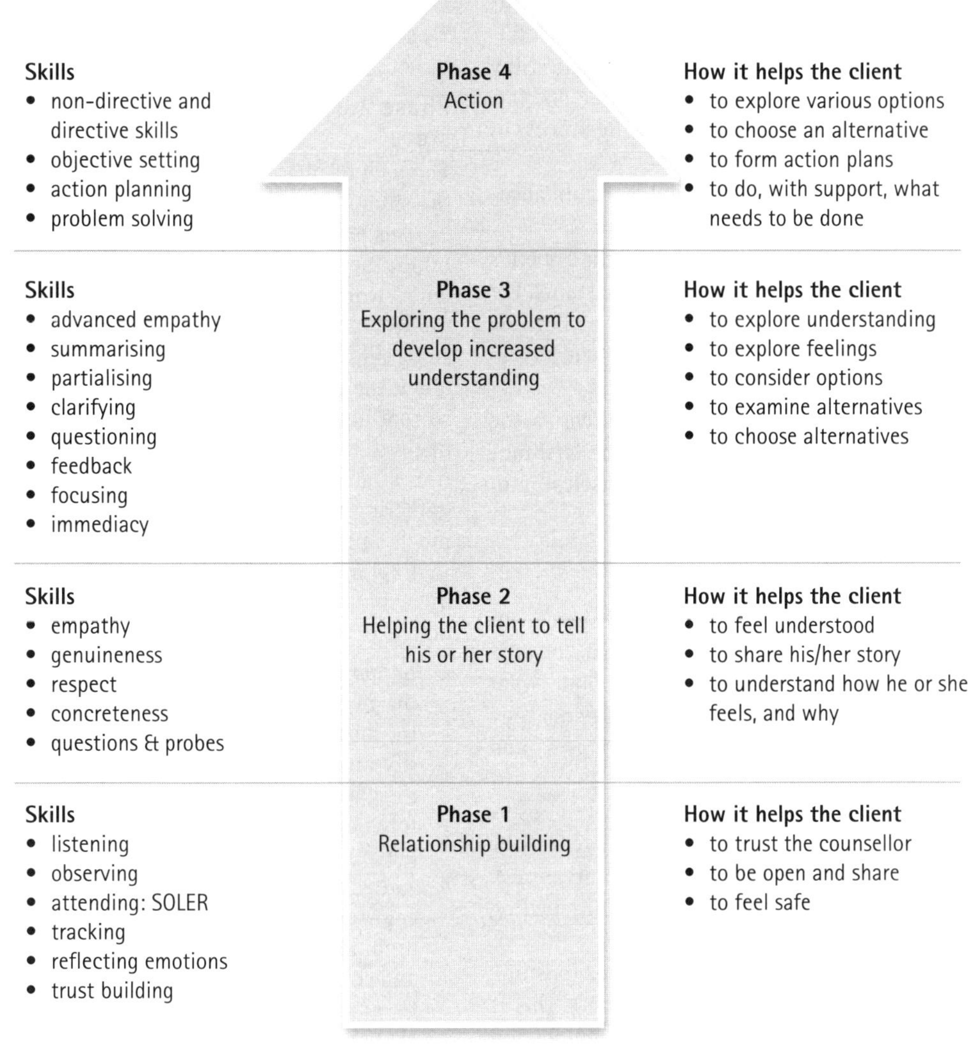

Figure 10.1
A counselling model

- Introduce yourself, the process and the context. Don't assume that your client knows what counselling entails. Brief the client as to the objectives and procedures of counselling, and give some idea of what is expected of the client, and what he or she may anticipate in return. The client must have no unrealistic expectations and should know that he or she is an active collaborator in the process.
- Allow the client to negotiate the definition of the relationship by listening, observing and confirming.
- Be sensitive to *how* and *what* you communicate. Convey the critical message of *trust* (i.e. that you are trustworthy), *acceptance* (by being non-judgemental), and *structure* (i.e. that you are skilled to facilitate the process of change).
- Assure the client that you will maintain absolute confidentiality.
- De-pathologise or normalise the client's response to his or her HIV-positive status. For example, if the client refers to a 'horrible affliction', respond by referring neutrally to 'HIV-positive status'.
- Do not be judgemental about others in the client's life. Convey your neutral understanding of people's reactions to the disclosure of the client's status.

Counselling skills central to phase 1

- *Listening skills.* Listen for and observe your own feelings (self-awareness), clients' experiences (what happened), their behaviour (what they do or fail to do), their feelings (what they feel in relation to their experiences and behaviour).
- *Observation skills.* Distinguish between observation (what you observe) and inference (the sense that you make of your observations). *Inference* is inevitably the source of labelling and blaming.
- *Sensitivity to non-verbal behaviour* (posture, direction, initiative and eye contact). This is achieved by applying of the communication skill of attentiveness (see 'Attending' on page 185).
- *Tracking skills.* Observe the client's initiatives and connect with the client at that level. Don't follow your own agenda.
- Being *responsive to the emotional tone* of the client's story. Show the client that you have understood him or her by reflecting his/her emotions in your response.
- *Trust building* through the counsellor's warmth, empathy, dedication, respect, acceptance and genuineness.

The counselling skills should help the client to:

- trust the counsellor; and
- feel safe to disclose information to the counsellor.

Phase 2: Helping the client tell his or her story

The *goal* of phase 2 is to help the client explore the situation and tell his or her story.

This phase is very important because it determines the counsellor's understanding of the client's world. This phase is often called the 'information-gathering phase' because the counsellor might spend considerable time finding out about the client's current and preferred scenario so that both can understand the problem(s) and begin to think about planning possible intervention strategies. How the counsellor goes about gathering information determines what and how much he or she understands of the problem.

Exploration of the client's story is facilitated by a supportive, client-centred approach and an active, benevolent curiosity.

- *Supportive client-centred helping* means that the needs of the client are central, and that the ultimate purpose of the process is to identify and implement actions that will improve the client's situation (Egan, 1998). It is therefore important to allow the client to tell his or her story in his or her own way.
- *Active, benevolent curiosity* relies on the counsellor's observation, questioning and probing. By using active listening techniques and communication skills, the counsellor tries to gain an accurate understanding of the client's problems, the way in which he or she is experiencing these problems, and what the client needs for a better future. The counsellor

should keep the following points in mind when exploring the client's story:

- o Learn and adopt the client's 'language'. To speak the client's 'language' is a vital source of understanding and communicates empathy and acceptance.
- o Use facilitative, open questions and not only closed questions. (See 'Probing or questioning' on page 190.)
- o Be sensitive to feedback about specific content.
- o Be respectful.
- o Be patient and revisit topics if it is necessary.
- o Avoid suggesting solutions and giving advice. Allow yourself time to develop your understanding of the client's world.
- o Deal with multiple levels of understanding. Focus on content or experience (what happened to the client?), behaviour (what did he or she do?), feelings (how did he or she feel?) and cognition (what does the client know or believe about an issue?).
- o Involve context in your enquiry.
- o Focus on *process over time*. The counsellor should attempt to understand patterns and trends rather than diagnostic entities (we do not only want to understand *that* the client is depressed, we also want to understand *how* he or she is depressed in terms of context and process).

The counsellor should resist the temptation to move to the intervention or action phase before the client's story has fully been explored.

Counselling skills central to phase 2

- *Accurate empathy*. Try to understand the client's world as he or she experiences it. Accurate empathy establishes trust and rapport and encourages self-expression. (See 'Basic empathy' on page 188.)
- *Genuineness*. Be yourself, be congruent, role free, consistent, spontaneous and non-defensive.
- *Respect*. Be non-judgemental and accept the person and his or her individuality.
- *Concreteness*. Identify specific feelings, experiences and behaviours. Avoid rambling, evasions and generalisations. Vague problems lead to vague solutions and vague actions.
- *Minimal verbal responses* such as 'mmm ... mmm' and 'uh-huh' can be used effectively to let the client know that you are still listening. The way the counsellor uses minimal verbal responses should convey patience, support, encouragement, warmth and caring.
- *Questions and probes*. Use questions and probes to elicit more information, but use them sparingly. Rather ask open than closed (yes or no) questions.

The counselling skills should help the client to:

- feel understood;
- open up and share his or her story with the counsellor; and
- better understand how he or she feels and why.

Phase 3: Developing an increased understanding of the problem

The *goal* of phase 3 is to gain, together with the client, a deeper understanding of the problem and to form the basis for specific action.

The depth of the counsellor's understanding of the client's world will depend on how well the client's story is explored. This will, in turn, determine the efficacy of the interventions. To gain a deeper understanding of a client's problem, the counsellor needs to look beyond the information gained in phase 2 by intensive listening and reflection of feelings. The counsellor must help clients break through 'blind spots' that prevent them from seeing themselves and their problems as they really are. Because clients often present with a whole range of problems and issues, it is up to the counsellor to help the client identify and work on *those issues that will make a difference*. The counsellor can help the client make sense of his or her world by expressing what is implied; focusing scattered thoughts; exploring and identifying themes in the client's story; and linking feelings, behaviours and experiences. To move from less understanding to more understanding, the counsellor should restate clearly what is hinted at, and restate clearly what is said confusedly. But remember to be tentative and cautious.

The counsellor's increased understanding of the client's world should be shared with the client. When the counsellor shares what he or she understands with the client, the counsellor conveys congruence, transparency and respect for the client's ability to resolve personal issues by themselves. By *not* describing his or her understanding, the counsellor introduces a power-political dimension into the counselling relationship. This 'power-political dimension' means that the counsellor uses his or her expertise, experience and (secret) superior knowledge to control and manipulate the client. Such an approach obviously constitutes an implicit but serious breach of ethics.

An increased understanding of the problem does not imply that the problems are more important than the solutions. But without a comprehensive understanding of the problems, the interventions or actions may be misguided and useless.

Counselling skills central to phase 3

- *Advanced accurate empathy.* This is the process whereby a counsellor helps the client to explore themes, issues and emotions that are new to the client's awareness. Advanced empathy challenges the client to explore deeper feelings. (See 'Advanced empathy' on page 192.)
- *Summarising.* This requires a sifting out of less relevant material. It clears the agenda of items that have been adequately discussed so that the focus can move on. It indicates that the counsellor has been listening attentively, and it provides structure and suggests patterns and themes.
- *Partialising.* This is the skill of looking at one big problem and dividing it into its various parts.
- *Clarifying.* Mirror what the client has said, rephrasing it in familiar language. This helps the client restructure his or her perceptions.
- *Questioning* extends the range and depth of the session; it helps in problem solving; it encourages the client to talk; and it allows for clarification and explanation.
- *Feedback or challenging* deals with discrepancies, e.g. between what is said and how it is said; it helps make communication clear and visible; and it makes denial more difficult.
- *Immediacy* refers to focusing on the here and now, and discussing directly and openly what is happening in the session (e.g. if the counsellor experiences the client as being provocative, this should be stated). This technique is valuable when a session seems to lack direction – reflect on and explore with the client what the reasons might be.

The counselling skills should help the client to:

- explore and understand the problem;
- explore feelings;
- explore previously hidden (or suppressed) feelings, emotions, attitudes or behaviour; and
- start considering options and examining alternatives.

Phase 4: Intervention or action

The *goal* of phase 4 is to explore intervention options and to take action to solve the client's problem.

Intervention is *not* offering a solution. It is a *process* in which the client becomes involved in order to improve the quality of his or her life. This is the phase in which the client answers the questions 'What can I do to solve my problems?' and 'How do I make it happen?' In some cases the relief of having shared pressing emotional discomfort with a counsellor is resolution enough for the client. In other cases clients need to adopt a specific problem management approach to be enabled to significantly practise problem management discipline or techniques. The counsellor gives supportive, client-centred counselling, and acts as an agent of change by facilitating the process in which the client envisions a better future, sets realistic goals and decides on methods to achieve them. The counsellor then monitors and evaluates the results by follow-up counselling. At the end of this phase of counselling the client should feel less confused and overwhelmed, and more empowered, enabled and focused. The client should be able to focus on an action or intervention that is realistic, motivational and obtainable within his or her own frame of reference.

Counselling skills central to phase 4

- *Non-directive counselling skills* such as basic empathy, advanced empathy, self-disclosure, immediacy, reflection and interpretation.
- A more *directive stance*, in which the counsellor attempts to influence a client's behaviour in a specific context, also has its place in HIV/Aids counselling. Directive counselling is helpful when the focus should be on practical, accessible aspects of the client's response to HIV/Aids. A client's concerns about infecting a partner with HIV could for example be laid to rest only by taking a directive stance and giving information about safer sex practices.

Enrichment

The problem-solving model

The following seven-stage process of solving problems may be useful to share with your clients (based on Brouard, 2002:128–130; Gillis, 1994:47–48).

1. *Defining the problem.* The most important step in the problem-solving model is defining the problem accurately and clearly. This often requires more time and effort than the other steps. Define the problem in terms of needs rather than solutions. Use reflective listening in order to understand what the client's needs may be.
2. *Brainstorming.* This stage entails the rapid generation and listing of possible solutions. Encourage your client to think of as many solutions as possible, as quickly as possible. Do not stop to evaluate the ideas as this will break the creative flow of ideas. Do not ask for clarification if you do not understand what the client means – there's time for that later. Encourage the client to think of even bizarre and crazy ideas as this stimulates creativity and at the same time helps to relax the client with humour. Continue until all ideas are exhausted. It is important for the client to realise that a problem does not necessarily have only one solution. In certain cases it is acceptable for the counsellor to suggest solutions. But always wait until the client has made his or her contributions.
3. *Weighing up each solution.* This stage entails reviewing each brainstormed solution and looking at its possible consequences. Ask the client to draw up a 'balance sheet' and write down the advantages and disadvantages of each solution. Usually the best solution is the one with the greatest number of good outcomes.
4. *Selecting solutions.* Now that the client has produced a long list of solutions and possible outcomes, it is time to select one of them according to its feasibility, practicality and acceptability. Often one solution will stand out as clearly superior. If not, ask the client to choose the most favourable solutions. Remember that many clients struggle with making choices because they lack confidence or self-esteem, or because they have made bad choices in the past. Be patient, give support gently and encourage the client to learn the skill of making choices. Keep in mind that the client may choose a particular solution that does not seem the obvious choice to you, but this option might work better for the client.
5. *Making an action plan.* Now that a solution has been chosen, it is necessary to think about how to put this into practice. Ask the client 'who, what, when, how, where' questions so that the plan is specific, manageable, achievable, realistic and has steps and a time frame. Encourage the client to write the plan down.
6. *Taking action.* The client must now put the plan into practice. Many clients will be anxious about this. Acknowledge this normal fear. Some clients may resist taking action. This resistance should be explored. Some people develop entrenched patterns which they are afraid to change. Others have 'gained' something from their dysfunctional behaviour, such as attention or control, and are reluctant to give this up. In this case, explore these 'rewards' and gently steer the client in the direction of change, if possible.
7. *Reviewing.* If the client returns to counselling for a follow-up visit, review the actions he or she has taken. This is an important opportunity to see what worked and what did not and why. Support positive outcomes and behaviours and explore negative outcomes. If there will not be a follow-up session with the client, encourage him or her to review actions and to go back into the problem-solving steps if it is necessary to find another solution.

- *Problem-solving skills* involve understanding the problem; discussing alternatives and possible solutions to the problem through brainstorming; exploring the consequences of all alternatives discussed; deciding on the best option; looking at how to go about doing it; and taking action. Talk about the action taken, and evaluate it in a follow-up visit.

The counselling skills should help the client to:
- explore various options and examine intervention alternatives;
- choose an alternative;
- form an action plan or plans; and
- do, with support, what needs to be done.

Termination of the counselling session

A counselling session is often terminated naturally without much prompting or planning. Before termination, it is important to summarise meaningfully; to reiterate the plan of action; to clarify referrals if necessary; and to diarise follow-up sessions.

Counsellors (especially lay counsellors) often find it difficult to terminate or to end a counselling relationship. This can be harmful to the client. By purposefully ending a counselling relationship the counsellor sends a clear message to the client that he or she is capable of continuing with the work initiated in the counselling session. Keeping the relationship open indefinitely conveys the message that the client cannot change or grow without the counsellor (Kluckow, 2004). Termination should be discussed at the beginning of the counselling relationship so that the client knows what to expect.

There are a number of reasons why counsellors often find it difficult to terminate a counselling relationship. Here are some that should be avoided (Kluckow, 2004):
- The counsellor gets more out of the counselling relationship than the client (in terms of self-esteem and sense of self-worth).
- The counsellor has a rescuing mentality, and needs to believe that the client will not make it without help.
- The client wants to maintain contact with the counsellor in a dependency-type relationship, and therefore does not make progress.

Note: According to the Health Professions Council of South Africa, a registered counsellor may see a client for a maximum of four sessions (or six hours) in total. Thereafter the client must be referred to a registered psychologist for further counselling or therapy. Lay counsellors should apply the rules of the service providers they work for – which is usually a maximum of three sessions.

10.5 ETHICS AND VALUES IN THE COUNSELLING PROCESS

The counsellor's values and attitudes play a critical role in the helping process. The way counsellors see themselves, their clients, the helping process, and the world around them will affect the way in which they counsel.

Counsellors deal with the most intimate part of a client's being. Counsellors should therefore enter the helping process with a sincere *respect* for their clients, an open and genuine *attitude*, the *intention* of helping their clients *empower* themselves and take *responsibility* for their own lives, and respect for observing *confidentiality*.

Respect

Respect is an *attitude* that portrays the belief that every person is a worthy being who is competent to decide what he or she really wants; has the potential for growth; and has the abilities to achieve what he or she really wants from life. Respect is fundamental to the helping relationship. 'Without the attitude and belief that every person is worthy of our respect and esteem, the counsellor cannot communicate empathetically or facilitate growth because he or she will not be able to create an atmosphere of acceptance and freedom in which the client can reveal his or her deepest, darkest and most painful experiences without fear of rejection' (Du Toit et al., 1998:77).

A counsellor can show his or her respect to clients in the following ways (Du Toit et al., 1998; Egan, 1998; Long, 1996):
- Accept the client by showing *unconditional positive regard*. This means that you as counsellor accept the client as he or she is, irrespective of the client's values or behaviour

and of whether you as counsellor approve of those values and behaviour. It does not mean that the counsellor has no own values or aims; only that during counselling the client's values come first. Giving unconditional positive regard is extremely important in the HIV/Aids field. A judgemental counsellor who condemns clients or shows offence at their sexual behaviour will only cause harm. Such a counsellor will not be able to facilitate healing.

- Respect the client's *rights*. Individuals have a right to be *who they are* – a right to their own feelings, beliefs, opinions, and choices.
- Respect the *uniqueness* of each client. The counsellor should not generalise. Although we have a lot in common, everyone is different and every problem is experienced differently. The counsellor should work with the specific characteristics, behaviour and needs of each client.
- Refrain from *judgement*. Counsellors are there to help their clients, not to judge or to blame them. HIV-positive people often already feel 'guilty' or 'bad', so a non-judgemental attitude from the counsellor is essential to understanding and growth because it encourages clients to be more accepting of themselves.
- Remain *serene* and *imperturbable*, and never react with embarrassment, shock or disapproval when people discuss painful situations or their sexual practices with you.
- Realise that respect is always both *considerate* and *tough-minded*. Although the counsellor should 'be for the client', this does not mean that the counsellor will always take the client's side or act as the client's advocate. 'Being for' means taking the client's point of view *seriously* – even when it needs to be challenged.
- Inherent in respect is acknowledgement and honouring of individual *diversity* in culture, ethnicity, spirituality, sexual orientation, family, educational level and socio-economic status. Avoid stereotyping while respecting people's *customs and choices*.
- When doing group counselling (e.g. in the workplace, or when seeing a family), accept the values of the group as well as the differences within the group. A counsellor shows respect in a group by carefully listening, understanding and accepting what group members are saying within their context or frame of reference.

Genuineness or congruence

Genuineness or congruence refers to a counsellor's attitudes to and behaviour with clients. A *congruent* person is honest and transparent in the counselling relationship because he or she surrenders all roles and facades (Rogers, 1980). A genuine or congruent counsellor demonstrates the following values or behaviour in dealings with clients (Egan, 1998; Gladding, 1996; Okun, 1997):

- Be *yourself*. Be real and sincere, honest and clear. Speak and act congruently in the helping relationship – practise what you preach.
- Be *honest* with yourself and your clients.
- Don't *overemphasise* the helping role and don't take refuge in the role of counsellor. Helping other people should be an integral part of your lifestyle. It is not a role that you should play only when you need to.
- Don't be *patronising* or *condescending*.
- Keep the *client's agenda* in focus. Don't pursue your own agenda or inflict yourself on others.
- Don't be *defensive*. Know your own strengths and weaknesses.
- Strive towards achieving *openness* and *self-acceptance*. This will help you to accept people whose behaviour conflicts with your values. Remember that it is impossible to hide negative feelings from clients – they will sense your incongruence.
- Develop *self-awareness*. Identify and reflect on personal qualities, life experiences, helping style, vulnerabilities and value conflicts that may affect your work with clients. Express your personal strengths in your counselling work, but also ensure that struggles or conflicts you may be experiencing do not compromise the counselling relationship.
- When a client reacts negatively to you or criticises you, examine the behaviour that might have caused the client to think nega-

tively. Try to understand the client's point of view and continue to work with him or her. To be able to help others you need to be at ease with yourself and able to examine negative criticism calmly, objectively and dispassionately.

Empowerment and self-responsibility

One of the values underlying counselling should be the desire to empower clients to take responsibility for themselves and to identify, develop and use resources that will be effective agents of change. This should take place in their everyday lives as well as in the counselling sessions. The empowerment of clients should be based on the following values (Egan, 1998:52–53):

- Believe in your client's pursuit of *growth, self-actualisation* and *self-determination.* View this pursuit in terms of the *client's* frame of reference and accept that you as counsellor cannot decide what the client's goals should be or what would be best for him or her. Accept the principle that clients know themselves better than anyone else, and that they are therefore in the best position to explore, expose and understand themselves.
- Believe in clients' *ability to change* if they choose to. Clients have more resources for managing problems than they, or sometimes their helpers, assume. The counsellor's basic attitude should be that clients have the resources both to participate in the counselling process and to manage their lives more effectively. Since these resources may be blocked or disabled in a variety of ways, it is the task of the counsellor to help clients identify, free and utilise these resources. This is one of the main aims of counselling.
- Refrain from *rescuing* the client. Rescuing means the voluntary, *unnecessary* assumption of responsibility for another person's feelings, choices or actions. Rescuing is implicitly disrespectful of the other person's ability to take responsibility for himself or herself. Rescuing reflects the *rescuer's* needs. It is typically motivated by lack of confidence in the capability of the person being rescued, a need to feel important, or a need to be needed (Long, 1996).
- *Share* the helping process with clients. Clients have the right to know what they are getting into. Explain to them exactly what the helping process entails, what they can expect from you, and vice versa.
- Help clients to see counselling sessions as *work sessions.* Only the client can make change happen. The counsellor can merely facilitate the process of change.
- Help clients become *better problem solvers.* Help them apply problem-solving techniques to their current problem situations, and help them to adopt more effective approaches to future problems.

Confidentiality

Confidentiality in the counselling context is non-negotiable. A counsellor may not, under any circumstances, disclose the HIV status *or any other information* to anybody without the express permission of the client. Confidentiality is an expression of the counsellor's respect for the client.

Confidentiality in the HIV/Aids field is controversial. Counsellors often become involved in endless debates about the rights of HIV-positive individuals as opposed to the rights of their partners and the rights of the community in general. HIV/Aids is, after all, a very serious and life-threatening condition. However, it is not the task or responsibility of the counsellor alone to solve these moral dilemmas. Counselling is a *partnership* and a relationship of *shared* responsibility between counsellor and client (Du Toit et al., 1998).

Whenever the counsellor feels overwhelmed by moral demands or a sense of responsibility, he or she should fall back on this partnership, and decide on a course of action together with the client. If a counsellor feels that it is necessary to disclose a client's HIV-positive status to a third party (e.g. for referral purposes or to protect a sex partner if the client refuses to use condoms), the reasons for the disclosure must be explained to the client. The counsellor must convince the client that the disclosure will be in everybody's best interest. However, the information may be disclosed only with the express permission of the client. If the client still refuses, the counsellor has to respect this decision.

10.6 BASIC COMMUNICATION SKILLS FOR COUNSELLING

Counselling is a *conversation* or *dialogue* between the counsellor and client, and the counsellor needs certain communication skills in order to build a relationship and facilitate change. These include attending, listening, basic empathy, probing, clarification, reflective commenting and summarising (Egan, 1998).

Attending

Attending refers to the ways in which counsellors can be 'with' their clients, both physically and psychologically (Egan, 1998:62). Effective attending (the way you relate physically and psychologically to clients) tells clients that you are with them and that they can share their world with you. Effective attending also puts you in a position to listen carefully to what your clients are saying.

Counsellors can use certain non-verbal skills when attending to their clients. Egan (1998:63–64) summarises these skills under the acronym SOLER. The counsellor should, however, be sensitive to the individual and cultural differences that manifest in the way people show and react to attentiveness (see 'Attending skills' on page 198). These skills are only external *guidelines* to help you show your inner attitudes and values of respect and genuineness. There are also other ways to show these attitudes. It is important for both the counsellor and the client to feel comfortable with the way in which attentiveness is expressed.

S Face the client *Squarely*. Adopt a posture that indicates involvement. The word *squarely* may be taken literally or metaphorically to mean that the bodily orientation you adopt should convey the message that you are involved with the client. If facing a person squarely is threatening to that person, a more angled position may be preferable – as long as you pay attention to the client. A desk between you and your client may, for instance, create a psychological barrier between you.

O Adopt an *Open* posture. Ask yourself to what degree your posture communicates openness and availability to the client. Crossed legs and crossed arms may be interpreted as diminished involvement with the client or even unavailability or remoteness, while an open posture can be a sign that you are open to the client and to what he or she has to say. The word *open* can also be taken literally or metaphorically. This means that you can still be attentive – even if you cross your legs.

L *Lean* towards the client (when appropriate) to show your involvement. A slight inclination towards the client might be a way of signalling that you are listening with empathy, while leaning back can convey the opposite message. Egan (1998) warns that leaning too far forward, or doing it too soon after meeting a client for the first time, may frighten the client because the client may interpret it as a demand for some kind of (premature) closeness or intimacy. If you read the client's body language, you can prevent yourself from making mistakes.

E Maintain good *Eye* contact, but don't stare. Eye contact with a client conveys the message that you are interested in what the client has to say. If you catch yourself looking away frequently, ask yourself why you are reluctant to get involved with this person or why you feel so uncomfortable in his or her presence. Be aware that direct eye contact is not regarded as acceptable in all cultures (see 'Attending skills' on page 198).

R Try to be *Relaxed* or natural with the client. Don't fidget nervously or put on distracting facial expressions. The client may wonder what it is that makes you so nervous! Being relaxed means that you are comfortable with using your body as a vehicle of personal contact and expression and for putting the client at ease.

Effective attending puts counsellors in a position to listen carefully to what their clients are saying or not saying. Attend to the client's body language, and not only your own.

Activity

> Watch two people in a public place, intimately engaged in conversation. How many of the skills of attending (SOLER) do they show? Can you see that the skills of attending are natural skills, and that all people who really care for others display them?

Listening

'Listening' refers to the ability of counsellors to capture and understand the messages clients communicate as they tell their stories, whether those messages are transmitted verbally or non-verbally, clearly or vaguely (Egan, 1998:62). Clients want more than the physical presence of the counsellor: they want the counsellor to be present psychologically, socially and emotionally.

According to Egan, active listening involves the following four skills:

- Listening to and understanding the client's *verbal* messages. When a client tells you his or her story, it usually comprises a mixture of experiences (what happened), behaviours (what the client did or failed to do), and affect (the feelings or emotions associated with the experiences and behaviour). The counsellor's first task is to listen carefully to what the client has to say. Listen to the mix of experiences, behaviour and feelings the client uses to describe the problem situation. Also 'hear' what the client is *not* saying.
- Listening to and interpreting the client's *non-verbal* messages. Counsellors should learn how to listen to and read non-verbal messages such as *bodily behaviour* (posture, body movement and gestures), *facial expressions* (smiles, frowns, raised eyebrows, twisted lips), *voice-related behaviour* (tone, pitch, voice level, intensity, inflection, spacing of words, emphases, pauses, silences and fluency), *observable physiological responses* (quickened breathing, a temporary rash, blushing, paleness, pupil dilation), *general appearance* (grooming and dress), and *physical appearance* (fitness, height, weight, complexion). Counsellors must learn how to 'read' these messages without distorting or over-interpreting them. They must also learn to listen to the whole context of the helping conversation – to verbal and non-verbal messages – without becoming fixated on specific details.
- Listening to and understanding the client in *context*. 'People are more than the sum of their verbal and non-verbal messages' (Egan, 1998:72). The counsellor should listen to the whole person in the context of his or her social settings.
- Listening with *empathy*. Empathic listening involves attending, observing and listening ('being with' the client) in such a way that the counsellor develops an understanding of the client and his or her world. Empathic counselling is *selfless* because it requires helpers to put their own concerns aside to be fully 'with' their clients. Skilled helpers also listen to any 'slant' or 'spin' that clients may give their story. While clients' feelings about themselves, others and the world are real, their *perceptions* are often distorted. 'Tough-minded' listening is needed to detect the gaps and distortions that are part of the client's experienced reality (so that it can be challenged at a later, more appropriate stage, if necessary). According to Egan (p. 75), 'to be client-centred, helpers must first be reality-centred'.

Roadblocks to effective listening

Active listening is unfortunately not an easy skill to acquire. Counsellors should be aware of the following hindrances to effective listening (Brouard, 2002; Egan, 1998:75–78):

- *Inadequate or on-off listening.* It is easy to be distracted from what other people are saying if you allow yourself to get lost in your own thoughts or if you begin to think about what you intend to say in reply. Counsellors are also often distracted because they have problems of their own, feel ill, or become distracted by social and cultural differences between themselves and their clients. All these factors make it difficult to listen to and understand their clients. The counsellor can overcome on-off listening by paying attention to more than the words (trying to pick up on the feeling level) and by watching non-verbal signs like gestures, facial expression and hesitation.

- *Evaluative listening.* Most people listen evaluatively to others. This means that they are judging and labelling what the other person is saying as right/wrong, good/bad, acceptable/unacceptable, relevant/irrelevant, etc. They then tend to respond evaluatively or with criticism as well. Criticism may leave a client feeling incompetent and it may diminish his or her self-esteem.

Enrichment

The art of listening – questions to ask yourself

- Do I concentrate fully and tune out all other distractions and thoughts?
- Do I make an effort to become truly interested in what the client is saying? Faking attention or pretending to listen are blocks to good communication.
- Do I try to see the world from the client's point of view?
- Do I listen 'between the lines' to the meaning behind the person's words? Listening for understanding helps decoding of the underlying message.
- Do I listen actively or passively? Active listening requires keeping up with the person, asking questions, giving feedback, etc.
- Do I hear the person out completely and calmly, or do I have a 'waiting to pounce' tendency? Interruptions with comments such as 'Yes but' indicate an impatient listener.
- Do I have preconceived notions of what I am going to say? Is my mind made up in advance about my answer or do I listen well with an open mind? If I am a 'case-is-closed' listener, I will be a poor communicator.
- Am I tuned in to non-verbal communication? Connecting to the non-verbal ensures a more accurate understanding.
- Am I aware of the emotions and feelings stirred up in me as I listen? Are certain words and topics loaded with special meaning for me? If 'trigger words' are allowed to bug me (red-flag listening), my judgement and listening effectiveness will diminish in value.
- Do I wait for the person's full stop before I respond?
- Do I have the time needed for good listening?
- Do I treat what is shared with me as privileged information? This includes confidentiality, respect, and a non-judgemental attitude.

(Life Line, 1997:29.)

- *Filtered listening.* We tend to listen to ourselves, other people and the world around us through biased (often prejudiced) filters. Filtered listening distorts our understanding of our clients.
- *Labels as filters.* Diagnostic labels can prevent you from really listening to your client. If you see a client as 'that women with Aids', your ability to listen empathetically to her problems will be severely distorted and diminished.
- *Fact-centred rather than person-centred listening.* Asking only informational or factual questions won't solve the client's problems. The client may also feel interrogated and harassed and become defensive if you ask too many questions. Rather listen to the client's whole story and focus on themes and core messages.
- *Rehearsing.* If you are rehearsing your answers mentally, you are not listening attentively. Counsellors who listen carefully to the themes and core messages in a client's story always know how to respond. The response may not be a fluent, eloquent or 'practised' one, but it will at least be sincere and appropriate.
- *Red-flag listening.* To some people, certain words act like red flags, putting them on immediate alert – they get unsettled and stop listening. These terms vary between groups, societies or organisations. Examples are: 'rapist', 'alcoholic', 'capitalist'. The first step to overcoming this barrier is to find out which words are your red flags, and try to explore the reasons why. It may also be helpful to talk to and listen attentively to someone who is more sensitive to the particular issue (e.g. alcoholism).
- *Sympathetic listening.* Although sympathy has its place in human transactions, Egan (1998) warns that the 'use' of sympathy is limited in the helping relationship because it can distort the counsellor's listening to the client's story. To sympathise with someone is to become that person's 'accomplice'. Sympathy conveys pity and even complicity, and pity for the client can diminish the extent to which you can help the client.

Basic empathy

According to Egan (1998:81), basic empathy involves *listening* to clients, *understanding* them and their concerns as best as we can, and *communicating* this understanding to them in such a way that they might *understand themselves* more fully and *act* on their understanding. In order to do this, the counsellor must set aside his or her own frame of reference and try to see the world from the client's point of view. Empathy is the ability to *recognise* and *acknowledge* the feelings of another person without *experiencing* those same emotions – it is an attempt to understand the world of the client by temporarily 'stepping into his or her shoes'. This understanding of the client's world must then be shared with the client in either a verbal or non-verbal way.

The key elements of basic empathy

Egan (1998:84–95) identifies and describes the key components of empathy. A simplified description is given below.

- *Formula for basic empathy.* Basic empathy can be expressed by restating what the client has implied using the following 'formula':

  You *feel* . . . [name the relevant emotion expressed by the client] . . . *because* (or *when*) . . . [indicate the relevant experiences and behaviours that gave rise to the feelings] . . .

  Example: 'You *feel* furious *because* he didn't tell you that he was HIV positive.' The counsellor does not 'solve' the client's problem with this response, but it demonstrates an understanding of the client's problem that will prompt the client to share more of her feelings or experiences.
- *Experiences, behaviours and feelings as elements of empathy.* An empathic response has the same key elements as the client's story: experiences, behaviour and feelings. The counsellor should respond to the client's feelings by referring to the correct *family* of emotions and to the correct *intensity* of emotions. Egan names four main families of emotions: *sad, mad, bad,* and *glad. Fear* can also be included. These feelings may vary in intensity. For example, the client can feel *sad, very sad*, or *extremely sad.* Keep the following in mind about the expression of feelings or emotions:
  - Clients don't always name their feelings and emotions verbally – they often express feelings non-verbally. These non-verbal expressions convey a vital part of the message and the counsellor should try to understand what is being conveyed.
  - Be cautious. Some clients feel threatened if the counsellor names and discusses their *feelings.* If this is the case, concentrate on *experiences* and *behaviours* and then *gradually* introduce actual named feelings into the discussion. Encouraging clients to talk about their physical reactions to emotions can be helpful.
  - Some clients can talk about some feelings (e.g. anger), while avoiding others (e.g. hurt). The empathic counsellor will be able to pick this up and deal with it accordingly.
  - Neither overemphasise nor underemphasise feelings or emotions. Remember that emotions go hand in hand with experiences and behaviours.
  - Use your own words, phrases or statements to express empathy. Be true to yourself. Egan warns that your responses to your clients should come from *you.* They should not be canned responses from a textbook (1998:87).
- *Principles of basic empathy*
  - Empathy should be used in *all the phases* of the counselling process. Empathy offers support, builds trust, paves the way to more effective participation from the client, and creates the atmosphere for stronger interventions by the counsellor.
  - Respond to the *core messages* in a client's conversation. Because it is impossible to respond to everything a client says, it is necessary to identify and respond to the core messages.
  - Respond to the *context* of what is said, and not only to the words or non-verbal behaviour of the client. The context of what is said includes everything that surrounds the client's words, such as his or her socio-economic background.

- Show empathy to stimulate *movement* in the helping process. For example, a client moves forward when empathy helps him or her to explore a problem situation in more detail or to investigate possible interventions or actions. Empathetic statements that accurately reflect how a client feels encourage the client to move forward.
- Empathy is also a tool to *check* whether you understood the client correctly. Allow the client to correct you. Remember that the client understands his or her world far better than you do. If your response is correct, the client will usually acknowledge it verbally or non-verbally, for example, by nodding, by using an affirmative word or phrase, or by moving forward in the helping process. If your response to your client's story is wrong, he or she will either say so, fumble, stop dead, or change the conversation. Be alert to the client's cues and get back on track.
- *Don't pretend* to understand. Admit if you have 'lost' the client, and work to get back on track. A counsellor may lose a client because the client becomes confused and emotional, or because the counsellor gets distracted.

The DON'Ts of empathy

The stumbling blocks to effective empathy include:

- *No response.* Although clients differ in how they deal with silence, they may think that what they have just said does not deserve a response from the counsellor. A brief response ('mmm', 'I see', 'yes', 'uh-huh' is usually better than silence. Even a somewhat inaccurate, tentative response is better than no response, or questions or clichés. (See 'The use of silence' on page 190 for the difference between meaningful and non-working silences.)
- *Distracting questions.* Counsellors often ask questions to get more information from the client in order to pursue their own agendas. They do this at the expense of the client, i.e. they ignore the feelings that the client expressed about his or her experiences.
- *Clichés.* Avoid using clichés. Clichés are hollow and they suggest that you're not taking the client's problems seriously. Don't say 'I know how you feel', because you don't.
- *Interpretations.* Empathy is not interpreting. The counsellor should respond to the client's feelings and should not distort the content of what the client is telling the counsellor.
- *Advice.* Although giving advice has its place in HIV/Aids counselling, it should be used sparingly to honour the value of self-responsibility (see 'Empowerment and self-responsibility' on page 184).
- *Parroting.* Merely repeating what the client has said is not empathy but parroting. Counsellors who 'parrot' what the client said, do not understand the client, are not 'with' the client, and show no respect for the client. Empathy should always *add* something to the conversation.
- *Sympathy and agreement.* Empathy is not the same as sympathy. According to Du Toit et al. (1998), sympathy stems from the facilitator's experiential world rather than from the client's. To sympathise with a client is to show pity, condolence and compassion – all well-intentioned, but not helpful in counselling. According to Egan (1998.97): sympathy denotes agreement, whereas empathy denotes understanding and acceptance of the person of the client. For example: If Mary is angry with her previous partner who infected her with HIV, an *empathic* counsellor will be able to understand Mary's feelings towards her ex-partner. A *sympathetic* counsellor will experience emotions of anger towards Mary's ex-partner.
- *Confrontation and arguments.* Avoid confrontation and arguments with the client. A counsellor who argues with a client is not showing empathy but approaching the client from his or her own frame of reference. This may put the client on the defensive (Du Toit et al., 1998).

Hints for communicating empathy

Egan (1998:97) suggests the following ways for the novice counsellor to improve empathic responses:

- *Give yourself time to think.* Assimilate and reflect on what the client has said in order to identify the core message.
- *Use short responses.* Don't make speeches. Keep your responses short, concrete and accurate and base them on the core message.
- *Gear your response to the client, but remain yourself.* Part of being empathic is to share your client's emotional tone (e.g. tone of voice). If a client speaks excitedly about successes, it is not empathic of the counsellor to respond in a dull, flat tone. But the counsellor must be true to his or her own nature – saying and doing things just to be on the client's wavelength is phoney, not empathic.

The use of silence

Silences can be meaningful in an atmosphere of trust and rapport between counsellor and client. A silence can be comfortable, and it can be invaluable if it becomes a time of *reflection* (contemplation) and gathering of thoughts and feelings. Silences allow the client to absorb or work with the experiences of the counselling session.

Non-working silences, however, can be uncomfortable and even destructive. If there is a lack of trust, silences can give the client the impression that the counsellor is floundering, or even being judgemental or non-accepting of what has been shared. A sensitive or experienced counsellor develops a feeling or an inner knowledge of when silence is working – giving the client the time and space to become aware of and sort through the feelings, insights, choices and decisions he or she is facing (Life Line, 1997:35).

Probing or questioning

Probing involves *statements* and *questions* from the counsellor that enable clients to *explore more fully* any relevant issue of their lives (Egan, 1998:81). Probes can take the form of statements, questions, requests, single words or phrases and non-verbal prompts. Egan (p. 112) gives the following advice about probes.

- Keep in mind that probes:
    - encourage non-assertive or reluctant clients to tell their stories;
    - help clients to remain focused on relevant and important issues;
    - help clients identify experiences, behaviours and feelings that give a fuller picture to their story (in other words, fill in the missing pieces of the picture);
    - help clients to move forward in the helping process; and
    - help clients understand themselves and their problem situations more fully.
- Use a mixture of probing statements, questions and interjections.
- Be careful with questions. Don't ask too many – the client might feel that you're grilling him or her, or that you don't know what else to do. Don't ask a question if you don't really want to know the answer! If you ask two questions in a row, it is probably one question too many.
- Although there is a place for closed questions, avoid questions that begin with 'does', 'did', or 'is'. Ask open-ended questions: questions that require more than a simple *yes* or *no* answer. Start sentences with 'how', 'tell me about', or 'what'. Open-ended questions are non-threatening and they encourage description.
- If a probe helps a client to reveal relevant information, follow it up with basic empathy (e.g. reflecting the feeling) rather than with another probe.
- Avoid leading questions that suggest the acceptable or desired answer. Clients tend to respond according to what they think the counsellor wants to hear. This is no good – it gives the counsellor too much control and the client too little space to explore.
- Use a mixture of empathy and probing to help clients clarify problems, identify blind spots, develop new scenarios, search for action strategies, formulate plans, and review outcomes of actions.

Clarification

Clarification means making sure that you've understood the client correctly. Someone who is distressed might give a confused explanation of what is happening. The counsellor then has to clarify to make sure that what he or she is hearing and understanding is actually what the client is trying to put across. For example: 'Do I understand correctly? You are saying that . . . ' or 'Do you mean that . . . ' (Life Line, 1997:34).

Reflective commenting

Reflective commenting (or paraphrasing) can be defined as mirroring or reflecting back to the client exactly what he or she is conveying to the counsellor. The reflective comment includes not only the specific *content* of the message but also the implied, stated or underlying *feelings*. In order to reflect, the counsellor needs to listen to the feelings behind the words of the client, and not only to the words. The reflective comment facilitates an atmosphere of understanding and makes people feel heard, valued and safe enough to share more of themselves, often on a deeper level. An example of a reflective comment is the following (Life Line, 1997:37):

Client: My life is a mess. I don't know how to get out of where I am. Everything I do seems to end in disaster.

Counsellor: Everything you do seems to be going wrong and you feel trapped in this mess.

The reflective comment of the counsellor in the example reflects both *content* and *feeling* (trapped).

Activity

Reflective commenting (or paraphrasing) requires correct identification and reflection of the client's *feelings*. Develop your own *feeling vocabulary* by taking a dictionary and listing all the words that describe feeling. For starters: *A*bandoned, accepted, aching, accused, adventurous . . . *B*adgered, baited, battered, beaten . . . *C*alm, careful, carefree, careless, caring . . . etc.

Summarising

It is sometimes useful for the counsellor to summarise what was said in a session so as to give focus to what has been discussed, and challenge the client to move forward. Summaries are particularly helpful under the following circumstances:

- *At the beginning of a new session.* A summary at this point can give direction to a client who does not know where to start; it can prevent a client from merely repeating what has already been said; and it can motivate a client to move forwards.
- *When a session seems to be going nowhere.* Summarising the main content along with the feelings the client is experiencing often helps the client focus on the most important areas and feelings that need to be worked with.
- *When a client gets stuck.* In such a situation, a summary may help the client to move forward and investigate other parts of the story.

Activity

Ask a colleague or friend to role-play a counselling session (or an interview) with you. Ask the friend to play the role of the client and to think of a specific problem that he or she would like to discuss with you. (Taking a real problem that has already been solved works best in role-play.) Ask a third person to listen to the counselling session and to make notes to indicate how you fared on the following aspects:

- Did you move through all four phases of the counselling process (relationship building, helping the client to tell his or her story, developing an increased understanding of the problem, and intervention or action)?
- Did you show respect, warmth, genuineness and acceptance?
- How were your counselling skills of attending, listening and showing empathy?
- Did you explore the client's experiences, behaviour, feelings and thoughts?
- Did you ask (too) many questions? Were they open-ended or closed?
- Did you explore possible interventions or actions with the client?

Reflect on how the counselling session was for you as counsellor. Ask the 'client' to reflect on how it was for him or her to be the client.

- A summary is also useful to *introduce a new phase* or to *terminate the session.*

The counsellor can also help the client to summarise. This helps the client to 'own' the process and to move on (Egan, 1998).

Integrating communication skills

Communication skills should be integrated in a natural way in the counselling process. Skilled counsellors continually attend and listen, and use a mix of empathy and probes to help clients come to grips with their problems. The client, the needs of the client, the problem situation, and the phase of counselling will determine the choice of communication skills and their application.

10.7 ADVANCED COMMUNICATION SKILLS

Basic communication skills are needed to observe and hear clients, to understand them and to communicate this understanding to them. Advanced communication skills require a different kind of understanding – challenging the client to talk about what has been hidden, distorted or repressed. These skills include: advanced empathy, immediacy, helper self-disclosure and information sharing, suggestions and recommendations. Advanced communication skills are important in the third phase of counselling to improve understanding of the problem.

Advanced empathy

Advanced empathy encourages the client to explore new themes, issues and emotions (Johnson, 2000). It involves the 'message behind the message' or the 'story behind the story'.

The following questions can help counsellors to probe deeper as they listen to their clients (Egan, 1998:170):

- What is the client only half-saying?
- What is the client saying in a confused way?
- What is the client hinting at?
- What covert message is hiding behind the explicit message?

For example, if you say to a client who is furious because her partner did not tell her that he was HIV positive: 'You feel angry because he did not tell you, but perhaps you also feel a bit hurt' – this may bring a new dimension to the fore. This client was prepared to talk about the anger, while the *hurt* – although a very real problem – was lurking in the background.

Egan (1998:171) warns that advanced empathic listening deals with what the client is actually trying to say, and not with the counsellor's *interpretation* of what the client is saying. 'Advanced therapy is not an attempt to *psych the client out*' (in other words, you're not trying to be cleverer than the client about interpreting what's really going on).

Advanced empathy can be used in the following ways (Du Toit et al., 1998:169–185; Egan, 1998:172–175):

- *Help clients make the implied explicit.* There is usually more than one intended message encoded in the explicit message. The counsellor must search for those deeper messages embedded in something the client said earlier, or in non-verbal behaviour such as tone of voice or facial expression.
- *Help clients identify themes in their stories.* Stories usually consist of many themes that might refer to feelings (such as themes of anxiety or depression), behaviour (such as themes of avoiding intimacy), or experiences (such as themes of being a victim). These themes are usually *implicit* in the story of the client, and the counsellor has to listen very carefully to identify them. Clients are often unaware of these themes. If they are pointed out, the client may begin to understand his or her story in a completely new light. Egan (1998:173) warns counsellors, however, 'to make sure that the themes they discover are based on the client's story and are not just the artefacts of some psychological theory. Advanced empathy works because clients recognise themselves in what you say.'
- *Avoid negativity and blaming.* Themes should be pointed out to clients without blaming anyone and without making value judgements about anyone's behaviour. The *way* in which the theme is communicated to the client is very important. Du Toit et al. (1998:175) give the following example: A counsellor

might say: 'Correct me if I have misheard, but what I seem to be hearing is that you've been experiencing a need for closeness.' Don't say: 'What I hear is your need for closeness, but I sense that your husband maintains his distance.' Du Toit et al. go further to say that 'such a statement implies a reproach against the husband. If the theme of closeness is identified, the client will make the connection herself.'

- *Help clients to make connections.* Clients often tell various stories without making connections between them. Egan calls these various stories 'islands' and proposes that counsellors should try to see how these 'islands' (stories, statements, experiences, problems and contexts) can be connected. The counsellor should try to determine which of the things that occur on island A might also be on islands B, C and D. It is the task of the counsellor to give feedback to the client and to help the client build a bridge between these islands. This bridge is built with empathy, and it is not merely an interpretation by the counsellor.
- *Share hunches with clients.* Advanced empathy means sharing with clients educated guesses or hunches (about them and their overt and covert experiences, behaviour and feelings) in the hope that this will help them see their problems more clearly. Such guesses and hunches will require active listening, understanding, empathy and effective probing. Communicating these hunches to clients can help them see the bigger picture; become aware of what they had merely implied or hinted at; see things they had overlooked; and identify themes.

Immediacy

Immediacy is the skill of communicating what is happening in the counselling relationship while it is happening. Immediacy improves the working alliance in counselling, and it will also influence the client's parallel processes or relationships outside the counselling relationship. For example, some of the difficulties clients have in relationships in general may appear in the counselling relationship too. If a client tends to be dependent and indecisive in relationships generally, this is likely to be true in the counselling relationship as well. Immediacy enables the counsellor to help the client move beyond this problem – in the counselling sessions as well as in everyday life.

Du Toit et al. (1998:190) state a golden rule of immediacy that the counsellor should never forget – the *I* rule: always comment in the first person. 'I sense that . . . ', or 'I'm wondering whether . . . ', or 'I am a bit confused . . . '. The *I* rule includes the counsellor in the situation, making it more difficult to blame the client. Never start a sentence with 'You are' when you apply immediacy.

According to Egan (1998:183), the skill of immediacy can be useful in the following situations:

- When a session is *directionless* and no progress is being made. For example: 'I feel that we are stuck here. Perhaps we should stop a moment and take a look at what we are doing.'
- When there is *tension* between client and counsellor: 'I have the feeling that we seem to be getting on each other's nerves. It might be helpful to stop for a moment and clear the air.'
- When *trust* seems to be a problem: 'I see your hesitancy to talk to me . . .'
- When *diversity* or some kind of *social distance* between the client and counsellor gets in the way: 'I get the feeling that the fact that I am black and you are white . . .'
- When *dependency* interferes with the helping process: 'I feel as if I must give my permission every time before you are willing to . . .'
- When *counterdependency* blocks the relationship: 'It seems that we are letting this session turn into a struggle between you and me . . .'
- When *attraction* between the counsellor and client is sidetracking the helping relationship: 'I think we like each other . . . This might be getting in the way of the work we are doing.'

Immediacy is a complex skill because it demands competence in a variety of skills such as empathy, self-awareness and advanced empathy. It should be used with care by more experienced helpers.

Helper self-disclosure

Self-disclosure literally means 'to disclose yourself to another person'. A certain amount of indirect self-disclosure automatically occurs in counselling when a client experiences some of the characteristics of the counsellor (such as warmth, congruence, etc.). Direct self-disclosure is the purposeful sharing of information about yourself that the client wouldn't otherwise know (Long, 1996). Self-disclosure therefore involves the ability of the counsellor to share with the client, in an appropriate and constructive manner, information about his or her own feelings, experiences or behaviour. Correctly used, self-disclosure can enhance the helping relationship and aid in problem solving. In a sense, the counsellor becomes a positive role model who indirectly challenges the client with 'If I could do it, you can do it too'.

However, self-disclosure is a controversial issue and it should be used only by experienced counsellors, and only if it will help a client to reach a treatment goal. Okun (1997:274) sets the following guiding principle for self-disclosure: 'The helper's self-disclosure should be for the client's benefit. This means the helper does not burden the client with his or her problems but instead regulates the quality and timing of self-disclosure to help the client focus more on his or her concerns and to encourage exploration and understanding.' Clients are not interested in rambling stories about the counsellor's own life, and these can make them very uncomfortable. They may start wondering which of you is the client!

Self-disclosure is used very effectively in the HIV/Aids context where HIV-positive co-helpers are used to tell their stories. Clients often appreciate this because it brings them into contact with HIV-positive individuals who have worked through many of the problems that they are still struggling with.

Information sharing, suggestions and recommendations

Sometimes clients are unable to explore their problems fully and take action because of a lack of information (Egan, 1998). It is therefore often necessary for counsellors to provide their clients with the necessary information, or to help them search for it, in order to move forward in the helping relationship. Information sharing is especially important in the HIV/Aids field. Although information often does not 'solve' clients' problems, it can give them new perspectives on how to handle these problems. Information sharing includes giving information as well as correcting misinformation. Egan (p. 177) warns that counsellors should take care when giving information.

- When information is challenging or shocking (e.g. an HIV-positive result), be tactful and know how to help the client handle the news. (See 'Counselling after a positive HIV test result' on page 209.)
- Do not overwhelm the client with information.
- Make sure that the information you give is clear and relevant to the client's problem situation.
- Don't let the client go away with a misunderstanding of the information.
- Be sure not to confuse giving information with giving advice. Giving advice is seldom useful.
- Be supportive and help the client to process the information.
- Don't tell clients what to do, and don't try to take over their lives. The values of respect and empowerment should always be kept in mind, and clients should be supported to make their own decisions. Nevertheless, if offered without intruding on the client's autonomy, suggestions and recommendations do have a place in counselling (especially HIV/Aids counselling), because they identify ways in which the client can manage problems more effectively.
- Factual information should be offered in a warm and caring way to allow movement from intellectual fact giving to communicating at a deeper emotional level. It is not uncommon for a client to seek factual information as a pretext for getting counselling (Life Line, 1997:35). For example, if a client asks you whether HIV can be transmitted by mosquitoes, your answer could be: 'No, HIV is only transmitted via blood, sex and from a

mother to her baby. You sound somewhat worried . . .' This response can open up new opportunities for action.

10.8 REFERRAL SKILLS

It is sometimes necessary to refer clients to another professional for specialised help. Referral should be done with great sensitivity to the feelings of the client. A special relationship usually develops between the counsellor and the client, and HIV-positive people who are confronted by many losses may experience the referral as a termination of the counselling relationship – in other words, just another loss that has to be coped with. The client may also experience the referral as a rejection.

Referral should never be seen as passing the buck. It should not be seen as terminating the counselling relationship, but as co-opting of *additional* helpers into the counselling process (Johnson, 2000:18). If, for instance, the client has specific spiritual needs in counselling, a spiritual counsellor or minister can be co-opted into the counselling process. According to Johnson, the 'family of caring professionals is thus extended, rather than having the client migrate from one counsellor to another'. The different counsellors involved in a client's care should define their separate involvements so as to prevent duplication or contradiction of the counselling activities.

10.9 COUNSELLING IN A TRADITIONAL AFRICAN SOCIETY

For a century or more, traditional healing and Western forms of counselling and psychotherapy have operated side by side in Africa, but mostly in mutual isolation. Despite the differences between traditional healing and Western counselling they share certain similarities that are universal to counselling. Nevertheless, Western counsellors* must be aware of these differences if they want to render a helpful service to clients from a traditional background. To ignore a client's cultural background not only leads to misunderstanding, but can be anti-therapeutic and harmful (Beuster, 1997). The following are some of the issues the Western counsellor should bear in mind.

Differences between traditional African and Western beliefs and assumptions

One of the most important differences between Western thinking and some traditional African approaches is the holism of the traditional outlook, integrating the biological, psychosocial and transpersonal aspects of illness. Traditional philosophies do not necessarily distinguish between physical and mental illness, but see illness as affecting the whole human being – including the person's relationship with his or her ancestors and the community. Physical, mental and social systems are seen as interconnected – changes in one system inevitably effecting changes in the others.

The individual is not regarded as being more important than the group (the West's high value on individualism is not universal) and the important role of social factors in the causation, maintenance and cure of illness is recognised. Whatever affects the individual also affects the group, and vice versa. Collective societies stress a joint 'we' consciousness, emotional dependence, collective identity and group solidarity (Bodibe & Sodi, 1997). People do not generate knowledge by introspectively examining their own feelings, their own thinking or their own intelligence (the ancient Western tradition of self-analysis), but acquire knowledge from their relationships with the sky, the land, their families, their communities and their ancestors (Beuster, 1997; Bührmann, 1986; Hammond-Tooke, 1989; Mbiti, 1969).

In contrast to this emphasis on group identity, Western societies are saturated in a tradition of individualism and the rights of the individual. This tradition emphasises personal autonomy and individual initiative: an 'I' rather than 'we' sense or mode of self-consciousness. In contrast, many non-Western cultures regard a focus on

* By 'Western counsellors' we do not necessarily mean white counsellors, but rather counsellors trained in the Western-European philosophical or psychological tradition.

the *self* as irrelevant and even as deviant. Skilled Western helpers should take the following quotation to heart and remember it when helping people from cultures that differ from their own:

> A trend that has swept the Western world in recent years has been the idea that individuals should be self-sufficient, autonomous, independent, self-directed and governed principally by what is best for them as individuals. Such qualities are often equated with mental health, but an African with such qualities would be regarded as extremely unhealthy.
>
> (Durie & Hermannson in Bodibe, 1992:151)

Western counsellors sometimes overemphasise the rational, logical and intellectual while neglecting the unconscious, intuitive and transpersonal sides of the psyche (Beuster, 1997; Bodibe, 1992; Bodibe & Sodi, 1997).

Similarities and differences between traditional healing and Western counselling

Bodibe (1992:155) discusses the following similarities and differences between traditional healing and Western psychotherapy or counselling.

Traditional healing and Western counselling display the following *similarities*:

- Both approaches emphasise the importance of building a relationship that is based on *trust*.
- Both aim at personality *integration* (wholeness) and *positive growth*.
- Both approaches emphasise the expression of *feelings* (although the ways of expressing feelings differ).
- Both rely on the *communication skills* of observation, active listening and probing to establish the problem dynamic. The traditional healer usually bases a diagnosis (problem dynamic) on careful *observation* of physical symptoms or strange behaviour; on *listening* to the client's story as told by the client and family members; on asking *questions* (probing) relating to ancestral influences, marital harmony or discord, sexual functioning, the nature, content and frequency of dreams, financial matters, the situation at work and relationships with superiors; and on *exploring* these areas carefully. A diagnostic tool not used by their Western counterparts is *divination* – which can be done by bone-throwing (*impamba*), the involvement of ancestral spirits through psychic abilities, and the interpretation of dreams and visions as a form of divination (Bodibe, 1992; Felhaber, 1997).

There are, however, also many *differences* between traditional healing and Western psychotherapy:

- The traditional approach is symbolic, intuitive and integrally part of traditional beliefs and cosmology. Western counselling is based largely on scientific and logical principles that have no direct link with symbolism.
- The traditional healer's approach is likely to be directive, giving advice by functioning as the mouthpiece of the ancestors who possess superior wisdom. Western counselling is based on the principle that the client has to take responsibility for his or her own actions and decisions. It is therefore mainly non-directive.
- Traditional healing emphasises the unity of body and mind in diagnosis and treatment. In Western counselling, the *psychological domain* is given preference (i.e. the person's feelings, thoughts and experiences). Not all people *talk* (or want to talk) about their feelings in the way that Western people do; instead they might *express* their feelings through song and dance.
- Traditional healing emphasises the unity of the person and the community. Western counselling tends to emphasise the individual and the self.
- Traditional healing often includes song and dance, being an emotive and active experience of participation. Western counselling is usually more cerebral, abstract, sedentary and sedate.
- The tools of traditional healing might include divination, dream interpretations, rituals, music, dance and drumming. Western therapy uses psychotherapeutic interviewing, testing (both assessment/diagnostic and projective) and (in some cases) hypnosis.

- A traditional healer might explore the client's relationship with neighbours and ancestors on the grounds that human conspiracies with witches and sorcerers might be behind some problems (see 'Witches and sorcerers as causal agents of illness' on page 116). Western counsellors often concentrate on the exploration of feelings, the promotion of insight, and reconstruction of reality.
- Traditional healing might try to restore harmony between the client and the ancestors. Western counselling will be aimed at developing inner resources to deal effectively with external factors and internal conflict.

The person-centred approach in Africa

The person-centred approach of Carl Rogers has had a tremendous influence on counselling in the Western world. Although most of the values and principles of the person-centred approach (such as empathy, warmth, caring, respect, congruence, unconditional acceptance and growth) are universal to people of all cultures, the person-centred approach should be adapted to take local cultural and philosophical differences into account. In many traditional societies change is not directed by the self (what the 'self' wants – an *internal locus of control*), but by the group (an *external locus of control*). In such a society, the focus should shift from the individual to the group in order to create change.

Du Toit et al. (1998:199–200) suggest that therapists working cross-culturally should take into account the following implications of a person-centred approach:

- The counsellor should respect the client and the client's culture and be led into the client's frame of reference.
- Cross-cultural counselling is a learning process, both for the counsellor and for the client. It is a process of finding common ground and understanding.
- To *assume* is to *stereotype*. Admitting your own ignorance is the only way to understand and appreciate the wisdom and subtleties of another culture.
- If we listen, ask, explore and learn, clients will show us how we can collaborate with them in their efforts to grow and develop.

Practical guidelines in cross-cultural counselling

The following practical guidelines may be helpful in cross-cultural counselling (based on material from Du Toit et al., 1998:201–207; Gillis, 1994:177–179; Nefale in Van Dyk et al., 2000; Seepamore, 2000; Sue & Sue, 1999):

The counselling process

- Although the *four phases of counselling* also apply to cross-cultural counselling, the ways in which they are presented may differ slightly to accommodate the client.
- The *four questions* that you want your client to answer during the counselling process (current scenario, preferred scenario, what do I need to do, and action – see page 175) may also vary, because your client might not think in terms of what 'I' prefer (preferred scenario), or make decisions as an individual (what 'I' need and want). The client may have to go back to the group or family to decide what will be best for the group. 'The counsellor may think badly of me – think that I can't make up my mind because I cannot answer him. What he doesn't understand is that I cannot make these decisions on my own. I have to discuss them with my family first' (Seepamore, 2000). A solution may be to send the client home with 'homework' to discuss the questions of current scenario, preferred scenario, and possible interventions with the group. Some clients even prefer to bring the family along for counselling.
- *Insight* into personal feelings or emotions is not highly valued in group-orientated cultures. It might instead be seen as a symptom of individualism benefiting the individual as opposed to the group.
- If you (or the client) feel uncomfortable because you come from different ethnic groups, bring it up in the first session. You can, for example, use a statement like: 'Sometimes clients feel uncomfortable working with

a counsellor of a different race. Would this be a problem for you?'

- Identify the client's expectations and world-view. Find out what the client believes counselling is, and explore his or her feelings about counselling.
- Strive to work within the client's cultural frame of reference, and encourage the client to correct 'cultural' misunderstandings on your part.
- In the *intervention* or action phase it may be necessary for the counsellor (at least in the beginning) to take a more *directive role* than usual, particularly if the client's traditional helpers are normally directive (giving advice). But the counsellor should gradually involve the client in goal-setting and empower the client to make his or her own choices (often with the approval of the group or significant others).

Attending skills

- Make sure that the way you orientate yourself to be with your client (attending*)* does not affront instead of reassuring your client. Read your client's body language and be guided by it.
- Familiarise yourself with traditional forms of greeting, and make sure you can pronounce and spell the client's name correctly. Don't make judgements based on stereotypes such as the client's hairstyle or dress.
- Bear in mind that people from different cultures may have different attitudes to matters such as personal communication distance, punctuality and time schedules.
- It may be a problem if you are much younger than your client, or of the opposite sex. In many cultures elderly people customarily don't discuss their problems with younger people because 'they are children'. Discuss this potential problem with your client.
- Respect the client's customs and ways of communicating. These may include making or avoiding of eye contact, who should sit, stand or walk first, how a man should act towards a woman and a woman towards a man, and how adults and children should behave towards one another.
- Be aware that direct eye contact is not an admired form of behaviour in all cultures. Many cultures regard it as rude, a challenge, or even as confrontational. In some cultures it would be regarded as ill-mannered if a young person were to look directly at an older person. Let the client be your guide – observe him or her and be sensitive to what is comfortable for him or her.
- Many counsellors have the habit of touching their clients as a way of showing empathy. But touching may not be appropriate in all cultures. It could be seen as degrading (you touch a child out of sympathy, not an adult) or, if the touching involves a person of the opposite sex, it may be seen as an expression of sexual attention.
- Bodily distance may also be important to the client. Use your client's body language and do not offend your client by sitting too close or too far away. It is a good idea to invite the client (and his or her family) to choose where they would like to sit or stand. Allow *them* to select a comfortable distance.
- Be sensitive to the client's needs and feelings before you close the door when other clients are sitting in a waiting room – especially when you are counselling somebody of the opposite sex. 'If the counsellor closes the door, it makes the other people very uncomfortable. They will ask each other: "What are those two doing in there?"' (Seepamore, 2000).
- Using first names may be regarded as an expression of over-familiarity, especially if the client is an older person. In many cultures first names are reserved for close friends, and clients will often say or think (without any malice), 'You are not my friend'.

Listening and probing skills

- The skill of *active listening* is extremely important in cross-cultural counselling. The counsellor can become a part of the client's world only by listening carefully to what the client says and doesn't say.
- Cross-cultural work sometimes offers the advantage that counsellors know that they will be at a disadvantage unless they *listen*

and *explore the problem dynamic* properly. If counsellors are aware that they do not know the meanings that clients attach to particular situations, they will try harder to explore meanings with their clients.

- Try to use the client's own words and expressions whenever possible. Encourage your client to ask for clarification when something is not clear, and to correct you if you have misunderstood something.
- Be careful how and what you ask when you explore the client's story. An older client (older than you) might not want to discuss his or her sex life with a younger counsellor. The counsellor should accept that this is not a question of trust, but of custom.
- Where appropriate, enquire about the client's traditional family structures and support systems, as these may differ from culture to culture.

Empathy

- *Empathy* can be used to bridge diversity gaps. According to Egan (1998), it is impossible for a counsellor really to understand the world of clients who differ from him or her in significant ways. Empathy based on effective attending and listening is one of the counsellor's most important tools for getting as close as possible to understanding the client's world.
- The counsellor should be sensitive to differences, but not assume differences where there may be none. When working cross-culturally the basic theory, values and communication skills are exactly the same as for working with people from the counsellor's own cultural group. Empathy is empathy in any culture or language – it is a way of being, regardless of the people we are in contact with. We simply might have to adapt the phrasing or our method of expressing feelings.
- Metaphors and stories work very well in communicating empathy in a traditional context. Wildervanck (in Du Toit et al., 1998:203) mentions that the following metaphors were used very effectively by counsellors to convey empathy in the African context:
    - To empathise with somebody who had missed a wonderful opportunity: 'The steenbok jumps out of the cooking pot.'
    - To convey the understanding that a child takes after her mother: 'She comes from the breast milk.'
    - To empathise with a person who has many problems and frustrations: 'You have grabbed the clay cooking pot by its hot side.'
- Be true to yourself. Don't do or say things that you feel uncomfortable with. If you talk to a client from the heart, on a person-to-person basis, using the skills of attending, listening and empathy to demonstrate your openness, honesty and genuine desire to help, trust and rapport will develop between you and the client.
- Keep in mind that some traditional people may find it difficult to talk about their *feelings*. The concepts of what you might think of as everyday feelings might even be alien to the client's culture or language. Counsellors should be creative and allow clients to express their feelings in traditional ways such as singing, dancing, miming ('*Show* me how you feel') and writing poetry.
- Some cultures associate maturity and wisdom with the ability to control emotions and feelings, and people from these cultures will not feel comfortable expressing their emotions in a counselling setting. Counsellors who are not aware of this might misinterpret their behaviour.
- Be careful with *silence*. Acceptance and trust are paramount in a counselling environment, and nothing undermines the helping relationship more quickly than enforced silences. A short, emphatic response is better than silence – especially if the relationship between counsellor and client is not yet established.

Self-disclosure

- Use *self-disclosure* (you disclosing to the client) at appropriate times. This is often an important means of establishing trust because it may be seen as a sign that the counsellor accepts the client.

- Keep in mind that clients from other cultures may find it difficult to disclose their intimate details to you in a counselling context. Cultures that do not believe in the appropriateness of intimate revelations of personal or social problems often see disclosure as not only exposing the *individual* in counselling, but also as exposing the *whole family* because the individual is regarded as an integral part of the family system.

General cultural considerations

- When counselling cross-culturally, the counsellor should take great care to avoid being perceived as being in any way condescending or patronising.
- Explore, actively challenge and acknowledge your prejudices, stereotypes and cultural assumptions about other groups.
- Recognise the limitations that cross-cultural counselling imposes on helpers. If you find it difficult to be genuinely accepting and non-judgemental, or if it becomes clear that further progress is impossible because of perceived or real cultural differences, suggest another helper with whom the client may feel more comfortable.

When working cross-culturally, the counsellor and the client have to cross certain borders. This does not mean invading the physical territory or personal space of others, but rather going beyond our own mental and social borders and reaching out to others' worlds in a gentle and non-threatening way. Borders are not seen as obstacles, but as a learning experience (Du Toit et al., 1998:204).

Language barriers – the use of a translator or interpreter

Language barriers between counsellors and clients can cause severe difficulties, especially in South Africa with its 11 official languages. Unfortunately there are not always trained counsellors available to address clients in their own language. Counsellors often have no choice but to use translators or interpreters to rephrase what they have said in a way that is understandable to the client. This is far from ideal, and counsellors should be aware of the problems of using the services of a third person in the counselling process. Translators often translate according to their own frames of reference; they may add their own experiences, interpretations, prejudices, and comments in the message to the client; confidentiality may be violated; and the relationship between the counsellor and the client may be jeopardised in favour of a relationship between the translator and the client. Keep the following precautions in mind when using the services of an interpreter or translator (Wong et al., 1999:208):

- Using a child as an interpreter might be considered an insult to an adult in a culture in which children are expected to show respect by not questioning their elders.
- In some cultures class differences between the interpreter and client may cause the client to feel intimidated and less inclined to offer information. Choose the translator or interpreter carefully and provide time for the interpreter and client to establish rapport.
- If informed consent is obtained through an interpreter, make sure that the client is fully informed of all the aspects of the procedure (e.g. testing) to which he or she is consenting.
- Communicate directly with the client when asking questions to reinforce interest in the client. Observe non-verbal responses but don't ignore the interpreter.
- Ask one question at a time.
- Don't interrupt the client and interpreter while they are conversing.
- Don't make comments to the interpreter about the client, because the client may well understand at least some of the language in which you are conversing.
- Be aware that some words (e.g. medical words) may not have equivalents in the other language. Avoid medical and psychological jargon.
- Allow time after the interview for the interpreter to share something that he or she felt could not be said earlier and ask the interpreter about his or her impressions of non-verbal messages.
- Arrange for the client (if possible) to speak to the same interpreter on subsequent visits.

10.10 CONCLUSION

HIV/Aids forces all of us in the helping professions to be counsellors. Counselling is no longer only the task of the psychologist. The task may be daunting, but if you keep the aims of counselling in mind, and if you use the qualities that drew you to the helping professions in the first place, you can render a very important service to those in need.

To further assist youin your task, the counselling skills that you have encountered in this chapter will be applied to specific contexts in the following chapters. Chapter 11 gives guidelines on pre- and post-HIV-test counselling; chapter 12 deals with specific considerations in counselling people living with HIV/Aids and their significant others; and chapter 13 discusses bereavement and spiritual counselling.

chapter

11 Pre- and Post-HIV-Test Counselling

Worrying about the beast
That night the fires burnt high
and glimmered through the poles,
separating them from the bush . . .
and nobody slept because of the darkness
that threatened to engulf them.

The HIV test is different from all other tests. It has enormous emotional, psychological, practical and social implications for the client. HIV testing should therefore *never* be done without thorough pre-test counselling. Pre-test counselling done in a proper and comprehensive way prepares the client and counsellor for more effective post-test counselling. Because clients are often too relieved or too shocked to take in much information during post-test counselling, the health care professional should make use of the educational opportunities offered by pre-test counselling.

The basic principles of counselling, and the values and communication skills discussed in chapter 10, should form the basis of pre- and post-HIV-test counselling. Pre- and post-HIV-test counselling are specific counselling contexts in which these principles and skills should be applied.

11.1 PRE-HIV-TEST COUNSELLING

The purpose of pre-test counselling is to give someone who is considering being tested for HIV all the necessary information and support to make an informed decision. Information on the technical aspects of testing and the possible personal, medical, social, psychological, legal and ethical implications of being diagnosed as either HIV positive or HIV negative should be provided. The purpose of pre-test counselling is also to find out the reasons why individuals want to be tested; the nature and extent of their previous and present high-risk behaviour; and the action required to prevent them from becoming infected or from transmitting HIV infection.

The following guidelines should be used for the pre-test interview.

Relationship building

It is often not easy for a client to share intimate details of his or her life with a counsellor. It is therefore important to create an atmosphere of safety and trust and to help the client tell his or her story. Assure privacy and welcome the client. Introduce yourself and explain what your role is (e.g. are you doing only the counselling, or will you also carry out the testing?). Explain the reason for pre-test counselling: that it is a legal and ethical requirement; that the test may have vast implications; that the client needs to be sure about having the test; and that it remains the client's choice to be tested or not. Assure the client of confidentiality (see below). Find out more about the client, e.g. age, occupation, relationship status and family background.

Confidentiality

Assure clients that their right to confidentiality will be respected at all times. If individuals choose not to disclose their status, they must be reassured that no information will be communicated to anyone without their prior permission. Discuss the concept of group confidentiality when necessary. Group confidentiality applies where the counsellor is not qualified to do the HIV test and a third party, usually a nurse, will be required to administer and interpret it (Blom, 2001). (Note that only trained health care professionals such as nurses and doctors may perform an HIV rapid antibody test, or may draw blood for an ELISA test.)

Enrichment

Confidentiality

Health care professionals are ethically and legally required to keep client information confidential. Giving out information on a patient's illness or treatment requires the patient's consent. The right of HIV-positive people to be treated fairly and confidentially should be recognised and accepted. If clients do not have the assurance that health care professionals will keep their diagnosis confidential, they might be afraid to go for treatment. Because people living with HIV often face discrimination and prejudice, it is even more important to keep the information about their infection confidential.

Reasons for testing

Explore why clients want to be tested. Is it for insurance purposes, because of anxiety about lifestyle, or because the person has been forced by somebody else to take the test? What makes the client feel that he or she might be infected? What particular behaviour or symptoms are causing concern to the client? Has the client sought testing before and, if so, when? From whom? For what reason? And with what result? These questions give the counsellor insight into individuals' perceptions of their own high-risk behaviour, the urgency of having the test, their knowledge of HIV, and their emotional state. If the client is being tested because you as a counsellor had suggested it, explain why you think it is advisable (e.g. for treatment purposes). Also explain to the client that the test is voluntary and that he or she may refuse to be tested.

The following are some of the reasons often given for wanting to be tested:

- Their partners requested it.
- They want to determine their HIV status before starting a new relationship.
- They want to be tested before getting married.
- They feel guilty and concerned about having had multiple sex partners.
- They have had recent sexual encounters in which they did not use condoms.
- They have symptoms that are giving them cause for concern.
- They have been referred by an STI or TB clinic because they have TB or a sexually transmitted infection.
- They have come to confirm a positive HIV test.
- Their current partner is HIV positive, or they have been involved with a partner who was HIV positive.
- They plan to become pregnant and want to check their HIV status before they do.
- They have been raped or assaulted.
- They need to be tested after an occupational exposure (e.g. a needle-stick injury).
- They are simply curious.

The reason why a client wants to be tested is important because it sets the scene for the rest of the pre-test counselling session. The counsellor should not make any judgemental comments about the client's reasons for testing. People are afraid of HIV and may not necessarily be prepared to share with you their personal reasons for wanting to be tested. Support the client with empathy and convey understanding of what they do tell you of their story. Allow space for personal expression and encourage the client to talk about their feelings and insecurities.

Activity

Frances comes to you for an HIV test. She works as a nanny and her employer wants her to be tested for HIV. Frances is afraid of the test, she does not really know what to expect, and she is uncertain whether she really wants to be tested or not. She also tells you that she is three months pregnant. How would you counsel Frances?

Assessment of risk

Assess the likelihood of whether the client has been exposed to HIV by considering if and how frequently he or she has been exposed to the following risk factors and lifestyle indicators:

- What is the client's sexual risk history in terms of frequency and type of sexual behaviour? Has the client been involved in high-risk sexual practices such as vaginal or anal intercourse with more than one sex partner without the use of condoms? In the case of anal sex, was it anal-receptive or anal-insertive sex? Did the client have sex with a sex worker (prostitute)? Is the client's sex partner HIV positive?
- Are there any other risks involved? Is the client an injecting drug user, a prisoner, a migrant worker, a refugee or a sex worker? Did the client at any time receive money, gifts or drugs for sex? Has the client ever been raped or coerced into having sex with another person? Does the client have another sexually transmitted infection or show signs and symptoms of tuberculosis?
- Has the client received a blood transfusion, an organ transplant or blood or body products? (Testing transfusion blood for HIV may not take place in some developing countries.)
- Has the client been exposed to possibly non-sterile invasive procedures such as tattooing, piercing or traditional procedures such as male circumcision, genital mutilation (female circumcision) and scarification?
- Has the client been exposed to HIV-infected blood in the work situation, or was the client in an accident?

If exploration reveals that the client has been at risk for HIV infection, share this with the client. If the client is pregnant, discuss the possibility of HIV transmission to her baby during pregnancy, during birth or during breastfeeding, as well as ways to prevent mother-to-child transmission.

Activity

What questions will you ask Frances to assess the likelihood that she has been exposed to HIV?

Beliefs and knowledge about HIV infection and safer sex

Determine exactly what your client believes and knows about HIV infection and Aids, and correct errors and myths by providing accurate information about what HIV infection and Aids entails, the modes of transmission, prevention, symptoms, the progression from HIV to Aids, and so on. The amount of information given will depend on the clients' needs and their knowledge and level of comprehension.

Ask your clients questions about their past and present sexual behaviour and provide information about safer sex practices and a healthier lifestyle. Find out whether they know how to practise safer sex, how to use a condom correctly, and where to get hold of condoms. Give them condoms if necessary.

Information about the test

It is important to ensure that your clients know what the HIV test entails (see 'HIV testing as diagnostic tool' on page 64). Explain the test procedures as well as the meaning of the test results. The following points should be discussed (based on Blom, 2001):

- *The testing procedure*. If the rapid HIV antibody test is done, explain to the client that his or her finger will be pricked to collect a drop of blood for the test. Also explain that the results will be available within 10–15 minutes. Explain that a confirmatory test will be done. If you are not qualified to do the test yourself, make it clear to the client that a nurse will be called in to administer the test. If blood is needed for an ELISA test, explain to the client that blood will be drawn (usually from a vein in the arm) and that it will be sent away to a laboratory for testing. The results of the ELISA test will not be available until 2–14 days later, and the client will have to come back for the results.

- *The role of a confirmatory test.* If the result of a rapid test is positive, a second confirmatory rapid test will be done. If the confirmatory test is also positive, the client has HIV antibodies in the blood, and he or she will receive post-test counselling accordingly. If the result of the rapid test is positive and the result of the confirmatory test is negative, the result is *inconclusive* or *discordant.* In this case blood from a vein will be taken and sent to a laboratory for an ELISA test. Explain to the client that the results of the ELISA will not be available until 2–14 days later.
- *Immediate results in the case of rapid testing.* The results of rapid HIV antibody tests are available almost immediately. Make clients aware of this and ask whether they are ready for the result on that particular day, or whether they might prefer to come back for the test on another day.
- *The difference between being seropositive and having Aids.* Explain to the client that the HIV antibody test is not a 'test for Aids'. It indicates that a person has HIV antibodies in the blood and is infected with HIV. It does not say when or how the infection occurred, or in what phase of infection the person is.
- *The presence of HIV antibodies* in the blood does not mean that the person is now immune to HIV. On the contrary, it means that he or she has been infected with HIV and can pass the virus on to others.
- *The meaning of a positive and a negative test result.* See 'What is meant by a positive (or reactive) HIV antibody test?' on page 68, and 'What is meant by a negative (non-reactive) HIV antibody test?' on page 68.
- *The meaning of 'window period'* (see 'The window period' on page 66). Stress the need for further testing if the person has been having high-risk sex *and tests negative.*
- *The reliability of the testing procedures.* A positive HIV antibody test result is always confirmed with a second test. The test results are very reliable, with only rare occurrences of false-positive or false-negative results (e.g. a false-negative test result for a client in the window period).

Activity

Don't overload your clients with information during the pre-test counselling session. Discuss all the important issues, and send them home with additional reading material. Design a pamphlet in which you explain everything they need to know about the HIV antibody test.

The implications of an HIV test result

The possible personal, medical, social, psychological, ethical and legal implications of a positive test result should be discussed with clients before testing. Explore with clients all the possible advantages and disadvantages of testing, and explore the implications of each result (positive, negative and inconclusive) for the individual, for the partner/s and for the family. Taking the test can have the following advantages:

- Knowing the result may reduce the stress associated with uncertainty.
- Rational plans can be made for emotional and spiritual preparation for living with HIV.
- Symptoms can be confirmed, alleviated or treated.
- Prophylactic (preventive) treatment can be considered (such as treatment for TB).
- Antiretroviral treatment can be considered (if the client is a candidate for treatment).
- Adjustments to lifestyle and sexual behaviour can protect the individual and sex partners from infection.
- Decisions about family planning and new sexual relationships can be made.

- Plans for future care and orphan care can be made.

The disadvantages of taking an HIV test (especially if the result is positive) include:

- Possible limitations on life insurance and mortgages.
- Having to endure the social stigma associated with the disease.
- Problems in maintaining relationships and in making new friends.
- Possible refusal by uninformed medical and dental personnel to treat an HIV-positive person. (Refusal to treat HIV-positive individuals is contrary to the South African Constitution.)
- Possible dismissal from work (although it is illegal to dismiss people because they are HIV positive).
- Possible rejection and discrimination by friends, family and colleagues.
- Emotional problems and a disintegration of the individual's life.
- Increased stress and uncertainty about the future.
- The stress and negative effects of maintaining secrecy for those who decide not to disclose the test results.

Assure clients who test positive that medical treatments are available that can help them stay healthier for longer.

Anticipate the results

It is important for the counsellor to anticipate a negative as well as a positive HIV antibody test result and to talk about how the client will deal with the test outcome. Ask the client how he or she will feel about a negative test result. Cover the window period and its implications and the importance of staying HIV negative through safer sex and blood practices, and give a condom demonstration if necessary.

Anticipating a positive result helps the counsellor ascertain the client's ability to deal with and adjust to a positive result. The counsellor gains insight into some of the potential problems associated with a positive test outcome. Preparing the client for the possibility of a positive result paves the way for more effective post-test counselling. Albers (1990) suggests that in order to prepare the client for the test result, the following questions should be asked.

- How would you feel if you tested negative? How would you feel if the test were negative but you were advised to be tested again in three or six months' time because you may still be in the window period?
- What would your reactions and feelings be to a positive test? Would a positive test change your life? How? What negative changes would you anticipate? What positive changes can you imagine?
- Do you intend telling others if you test positive? Who would you tell? Why that person? How would you tell them? Why would you tell them? Clients must be warned about people's possible reactions. Often those closest to the client cannot cope with the news. The counsellor must help clients to think not only of themselves but also of those who are to be told. (For example, if the client says to you: 'The news will surely kill my old and frail mother,' you may ask: 'Why do you want your mother to know?') Clients must also be warned that some people may not keep the information to themselves, and that this might have harmful effects for the client. Disclosure should always be in the best interest of the client.
- How would you tell your sex partner? If the test result is positive, the sex partner also needs to be tested.
- How would a positive test result change your relationships and the circumstances of your family? Would your relationships be improved or hindered by telling people you are HIV positive? What do you believe their reactions would be?
- What would the implications of an HIV-positive test result be for your job? Explore issues around employment and explain that termination of employment on the grounds of HIV status is not legal; that pre-employment testing is not legal; and that there is no legal requirement on employees to inform their employers of their HIV status (but disclosure might become necessary when an individual becomes too sick to work). Clients who have

medical aid should check for HIV-specific provisions.

- Where would you seek medical help? How do you feel about a disease that requires a lot of care, lifestyle changes, commitment and discipline? Will family members or friends be able to help you to be disciplined about your health? Could you take medication every four hours if necessary?
- Who could provide (and is currently providing) emotional and social support (family, friends, others)?
- How did you cope with previous crises? What did you do in a time of crisis to overcome the problem? Emphasise that support is important and that there are groups and organisations that can help.

The choice to be tested remains the client's. The advantages and disadvantages of testing can be explained to clients, but clients should not be pressured into testing if they feel that they will not be able to deal with the results. The mere *knowledge* of your HIV status will not necessarily protect you or your loved ones from infection, but it does make it easier to access treatment and support. People who prefer not to be tested should practise safe sex at all times. People who suspect that they are HIV positive should refrain from donating blood, and they should observe the guidelines for positive living (see 'Positive living' on page 299).

Activity

After discussing her extramarital affairs with you, Frances decided that she should be tested. She is very worried about what and how she is going to tell her husband if her test result comes back positive. She is also afraid that she might lose her job. Illustrate in role play how you would handle this situation. Ask a friend to play the role of Frances while you counsel her.

Information about giving the results and ongoing support

Explain to clients when, how and by whom the test results will be given to them. Assure clients of personal attention, privacy, confidentiality and ongoing support and advice if needed. If blood samples are sent away for ELISA tests, arrange follow-up interviews where the results will be made available. Some people might prefer to bring along a friend or family member when they come back for the results. The counsellor should accommodate such preferences when clients require them, but remember to discuss issues of confidentiality and disclosure with the client.

Support networks and the waiting period

Identify clients' support networks. Ask them who else knows that they are enquiring about HIV testing. What will they do after leaving if the result of the HIV test is positive? Where will they go? Who will be with them? How did they cope with crises in the past? Who supported them then? Will those people be available now?

Waiting for the results of an HIV antibody test (e.g. in the case of the laboratory-based ELISA) can be extremely stressful for the client. This waiting period can last from 2 to 14 days, depending on where the test is done (whether by a private practice, a government health service or a rural clinic). If the client has to wait for the test results, the counsellor should anticipate the difficulties of this period by discussing the following points with the client:

- Find out the names of people who clients might contact for moral support while waiting for the results.
- Encourage clients to contact you or a colleague if they have questions.
- Counsel clients on how to protect sex partners (e.g. by using condoms) in the interim period.
- Explore infection control measures if necessary.
- Encourage clients to do something enjoyable to keep occupied while waiting for the results (e.g. hiking, going to the movies or playing soccer with friends).

Informed consent

The decision to be tested can be made by the client only, and informed consent must be obtained prior to testing. Consenting to medical testing or treatment has two elements: *information* and *permission*. Before an HIV test can be done, the client must understand the nature of the test, and he or she must also give permission – preferably written permission – to be tested. A client may never be misled or deceived into consenting to an HIV test.

Enrichment

Informed consent

By law, health care professionals may not do an HIV test on a person unless that person clearly understands what the purpose of the test is; what advantages or disadvantages testing may hold for him or her; why the health care professional wants this information; what influence the result of such a test will have on his or her treatment; and how his or her medical protocol will be altered by this information. The psychosocial impact of a positive test result should also be discussed with the client.

(Fine et al., 1997)

Conclusion

Pre-HIV test counselling is extremely important. It should be seen not only as preparation for the HIV test, but also as an opportunity to educate people about HIV/Aids and safer sex. Remember that this may be the one and only time that you will see the client, because he or she might decide not to be tested, or not to come back for the test results after all.

Activity

How would you handle the following phone call? 'Hello, my name is Mrs Johnson. I sent my nanny, Frances, to you a week ago for an Aids test. I am just phoning to get her results.'

Note: Don't be abusive or angry. Use this as an educational opportunity for Mrs Johnson.

11.2 POST-HIV-TEST COUNSELLING

Not many things in life could be as stressful as waiting for HIV test results. For many clients it feels as if the counsellor holds the key to the future in his or her hands.

Although the post-HIV-test counselling interview is separate from the pre-test counselling interview, it is inextricably linked to it. The pre-test counselling interview should have given the client an idea of what to expect in post-test counselling. Pre- and post-test counselling should preferably be done by the same person because the established relationship between client and counsellor provides a sense of continuity for the client. The counsellor will also have a better idea of how to approach the post-test counselling because of what he or she experienced in the pre-test counselling.

Counselling after testing will depend on the outcome of the test – which may be a negative result, a positive result or an indeterminate or inconclusive result.

Counselling after a negative HIV test result

For both the client and the counsellor, a negative HIV result is a tremendous relief. However, a negative test result could give someone who is frequently involved in high-risk behaviour a false sense of security. It is therefore extremely important for the counsellor to counsel HIV-negative clients in order to reduce the chances of future infection. Risk reduction and safer sex practices must be emphasised (see chapter 8).

Some people who practise high-risk behaviour and test negative believe that they are 'immune' to HIV and that precautions are therefore unnecessary. This dangerous assumption must be rectified. Explain to clients that nobody is immune to HIV and that they risk being infected if they do not, for example, practise safe sex.

The possibility that the client is in the window period, or that the negative test result may be *false negative*, should also be pointed out. If there is concern about the HIV status of the person, he or she should return for a repeat test 3–6 months

Don't underestimate the extreme importance of counselling a client who tested HIV negative. This may be your only chance to explore the person's sexual practices, potential drug abuse and other risk behaviours, and to discuss safer sex practices. Free condoms can be given out at this session together with a demonstration on how to use them and information on where to get more when needed. Use this counselling session to prevent a future situation where somebody else has to give the client a positive HIV test result.

later, meanwhile taking appropriate precautions to protect him- or herself and sex partners.

Counselling after a positive HIV test result

The health care professional needs to be tremendously responsible in how to communicate positive test results to clients. People's reactions to test results depend largely on how thoroughly their counsellors have educated and prepared them before and after testing. Although it is good to encourage clients to ask questions, one should not bombard a client with information that he or she is unable to absorb at that moment. Learn to be comfortable with silence. Counsellors don't always have to say something.

There is no recipe or ten-point plan for telling a person that he or she is HIV positive. The best the counsellor can do is to be there for the client and to respond to the needs of the client. Let the client lead you in your response and care. The following guidelines may prove useful (Albers, 1990; Blom, 2001; Brouard, 2002; Eastaugh, 1997; Van Dyk, 1999).

Prepare yourself before giving the results

The counsellor should prepare him- or herself before giving a client the results (positive or negative) of an HIV test.

- Make sure that you have the right results. Check the name of the client against the formal results.
- Make sure that you understand what the results mean.
- Make sure that you have time to spend with the client.
- Make sure that you are emotionally ready to give the results to the client.

Sharing the results with the client

Positive (as well as negative) test results should be given to the client personally. Feedback should take place in a quiet, private environment, and enough time should be allowed for discussion. Greet and welcome the client and ascertain that the client is ready for the results. A positive result ought to be communicated calmly, professionally and empathically. Simple and straightforward language should be used. Do not give the individual false hopes and do not paint a hopeless scenario. Choose neutral words when conveying a positive HIV test result. Don't attach value to the results by saying 'I have bad news for you'. Such an attitude reflects a hopelessness in the mind of the counsellor. Rather say: 'Mr Peterson, the results of your HIV test came back, and you are HIV positive.' Nowadays, HIV infection is a chronic, manageable infection and the counsellor's task is to convey optimism and hope.

There are a few DON'Ts that we need to observe when sharing a positive HIV test result with a client.

- Don't lie or dodge the issue.
- Don't beat about the bush or use delaying tactics. Come to the point.
- Don't present the client with the formal printed laboratory report to 'see for themselves' without saying anything. These reports are difficult to understand at the best of times. Give the client the printed results *after* telling him or her what the result is.
- Don't break the news in a corridor or any other public place.
- Don't give the impression of being rushed, distracted or distant.
- Don't interrupt or argue.
- Don't say that 'Nothing can be done', because something can always be done to ease suffering.

Enrichment

Sensitivity to the client's needs

The counsellor should be sensitive to the individual and cultural needs of each client. Nomsa, a black woman, relayed her experience as follows: 'The counsellor looked very nervous, made small talk, and offered me some tea. I thought: "Now why is she offering me tea? What is wrong?" I got cross with her because I'm not here for tea. I'm here for my test results.'

On the other hand, Maria, a white Afrikaans-speaking woman, would have loved a cup of tea. She said: 'Everything was so correct and clinical. I would have loved a cup of tea to calm my nerves. My mother always made us some tea when things in life went wrong.'

- Don't react to anger with anger.
- Don't say 'I know how you feel', because you don't.
- Don't be afraid to admit ignorance if you don't know something.

Client reaction to a positive HIV test result

It is never easy to tell people that they are HIV positive. Counsellors have to work through their own feelings about the results before they counsel. Clients' responses to the results usually vary from one person to another, and may include shock, disbelief, numbness, crying, agitation, stress, guilt, withdrawal, anger and outrage. Some may respond with denial, indifference or even relief. The counsellor should not take any reactions personally, and he or she should show empathy, warmth and caring. Allow clients to deal with the results in their own way and give them the opportunity to express their feelings. Accept and normalise any responses and feelings that have been evoked. Reflect the feelings that are demonstrated and talk about the expressed feelings, concerns and reactions. Maintain neutrality and respond professionally to outbursts. Don't show surprise or make value-laden comments such as 'There is no need to be upset with me!' Keep in mind that the client is facing multiple losses (such as a loss of health, sexuality, and a future) and that the client may manifest all the components of bereavement such as denial, anger, bargaining, depression and acceptance. The counsellor must respect the personal nature of an individual's feelings. The counsellor should also keep the mode of infection in mind, because this may have implications for coping strategies. Being infected through rape, a needle-stick injury, an infidelity or a loving relationship will each create its own unique dynamic (Brouard, 2002:60).

Responding to the client's needs

People's needs after receiving HIV-positive test results will vary, and the counsellor has to determine what those needs are and deal with them accordingly. Not all these needs will necessarily come to the fore or be discussed in the first session. Some needs will be addressed during the second or follow-up counselling session. Allow the client to lead the session and to introduce his or her needs. As counsellor you have to provide a safe and caring environment for the client to explore his or her needs.

The following issues usually come to the fore, or can be discussed at the client's pace:

- Fear of pain, and death are often the most serious and immediate problems for a client. Helping clients to explore their fears for the future is one of the most important therapeutic interventions that the counsellor can provide. Counsellors don't have to have all the answers; it is often enough just to be there for the client and to listen.
- Some clients need information. Answer questions compassionately and appropriately but be careful not to over-intellectualise. Rather work with the clients' feelings. Give them written information to take home. Clients often ask questions about antiretroviral medication (convey hope by explaining that antiretroviral therapy may reduce the viral load in the blood, but also be honest and tell them that it is not a cure for HIV infection) and about diseases or symptoms that they are now vulnerable to. Explain that opportunistic infections can be successfully treated and prevented with medication.
- One of the major concerns for HIV-positive people is who to tell about their condition and how to break the news. Discuss disclosure to at least one supportive person who will be there for the client, and ascertain whether there is a partner involved. If necessary, discuss how this person will be told, and if the client is not ready to disclose to the sex partner, how to negotiate safer sex until disclosure has taken place. It is often helpful at this point to use role-play situations in which the client can practise communicating the news to others. (See 'Disclosure of HIV-positive status' on page 220.) The client may also ask the counsellor to convey the news to loved ones, and the counsellor should be prepared to be there to give support during disclosure. (See 'Confidentiality and privacy' on page 335 for the legal implications of confidentiality and conveying the news to sex partners.) Explore other disclosures to past or future sex partners,

health care providers, insurers, family and friends, and the employer.

- Some clients may fear the loss of their jobs. Discuss the legal rights of HIV-positive people, and stress that rights go with responsibilities.
- Financial problems may be a concern for some clients. Discuss welfare options including disability grants and how these are accessed.
- Concerns around children should be discussed. Explore pregnancy and its risks, prevention of mother-to-child (vertical) transmission, termination of pregnancy, family planning, guardianship of orphans, and decisions about testing children. (See 'Counselling HIV-positive pregnant women' on page 231.)
- Discuss medical options such as follow-up tests and what they mean; the development of a health care plan with a state clinic or private practitioner; available treatments and cost; alternative health options (including traditional healers); and the importance of regular medical check-ups.
- Inform the client of the increased risk of TB in people who are HIV positive. Tell them the symptoms of TB and encourage them to seek treatment if they develop symptoms.
- Lifestyle changes such as cutting down on alcohol and substances, stopping smoking, getting sufficient sleep and rest, appropriate exercise, dealing with stress, eating a proper balanced diet, use of supplements and immune boosters, safer sexual behaviour and re-infection, safer blood practices and infection control should be discussed.
- Find out what support groups are available to clients. Refer them to support groups where people meet regularly to talk about their difficulties or simply to relax and enjoy each other's company. Information about support groups is usually available at the nearest Aids centre or from the offices of non-governmental organisations working in the community.
- Help the client develop a problem management plan (see enrichment box 'The problem-solving model' on page 181). A useful starting point is to ask the client to compile a list of his or her good qualities and possible limitations (e.g. coping skills, self-esteem, personality style, communication style, sense of humour).

Enrichment

Shared confidentiality as opposed to secrecy

HIV-positive individuals often battle with the question of 'who to tell'. Some people decide to share the information with a selected few who will keep it confidential; others decide to keep their HIV-positive status a secret. Shared confidentiality is encouraged. This means sharing the information (on a confidential basis) with family, loved ones, caregivers and trusted friends who are willing to give support. Clients should consider withholding the information from those who do not have their best interests at heart. Some clients prefer to keep their HIV-positive status a total secret. Although it remains the client's choice, secrecy may have very negative consequences. It may isolate and alienate the client from a support system that is desperately needed. The kind of social support generally given to families with terminally ill members cannot openly be given to families who keep the HIV diagnosis a secret. Bereavement may ultimately also be very difficult to handle in these families because the bereavement will be the culmination of a long process of denial.

- Identify the ways in which clients have dealt successfully with their problems in the past, and help them (if necessary) develop new coping skills.

According to Brouard (2002), the counsellor should work with *hope* and *empowerment* when responding to a client's needs, by:

- supporting the client's realistic hopefulness and being encouraging without discounting the client's concerns or avoiding talking about death and dying;
- focusing on promising research;
- focusing on quality-of-life issues;
- encouraging the client to take control of his/her health;
- encouraging the use of resources; and
- stressing that people with HIV are living productive lives.

A plan for the next 24 hours

Help the client to plan clearly and concretely how he or she will manage the next 24 hours. Simplify the options and help with the immediate and most pressing concerns if possible. Identify the next steps and let the client tell you exactly what he or she is going to do within the next few hours or days. Check the client's plan for feasibility, including time lines. Although it is better for the client not to be alone, personal needs should be taken into consideration: some people *prefer* to be alone and to work through a crisis all by themselves. Give appropriate contact numbers and arrange a follow-up appointment, for the next day if possible. Before the client has left, assess their suicide risk and respond accordingly.

Activity

If you really want to know what your clients are going through while waiting for their HIV test results, go for testing yourself. Make notes of your feelings and emotions while going through the process and ask yourself the following questions: Was the pre- and post-test counselling properly done? How did it make you feel? How would you do the counselling differently? How did you feel while waiting for the results? What did you do while waiting? Who did you tell? Who supported you while you were waiting for the results? Will your own testing experience influence your counselling of a client? How?

Activity

Create a user-friendly pamphlet or booklet for HIV/Aids counsellors to use as a handout after post-HIV-test counselling. The pamphlet should include information for people who test HIV negative as well as for those who test positive. Include information (names, telephone numbers and addresses) of available resources, support services and Aids centres. Please note that a handout should never take the place of personal pre- and post-HIV-test counselling!

Follow-up visits

When people hear that they are HIV positive, they usually experience so much stress that they absorb very little information. Follow-up visits are therefore necessary to give clients the opportunity to ask questions and talk about their fears and the various problems they encounter. Significant others, such as a lover, spouse or other members of the family, may be included in the session.

If health care professionals are not in a position to do follow-up counselling, information about relevant health services should be given. If there is a concern that the person might not return for follow-up counselling, information about available medical treatments such as antiretroviral therapy, treatment of opportunistic infections (including information about TB), and social services for financial and ongoing emotional support should be given. Give the client a handout with whatever relevant information he or she may need (such as the telephone numbers and addresses of Aids centres and other social services).

Crisis intervention

Crisis intervention is often necessary after an HIV-positive test result is given. This is especially necessary if the client shows tendencies to or talks about suicide. The possibility of suicide can usually be identified in the pre-test counselling session. The counsellor has to take a more active role in crisis intervention to help the client contain his or her anxiety or despair, to identify and evaluate any immediate threats to safety, and to take active steps to increase the safety of the client. The counsellor should focus on options to access immediate informal support, professional help or emergency services. Contact a friend or family member of the client who can fetch them from your office and who will be able to stay with them, or arrange for somebody to be with them until the immediate crisis is over. If a friend or family member cannot be with the client, emergency hospitalisation should be arranged (see 'Crisis intervention' on page 234 and 'Suicide' on page 226).

Counselling after an inconclusive HIV test result

If a test result is inconclusive, the counsellor must explain to the client what such a result means: it is ambiguous or indeterminate, and it is not possible at that stage to say whether or not that person is HIV positive. The test result may be inconclusive because the test is cross-reacting with a non-HIV protein or because there has been insufficient time for full seroconversion to occur after exposure to HIV.

When a test result is inconclusive, other methods may be used to try to achieve a reliable result. The test can also be repeated after two weeks. If it is still inconclusive, it should be repeated at three, six and twelve months. If still inconclusive after a year, it should be accepted that the person is not infected with HIV.

Waiting for further tests to be done after inconclusive results can induce acute and severe

Activity

Devise a form that can be used for the pre- and post-HIV-test interview. Include the following information:

- Biographical details of the client
- Pre-test counselling:
  - Reason for testing
  - Medical history (STIs, TB, other symptoms, previous testing, results)
  - Sexual history
  - Sexual practices (safe or unsafe?)
  - Beliefs and knowledge about HIV/Aids (transmission, window period, etc.)
  - Information about the test
  - Implications of results (does client understand implications?)
  - Support network
  - Does client understand concepts of confidentiality and informed consent?
- Permission to be tested for HIV
  - Does the client want to be tested for HIV (Yes/No), or does he or she need time to think about it?
  - Is the client fully informed about the nature, procedure, aim, importance and consequences of HIV testing?
  - Did the client give written permission that a blood sample can be taken and tested for HIV?
- Post-test counselling:
  - What was the result of the HIV test? Positive, negative or inconclusive?
  - If negative: Safer sex practices, window period, re-testing
  - If positive: Issues discussed
  - Any special problems? (e.g suicidal tendencies?)
  - Support network
  - Immediate plans for next 24 hours
  - Referral and follow-up

psychological effects in people. Clients should be supported while waiting for the results. They should also be encouraged to use safer sex practices while waiting.

11.3 CONCLUSION

An HIV-positive test result makes a tremendous and irreversible impact on a person's life. Important decisions and changes have to be made by the client and loved ones to live within the constraints imposed by the virus. The counsellor must therefore undertake the very important task of helping the client to live a healthy and happy life after diagnosis. Chapter 12 discusses counselling in various contexts, as well as specific themes in the counselling needs of people living with HIV/Aids and of the loved ones affected by their illness. The ethical and legal aspects of HIV testing are discussed in Chapter 19.

Activity

- Ask a friend to role play a post-HIV-test counselling session with you. Counsel the friend on the results of his or her HIV test if the test result is positive. Remember that role play can be very draining and disturbing and that it is always necessary to debrief afterwards. Say to your friend: 'Thank you Peter for doing the role play with me. This was only a make-believe situation. I am not really a counsellor, you are not my client and you are not HIV positive.'
- Ask a friend to play the role of a sex worker who tested HIV negative. Counsel her on the results of her HIV test.
- You are a social worker working in an Aids unit established by the Department of Social Development. You have a very heavy daily case load. Some mornings when you arrive at your office, 30 people are already waiting, either to be tested or to get their results. You feel dispirited because it is almost impossible in the limited time available to do proper pre- and post-test counselling. Organise a workshop with colleagues who experience the same problem and try to find solutions for this problem.
- What do you do if a client does not want pre-test counselling before taking a test? (See 'What if a person refuses pre-HIV test counselling (and HIV testing)?' on page 338.)

chapter

12 Counselling in Various Contexts

Listening to the fear

And then the listening women saw the fear
embedded deep in the words of the men.
Hidden among the reeds,
below the smooth surface of the water.

'Aids is the stuff of all our nightmares, triggering many of our deepest fears' (Watts, 1988). These words – spoken by an HIV-positive client – aptly express why Aids is different from any other life-threatening disease. The diagnosis of HIV infection or Aids evokes severe emotional reactions – not only in the *infected* person, but also in his or her *affected* significant others. The counsellor can help those who are infected and affected by HIV/Aids to *live beyond* the diagnosis only if he or she has an understanding of what the person living with HIV/Aids and his or her loved ones are going through. But it is also important to realise that, if you are an HIV/Aids counsellor, you too are an *affected other*, and you should therefore be aware of your own feelings and work through them if you want to be able to counsel effectively.

12.1 THE PSYCHOSOCIAL EXPERIENCES OF A PERSON LIVING WITH HIV/AIDS

Being HIV positive affects people mentally, socially and emotionally. The following case study describes the psychosocial experiences of a person with Aids after he was diagnosed with the illness in 1986 (Palermino, 1988:63):

One person's experience of Aids

My doctor gave me the news. My first reaction was one of relief. The years of uncertainty had ended. The myriad of symptoms could all be explained. No more worries about if I would develop Aids. I now had it.

The next day, I lay in bed exhausted and began to realise the full meaning of the diagnosis. What may lie ahead? I had moments of denying it was really happening; I wanted to believe I would be well in a few days. I phoned my supervisor at work and told her I would be back in two days. I only briefly wondered if there had been some mistake. Maybe I had been misdiagnosed. My mind was racing. I could not concentrate on anything for more than a few seconds. Ninety per cent of my thoughts were death-related or reflections on what life choices I had made. Mistakes, broken dreams . . . What would my funeral be like? My obituaries? What infection would finally kill me?

Suffering and grief were what I felt. Imagine losing your job, your love relationship, your home, and all of your friends. On top of that you feel you have no future, you will not feel the wind against your skin, or watch snow fall. You will not hear music or go sailing with friends. And you will not love or be loved.

I had crossed the line. The line between the living and the dead. I feared being alone and yet needed to be alone. In my 20s I grew to believe in God, or my higher power, as I prefer to call him. Had he betrayed me? I felt ripped off. Yet I also had a sense of universal truths, of my own connection with all that I feared losing. And I do believe that on some level I have always been a part of this world and always will be.

Through the first week, my biggest concern was telling my parents. They are both in their 70s. One cannot know for sure the reactions of friends and loved ones. I didn't expect it, but my oldest brother Paul has become one of my main sources of support since my diagnosis. One friend sent a card with the following note: 'I know there is nothing I can say or do to change your diagnosis. My heart is with you. I love you. If you need anything, call. I am here for you if and when you're ready. Take things slowly, be gentle with yourself, meditate, scream, cry, laugh. Be yourself.' In the height of the crisis of being diagnosed her words were of great comfort.

The early weeks of my diagnosis were the most challenging so far. The week after I was diagnosed with Pneumocystis, the doctor found a Kaposi's sarcoma lesion in my mouth. I was afraid to see my doctor. What else might he find? I was terrified I would die if he did not keep a close watch, and yet I feared he would continue to find other infections. He and his staff were excellent when I needed them the most. He is a model doctor because when I need things explained, he always takes the time to do so. One day his office staff needed to take several tubes of blood. One drew blood while another massaged my belly. A personal touch is so important when you are being assaulted by so many needles and so much machinery.

Second to facing death, I believe financial concerns are the major issue for most people with Aids. The bureaucracy and intricacies of disability and medical coverage are astounding and infuriating. Loss of career status has also been a difficult transition.

I have experienced varying periods of depression, grandiosity, rage, and gratefulness. I had thoughts of suicide several times during the first weeks. Looking back, I see it as an attempt to control what was happening to me.

If I am going to die, I want to say when and how. I had seen all the horrible possibilities of the disease and wondered what would befall me. I started to bargain: I can accept weight loss and chills, but not fevers. Skin lesions? Yes, but not constant vomiting or diarrhoea. And I was most terrified about going insane due to neurological infections.

One friend who had been diagnosed the year before told me: 'Things will fall into place, it gets easier.' He was right. Eight months have passed since my diagnosis. I continue to experience the roller coaster effects of having a life-threatening illness, but the peaks and valleys are less dramatic. For now my health is relatively good and I can go on with living. I have grown to accept what I can and cannot do each day, to enjoy that which I can do and appreciate the mere fact that I am alive today. I try to do something joyous every day.

Activity

When you have read the case study, answer the following questions:

- List the psychosocial experiences, feelings and concerns that the client had.
- What were the client's concerns about his significant others?
- What positive experiences or feelings did the client have after his diagnosis?

The case study on the preceding pages shows that HIV-positive people often experience the following psychosocial, spiritual and socio-economic feelings and needs.

Fear

HIV-positive people have many fears. They are particularly afraid of being isolated, stigmatised and rejected. They fear the uncertainty of the future: will there be pain or disfigurement, and who will look after them? They are afraid of dying – and particularly of dying alone and in pain. Many HIV-positive people have experienced the pain and death of loved ones and friends who have already died of Aids, and they know and fear what awaits them. Fear may also be caused by not knowing enough about what is involved in being HIV positive and how the problems can be handled.

Loss

HIV-positive people often feel that they have lost everything that is important and beautiful to them. They experience loss of control, loss of independence, loss of their ambitions, their physical attractiveness, sexual relationships, status and respect in the community, financial stability and independence. They fear the loss of their ability to care for themselves and their families, and they fear the loss of their jobs, their friends and family. They mourn the loss of life itself. People with Aids also feel that they have lost their privacy and their control over their lives once they begin to need constant care. But perhaps the most commonly experienced loss is the loss of confidence and self-worth caused by the rejection of people who are important to them – people who were once friends but who now reject them because of the physical impact of HIV-related diseases that cause, for example, physical wasting and loss of strength or bodily control.

Grief

People with HIV infection often have profound feelings of grief about the losses they have experienced or are anticipating. They grieve for their friends who die from Aids, and they grieve with and for their loved ones – those who must stay behind and try to cope with life without them.

Guilt

Guilt and self-reproach for having contracted HIV and for having also possibly infected others are frequently expressed by HIV-positive individuals. They often feel guilty about the behaviour that may have caused the infection. Feelings of guilt may be associated with a person's unresolved conflicts about homosexuality or about sexuality in general. Having to tell family members and friends that one is HIV positive often means that one also has to tell them for the first time about one's sexual preferences or sexual behaviour. There is also guilt about the sadness that the illness will inflict on loved ones and families – especially children. Previous events that may have caused others pain or sadness but which still remain unresolved will often now be remembered and be the cause of even greater feelings of guilt and anguish.

Denial

Most HIV-positive people go through a phase of *denial.* Denial is an important and protective defence mechanism because it temporarily reduces emotional stress. Clients should be allowed to cling to their denial if they are not yet ready to accept their diagnosis, because denial often gives them a breathing space in which to rest and gather their strength. However, counsellors should confront this denial if it causes destructive behaviour such as refusing appropriate medical care or continued indulgence in unrestrained high-risk behaviour.

Anger

HIV-positive people are often very angry with themselves and others, and this anger is sometimes directed at those closest to them. They are angry because there is no cure for Aids and because of the uncertainty of their future. They are often also angry with those who infected them and with society's reaction of hostility and indifference.

Anxiety

The chronic uncertainty associated with the progress of HIV infection often aggravates feelings of anxiety. People with HIV/Aids often experience anxiety because of the prognosis of the illness; the risk of infection with other diseases; the risk of infecting loved ones with HIV; social, occupational, domestic and sexual hostility and rejection; abandonment, isolation, and physical pain; fear of dying in pain or without dignity; inability to alter circumstances and consequences of HIV infection; uncertainty about how to keep as healthy as possible in the future; fears about the ability of loved ones and family to cope; worries about the availability (or unavailability) of appropriate medical treatment; a loss of privacy and concerns about confidentiality; future social and sexual unacceptability; their declining ability to function efficiently; and their loss of physical and financial independence. One can see the raw anxiety in this client's moving plea ('An open letter', 1988):

> A telephone call is not contagious and no one will die from visiting me occasionally. I'm not going to infect anyone if they hug me once in a while. I'm not asking for miracles, or approval, or sympathy. But this is only the beginning of the nightmare. What will happen when I get seriously ill? When I am in hospital, too weak to help myself, emaciated, fighting for life, and scared? I'm going to need friends. Please, don't let me die alone!

Low self-esteem

The self-esteem of HIV-positive people is often severely threatened. Rejection by colleagues, friends and loved ones can cause loss of confidence and loss of one's sense of social identity, leading to feelings of reduced self-worth. The inability to continue in a career or to participate in social, sexual and loving relationships also diminishes the client's self-esteem. The physical consequences of HIV infection such as physical wasting and the loss of strength and bodily control contribute even more to a lowering of self-esteem.

Depression

People with HIV/Aids often experience depression because they feel that they have lost so much in life and that they themselves are to blame for it. The following factors all serve to increase depression: the absence of a cure and the resulting feeling of powerlessness; knowing others who have died of Aids; the loss of personal control over their lives; and self-blame and feelings of guilt. It is important for counsellors to recognise signs of depression, and to refer their clients to a professional psychologist if necessary. (See 'Depression' on page 225 for a more complete discussion.)

Suicidal behaviour or thinking

Inwardly directed anger may manifest as self-blame, self-destructive behaviour or (in its most intense form) suicidal impulses or intention. Suicide may be construed as a way of avoiding pain and discomfort, of lessening the shame and grief of loved ones, and of trying to obtain a measure of control over one's illness. Suicide may be either *active* (deliberate self-injury resulting in death) or *passive* (concealing or disregarding the onset of the possibly fatal complications of HIV infection or disease). The counsellor should be aware that there is a significantly higher risk of suicide among people with HIV/Aids. (See 'Suicide' on page 226 for a more complete discussion.)

Obsessive conditions and hypochondria

Some HIV-positive individuals become so preoccupied with their health that even the smallest physical changes or sensations can cause obsessive behaviour or hypochondria. This may be temporary and limited to the time immediately after diagnosis, or it may persist in people who find it difficult to adjust to or accept the disease.

Spiritual concerns

HIV-positive people who are confronted with death, loneliness, and loss of control often ask questions about spiritual matters in their search for religious support. They may want to discuss the concepts of sin, guilt, forgiveness, reconciliation, and acceptance. (See 'Spiritual counselling' on page 249.)

Socio-economic issues

Socio-economic and environmental problems such as loss of an occupation and income, discrimination, social stigma (if the client's diagnosis becomes commonly known), relationship changes, and changing requirements for sexual expression, may contribute to psychosocial problems after the diagnosis of HIV infection. Because many HIV-positive people also have financial problems, they often cannot afford to buy the antiretroviral therapy that might give them a longer lease on life.

The client's perception of the level and adequacy of social support is very important. Perceived lack of support when it is most needed may become a source of pressure or frustration.

Hope and equilibrium

With the help of counsellors and the support of their loved ones and friends, many HIV-positive individuals come to a point where they realise that HIV infection is a manageable disease. They access health care when necessary and they realise that antiretroviral therapy and other medications are available should they need it. *Positive living* has become the dictum of many people living with HIV and Aids around the world. Although not all days are good, they learn to cope with the bad days and live in hope.

12.2 THE IMPACT OF HIV INFECTION ON AFFECTED SIGNIFICANT OTHERS

The significant others in the life of a person living with HIV/Aids play an important role in that person's physical and psychological care. But significant others themselves often need help to come to terms with their own fears and prejudices and the implications and consequences of their loved one's sickness and ultimate death. The counsellor can play a tremendous role in counselling the partners, friends and family of the HIV-positive person in the practicalities of physical and emotional care.

Counsellors should be open-minded about what might constitute a 'family' in these circumstances. 'Family members' may include families of choice (lovers and friends – especially when the infected person is gay or lesbian) as well as families that are related by birth or marriage. Sometimes the 'real' family of an infected person will reject him or her completely. In such circumstances it is often only the family of choice (the lover and friends) who will care for the loved one until the end. It is important for the counsellor to respect these extralegal relationships.

Affected significant others experience more or less the same psychosocial feelings as do their HIV-positive loved ones – the same feelings of depression, loneliness, fear, uncertainty, anxiety, anger, emotional numbness and, at times, hope. The impact of HIV infection on affected others can be summarised as follows (Johnson in Van Dyk et al., 2000:12):

- Affected others often experience fear and anxiety about their own risk of infection as a function of their relationship with the HIV-positive person. They scrutinise the relationship or contact for possible risk situations in the past and this places a huge strain on the relationship.
- Affected others (especially the partner of the HIV-positive person) are often furious with the infected person for 'bringing this onto them'.
- Affected others begin to anticipate the loss of the HIV-positive person, and issues of loss, bereavement and uncertainty are introduced into the relationship at a time when this may not be appropriate.
- Affected others, especially if they are very close to the infected person, often feel unable to cope with the new demands that the infection places on them. They feel incompetent, unqualified and powerless in their interaction with the HIV-positive significant other. These feelings contribute to a need to distance themselves from the disease process as well as the person. '*Denial* of the illness becomes a negation of the person, accounting for much of the isolation experienced by the HIV-positive person' (Johnson in Van Dyk et al., 2000:12).

- The HIV-positive status of a significant other sadly often acquires a certain *relational currency*. This means that friends, relatives and colleagues tend to 'use' the infected person's seropositive status as an issue in their ongoing relationships with each other. Old scores are settled, new disputes are initiated, and relationships are redefined around the issue of the HIV-positive person's illness. Interactions often take place around – rather than *with* – the HIV-positive person.
- Disclosure of a loved one's seropositive status is always a shock, and no two people react in the same way to the news. Affected others' responses can range from involvement, caring and support on the one hand, to abandonment, indifference, and antagonism on the other. Sadly, HIV-positive people are often rejected by their significant others because of the stigma that still surrounds this disease in many societies – including our own.
- Affected others suffer in many ways as a result of untimely deaths. People who die of Aids are usually young (between 20 and 35 years old), and this leads to the unnatural situation of parents outliving their children. Grandparents who are preparing themselves for a quiet and contented old age now find themselves nursing and caring for sick and dying children and taking care of the grandchildren.
- Children suffer tremendously when their parents are infected, and the needs of children with infected parents are often neglected. In many African societies there is no tradition of talking to children as equals and on an intimate basis, and caregivers often report seeing 'the suffering of children, who are too often hovering in the shadows of a sick room, seeing and hearing everything but never addressed directly' (UNAIDS, 2000a:33). Children are largely excluded from the counselling process in Africa because (among other reasons) caregivers often simply do not know how to talk to children.
- Significant others often have to fulfil a role for which they are not trained, namely that of *caregiver*. They have to look after seriously ill loved ones. This can be an arduous, disconcerting and all-consuming task that utterly drains all the caregiver's physical, emotional and (often) financial resources. If there are unresolved relationship issues in such circumstances, they can quickly become acutely aggravated.
- Neurological complications and deterioration in mental functioning in the patient can be extremely disturbing to significant others. They may feel that they are already losing their loved ones and this can precipitate an early grieving process.
- The *needs* of affected significant others are similar to those experienced by the HIV-positive person. These needs are acceptance, respect, certainty, affiliation, support, love and caring.

12.3 SPECIFIC ISSUES IN HIV/AIDS COUNSELLING

HIV/Aids brings very specific and unique issues out into the open, and counsellors should spend time exploring these issues with their clients. The following prominent themes tend to emerge repeatedly in HIV/Aids counselling:

- uncertainty about the progress of the disease, especially as current treatment options lengthen life expectancy;
- relationship problems with significant others;
- issues surrounding the disclosure of HIV-positive status;
- dealing with the fear, stigma and stereotypes associated with HIV infection;
- pregnancy;
- career and financial concerns;
- sexual relationships;
- stress and anxiety;
- depression and suicidal thinking;
- spiritual and existential matters; and
- issues about death and dying.

Some of these themes are discussed in other parts of the book. This chapter will deal with disclosure, pregnancy, stress, anxiety, depression and suicide. If clients present with serious problems (or need more than three counselling sessions), counsellors should refer them for professional help.

Disclosure of HIV-positive status

The decision whether or not to disclose being HIV positive is difficult because disclosure (or non-disclosure) may have major and life-changing consequences. Counsellors should help their clients to consider carefully the benefits and the negative consequences that disclosure may have for them as individuals. Because disclosure is a very personal and individual decision, all relevant personal circumstances should be taken into account. Clients should decide whether they want *full disclosure* (i.e. publicly revealing their HIV status) or *partial disclosure* (i.e. telling only certain people, such as a partner, spouse, relative or friend). Disclosure can be accompanied by the following benefits (Southern African AIDS Trust, 2000):

- Disclosure can help people accept their HIV-positive status and reduce the stress of coping on their own.
- Disclosure can ease access to medical services, care and support, including access to antiretroviral therapy.
- Disclosure can help people protect themselves and others. Openness about their HIV-positive status may help women to negotiate safer sex practices.
- Disclosure may help to reduce the stigma, discrimination and denial that surround HIV/Aids.
- Disclosure promotes responsibility. It may encourage the person's loved ones to plan for the future.

Disclosure can also be accompanied by negative consequences such as problems in relationships (e.g. with sexual partners, family, friends, community members, employer or colleagues), rejection, and the conviction that people are constantly judging one. The following case studies illustrate some of the different experiences people have had after disclosing their HIV-positive status.

Case studies on disclosure

- *Testimony 1 – Disclosure and a new lease of life:* 'I was tested unknowingly in 1988 and the result was disclosed in the ward where everybody heard. I was shocked and felt humiliated. When I got home, I only told my husband. I hoped he would support me but he accused me and after a short while he abandoned me. I suffered alone for the next five years without telling anybody. I wasted away because there was nobody to advise me on what to do. I did not tell my parents and sisters about my HIV status because they were very negative on the issue of HIV. The miraculous change came in 1993 when I got my first counselling at The Centre in Harare. It was like I started living again. I stopped mourning for myself and started getting confident. I now knew the right foods to eat and how to avoid stress. I became a happy person and started gaining back my weight. I was introduced to other people living with HIV and Aids and started feeling comfortable talking about the illness' (Southern African AIDS Trust, 2000:5).
- *Testimony 2 – Fear, love and support:* 'I tested HIV positive in July 1990. What made me disclose? I believe it was fear. Fear of illness. Fear of the unknown. I felt so alone and needed to talk to someone. I just could not handle it on my own. Love and support from everyone around me made it easier. Their acceptance gave me strength and courage to keep telling more people. I wouldn't have told so many if the first people had rejected me. If I had to do it again, I wouldn't do it differently. My friends have always given me support, so I guess I'd still tell them first' (Southern African AIDS Trust, 2000:3).
- *Testimony 3 – Life needs courage:* 'I decided to come out publicly because a lot of Swazis are dying and they think HIV is a problem in other countries but not ours. I have had problems with my wife's family. They accuse me of being unfeeling and insensitive – to them it was humiliating that everyone knows my status. But my wife stood by me and we are still together. In the long run I feel good about my choice. Just talking about my situation has helped a lot of HIV-positive people and their relatives. My advice is to remember that life needs courage' (Southern African AIDS Trust, 2000:7).

Clients should think through all the pros and cons very carefully and plan ahead before they disclose their HIV-positive status. The counsellor can support the client by using the following guidelines (Southern African AIDS Trust, 2000:6–7):

- Help the client to take time to think things through. Explore the implications of disclosure fully so that the person has an opportunity to consider in advance what the reaction of family, friends, colleagues and others might be. Make sure it is what the client *wants* to do and assist him or her to plan how he or she is going to do it.
- The client should feel comfortable with his or her diagnosis before disclosing it to others.
- Provide support and reassurance to the client and help them to accept themselves.
- Be practical. Help the client to develop a 'plan' for disclosure. Such a plan will include preparations that need to be made before disclosure, who the client will inform first, how and where the disclosure will take place, and what the level of disclosure will be.
- Share the idea with the client that there are two kinds of disclosure: *disclosure for support*, where talking to a trusted person can help the client to deal with his or her feelings, and *disclosure for ethical reasons*, where there is another person who is at risk of contracting HIV (such as a sexual partner, or a health care professional).
- Identify sources of support, such as groups for people living with HIV and Aids, church members and counselling organisations.
- Suggest to the client that it is perhaps better to disclose gradually rather than to everyone at once.
- Prepare the client for a shocked and even hostile reaction from other people. Reassure clients that people close to them will probably learn to accept their HIV status over time.
- Help clients to realise that, once a decision to disclose has been made, it may be easier to begin with those nearest to them: relatives, family, friends, or someone to whom they are very close and whom they trust.
- Help the client to think about the likely response of the person to whom he or she has decided to disclose. Help the client to assess how much the person he or she plans to disclose to knows and understands about HIV and Aids. This will help the client to decide what they need to tell the person and how to tell them. Such preparation will make disclosure less traumatic for both of them. Suggest that the client choose somebody to disclose to who is mature, accepting, empathic and supportive.
- Remind the client that the right time and place for disclosure is important.
- Role play to help the client prepare for disclosure.
- It is important for a client to be strong enough to allow others to express their feelings and concerns after their disclosure. Assist the client to work on these issues over time.
- Counsellors should protect their clients against undue pressure to disclose.
- The counsellor should be willing to mediate the disclosure process if the need arises (e.g. if the client asks the counsellor to be present when he or she discloses his or her HIV-positive status).
- Provide the client with information and support to 'live positively' and give information on safer sex practices to protect sex partners.

How to disclose a parent's HIV-positive status to a child

Research conducted by Stein and colleagues (2004) in Khayelitsha, a township in South Africa, indicated that HIV-positive mothers often indefinitely delay disclosure to children on the grounds that their children are too young to understand the nature of HIV/Aids, and because they believe that disclosure is not in the best interest of their children. In another study in KwaZulu-Natal, it was found that children are frequently excluded from discussions about the imminent or recent death of a parent, on the grounds that death is not an appropriate topic for children to discuss (Marcus in Stein, 2004). Keeping silent about the HIV status of a parent does an injustice to any child. A study by Rosenhein and Reicher (1985) found that children who were informed of their parents' terminal illness showed significantly less anxiety than children who were not told. It was also noted that children who were not explicitly told are seldom wholly oblivious to the terminal nature of the parents' disease. To be kept in the dark made them feel guilty, anxious, depressed, isolated and lonely. Through informal discussions with South African youth, Stein (2004) found that children feel betrayed when they are finally told about a parent's HIV infection in adolescence, even if this disclosure occurs prior to illness or to death of the parent.

Counsellors should appreciate the psychological, emotional and practical difficulties attached to the task of disclosing a terminal disease to children. A few points to consider in facilitating the process of disclosure are:

- Empower parents to deal with their feelings of guilt and shame. Parents often feel guilty and anxious about 'abandoning' their children when they die.
- Make use of practical resources such as a memory book or a memory box to support parental disclosure to children (see enrichment box 'Memory projects' on page 277).
- Include children in the care of the sick parent and explain to them what you are doing in a language that they will understand.
- Disclosure is not a once-off experience. It takes time, and the age of the child should be kept in mind. Tell children what they need to know and build onto that (also see the next section on how to tell a child that he or she is HIV positive).
- Allow children to participate in grieving, and discuss it with the child. Allowing children to say goodbye and exchange wishes and thoughts regarding death leaves less unfinished business for children to manage after the death (Stein, 2004:17).
- Share the plans that you have made for the child's future with him or her. The child may be concerned about who is going to care for him or her after the parent's death.

The way in which children deal with their parents' illness often depends on how caregivers deal with the situation. Stein (2004:19) quotes Tanchel who argues that 'children need to be supported through, rather than protected from emotional pain, including illness and death: What is most frightening for children is when they know something unspoken is terribly wrong.'

How to tell a child that he or she is HIV positive

To disclose to a child that he or she is HIV positive is possibly one of the greatest struggles that a parent could have. Not only is the parent disclosing a life-threatening disease to a child, but he or she probably also battles with feelings of guilt, sadness, depression, hopelessness, fear and feelings of loss. However hard it is for parents to disclose to children, evidence suggests that children may suffer more from the silence around HIV. Some children have known for a while that they are positive and feel angry, hurt and confused by the time they are officially told. They also see the silence as a message that they should be worried or ashamed. The fear of parents is also understandable: They fear the loss of the child, they fear that the child will tell others, and that the child will blame and hate them. While it is ideal for parents to tell a child that he or she is HIV positive, they must be ready to do so, and not be forced. The following guidelines might be helpful in disclosing their HIV status to children or adolescents (based on guidelines given by the Pediatric HIV Psychosocial Support Progamme at the National Institute of Health).

- Keep in mind that disclosure is a 'process and not an event'. You don't have to tell everything at once. Keep the child's age and developmental stage in mind. For example, for a very young child (pre-school), what is happening to him or her can be explained without using the words 'HIV' or 'Aids'. That can be added at a later stage when a child is old enough to understand the concept.
- The amount of information given can vary according to need and circumstance. Give enough information to help the child understand his or her day-to-day experiences and add information as it becomes necessary.
- Don't ever lie to a child. Be honest, keep communication lines open and don't lose the trust of the child. Children often feel betrayed

if a parent has lied to them, and they will then mistrust other parent communications.

- Be prepared for reactions, feelings, questions and thoughts for a long time after disclosure.
- Prepare yourself for disclosure. How are you going to tell? On your own or with someone's help? With the help of pictures, a book or a video? Is there someone who can help the child deal with his or her feelings? It may help to write down what you would like your child to know.
- Reassure the child that he or she is not to be blamed. Children often believe that sickness is their fault and that they did something wrong.
- Assure the child of your love. That is often all they want to hear – that you love them and that you will take care of them.
- Assure the child that the virus is not contagious (and that his or her friends or siblings won't get it).
- Let the child lead you. He or she will show you in all kinds of ways if you are telling too little (by asking more questions) or too much (by changing the subject).
- The general rule is: be simple, clear and honest.
- There is no 'right' or 'wrong' time to tell a child that he or she is HIV positive. When to tell depends on the parent, the child and the family circumstances. Look for clues from children, e.g. do they ask direct questions that indicate that they sense something? Are there signs of behaviour change such as clinging or fighting? Did something happen that creates the need to tell? But don't wait for the child to give you a clue!
- Choose a place that is comfortable for you and for the child, and where you will have time and privacy (e.g. a park, a garden or a bedroom).
- Decide who else should be told. The child will probably tell his or her siblings, grandparents, friends or teacher. Don't instruct the child to 'keep it a secret', because this may create feelings of guilt, shame and isolation.
- Once the disclosure has taken place, monitor the child's behaviour – for example sleeping, school problems and withdrawal. Changes in behaviour might indicate a need for more support or intervention.

Although it might be very difficult for a parent to disclose a child's HIV-positive status to him or her, it is the best thing to do for all concerned. To keep a secret places a huge burden on a family. Telling the child themselves give parents control over how it happens. And however hard it is, parents should realise that the child may need to prepare for tasks ahead such as sickness, painful procedures, discrimination and death.

Stress

All of us experience some stress and anxiety in our day-to-day encounters with difficult situations at work, financial concerns, family demands and social interactions. Moderate amounts of stress are usually not harmful, and can even be stimulating, but excessive stress can be detrimental to one's health.

Research has shown that many diseases are caused or aggravated by an interaction of social, psychological and biological factors. Chronic stress was found to create greater susceptibility to many diseases such as flu, dermatitis and the recurrence of herpes symptoms (Sue et al., 2000). Psychological factors such as stress, emotional inhibition (e.g. keeping the fact that you are gay a secret), a negative self-concept ('I am responsible for the bad things that happen to me'), and a lack of social support have been shown to contribute to a more rapid progression from HIV

Enrichment

Stress and the immune system

While stress does not cause infection or diseases directly, it may decrease the efficiency of the immune system and thereby increase a person's susceptibility to disease. Stress produces physiological changes in the body. For example, part of the stress response involves the release of neurohormones such as corticosteroids and endorphins, and these can impair immune functioning in cases of severe stress. Endorphins, for instance, decrease the natural ability of killer-T cells to fight tumour development. A deficient immune system may further fail to detect invaders or to produce antibodies to protect the body against these invaders (Sue et al., 2000).

infection to Aids (Cole et al., 1997). Self-efficacy and an ability to cope with stressors, on the other hand, were associated with a slower deterioration of the immune system in HIV-positive individuals. It was also found that psychological and social stressors such as looking after a partner with dementia – especially without social support – as well as the loss of a partner (bereavement), weakened the immune system of the affected other significantly.

There are also indirect links between stress and immune depression. People who experience a lot of stress or who are depressed also tend to sleep less, eat less nutritiously, consume more alcohol, and give less attention to their physical care. All these factors can decrease immune functioning.

Treatment

Treatment for stress can include medication for the physical symptoms of stress, stress management or facilitation of lifestyle changes to actively reduce stress. Relaxation training is an important component of stress management, and clients should be taught the ability to relax the muscles of the body in any stressful situation. The relaxation technique is based on tensing and relaxing muscles. Clients are taught to contract (tense) and then relax specific muscle groups (e.g. first the hands, then the arms, the legs, etc.) for several minutes at a time until they learn to monitor their own relaxation. Relaxation exercises can be combined with mental imagery which enables clients to imagine being in peaceful, beautiful and calm places.

Counsellors should also help people to change their lifestyles to prevent illness and to enhance the quality of their lives. Clients should, for instance, be encouraged to avoid or change stressful situations, establish priorities, postpone low-priority tasks without feeling guilty, take time out for themselves, engage in relaxing and enjoyable activities, exercise regularly, eat nutritious foods, share their lives and problems with friends, meditate or do whatever helps them to be relaxed (Sue et al., 2000; Van Dyk, 1999).

Adjustment disorder

People often find it difficult to adjust to common life stressors such as the loss of a job, bereavement, divorce or separation. A person can be said to have an adjustment disorder if his or her response to a stressor is *maladaptive*: this means that the person experiences excessive distress and is unable to function as usual in his or her social, occupational or academic life (Carson et al., 1998; Sue et al., 2000). An HIV-positive diagnosis can be the cause of an adjustment disorder.

Adjustment disorders usually develop within three months after the stressful event and they usually disappear within six months. They are characterised by diverse symptoms such as anxiety, depression, a combination of anxiety and depression, and behavioural and/or emotional disturbances. Adjustment disorders are seldom very serious, and they usually decrease in severity or disappear when the stressor has subsided or when the individual learns to adapt to the stressor or to the new situation. Adjustment disorders can, however, become chronic and last for longer than six months when the stressor is chronic (e.g. a medical condition such as HIV infection).

Bereavement often causes adjustment disorders. Complicated or prolonged bereavement can occur when there has been an untimely or unexpected death – as is very often the case with Aids-related deaths. Those who feel resentment, hostility, or intense guilt towards the deceased may experience extreme adjustment disorders (Carson et al., 1998).

Acute stress disorder and post-traumatic stress disorder

Some people experience *acute stress disorder* after an HIV-positive diagnosis, or after the death of a significant other. An acute stress disorder is an anxiety disorder that develops in response to an extreme psychological or physical trauma. Overwhelming anxiety can seriously disrupt a person's social or occupational functioning (Sue et al., 2000).

Acute stress disorder is accompanied by the following symptoms (Carson et al., 1998; Sue et al., 2000):

- severe feelings of anxiety and helplessness;
- feelings of dissociation, emotional unresponsiveness, numbness, and withdrawal from social contact;
- persistent reliving or re-experiencing of the traumatic event through intrusive, recurring thoughts, repetitive dreams about the event, illusions and flashbacks;
- sleep disturbance, irritability, finding it difficult to concentrate or remember things, and restlessness; and
- avoidance of interpersonal involvement and loss of sexual interest.

A condition can be diagnosed as *an acute stress disorder* if the symptoms occur within four weeks of the traumatic event and last for two days or up to a month.

If the symptoms persist for more than a month, a diagnosis of *post-traumatic stress disorder* should be considered. The symptoms of post-traumatic stress disorder are similar to those of acute stress disorder, but they differ primarily in *onset* and *duration*. Post-traumatic stress disorder can occur at any time after the stressful event (acute stress disorder occurs within a month), and post-traumatic stress disorder always lasts for longer than a month (acute stress disorder lasts from a few days to a month). If the symptoms of post-traumatic stress disorder begin within six months after the stressful event, the reaction is considered to be acute. If symptoms begin more than six months after the event, the reaction is considered to be delayed.

Not all people who experience a traumatic event develop acute or post-traumatic stress disorder. Factors such as the person's individual characteristics, his or her perception of the event, and the existence of support groups also influence whether an acute or a post-traumatic stress disorder will develop (Sue et al., 2000). Counsellors should refer their clients for professional help if the clients cannot cope with their stress and anxiety.

Treatment

Treatment for anxiety symptoms often includes anti-anxiety medications, crisis-intervention approaches, debriefing, and cognitive behavioural approaches such as systematic desensitisation.

Systematic desensitisation relies on the principle that it is impossible to be both anxious and relaxed at the same time (Okun, 1997). Clients are first trained to relax (by tensing and then relaxing the muscles). If they are in a relaxed state, desensitisation follows by introducing the issue that usually arouses anxiety. Say, for example, that an HIV-positive person who has to visit the hospital frequently is absolutely terrified of hospitals. After teaching the client how to relax, the counsellor should introduce the anxiety-provoking (but not harmful) issues by starting with the least anxiety-provoking object or circumstance, and then work gradually up to the most anxiety-provoking stimuli. The counsellor could, for example, begin by showing the client a video of a hospital, then drive the client past the hospital in a car, then walk past the hospital with the client, then let him or her walk alone, then enter the hospital, and so on.

Debriefing sessions with peer support groups in which clients can express and release their anxious emotions are also beneficial in helping them cope with anxiety and stress. Discussion and support groups are very helpful in assisting clients in the adaptation process after a traumatic experience.

Depression

Depression is common in our society and is frequently experienced by HIV-positive individuals and their significant others. Anybody working in the HIV/Aids field should at least be able to recognise the symptoms of serious depression and refer clients for treatment and therapy if they are not able to assist clients themselves.

The symptoms of depression may be categorised as follows (Sue et al., 2000):

- *Affective symptoms*. The most striking symptom of depression is a depressed mood characterised by feelings of sadness, unhappiness, worthlessness, anxiety, and apathy. Depressed clients often say that they have lost the joy of living.

- *Cognitive symptoms.* Clients report feelings of futility, emptiness and hopelessness. They often have profoundly pessimistic beliefs about the future; they find it difficult to cope with daily life because of a loss of motivation, interest and energy. Suicidal thoughts, guilt, negative thinking and concentration problems are also common among depressed people.
- *Behavioural symptoms.* Lack of energy is one of the most common behavioural symptoms of depression. Other symptoms include neglect of personal appearance (dirty clothing, unkempt hair, lack of personal hygiene), crying, agitation, social withdrawal, slow or reduced speech, and passivity. Depressed people often have dull, mask-like facial expressions. They move slowly and they do not initiate new activities. These symptoms are called *psychomotor retardation.* Although psychomotor retardation is common in people with depression, some depressed people report states of agitation and restlessness.
- *Physiological symptoms.* Depressed clients often complain of a loss of appetite and weight (but some have an increased appetite and experience weight gain), sleep disturbance (difficulty in falling asleep, waking up early, waking up during the night, insomnia, nightmares), loss of libido or aversion to sexual activity, disrupted menstrual cycle in women (lengthening of the cycle, 'skipped' periods, decrease of menstrual flow), and constipation.

In order for a condition to be diagnosed as a *major depressive disorder*, the symptoms of depression should be present for at least two weeks and they should represent a radical change from the individual's previous levels of functioning. Counsellors should take note of cultural differences in the expression of depression – especially when these concern the duration of mourning after the loss of a significant other. Counsellors should also be aware of the fact that depression in children and adolescents often presents in 'disguised' forms such as boredom, restlessness, and feelings of worthlessness or even hostility.

Treatment

Depression can be treated with a combination of *biomedical* intervention (antidepressant drugs and electroconvulsive therapy) and *psychotherapy.* Psychotherapy is based on various psychological approaches and can, for example, focus on the cognitive (cognitive-behavioural therapy) or interpersonal (systemic therapy) aspects of depression. Interpersonal psychotherapy targets the client's interpersonal relationships and focuses on the conflicts and problems that occur in these relationships. The identification of role conflicts and improvements in the ability to communicate and use social skills should help clients to find relationships more satisfying.

Cognitive-behavioural therapy teaches the client to identify negative, self-critical thoughts; to note the connection between negative thoughts and depression; to examine each negative thought; and to try to replace these thoughts with realistic interpretations of each situation. Clients are asked to list their negative thoughts and to think of rational alternatives, and to do pleasant and rewarding things.

The treatment of depression will depend largely on the client's symptoms. It is easier to influence a depressed client's behaviour and cognition than it is to change his or her feelings. It is therefore a good idea to focus on behaviour or cognition. Encourage depressed clients to join support groups and try to involve their significant others. Don't ever ignore suicide threats!

Suicide

The belief that someone who threatens to commit suicide is not serious about it or will not actually try it, is unfounded. According to Sue et al. (2000), at least 80% of suicides are preceded by either verbal or non-verbal behaviour cues that indicate the suicidal person's intentions. More than two-thirds of people who committed suicide had communicated their intent within the three months preceding the act.

Mood indicators of suicide

Factors closely linked with suicide are hopelessness or negative expectations about the future, and depression. Although one cannot make the assumption that depression *causes* suicide, the correlation between depression and suicide is very high – in adults as well as children and adolescents. Counsellors should note that people very seldom commit suicide while they are severely depressed. Severely depressed people lack energy and their motor functioning is slowed down or retarded so that they are unable to reach the level of activity required for suicide. The danger period often occurs after some treatment when the depression begins to lift and when the person's energy and motivation begin to increase again. Researchers have found that most suicide attempts occur when depressed hospitalised patients go home for the weekend, or soon after discharge (Sue et al., 2000:370).

Other mood indicators of suicide are sadness, heightened feelings of anxiety, anger, guilt and shame. Long-term stress and the consumption of alcohol and drugs are also associated with suicide.

HIV/Aids and suicide

HIV infection and Aids are associated with an increased likelihood of suicide (Sherr, 1995). Some studies report the risk of suicide as being 36 times greater in individuals with HIV/Aids. It seems that suicidal thoughts and acts in association with HIV/Aids tend to concentrate around the time of *diagnosis* and again at the *end stage of disease*.

According to Sherr (1995:22) the reasons for suicide may differ for the two 'peak periods' in the life of the HIV-positive individual. Suicide ideation (fantasising about suicide) or suicidal acts at the time of diagnosis may be triggered by factors such as the way in which testing was carried out; a lack of social support at the time; the individual's inability to cope; and inadequate emotional resources. Suicide in the later phase of Aids is usually associated with deterioration of health; physical illness associated with pain; disability or disfigurement; a decrease in the quality of life; and a feeling that one at least wants to control the way one dies (Pugh, 1995). Those whose loved ones die as a result of suicide are particularly vulnerable to committing suicide themselves, especially if they themselves are HIV-positive.

In clients who have to wait for test results there is a disturbing correlation between HIV testing (before the results are known) and thinking about suicide. Studies have found that anxiety and suicidal thoughts were very high at the time of HIV testing, but dropped ten weeks later – regardless of the results of the HIV test (Pugh, 1995:48). It seems that the negativity and suicidal thinking are related to the stress and uncertainty of HIV testing, rather than to serostatus when asymptomatic. Proper, conscientious and thorough pre- and post-HIV-test counselling is therefore extremely important.

Enrichment

Signs of depression and suicide risk

Be alert and recognise the following signs:

- Change in personality: sad, withdrawn, irritable, anxious, tired, indecisive, apathetic.
- Change in behaviour: can't concentrate on school, work, routine tasks.
- Change in sleep pattern: oversleeping, insomnia, sometimes with early waking.
- Change in eating habits: loss of appetite and weight, or overeating.
- Loss of interest in friends, sex, hobbies, and activities previously enjoyed.
- Worry about money, illness (real or imaginary).
- Fear of losing control, going crazy, harming self or others.
- Feeling helpless and worthless; believes that 'nobody cares', 'everyone would be better off without me'.
- Feeling of overwhelming guilt, shame, and self-hatred.
- No hope for the future, 'it will never get better, I will always feel this way'.
- Drug or alcohol abuse.
- Recent loss through death, divorce, separation, broken relationship, or loss of health, job, money, status, self-confidence, self-esteem.
- Loss of religious faith.
- Nightmares.
- Suicidal impulses, statements, plans, giving away favourite things, previous suicide attempts or gestures.
- Agitation, hyperactivity or restlessness may indicate masked depression.

(Brouard, 2002)

Children, depression and suicide

Because suicide is on the increase in children and adolescents, it is important to know the warning signs of depression and suicidal thinking in young people. Parents and teachers should be on the lookout for warning signs such as depression, previous suicide attempts, significant changes in behaviour, or extremes in mood and behavioural patterns. These might include signs of increased anxiety or withdrawal; a decline in school attendance and achievement; inability to concentrate; lack of interest in hobbies and usual social activities; preoccupation with death or suicide; impulsive risk taking; marked changes in everyday living habits such as eating, sleeping and hygiene; and repeated running away from school (Gillis, 1994).

Van den Boom (1995) reported a study by Weller and colleagues on the impact of bereavement on children. They evaluated a group of children between the ages of 5 and 12 years who had recently lost a parent. From the group evaluated, 37% displayed symptoms of major depression and 47% of those reported morbid and suicidal ideation. The researchers concluded that physical and emotional support; an environment in which the child feels able to express distressing or conflicting thoughts; feelings and fantasies about the loss; and stability and consistency in the child's environment are all extremely important in helping the child to work through the experienced loss.

Prevention of suicide

According to Sue et al. (2000) the successful prevention of suicide is a three-phase process: knowledge and identification of the risk factors and warning signs of suicide; evaluation of the probability (high, moderate or low) that the person will commit suicide; and implementation of action to prevent suicide. Prevention can be based on crisis intervention, psychotherapy and hospitalisation. The following aspects of suicide prevention should be borne in mind.

- Counsellors should feel comfortable about discussing suicide with their clients. Discussing suicide with clients will not encourage a suicide attempt (as is wrongly believed by some people). Clients are often relieved to be able to discuss suicide openly with their counsellor. Direct questions (such as the following) should be asked if they are appropriate or necessary (Sue et al., 2000:382):
    - 'Are you feeling unhappy and down most of the time?' If the answer is yes, then ask:
    - 'Do you feel so unhappy that you sometimes wish you were dead?' If the answer is yes, then ask:
    - 'Have you ever thought about taking your own life?' If the answer is yes, then ask:
    - 'What methods have you thought about using to kill yourself?' If the client specifies a particular method, then ask:
    - 'When do you plan to do this?'
- The amount of detail involved in a suicide threat can indicate the level of its seriousness. A person who provides specific details such as method, time and place is at much greater risk than the person who describes such factors vaguely.
- Suicidal potential increases if the person has direct access to a means of suicide such as a loaded pistol.
- If you believe that the risk of suicide is very high, take action to influence the client's immediate environment. Don't let the client leave your office without a clear treatment plan and the involvement of significant others. Don't hesitate to involve other health care professionals in the prevention plan. (See 'Crisis intervention' on page 234.)
- Some counsellors use a 'contract' as a means of preventing suicide. This means that they ask the client to agree or promise – verbally or in writing – not to commit suicide within, for instance, the following week, or before the next counselling session. Such an agreement can be a very powerful means of blocking suicidal attempts.
- The prevention of suicide depends on the counsellor's ability to recognise the signs and precipitating events. In almost every case of suicide, there are certain hints that the person is about to commit suicide. Suicide is also often preceded by a precipitating event such as the loss of a loved one, family discord, or a chronic or terminal illness such as Aids.

- A person may verbally communicate his or her intention to commit suicide. These communications can be direct ('I want to die'; 'I'm going to kill myself') or indirect ('You will be better off without me'; 'I won't see you again').
- Behavioural clues can be communicated directly or indirectly. The most direct clue is an actual suicide attempt. Even if the act was incomplete, it should be taken as demonstrating a very serious intent to commit suicide. Indirect behavioural clues include actions such as putting one's affairs in order, giving away one's possessions, buying a casket, saying goodbye to people, and making a will. The counsellor should be able to distinguish between this behaviour as an indicator or sign of suicide, and the normal and rational behaviour of someone who knows that he or she is about to die from a fatal condition such as Aids. (In the second case, it is only natural for those who have a fatal illness to wish to get their affairs in order, because they know that their death is impending.) If the situation appears strange or unusual, the counsellor should keep the possibility of suicide in mind.
- Detect and treat depression immediately.

Activity

If you work in the HIV/Aids field, it is almost inevitable that you will have to cope with a suicide threat at some time. Do you know how to handle it? There are many crisis management centres that also offer suicide prevention services. Make a list of the services (such as Life Line, the Aids helpline, FAMSA, Telefriend, or the Depression and Anxiety Support Group) offered in your community. Contact one or more of these centres and find out what services they offer, how they handle suicide threats, who offers the services, and what training their counsellors have received. If you have the time, and want to do something for your community, why don't you volunteer to work for one of these services?

12.4 SPECIFIC COUNSELLING CONTEXTS

Family counselling

No one lives in a vacuum. An individual's seropositive status has a tremendous influence on the systems in which he or she exists, and the infected person is simultaneously affected by these systems. The response of the affected others should therefore be seen by the counsellor as part of a relational process between the infected client and the affected significant others. This *relationship*, rather than the individual person, should become the focus of the counselling process (Johnson, 2000). The family relationship is seriously jeopardised by HIV, which brings issues to the fore such as role adjustments and role changes; multiple feelings such as anger, guilt, fear, and depression; issues of sickness, death and dying; disclosure and rejection; and loss of income, care, nurturing and stability.

The *ecological* or *systems* approach is often used by counsellors to improve observation, communication skills and the relationships within the system (e.g. the family). Techniques used may include the following (Okun, 1997; Sue et al., 2000).

- Rearrange the system by *reframing* the problem from a systems perspective (when, for example, the family is using the infected person's HIV status to defer the resolution of other underlying problems in the family).
- Teach verbal and non-verbal communication and problem-solving skills by providing feedback, new information and coaching (e.g. family members are trained to attend, to listen and to show empathy, and they are given opportunities to practise problem-solving skills).
- Assign direct and indirect behavioural tasks to different family members so that they can help to enhance the functioning of the family system.
- Give the family the guidance, support and practical information they need to help one another (e.g. by providing information about how to handle the infection in the family or cope with a family member who is depressed).
- Use bibliotherapy – supply reading material that teaches family members how to think positively and to overcome negative thinking.

According to Egan (1998), the same counselling principles that apply to individual counselling (see chapter 10) also apply to the family or systems approach. The only difference is that the *family* becomes the client. The counsellor should help the family to identify problems, concerns and issues about the virus in their system (*the current scenario*); to verbalise what they as a family want or need within the limits imposed by the virus (*the preferred scenario*); to identify what they as a family need to do (*strategies*); and to implement strategies that will improve communication within the family and so enable them to live more effectively with the problems created by the virus (*action*).

The following guidelines may help the lay counsellor in working with a family (based on Brouard, 2002):

- Start with where the family is and help each member deal with his or her feelings (keep in mind that people may experience the same issue differently).
- Be aware of who the key role players are, and look at the relationships in the family (who is the client closest to or least close to).
- Try to get everyone to talk.
- Get the family members to talk to one another about their feelings and ensure that they also include the HIV-positive person in the talking.
- Look at past and current stresses and how past crises were dealt with.
- Help family members to come to terms with the diagnosis.
- Help the person living with HIV/Aids to feel more positive about him- or herself and the role he or she has to play in the family.
- Try to help the family to let the sick person keep his or her role for as long as possible.
- Answer questions and give lots of information. Dispel fears regarding transmission risks, especially in the household, and discuss appropriate infection control.
- Discuss financial and practical concerns such as wills and insurance, and link the family with social service organisations if necessary.
- Discuss care arrangements and prepare for loss and bereavement if appropriate.
- Remember that families are resilient and that they can cope and be supportive.

Counsellors must have the self-knowledge to know when they are unable to help clients because of inadequate training in family therapy or because the family's problems are too serious (i.e. beyond the helping capacity of the counsellor). In such cases, HIV/Aids counsellors should never hesitate to refer clients for appropriate help.

Enrichment

How medical and psychological symptoms may affect the counselling process

The medical and psychological symptoms of HIV and Aids can affect the counselling process in a number of ways (Johnson, 2000):

- The symptoms of opportunistic infections and the side effects of medication may increase levels of pain and discomfort to such an extent that the continuity and progress of the counselling process may be adversely affected.
- In advanced stages of Aids, cognitive disorders like dementia may develop. Dementia may make it difficult or impossible for the client to participate in counselling. Neurological disease or dementia can be very disturbing to family members, loved ones and caregivers, and the counsellor should be prepared to communicate with and counsel them on the day-to-day management of the client.
- Psychological symptoms such as feelings of hopelessness, anger, suspicion, depression and isolation may negatively influence the client's attitude to counselling.
- Frequent hospitalisation may disrupt counselling.

Couple counselling

Couples (married, live-together or gay couples) often need to see a counsellor together because they are concerned about HIV-related issues that involve the relationship. Some of the issues that usually present in HIV couple counselling are: fear of infection and re-infection; discordant HIV status; disclosure to partner or others; feelings of guilt for bringing HIV into the relationship; survivor guilt; blaming and punishing each other; fear of relationship failure; sexual difficulties; relationship issues with the extended family; caring when illness comes; financial problems; and communication difficulties around issues such as sex, death, dying and loss.

The following principles and techniques might be helpful for lay counsellors working with couples (based on Brouard, 2002):

- Observe the couple's non-verbal behaviour and encourage them to look at each other when they speak.
- Use active listening skills, focus on interactions between the partners and encourage them to think of the process and not of individual incidents.
- Avoid getting bogged down in long histories and don't get hooked into one person's issues. While acknowledging past issues (previous relationships, family upbringing, relationship history, past hurts, etc.), for the purposes of lay counselling with couples try to focus more on the here and now.
- Acknowledge both points of view and do not listen for too long to one partner. If one partner dominates, try to include the other partner in the discussion by subtly leading away from the dominant partner. For example, ask the other partner if he or she has had similar experiences or feelings, or how he or she feels about the issue being discussed.
- Be alert to communication patterns and styles, for example *placating* (one person always gives in), *blaming* (not taking responsibility for own behaviour and issues), *distracting* (de-focusing and changing the subject), and *computing* (adding up hurts and keeping score).
- Encourage the couple to mirror, hear and empathise with each other. Communication should be respectful, understanding and sensitive and it should enhance connecting.
- Teach the couple empathy skills.
- Focus on negotiation styles of couples. They should aim to:
    - turn complaints and blaming into requests or wishes;
    - simplify requests;
    - ensure that requests are reciprocal and mutual (i.e. give both a responsibility and task);
    - turn requests into workable tasks;
    - communicate requests in keeping with good communication norms; and
    - implement and monitor their new negotiation skills.
- Affirm and acknowledge differences (partners do not have to think alike on everything).
- Explain to them that before pressurising each other to change, they might want to examine why that change is so important, and reframe the difference in positive terms.
- Encourage couples to make small, manageable changes, if change is desired and mutually agreed upon.
- Encourage couples to see that all relationship difficulties are co-created.
- Help partners to see that the difficulties they have with each other are often their own (projection): we tend to see in others what we don't like in ourselves.
- Use problem-solving skills: What are the problems? What do they want for the relationship? And what do they have to do to achieve this? (See 'The problem-solving model' on page 181.)
- Rebuild faith and trust.
- Use homework to give couples things to think about and practise.
- Be sensitive to issues around culture, race and sexual identity, and work on being non-judgemental.

Counselling HIV-positive pregnant women

As counsellors, you will often have to counsel HIV-positive pregnant women. Pregnant women are very concerned about the health of their unborn babies, and it is extremely important that counsellors support them emotionally. Women may also enquire about the termination of pregnancy. Give the woman all the emotional support and information she will need to make an informed decision about the pregnancy, but remember that the final choice of whether to continue or to terminate the pregnancy is hers and hers alone. Always ask the woman what she wants, and also ask her if there is anybody else who should be present during the interview. Discuss the following issues with her (Blom, 2001):

- What does she know about HIV and pregnancy?
- How far is she pregnant?
- Was she tested for HIV, is she definitively HIV positive, or should another test be done?
- Discuss the chances of HIV transmission from the mother to her baby *in utero* and during birth, as well as strategies to decrease vertical transmission.
- Discuss the risks involved in breastfeeding and advise her on bottle feeding versus exclusive breastfeeding. (See 'Breastfeeding' on page 32.)
- Discuss possible referral of the client to a doctor for consultation.
- Discuss the possibility of antiretroviral therapy for mother and baby.
- Discuss the woman's relationship with the father of the baby, as well as other relationships.
- Discuss the risks of termination of pregnancy.
- Discuss the woman's support systems.
- Inform the woman about her rights and about the time periods during which a woman has the right to termination of pregnancy (see 'Women's rights' on page 361).
- Provide non-directive, non-judgemental counselling for a woman who decides to go ahead with abortion. Pre-abortion counselling is intended to assist a woman to make an informed choice regarding termination of pregnancy.
- Possible alternatives to the termination of the pregnancy should also be explored with her, such as adoption.
- She should also be counselled about family planning and contraception (preferably using condoms, with or without another method) to prevent unwanted pregnancy in future.

Counselling HIV-positive and HIV-affected children

Children can be affected by HIV/Aids in various ways. They may be infected with HIV themselves; they may have one or two parents who are HIV-positive; or they may be orphaned because of the Aids-related deaths of their parents. The counsellor should keep the following points in mind when counselling children (Johnson, 2000; Wong et al., 1999:209–211).

- Parental or custodian consent should always be obtained before counselling children.
- Use the same phases of the counselling process as you do with adults (see 'Phases in the counselling process' on page 176) but take special care to make sure that the child *understands* what you are saying.
- Use the child's language, but never 'talk down' to the child. To adopt the child's language is a vital source of understanding and it communicates empathy and acceptance. Take a position at the child's eye level; speak clearly in a quiet, unhurried and confident voice; be specific; and use simple words and short sentences – especially with younger children.
- Be honest with children and allow them to express their concerns and fears.
- Children are very alert to non-verbal messages and they attach meaning to every gesture and move that is made. Children will *sense* your personal feelings, attitudes, and anxieties. Make sure that your non-verbal messages are consistent with your spoken words (or else the child will pick up the discrepancy).
- Keep the *child's* understanding of death and dying in mind when counselling children. (See 'Children and bereavement' on page 247.)
- Keep a child's age and developmental phase in mind when counselling him or her. (See enrichment box 'The child in counselling' on page 233.)
- Clarify the counselling process and your role in relation to the child. Explain the reason, aim and method of counselling.
- Provide a considerate counselling context and use a few age-appropriate props rather than an overwhelming 'toy-shop atmosphere'.
- Allow children time to feel comfortable and develop the relationship in a patient, caring manner. Avoid sudden or rapid advances, broad smiles, extended eye contact or other gestures that may be construed as threatening. Talk to the parent if a young child is

Enrichment

The child in counselling

The counsellor should keep the child's age and developmental phase in mind when counselling him or her.

- Children under five years are egocentric (in developmental terms), and see things only in relation to themselves; they think concretely and interpret words directly. Counsellors should therefore focus communication on them and avoid phrases that might be misinterpreted. Small children will, for instance, take your explanation of an injection as a 'little stick in the arm' literally to mean – a stick or branch in their arm.
- Younger school-age children want a reason and explanation for everything that the counsellor does, but they want no verification beyond that. School-age children are very concerned about bodily integrity and they are often worried that something may harm or injure them (or their possessions). The counsellor should help children to voice their concerns and should introduce activities to reduce their anxiety.
- Because adolescents often fluctuate between child-like and adult thinking and behaviour, they often tend to seek the security of the more familiar and comfortable expectations of childhood when they become anxious. The counsellor should anticipate these shifts in identity and adjust the course of interaction to meet the needs of the moment. In their communication with adolescents, counsellors should be supportive, attentive and try not to interrupt or to ask prying and embarrassing questions. They should also avoid comments or expressions that convey surprise or disapproval. Resist any impulse to give advice, and listen very carefully to everything the adolescent says. Confidentiality is of great importance when interviewing adolescents. Explain to parents and adolescents the limits of confidentiality – specifically the fact that the young person's disclosures will not be shared unless they indicate a need for intervention (as in the case of suicidal behaviour).

Enrichment

Creative ways to communicate with children

- *Storytelling:* Ask children to tell a story about an event (e.g. being in hospital). Show them a picture and ask them to tell a story. Cut out comic strips, remove the words and ask children to add words to the pictures.
- *Mutual storytelling:* Ask the child to tell a story. Then tell a story of your own. Base it on the child's story but change the negative events of the child's story to a positive outcome in your story.
- *Bibliotherapy:* Give the child a book to read (or read it to the child) and explore the meaning of the book with the child. Ask the child to retell the story, to draw a picture based on the story, to talk about the characters, or to summarise the moral or meaning of the story.
- *Dreams:* Ask the child to talk about a dream or nightmare, and explore the meaning that the dream might have with the child. Dreams often reveal unconscious and repressed thoughts and feelings.
- *'What if' questions:* Encourage children to explore potential situations and to consider different problem-solving options by asking 'what if . . .' questions. Children's responses indicate what they already know, what they don't know and what they are curious about, and this gives them the opportunity to practise coping skills.
- *Three wishes:* Ask the child: 'If you could have any three things in the world, what would they be?' Explore the child's wishes.
- *Rating game:* Use some type of rating scale (sad and happy faces, or numbers) to rate the child's feelings about an event.
- *Word association game:* Recite certain key words, and ask children to say the first word that comes into their minds when they hear this key word.
- *Sentence completion:* Present a partial statement and ask the child to finish it. For example: 'The thing in the world I like best is . . .'
- *Pros and cons:* Select a topic and ask the child to list five good things and five bad things about it. It is a very useful technique to use when focusing on relationships because it enables people to list things they like and dislike about each other.
- *Non-verbal techniques:* You may suggest to older children (and adults) that they keep a journal or diary. Ask them to write letters that are never posted, to draw and to play.

(Based on Wong et al., 1999:212–213)

initially shy, or communicate through objects such as dolls, puppets or stuffed animals before questioning a young child directly. Give older children the opportunity to talk without the parents being present.
- Be patient and revisit topics if necessary. Reflect the child's feelings and confirm your understandings with the child.
- Do not be discouraged by apparent inattentiveness when you talk about sensitive issues. This is often a child's way of coping with stressful issues.
- Use a variety of communication skills (see enrichment box 'Creative ways to communicate with children' on page 233).
- Be sensitive to ethical issues (obtain parental consent, maintain confidentiality, clarify liaison with other professionals with the parents as well as with the child, and avoid potentially ambiguous situations).
- Do not blame or discredit *any* of the adults in the child's world. Although these relationships may be painful to the child, adults are and remain significant people in the child's life.
- Do not enter into alliances with other people in the counselling process. Remain neutral.
- Be sensitive to the potentially 'abusive' aspects of counselling children. (You are an adult in a position of authority, and the child has limited say in what happens.)
- Avoid mindless, extended therapy. Focus on the presenting problem, and *work*. Children should not remain in counselling any longer than is necessary. Be aware of the fact that children often feel that being in counselling means that there is something wrong with them.
- Be sensitive to cultural issues in counselling children. Be prepared to learn from children from other cultures.

Crisis intervention

Crisis intervention is a form of emotional 'first aid' or a short-term helping process designed to provide immediate relief in an emergency situation (Gillis, 1994). Crisis intervention is active, direct and brief, and occurs shortly after a crisis has happened. The same phases of the counselling process (discussed in chapter 10) apply in these situations, and empathic listening is vitally important.

The crucial issue is not the actual crisis situation itself, but a client's *emotional reaction* to the situation and his or her *ability to deal with it*. Clients in crisis experience apathy, depression, guilt and loss of self-esteem. They find that the ways in which they used to solve problems in the past no longer work for them, and they find this very upsetting and frightening.

- The major goal of short-term crisis intervention is to give individuals and their families as much support and assistance as possible. This will help clients regain their psychological balance as quickly as possible (Okun, 1997).
- Keep the following points in mind when you are engaged in crisis intervention: Ascertain who and where to call for support in an emergency. Have the telephone numbers of crisis clinics, hotlines and suicide prevention centres ready at hand – as well as telephone numbers for referrals to professionals. You should not have to *begin* to fumble around for telephone numbers at the very height of a crisis.
- Crisis intervention is directive. The client is usually in no state to think straight, and he or she needs your advice and direction immediately.
- Immediate hospitalisation (voluntary or involuntary) for medical treatment, evaluation, and therapy by a psychiatric team every day until the crisis has passed is often necessary. Make sure that you know what hospitals and facilities are available.
- Enlist relatives and friends to help monitor the client when he or she leaves your office or the hospital. Provide the family (and client) with telephone numbers where they can reach 24-hour help if necessary. There are various organisations in the community (such as Life Line and the Aids helpline) that offer suicide prevention services and counselling. (See 'Websites and Toll-free Helplines' on page 369.)
- Ensure ongoing therapy.

Ethical concerns in counselling

Keep the following ethical concerns in mind when counselling HIV-positive clients (Johnson, 2000:17):

- It is preferable not to make notes during counselling sessions. Rather summarise the main themes of the counselling conversation after the session. It is very difficult to listen attentively to a client while making notes at the same time. However, if the counsellor prefers to make notes, he or she should do this discreetly and with the consent of the client.
- As was pointed out in chapter 10, confidentiality is non-negotiable.
- Referrals, reports and liaison with other people who are involved should be dealt with in a transparent manner.
- Avoid being drawn into alliances with specific individuals or factions.
- Never disqualify other counsellors or professionals or agencies.
- Guard against stereotyping.
- Find a competent supervisor or mentor for your counselling activities. Such supervision will ensure that you are on the right track. Proper supervision will also be a source of new ideas for you and it will prevent burnout. (See 'Mentoring and supervision' on page 330.)

To be an HIV/Aids counsellor is to be an activist (whether you like it or not). HIV-positive people still experience a lot of rejection and discrimination in society, and it is often necessary for the counsellor to assume the role of an activist in fighting such problems.

12.5 CONCLUSION

There are many different issues and contexts in HIV/Aids counselling. Counsellors often feel overwhelmed by the demands on them, but they cannot go wrong if they have a genuine concern and compassion for people and if they generate warmth, trust, acceptance and genuineness. Counsellors should simply be themselves and trust themselves. In responding to a client's needs, an attitude of non-judgemental empathic attentiveness is more important than doing or saying specific things. Listening is more important than talking, *being with* more important than *doing to* (Macfie, 1997).

chapter

13 Bereavement and Spiritual Counselling

by Prof. Peet van Dyk
School of Religion and Theology, Unisa

Who will save us?
And she kept her song soft,
her mourning for lost humanity.
Who will save them from the beast?
Who will prevent him from coming in to rule?

Aids has affected our world-view: it has undermined our optimism about knowledge, science and technology and brought us face to face with our neglect of the emotional and spiritual aspects of life. It has exposed the spiritual poverty underlying the ideals of rampant materialism and exploitative expansionism – ideals that characterise modern Western culture (Van Arkel, 1991).

HIV/Aids challenges all aspects of modern life, and counselling must adopt a holistic approach that takes all aspects of modern life into account. Clients need information and knowledge to cope with the disease (cognitive information), and they also need to be equipped to cope emotionally and spiritually with the ravages of the disease. Because one counsellor cannot realistically deal with all the ways in which the pandemic affects both individuals and society, it is preferable to have teams of experts, each of whom is skilled in one particular aspect of coping with the pandemic, to counsel those who are affected. In this chapter we will explore:

- how counsellors can facilitate the process of bereavement (of both the HIV-positive client and his or her significant others); and
- religious and ethical aspects of the disease.

13.1 BEREAVEMENT COUNSELLING

The bereavement experienced by a person who has lost a loved one and the bereavement experienced by a terminally ill or dying person are very similar. Both people experience a deep sense of loss: in the first case, the loss of your loved one, and in the second case, the loss of your future, your hopes, your loved ones, your health, self-esteem and well-being, and your dignity as a human being. In either case people are confronted with their own mortality. Terminally ill people are *directly* confronted by their own imminent death (the imminence becoming more pressing as the disease progresses), while people who have lost loved ones are *indirectly* confronted with the possibility of their own *future* death. It is therefore understandable that the process of bereavement is often very similar for both those who are dying and those who are forced to witness death. In all cases where HIV-positive people are still leading relatively normal and healthy lives for extended periods, the counsellor needs to facilitate a process of *reinvestment* in life. This is also an important element in the counselling of a person who has lost or is in the process of losing a loved one.

In the HIV/Aids scenario the counsellor is confronted with a dual process of bereavement: of the HIV-positive person as well as those who will be left behind when the client dies. It is important to realise that, in the case of a lengthy terminal disease (such as HIV infection), bereavement begins with the loss of some or all of the following features of normal, healthy human life: health, shared pleasurable activities (such as sex), relationships, family, the sense of the future, certainty, an understanding of the meaning of life, hope, energy, enthusiasm, employment (which confers the sense of identity) and personal independence (Perelli, 1991; Sherr, 1995). The significant others of the infected person also begin the process of bereavement as they are forced to witness how their loved one gradually loses all the features of normal health and active human existence. In the case of the sex partners of HIV-positive people, the partners may also have the added agony of worrying about whether they will become infected.

Attachment theory

Bereavement is triggered primarily by the sense of loss that occurs when we lose something or someone to which we have become attached. People make strong affectional bonds with others and react strongly when those bonds are threatened or broken (Worden, 1982). According to Bowlby's (1977) theory, we do not form these attachments primarily to satisfy our biological drives, but rather to fulfil our needs for security and safety. Forming attachments with significant others is normal behaviour for both children and adults.

Separation or loss initiates a process of grief. Grief is a very basic (and to a large extent an automatic and instinctive) biological reaction that may cause aggressive behaviour and stimulates attempts to regain the lost object (Bowlby, 1977). The extent to which human beings grieve a loss depends on how attached or close they were to the person or object of their loss. Grief is not always triggered by an *actual* loss. The mere anticipation of loss (as when a person is diagnosed with a life-threatening disease such as HIV/Aids) may be sufficient to initiate the grief process (Sherr, 1995). Mourning processes may be based on 'primitive biological processes', but they also display many uniquely human features, for example, the almost universal belief in an afterlife in which one can rejoin one's loved ones (Worden, 1982).

Many counsellors regard the process of mourning as being similar to the process of healing from an illness: mourning occurs until normal functions once more become predominant in the bereaved person's life. Among such functions, emotional and physical equilibrium are the most important.

Kübler-Ross stages of bereavement

Elisabeth Kübler-Ross (1969) examined the many and varied reactions to loss, and found similarities according to which she identified the various stages of grieving.

- *Denial and initial shock.* Often the first reaction to a loss is a feeling of numbness and disbelief. Denial is usually partial, but in some extreme cases a person may totally ignore or dismiss the loss.
- *Anger.* Although anger may seem inappropriate and in many cases comes unexpectedly to the grieving person, it is nonetheless one of the most basic reactions to a significant loss.
- *Bargaining and guilt.* Grieving people often bargain with God, themselves or, in the case of HIV, even with the virus. This usually involves (unrealistic) promises and the expec-

tation of a reward, for example, that the person will be cured or that he or she will remain healthy indefinitely. Feelings of guilt are also common. These may be based on real or imaginary reasons and can therefore be rational or in some cases totally irrational. In both cases the bereaved person may blame him- or herself for the loss.
- *Sadness and depression.* In the case of bereavement, depression is often anger turned inward (Kluckow 2004). It may involve withdrawal, losing interest in activities, apathy, tearfulness and lack of concentration.
- *Resolution and acceptance.* In time, and after going through some or all of the above stages, a person may come to terms with his or her loss. This involves some degree of acceptance and a return to normal life.

Counsellors sometimes over-simplify Kübler-Ross by seeing the stages of bereavement as separate phases that follow each other in strict order. They believe that it is impossible for a bereaved person to progress to a subsequent stage before the previous one has been adequately dealt with. This mistaken idea may cause counsellors to 'force' their clients through consecutive stages of bereavement without taking individual differences and the individuality of grieving into account (De Villiers, 1988). This view also does not take into account that most people tend to work through several phases simultaneously.

Tasks of mourning

Worden (1982) avoids the term 'stages' and uses the active term 'bereavement tasks' instead, emphasising that bereavement does not engulf or overwhelm the person, and does not have to be passively accepted. Bereaved people should actively *work through* their grief *in their own time*. The process of restoration requires the bereaved person to perform some of the 'tasks of mourning' before equilibrium can be re-established, and the process of mourning can be completed. Since these tasks form part of a process, they require effort – an effort which Freud called 'grief work'. Bereavement cannot be rushed or artificially expedited.

The tasks of mourning frequently overlap one another and do not necessarily follow in any specific serial sequence. The grieving person may therefore complete some tasks simultaneously – although in other cases the finalisation of one task may depend on the prior completion of a previous one. Thus, for example, one cannot process the emotional impact of a loss until one has accepted the *reality* of the loss (i.e. the fact that it has actually happened). In the discussion below we will follow Worden and talk about 'tasks of bereavement' in order to emphasise that dealing with loss is an *active* process.

Task 1: Accepting the reality of the loss

When a loss occurs, the first reaction is always a sense that it has not happened. This is often accompanied by a feeling of numbness, shock or unreality. This reaction is typical when a loved one dies (even when it was expected) *and* when a person hears for the first time that he or she is infected with HIV or is terminally ill. The first task of grieving is to face the reality of the death or the loss of health that will eventually end in death. For the person who has lost a loved one, this requires an acceptance of the belief that reunion is impossible – at least in this life. Part of this process involves typical searching behaviour – looking for the person, momentarily forgetting that the person is not there any more, or mistaking other people for the lost one. The equivalent behaviour for people diagnosed with a life-threatening disease (e.g. HIV/Aids) is to momentarily forget about the HIV-positive status and/or to live as though they were not infected.

Denial of the loss may vary from slight distortions of the reality of the situation to severe delusions. Delusions may range from the bizarre to the more natural. They may, for example, take the form of 'mummification' – the process that occurs when the bereaved person lovingly preserves all the possessions of the deceased loved one. Some people with a life-threatening disease may be reluctant to let go of a risky lifestyle and – in the terminal phases of the disease – they may begin to cling tenaciously to possessions that they will never need again. This is one of the primary reasons why people often die after a long illness without having taken care of their estate and without having made proper arrangements to distribute their possessions.

In the case of HIV-positive people (especially when they have been diagnosed as HIV positive at a relatively early stage of the infection), the process of accepting the reality of their status may be extremely difficult and drawn out. Because infected people initially show no symptoms (or only very mild ones), and because they may continue to remain healthy for many years after infection, the tendency towards denial of their illness is encouraged, and they may continue to carry on living as though nothing has happened.

When denial takes the form of mild distortions of reality, these may serve the temporary role of buffering the intensity of the loss. Even so, it is important that the distortions do not hinder the eventual acceptance of the reality of the disease and approaching death (Worden, 1982). It is also common for people to deny loss by minimising the importance of the loss or by removing from their lives all objects or people that may remind them of the loss. Selective forgetfulness and denying the irreversibility of the death or of the disease are also common. In the case of HIV-positive people it is especially difficult to distinguish between a healthy sense of hope (e.g. that a cure or effective treatment for Aids may be found) and a systematic denial or refusal to accept that they will eventually die.

Most counsellors nowadays agree that accepting death is at best only partial (Irion, 1985). Complete acceptance is an ideal that can probably never be reached completely. The degree of partial acceptance varies from person to person and will also depend on how close the deceased was to the bereaved person and how complicated their relationship may have been. Fully accepting one's own death is also not really possible – especially when relatively young, as is often the case with HIV-positive people. Some degree of denial will therefore always remain and may sometimes serve the important function of lessening the pain.

Unfortunately, certain unrealistic religious attitudes may sometimes transgress the boundary of offering reasonable comfort and hope to the individual and so become complicit in denying reality. Such unrealistic attitudes may take the form of refusing to accept that God is not going to heal the sick person, or denying the importance of this life and focusing entirely on life after death. When hope thus becomes denial, it may complicate the process of bereavement and make it more difficult to complete the bereavement process.

Worden (1982:12) evaluates this tendency as follows:

> It should be emphasised that after a death it is very normal to hope for a reunion or to assume that the deceased is not gone. However, for most people this illusion is short-lived, at least for this life, and this enables them to move through to Task II (i.e. to experience the pain of grief).

Counsellors can assist their clients in various ways to actualise (make real) their loss. Although it may seem inadequate to some, talking about one's grief is still one of the most important ways of getting to grips with it. In the case of survivors this may include talking about the following points:

- Where did the death occur?
- How did it happen?
- Where were you when you heard about it?
- Who told you about it?
- What were the funeral and service like?

In the case of an HIV-positive person, the above questions can be adapted as follows:

- Why and when did you go for HIV testing?
- How and by whom was the news revealed to you?
- How did you react to the news and what did you do immediately after receiving the news?

In addition to talking about the loss, many people need to process the loss by reviewing the events in their minds and by (ritually) visiting the grave of the deceased or other places associated with the loss. Going through these processes will help the bereaved person to actualise the loss and to accept the reality of it.

Task 2: Experiencing the pain of grief

Grief makes people experience emotional pain, and this may sometimes also manifest itself as physical pain. Parkes (1972:173) describes the necessity of experiencing and going beyond the pain by saying that 'anything that continually allows the person to avoid or suppress this pain can be expected to prolong the course of mourning'.

The intensity of pain depends on the personality of the bereaved person and on how precious the lost person or thing was to the bereaved person. The threat of losing (within the foreseeable future) one's health and everything that one has accumulated in one's life will inevitably cause most people to feel a severe degree of pain. Confronting the reality of HIV/Aids may generate a variety of *fears* that may cause severe emotional strain. These fears may include the following (Sunderland & Shelp, 1987):

- Fear of *impairment*. To admit illness is to arouse some feeling of inferiority to the general (healthy) community. It also raises the issue of mortality and causes some degree of social isolation as the illness prevents one from enjoying the normal pleasures of social life.
- Fear of *uncertainty* may be very acute – it may spur people on to take various measures to reacquire their earlier undisturbed state of mind or equilibrium. To test HIV positive initiates a major health crisis that severely threatens all our stabilities, hopes, certainties, life plans, ambitions and ordinary day-to-day capacities. This kind of crisis always causes profound emotional stress and is accompanied by associated changes in outlook and adaptive changes in personality. While such changes may be occasions for growth, they may also stimulate psychological and spiritual regression and deterioration.
- Fear of *stigmatisation and ostracism* are very real factors after being diagnosed HIV positive. It is the fear of *rejection and isolation* that causes Aids patients the greatest pain. Conditions such as STIs and Aids evoke self-righteous judgements in some – who may not hesitate to judge and blame the sick person for his or her condition. Fear, self-righteousness and herd instinct in some communities can be so great that they may regard the person with Aids as having committed a crime. Stigmatised people may therefore be denied the ordinary privileges of social life. If infected people are perceived as being guilty (for example, because they are known to be promiscuous or homosexual), the community might hold them responsible for the consequences of their actions and deny them sympathy, or even seek to punish them. These acts of hostility may include termination of employment, denial of access to medical schemes, and various other measures of exclusion that are sometimes presented as reasonable attempts to protect others. In Africa racism may also play a role in hostile and indifferent attitudes to infected people.
- Fear of *sexuality*. Because sexual transmission is the primary way in which people become infected with HIV, infection with HIV is surrounded by an aura of superstition, mystery, taboos, fear and the double standards common in all matters relating to sex. Consequently it may be very difficult to talk openly and rationally about the disease and to counsel people living with HIV.
- Fear of *death* is an extension of the fear of infection and impairment – sickness is proximity to death. Often the *anticipation* of dying carries with it the same emotional stress as the reality itself.

The experience of pain in the case of HIV-positive people and their significant others may be complicated by the fact that they may actually deny themselves the right to grieve – whether consciously or unconsciously. For example, by blaming either themselves or the deceased person for the loss, they may make it more difficult to accept the pain of loss or allow themselves to experience the pain. In many cases such an attitude will increase the intensity and continuity of the pain. Counsellors should therefore facilitate this grieving task by assuring people of their right to grieve (even though society may try to deny them this right). Various *forms* of guilt often cause difficulties in the bereavement counselling of the HIV-positive person and those affected by HIV-related losses.

Because society in general often views grieving as morbid, unhealthy and demoralising, a counsellor's work may be regarded by such people as wrongly stimulating a mourner's grief.

This is not so. The absolute avoidance of pain (i.e. the negation of the second task) is to feel nothing at all (Worden, 1982). Cutting oneself off from any feelings by implementing thought-stopping procedures and thereby short-circuiting unpleasant thoughts, or by deliberately stimulating pleasant thoughts, are both ways of avoiding legitimate pain. Examples of cutting-off behaviours may include compulsive travelling by bereaved people, or the adoption of an artificial, hyperactive lifestyle that is out of keeping with the bereaved person's previous way of life. Some people use such cutting-off behaviours (which may include alcohol and substance abuse, among many others) to stop themselves from thinking of or getting in touch with their pain.

Eventually the person should allow him- or herself to face the pain and all the emotions that go with it. Counsellors should assist their clients in realising and expressing their feelings. The most common of these feelings are described below.

Anger

Anger is probably the most common of the bereavement emotions – *but usually the least expected by the bereaved.* Clients should acknowledge their anger. Anger may be directed against the unfairness of life; against the person from whom the infection was received; against own indiscretions; or even against the deceased because his or her actions precipitated the loss and therefore caused all the grief with which the bereaved person now has to deal. Even when there is no obvious or rational reason for being angry with the deceased person, it is perfectly natural for a bereaved person to *blame* the dead person for having abandoned him or her. However irrational and illogical such emotions may seem to be, they are very widely experienced by bereaved people and are therefore part of the *reality* of bereavement.

Because it is not considered 'proper' or appropriate to direct anger at a deceased person, it is often redirected to other people such as a doctor, a social worker or a counsellor. Because people find it difficult to express anger at themselves or close partners, they may deny (suppress) such feelings. It then becomes the task of the counsellor to help grieving people to identify their anger and vent their feelings *by using indirect techniques*. You might, for example, use the following questions to help grieving people to get in touch with their feelings:

- What do you miss most about the deceased?
- What don't you miss about the deceased person?

or

- What do you miss most from the time before you knew that you were HIV positive?
- What don't you miss about the time before you received the news?

Guilt

There are many real and imaginary (often irrational) reasons why people feel guilty. It is the task of the counsellor to challenge unnecessary feelings of guilt by asking pertinent questions until the client comes to the recognition that the feelings of guilt are unfounded and groundless. If the feelings are based on real, justifiable guilt, it is important to emphasise to clients that nobody is perfect and that everybody makes mistakes. In these circumstances it is best to identify possible mitigating circumstances and also to emphasise the necessity for forgiveness (of self or others), for instance when HIV-positive people feel guilty about also infecting their partners. In such circumstances, the counsellor may want to ask the following questions:

- Did you *deliberately* or *unknowingly* infect your partner?
- Have you asked forgiveness from your partner?
- Is it possible to forgive yourself? (If the person holds religious convictions, it may also be helpful to encourage them to go to confession or/and ask God's forgiveness in whatever way is appropriate.)

Anxiety and helplessness

Anxiety and feelings of helplessness are very common in people who have lost loved ones and in those who have life-threatening diseases. Fear of death and a feeling that they can do nothing about their fate often overwhelm Aids patients. Similar feelings usually occur after the death of a loved one: witnessing the death of another reminds us of our own mortality. Bereaved people often have visions and dreams about the body of the deceased person enclosed by the dark and cold earth. Bereaved people are also prone to feel that life has no purpose and that they have no control over their destiny. All such feelings may give rise to severe anxiety attacks and bouts of depression. Helplessness is evidenced in feelings of being unable to survive without the departed person and unable to carry on living because of the ever-present threat of death.

Counsellors should take great care to explore such fears and anxieties with their clients and identify ways in which the person coped *before* the loss occurred. Discuss with them how they can regain their sense of purpose in life and, even more importantly, encourage them to engage in some new activities that will help them to find a new purpose in life. If we can get clients to realise *and experience* that they can do things to change their own lives and the lives of others for the better, we will have provided them with one of the best antidotes to anxiety and feelings of helplessness. Although HIV-positive people cannot change their HIV-positive status, they can (with the right attitudes and actions) begin to live in an optimistic, altruistic and healthy way. If they do manage to become more altruistic, caring, self-sacrificing and optimistic, HIV-positive people can add many healthy and creative years to their lives. Some clients may also find it helpful to see their HIV-positive status as a timely warning that they should begin to make the most of their lives. At least this disease gives people ample opportunity to prepare themselves for closure, to change things and (in many cases) to do the things that they always wanted to do but never had the chance of doing.

Sadness and depression

Sadness and accompanying crying are an integral part of mourning and should not be avoided. Crying should always be purposeful, and the counsellor should explore the changing meaning of crying and sadness during the mourning process with the bereaved person. Crying and sadness perform the function of acknowledging the pain of the loss. Bereaved people are expected to be sad and to grieve over the lost person or their lost opportunities, health, prospects and life expectancy (as in the case of HIV-positive people). Denying a grieving person the opportunity of crying or sadness (because of social pressure, anger or any other reason) may unnecessarily complicate and lengthen the grieving process. Counsellors should always emphasise that people who have suffered a loss have the right to cry and to feel sad about their losses – and that it is important and right that they should express these feelings.

Sadness and depression often go hand in hand. Depression may be reactive (relating to a past loss) or preparatory (relating to a future loss). In the case of grieving people, reactive depression can be dealt with by encouragement and reassurance, but in dealing with preparatory depression it may be more important to allow people to express their feelings (Brouard 2002).

Grieving openly is often difficult for HIV-positive people or for their loved ones because of the secrecy and stigma associated with sexually transmitted infections. Experiencing pain alone or secretly often makes the pain worse. Bereavement counsellors in HIV/Aids-related cases should therefore make a conscious effort to refer such people to support groups or help them to share their pain with others, especially if it is not possible for them to share their grief with their family and friends, or if they do not want to.

People who deny themselves conscious grieving usually break down at a later stage. Their breakdown may not be obvious, or it may manifest itself in the form of acute and chronic depression. One of the aims of grief counselling is to help people to process their painful experience so that they won't carry their pain with them throughout their lives.

In the case of HIV-positive people, the purpose of grief counselling is to prevent them from being so traumatised that they 'stop living' long before Aids develops or before their health starts to deteriorate. It is only by processing pain and undertaking grief work that the bereaved can slowly return to normal and begin to get on with the remainder of their lives. In cases where the task of experiencing the pain has not been properly or adequately completed, clients should be referred to therapists to work through the process in therapy and so prevent subsequent psychological problems such as chronic depression.

Conclusion

The mere *expression* of emotions is not enough. Emotions should always be *focused.* Sadness should be accompanied by an awareness of exactly what was lost. Anger should not merely be expressed as rage and indignation – the reasons for the anger should be carefully identified and considered. Guilt should be evaluated and resolved, and anxiety should be acknowledged, clarified and managed.

Task 3: Adjusting to a changed environment

Experiencing a loss may mean different things to different people, but everyone who experiences a loss is forced to adjust to the new circumstances and the new environment created by the loss. For example, people have to discover what it is like to live without the deceased person or what losing their health, prospects, lifestyle and future means in reality. Complete realisation of what the loss entails usually emerges only a few months after it has occurred. One might realise, for example, what it means to live alone, to sleep alone in an empty house or to manage household affairs and finances alone. Bereaved people sometimes discover the exact role that the deceased person played only after his or her death. Those who are left behind often appreciate the full implications of their loss by being forced to adjust to new circumstances, to learn new skills or even just to do things they never had to do before. Many people resent this process of adjustment and become deeply frustrated by small and irritating things that have to be attended to and that seem to take up a lot of their time.

Although the manner in which HIV-positive people experience loss when they first come to know their positive diagnosis is not very well defined, it is known to be an extremely painful experience because it ultimately means losing what is most precious – one's own life. What makes it even worse is the realisation that the HIV-positive diagnosis is just the first stage in a long and painful process of loss – inevitably culminating in death. This long and painful process may include losing partners, close friends, family support, employment, financial security, a previous (normal and healthy) lifestyle, health and even dignity. This series of painful, frightening and humiliating losses – to which the person *must* adapt – are even more stressful because they are often unanticipated and unpredictable.

We can illustrate this process with an example. Most HIV-positive people have been accustomed to leading very active lives and many have never been in hospital, undergone any extensive medical treatment or been required to take regular medication. Then suddenly, as Aids begins to manifest and opportunistic diseases begin to appear, they have to subject themselves to constant and expensive courses of treatment – which may make them feel very ill (due to the side effects) and which may also quickly deplete and drain their financial resources. Aids patients may receive chemotherapy, radiation treatment or begin to take antiretroviral drugs. Taking antiretroviral medication entails a strict regimen: some drugs have to be taken before meals and some after meals, and often the only way to get the timing right is by setting alarm clocks and rearranging one's whole daily schedule. This may be extremely difficult or even impossible for people with only a basic education or no formal education at all. But even people with higher education, high incomes and privileged lifestyles are often disturbed and disorientated by the daunting demands that HIV/Aids treatment imposes on them. Either way, HIV/Aids can easily disrupt all the accustomed patterns, habits, assumptions and rhythms of life – and this disruption and disorientation can increase anxiety.

Successful adjustment to the task of adaptation requires people to redefine their loss in such a way that *the positive aspects of the loss* can also be appreciated. For example, if an HIV-positive person begins to live a far less selfish life by helping other HIV-positive people in need, he or she may become more mature. Bowlby (1977) describes the task of adaptation to loss as a person's recognition of changed circumstances, and a redefinition of goals in life. In many cases the HIV-positive person may successfully learn to live life each day to its fullest and begin to enjoy the beauties of nature and creation – beauties previously taken for granted (Perelli, 1991).

What is certain is that adaptation to difficult situations will become even more difficult if people allow themselves to sink into a swamp of self-pity and if they intensify their helplessness by not developing the necessary coping skills or by withdrawing from the world (Worden, 1982).

The task of adapting to changed circumstances is probably an area in which bereaved people can be most proactive if they deliberately develop and train themselves in those practical skills that will enable them to cope successfully with the practical problems created by their loss. For example, if HIV-positive people get involved in hospice programmes and in informing others about the practical aspects of handling the disease, they may become well trained in the very skills that they themselves may later need in handling their own worsening health situation.

Counsellors can help their clients adapt to their changed circumstances by using a problem-solving approach and encouraging clients to work out their own solutions to problems. It may be necessary for the counsellor to equip the client with decision-making and coping skills. Counsellors may collaborate with their clients in exploring practical ways of solving their problems and coping with anxieties. However, clients should be discouraged from making major life-changing decisions while they are in the middle of the grieving process. Overhasty decisions that involve (for example) changing or resigning from jobs, selling property, moving to another neighbourhood or city/town, and so on, should preferably be delayed. Such changes are frequently unnecessary or may give rise to new (and serious) problems. Moving away from an old neighbourhood, for example, may separate an individual from friends and other support systems, and this may worsen feelings of loneliness. Good judgement is often affected during periods of acute grief (when some important decisions may present themselves), and it is generally a good rule for bereaved people to postpone important decisions until after they have worked through all the tasks of the grieving process.

Task 4: Withdrawing emotional energy and reinvesting it in another person or field of life

Emotional energy can be *reinvested* only after the focus has been withdrawn from the deceased. Mourning therefore entails the psychological task of detaching memories and hopes. The survivor must deliberately draw away from the pervasive influence of the dead person. But this may be extremely difficult because it may be perceived as dishonouring or disloyalty towards the deceased person (Worden, 1982).

For the HIV-positive person, this shifting of focus or acquisition of emotional detachment is more subtle and difficult to express. It may entail, for example, becoming less focused on death and more focused on the remaining period of life, which may last another decade or longer. Redirecting emotional energy towards living life to the fullest is vitally important and the only way to improve the quality of the remainder of life. Focusing exclusively on the negative aspects of the disease and on impending death will leave no emotional energy for living.

Failure to complete this task is described by Worden (1982:16) as 'the failure to love again'. Being obsessed with the past (a person or a previous healthy life) reflects a choice not to love. And choosing not to love makes happiness impossible. It is vital for people infected by HIV to rediscover *the ability to choose life*, despite feeling disappointed in life or in God because of perceived unfair treatment. Choosing life means not sinking down into depression and psychological deterioration long before physical death. The HIV-positive person must choose either immediate death-in-life, or a life lived to the fullest – a purposeful and deliberate investment of emotional and psychic energy into life.

The task of reinvesting emotional energy is difficult, and many bereaved people get stuck at this point (sadly only realising when it is too late that they allowed their lives to stop prematurely). Grief counsellors should therefore pay special attention to investigating how clients can reinvest their emotional energy.

Counsellors can facilitate the process of developing new relationships and redefining existing ones by emphasising to survivors that it is acceptable and desirable for them to find new friends and/or partners and explaining to them that the deceased person would have expected them to keep on living and be happy. Happy memories of the deceased should not prevent the person from developing new friendships. (But bereaved people should be equally careful not to rebound overhastily into new and ill-advised relationships.)

In the case of HIV-positive people, the loss (or potential loss) of sexual partners may be a source of severe emotional and physical stress. HIV-positive people should be counselled about safer sexual practices with a spouse. But if their uninfected partners or spouses feel uncomfortable about having sex, they should explore together other kind of intimacies (e.g. hugging, caressing and mutual masturbation) – all of which may also be pleasurable and fulfil the emotional needs of both parties.

As mentioned before, the tasks of bereavement cannot be rushed, and no short-cuts are available. Although people differ in how long they take to work through all the tasks of bereavement, most require at least twelve to eighteen months.

Practical techniques to facilitate the bereavement process

In their facilitation of the mourning process, counsellors may use various practical techniques. These may include the following (Worden, 1982; Nefale, 2000).

- *Objects and memorabilia.* The counsellor can help a client focus more clearly by using photographs and letters of the deceased or of people who were associated with the loss. Audio and video tapes, jewellery, pieces of clothing and other objects with which the client is comfortable can be used to facilitate talking and bringing the mourning process to closure.
- *Imagery.* Imagining the deceased or visualising certain situations can be very useful for coming to terms with difficult emotions and circumstances. These images should be clearly focused (not vague, arbitrary or erratic). If clients direct these images towards a specific person or process, they may begin to understand their emotions and reactions better.
- *Writing.* Writing letters to the deceased or to people who are involved in the loss may also be helpful. The main purpose of these letters is to focus the client. If the person addressed in the letter is still living, the letter need not actually be posted. The bereaved person could be encouraged to write a counselling letter to him- or herself, emphasising the need for a more optimistic and active engagement with life. Or a client could write a letter to ask for forgiveness from a former partner or somebody whom he or she may have infected with the HI virus (or has otherwise negatively influenced because of their illness). Some people may also find it helpful to write fiction or poetry that expresses and identifies feelings and blockages.
- *Drawing.* Suggest to children (or to adults who prefer to express themselves visually) that they draw pictures of some aspect of the disease or the death of the loved one. These pictures may reveal to the client and the counsellor some aspects of the grieving process that were opaque – or they may express feelings that were difficult to reveal otherwise.
- *Role playing.* Playing out situations from the past or rehearsing difficult future situations may help the client with future tasks and bring closure to past events. Role playing can also help establish positive behaviour.
- *Cognitive restructuring.* The assumption behind cognitive restructuring is that our emotions and feelings are influenced by what we think about. The counsellor should therefore try to help the client get rid of negative or destructive thoughts and adopt healthier and life-affirming thoughts. If people constantly denigrate and criticise themselves by repeating negative things about themselves, this will increase negativity, depression, hopelessness and anger. By helping clients to test the reality of generalisations, expose distortions and reveal irrational thoughts, counsellors can help them restructure their thoughts and change their negative feelings.
- *Memory books.* Memory books can help in the grieving process in the context of Aids losses and death (Nefale, 2000). Compiling books of photos, mementoes, poems and stories about the family or deceased person helps clients to come to terms with the magnitude of the loss

and bring closure and focus once again on the realities of life without forgetting the lost loved one. In many parts of Africa this technique is often used by HIV-positive parents to make the process of dying easier for themselves and life more bearable for the children who will remain behind after their death.

General guidelines for bereavement counselling

There is no fixed way of doing bereavement counselling. Counsellors will therefore have to adapt their approach to each specific case and person. The following general principles should be taken into account.

Expect grieving to take time, and make time for it

Mourning takes time. People should expect to go through a gradual process of cutting ties and making time to grieve. The client and the counsellor must be aware of critical times in the grieving process, and the counsellor must prepare the client for this. The first three months after the loss, and the first anniversary of the event, are especially critical – both counsellor and client should prepare properly for these periods by ensuring that the bereaved will have adequate support during these times. But all people differ, and some may experience totally different timetables of mourning, characterised by different critical dates and times that may be special or significant to the surviving person. These might include a wedding anniversary, Valentine's Day, Christmas, New Year's Eve, the birthday of the survivor or the dead person, or the period during which the affected people traditionally took their annual holiday. There can be many significant dates and times, and the counsellor must identify them and make sure that the client is adequately supported.

Interpretation of 'normal' behaviour

The counsellor and the bereaved person should know what 'normal' grieving behaviour is. Bereaved people must know that they are not 'going crazy', and that they may often have new experiences, feel strange feelings and find themselves behaving in ways that may be weird or frightening to them. Typical manifestations of grief may include some of the following behaviours, feelings, physical sensations and cognitions:

- *Behaviours.* Sleep and appetite disturbances; a tendency towards absent-mindedness; social withdrawal; dreams of the deceased; avoidance patterns that prevent being reminded of the loss; searching and calling out; sighing, restlessness; crying; an urge to visit significant places reminiscent of the loss or the deceased person; treasuring significant objects. Children may regress to behaviour that is typical of a younger child (e.g. thumb sucking or bed wetting). They may also become very active and excitable or (the reverse) withdrawn and clinging, or they may cry and seek attention in various other ways. Other children may become extremely well behaved (they may try to become 'the perfect child') while older children may begin to indulge in various forms of (uncharacteristic) reckless behaviour (Norton & Dawson, 2000).
- *Feelings.* Sadness, anxiety, numbness, guilt, shock, loneliness, fatigue, helplessness, yearning, anger, emancipation, relief. Children may blame themselves for their loss and feel guilty about it. They often feel extremely anxious and afraid of what may happen next and who will look after them. Shock may trigger a feeling of numbness which may manifest itself as the showing of no emotions at all (Norton & Dawson, 2000).
- *Physical sensations.* Hollowness in the stomach, tightness in the chest and throat, shortness of breath, weakness of muscles and lack of energy, dry throat, over-sensitivity and a sense of depersonalisation. Children at school will find it difficult to concentrate; they may become ill more often and get severe headaches. Children may also have nightmares and bad dreams (Norton & Dawson, 2000).
- *Cognitions.* Disbelief, confusion, preoccupation, hallucinations and mistaking (wrongly perceiving) objects and people. Children may manifest decreased levels of self-esteem with resultant problems. They may also begin to think in a way that is 'magical' and fantastical

– especially when such thinking is related to matters concerning death (Norton & Dawson, 2000).

If any of the above manifestations persist for too long (e.g. if debilitating depression lasts much longer than three months, and if the acute part of the bereavement process stretches over a period longer than a year to a year and a half), or if the grief does not diminish over time, these may be indications of complicated grief processing or pathology. Counsellors should be aware that unresolved grief can manifest as medical or psychiatric problems that may require psychological therapy or psychiatric treatment.

Take individual and cultural differences into account

Although many emotional experiences are common to all people who mourn, people may exhibit enormous variations in their manifestations of grief, in the behaviour they demonstrate, and in the ways in which they express their grief. For example, some people will talk at length about their grief, whereas others may prefer to remain silent while they work very hard at the tasks of processing their grief. The counsellor must be sensitive to cultural differences: it is customary in some cultures to be extremely emotional, other cultures may behave aggressively; and yet others may have a taboo about expressing public grief. In many traditional cultures grief is shared with the community. Consulting the ancestors through traditional healers may be essential for closure of the grieving process. The following case study of a mother's feelings after her son had died of Aids emphasises the importance of being sensitive and respectful towards other cultures' customs (Cochrane et al., 1988:17):

> She watched as her son retreated in coma into a fetal position in the hours before his death. As a mother, she knew that what he needed (and what she needed also) was for her to crawl into bed with him and hold him as he died. But she was deterred by her fears that [the] nursing personnel would not find this behaviour acceptable and would reprimand her. To this day, she berates herself for sacrificing her son's dying needs in order to maintain their family's ethnic dignity in the face of the predominantly non-black world of the hospital.

Ensure continuing support and address different defences and coping styles

Support for the bereaved should be continuous and not last only for the first few days. Sometimes survivors and people with life-threatening diseases need a lot of persuasion not to withdraw from life but rather to share their grief with others and accept support. The support may come from family and friends, organised support groups and regular counselling sessions. The counsellor and client should discuss all possible support systems and together ensure that they are available and that they serve their purpose.

Different styles of coping with mourning and the ways in which people defend themselves against unbearable pain should be discussed within the confidential and caring counsellor-client milieu. Counsellor and client should together evaluate practical strategies and their effectiveness in diminishing distress and solving problems. In some cases the temporary use of prescribed medication such as antidepressants may also be necessary.

Within the context of bereavement counselling two more aspects should be taken into account: the specific needs of grieving children, and the grieving caused to the counsellor by counselling other bereaved persons.

Children and bereavement

Many societies and cultures believe that children do not grieve or that they don't feel that strongly about losses. Scientific investigations have, however, shown that this is not the case. Although young children may not always know how to verbalise and express their feelings, they do have strong feelings and experience severe pain due to losses they have suffered (Klucow 2004). Children therefore have to go through the same tasks of grieving as adults, although their cognitive abilities should always be taken into account. Children only gradually come to a full understanding of death and dying.

- The preschool child (3–5 years) generally thinks of death in terms of separation and he or she regards it as temporary in nature – something akin to sleep (Gillis, 1994; Johnson, 2000). In the child's view, death is a reversible phenomenon and the child expects the deceased person (or someone similar) to return.

- A young child (6–9 years) might grasp the reality and finality of death, but does not see death as universal (affecting all people) or as personal (applying to him or her).
- Children older than 10 years understand that death is final, personal and universal (Johnson, 2000). It is at this stage that children start to realise that death may also apply to them and that it is a concrete fact of life that nobody can avoid.

When counselling children about loved ones who have died we should appreciate the limitations in children's understanding of death. It is futile to try and explain to a preschool child that his or her deceased father is never going to return. Do not deliberately mislead the child by saying (for example), 'Father is only sleeping', or by avoiding the term 'death' altogether, but be aware that the child will fully appreciate the finality of death only when he or she is older. It is equally futile to force a preschool HIV-positive child to understand what death really implies.

It is unwise to try to soften the reality or irreversibility of death by avoiding the subject or by using euphemisms that the child may misunderstand. This will prevent the child from confronting his or her grief and dealing with it (Gillis, 1994). Death should be openly discussed and presented as a normal part of the cycle of life. Be open, honest and gentle in describing death. Only offer details that children can absorb and do not overload them with information. Rather tell them a little bit at a time (Kluckow, 2004).

The child must be physically and emotionally comfortable and know that there is an adult who is prepared to share his or her grief. Children need extra affection and security during the grieving process. Memories about the deceased should be encouraged – the bereaved need to look back before they can once again look forward (Gillis, 1994). Check whether the child is feeling guilty, and offer constant reassurance that he or she has done nothing wrong (Kluckow, 2004).

Children must be allowed to participate in mourning rites and rituals. A good balance should be struck between shocking children with the gruesome details of death and totally excluding them from the funeral arrangements or barring them from the actual funeral. Children should participate in the rituals of death so that they can experience the concreteness of death and feel that they are not alone in their grieving (Gillis, 1994). The details of the funeral process should be explained in detail to the child.

Although some disruption is inevitable, the daily routine of children should be disrupted as little as possible by death in the family. Help the child to channel behaviour in healthy and appropriate ways and ensure that the necessary boundaries and limitations are maintained by caregivers. Also notify the school of the child's loss before he or she returns (Kluckow, 2004).

The counsellor's own grief

If they are to prevent burnout and be able to deal effectively with bereaved people, counsellors should also be able to look after themselves. If they are going to participate in bereavement counselling, counsellors should have come to terms with their own mortality and have accepted it in such a way that they can confront the realities of death and talk openly about it to their clients.

It may also be very painful to counsellors to witness and experience the pain and grief of others. Counsellors in the HIV/Aids field often find that they are constantly attending funerals and are being exposed to a variety of painful experiences. This may eventually become difficult for them to handle. By counselling HIV-positive people and their significant others, counsellors also become more aware of their own losses because they are regularly being confronted by the reality of the losses and bereavement of others. This relentless exposure may increase their own anxiety and stress, and if they are not properly debriefed or counselled themselves, they may eventually suffer burnout. By deliberately taking regular breaks, attending debriefing sessions and by ensuring that they have adequate support systems to cope with their own grieving process, counsellors can avoid emotional burnout.

Activity

Counsellors should perform the following exercise in order to explore their own grief. Ask yourself the following questions and try to answer them by exploring your own experiences and emotions (Van Dyk et al., 2000):

- What was the first death that you can remember? What was your age at the time? When did you attend your first funeral?
- What are the impressions that you remember best from the above experience(s) and events?
- When were you last bereaved and how did you cope with that loss?
- What was the most difficult death that you have ever experienced – and why was it so?
- Whose death from among your present family or friends would be the most difficult for you to handle? Why is this so?
- What is your primary style of coping with loss?
- How do you know when your own grief has been resolved?
- Under what conditions do you think it is appropriate for you to share your own experiences of grief with clients?

13.2 SPIRITUAL COUNSELLING

Researchers often refer to the importance of dealing with the spiritual and emotional needs of HIV-positive clients and their loved ones, but this process remains one of the most neglected aspects of counselling, especially within the HIV/Aids context. Counsellors must not force their own religious views onto their clients, but they should also not ignore the religious needs of clients or merely refer clients to their own religious leaders.

Unfortunately many clergy find it difficult to counsel HIV-positive people properly because they are themselves ignorant about the disease and all its ramifications. In any event, many HIV-positive people avoid approaching their religious leaders for advice or consolation because they fear that they may well be condemned rather than supported. Unfortunately this is sometimes true, but in many other cases it is totally unfounded. The fact remains that religious organisations will have to speak out much more openly about all aspects of HIV/Aids and facilitate an open and supportive milieu before HIV-positive individuals will trust them sufficiently to handle their religious needs. HIV/Aids counsellors should therefore identify clergy who are willing to become part of the counselling team or equip themselves to also handle the religious and emotional needs of their clients.

Why spiritual counselling of HIV-positive people is so difficult

Counselling HIV-positive clients is often extraordinarily difficult, especially counselling on emotional and religious issues resulting from the disease. One of the most obvious reasons for this difficulty is that HIV/Aids is largely *sexually transmitted.* Rational understanding of its origins, progress and ultimate effects is therefore often clouded by sexual taboos, denial, superstitions, stigmatisation and the irrational fears evoked in many people by sexuality and sexually transmitted infections (Sunderland & Shelp, 1987; Van Arkel, 1991). For this reason, and for many others, many HIV-positive people avoid counselling that addresses the religious or spiritual issues provoked by the disease (Van Arkel, 1991). This understandable but ironic situation means that many of the most urgent and troubling spiritual and existential questions that confront HIV-positive people often remain unanswered at a time when their need for spiritual comfort, consolation and understanding is more acute than it has ever been at any other time in their lives. Those who seek spiritual counselling are often deeply disappointed because many religious leaders find it difficult to deal with people who are infected with the HI virus. In addition, HIV-positive people are understandably reluctant to expose their true feelings and experiences in counselling sessions because of their expectation of being condemned and judged (Sunderland & Shelp, 1987).

Another revolutionary feature of the HIV/Aids pandemic is that it has undermined and eroded the most basic traditional features of spiritual counselling. The basic task of the spiritual counsellor has always been to deliver a message of *hope* to the person who is ill (both in a spiritual and physical sense). Even in the case of terminally ill cancer patients, the spiritual counsellor can usually offer some kind of consolation: he or she could always keep alive the hope 'that a miracle might still happen' – the hope that the disease might go into remission and that the patient might be healed (Goss, 1989). Although this ray of hope naturally diminishes as patients approach death, it is never totally absent from spiritual counselling. Even when there seems to be little hope of recovery, there is a 'silent agreement' or complicity between the patient and the spiritual counsellor. This agreement is that the counsellor will continue to express *hope* – a hope that becomes a shared form of denial that binds the counsellor and the sick person together.

Another feature of spiritual and religious counselling is that, as hope for *physical* recovery gradually diminishes, the patient's approaching death is counteracted by an increased emphasis on *eternal* hope – the hope that the person will continue to enjoy a spiritual life in another world after death.

The peculiar nature of HIV/Aids has drastically undermined these features of the traditional counselling process. These undermining factors include the length and erratic progress of the illness and its accompanying opportunistic infections; the stigma (the moral disgrace) that is frequently attached to HIV infection; the lack of social support (manifested as avoidance behaviour by loved ones and members of the community); untimely and multiple losses; protracted illness and disfigurements; and neurological complications (Sunderland & Shelp, 1987).

The next section gives some guidelines for spiritual counselling of HIV-positive people, their loved ones and the community at large. The section focuses on spiritual counselling, but it will also deal with the theological issues evoked by HIV/Aids.

Why does God cause/allow Aids?

One of the most difficult but nonetheless urgent and immediate questions of life is why God allows suffering to exist on earth. Would it not have been better for God to have excluded all suffering (such as illness, pain and death) from this earth? An associated question is: *Is illness caused directly by sin or some kind of transgression?* Although a person may accept that some agent (i.e. a germ or virus) may be the direct cause of disease, such an explanation is not adequate within a religious framework. Ultimately the question still remains: *Why did it happen to me? Why did this agent choose to attack me – and not somebody else?* In the following pages possible answers to these difficult questions are reviewed from different points of view or frames of reference.

A secular frame of reference

The above question can be answered quite easily from the perspective of a secular (non-religious) world-view: *there is no ultimate cause.* The agent attacked a specific person because he or she was accidentally exposed to it (and his or her immune system was vulnerable or unable to fight the organism), or because the person's behaviour brought about the exposure to the organism. For example, the person visited a malaria area without taking precautions and therefore increased the chances of contracting the disease.

In contemporary Westernised cultures this secular view of disease is very common. The advantage of this point of view is that it generates no guilt because it does not hypothesise about an ultimate cause (such as God or the ancestors) behind a condition such as Aids. People with such a world-view don't have to feel guilty about contracting the disease and cannot blame God for it, but they must accept that they are exposed to random processes of nature (e.g. disease-causing agents). All they can do is try to avoid certain dangerous situations or high-risk environments and take all the necessary precautions to prevent infection. If they contract disease in spite of this, they can only accept it in a fatalistic way – bad things can happen.

From the secular point of view, the question why someone was infected may be an expression of anger rather than a quest for a higher causative agent (such as God). From the HIV-positive person's point of view, the cause may simply be a high-risk lifestyle without sensible precautions.

If the counsellor comes to the conclusion that the client sees life in terms of this framework, he or she should deal with it by addressing the anger and frustration in an appropriate way. This may be done by emphasising the following:

- People are not machines. Nobody is perfect and therefore people sometimes do take risks or act ill-advisedly.
- We can choose to stay angry with other people (or with ourselves) and thereby spoil the rest of our lives, but that will not change what has happened to us. However, we *can* change the rest of our lives by choosing to be positive and by helping others.
- We should be *consistent* and honest with ourselves. If we believe that there is no higher power directing events on earth, there is no sense in being angry with life in general or in feeling guilty. Anger and guilt can then be directed only at other people or at ourselves – and that is not a productive or helpful way of living.

A Judeo-Christian framework

Within a Judeo-Christian framework we may extend the question 'Why does God allow Aids?' to the following:

- Is HIV/Aids God's punishment?
- Am I a bad person? Did I deserve to get ill because I sinned?

Four basic answers can be given to these two questions.

- Sickness and death came into the world because of sin (Genesis 6:3). However, this does not mean that we can attribute specific illnesses to specific sins. Unfortunately this is exactly what is often done by Jews and Christians. For those who think in terms of what theologians call 'rigid wisdom' (against which the book of Job protests), sin and illness are closely connected. That is, sin always causes sorrow (e.g. disease). In some cases the argument is even reversed. That is, if people get ill, they must have sinned and they should therefore confess and ask for forgiveness. In the book of Job this is the view of Job's friends, but the view is rejected by the book as a whole (Job 42:7). In the New Testament the close connection between sin and illness is also rejected in John 9:3. Although the view that illness is caused by sin is still very common among Jews and Christians, it is nonetheless unbiblical and causes much unnecessary guilt and pain in people with life-threatening diseases such as HIV/Aids. This perception should therefore be rejected in the strongest terms: 'bad' people do not become ill more often than 'good' people!
- A second possible view is to see the purpose of illness (or any suffering) not as punishment for sins but rather as a test of our faith and to make us better people. Suffering enables us to purify ourselves and to grow spiritually.
- Because of our limited insight and knowledge as human beings, we cannot on the whole make any sense of suffering. Although we accept that suffering may not be intended as punishment, we might believe that it fits into God's plans in some mysterious way – although we often do not know exactly what God's purposes and intentions may be. It is therefore problematic for any religious person (including counsellors) to try and 'play God' by explaining the purpose of suffering or disease.
- A fourth answer may be an alternative to the three lines of argument presented above. Although it is related to the secularised world-view, it is not necessarily agnostic or atheistic. This view emphasises that it was God's intention to give humans full freedom and that God therefore created a cosmos which is essentially neutral. Life is presented as a challenge to us to try and make the best of our lives without too much interference from God (Van Dyk, 2000). (Exactly how much a person may allow for God's intrusion into the course of daily life will depend on that person's world-view.) When something bad happens to the faithful, we should therefore not necessarily attribute it directly to the will of God because in a sense it may only fit into the *broader* framework of God's creation. God is therefore still acknowledged to be a force in human life, although God (in such a view) remains much more in the background and acts in much more mysterious ways than most Christians and Jews would usually affirm.

HIV-positive people are often plagued by the question whether their infection means that they are bad people. By extension this would imply that they will end up in hell. HIV-positive people are often reluctant to admit these concerns. Counsellors should therefore treat this issue in a sensitive way and rather deal with it indirectly by volunteering that this is *an unacceptable and false conviction* of many people within the community.

As noted earlier, sin and sickness have no demonstrable relationship with each other. This means that a person who is HIV positive is not *necessarily* a bad person (i.e. the person's moral status is not a causative factor in the disease). Those who affirm that diseases are caused by sin are reflecting an inappropriate, self-righteous and sanctimonious attitude to those in pain. Sadly, such attitudes do occur in faith communities. The people who hold them often have deep unresolved personal issues about sex, sexuality and sexually transmitted infections.

Even if people think that they have sinned (which, in any case, is true of all people), the spiritual HIV/Aids counsellor should emphasise forgiveness and reconciliation to God and other believers. The Old and New Testaments abound with examples of people who sinned and who were subsequently forgiven by God. These include great heroes of faith like Abraham, Moses and King David. Within a Christian framework the examples of the prostitute (John 8) and the robber whom Jesus pardoned on the cross (Luke 23:43) can be used as helpful examples of God's infinite desire for forgiveness (rather than for punishment and retribution).

Enrichment

Is disease 'good'?

People who are suffering often find it unacceptable and frustrating when counsellors offer them the cliché that everything will work out in the end or work out for the good of the faithful. An unqualified statement like this is problematic in many ways. The fact that sickness may be for the good of the sick person may not be immediately demonstrable and this may encourage counsellors to tie themselves in knots in their attempts to prove just how suffering can be beneficial to the suffering person. This answer also still does not answer the question: Why is it necessary for God to use suffering and pain to purify his children? This question is especially relevant when the person is suffering from a serious condition such as Aids or cancer, or when a baby is suffering from an incurable disease. It is therefore better to emphasise that we have less than perfect insight into God's plans and dealings, rather than to state in an unqualified manner that a disease is ultimately for our good.

Traditional religious frameworks in Africa

Many African people adhere to traditional beliefs, combining these with other religious systems such as Christianity. Although (mostly white) religious leaders often tend to be negatively inclined towards these forms of 'syncretism' (i.e. the combining of elements from different religions and belief systems), it is important for counsellors to recognise such systems and include traditional beliefs in their religious perspectives on HIV/Aids.

In the religious systems of some cultures, disease is attributed to natural agents, witchcraft or the displeasure of the ancestors. But even when a disease is attributed to an external agent (e.g. a germ or virus) there will still be a search for the ultimate cause of the disease – the person or agent who caused or sent the disease (see 'Witches and sorcerers as causal agents of illness' on page 116). Trying to persuade traditional people to change their views about illness and suffering would be offensive, insensitive, condescending – and doomed to failure, as would trying to persuade Christians, Jews or Muslims to abandon their faith. It is essential to work *within* the religious framework, whatever it may be, rather than try to challenge it. Counsellors who have no understanding of or tolerance for a given religious framework should either become better informed or desist from attempting to counsel clients of different faiths.

In some cases counsellors should advise HIV-positive people to consult traditional healers who may be better equipped to deal with religious issues within the client's religious framework. It must, however, be emphasised that HIV/Aids cannot be cured even though some traditional healers may claim that it is possible. Nevertheless, the religious rituals may improve the infected person's quality of life and resolve issues that could not be cleared by a Western counsellor.

Other religions

Forgiveness and ways of cleansing the mind and body are basic to all religions. By encouraging people to engage in purification rituals, to meditate and to restructure the remainder of their lives, they may be prepared for life after death or for reincarnation. It should be emphasised that HIV infection is not a condemnation or the end of the road for infected individuals. It may rather be an opportunity for them to prepare themselves properly for the remainder of their lives and for their transition to another world.

A religious perspective on death

One of the most important functions of religion is to provide coping strategies for accepting the inevitability of death. Death is difficult to accept when young people die (especially when they die from diseases such as HIV/Aids). In many African cultures, for example, the death of young people is seen as 'unnatural', and in modern Western societies people are alienated from death, partly

Enrichment

Children and religion

Religious counsellors should always take the developmental stage of children into account when talking to them about God, illness and death. The following few basic points should be taken into account when counselling children (Wong et al., 1999):

- Because toddlers' cognitive processes are undeveloped, they have only a vague (or 'concrete') idea of what God and religious teachings mean. Religious routines and rituals (e.g. prayers) may however be comforting to a sick child or a child who has to deal with serious illness in a close relative.
- Older preschool children begin to develop a capacity for understanding religious teachings. At this stage they have a concrete conception of God and begin to imagine him physically (like an imaginary friend).

  Although young children enthusiastically participate in religious rituals, they still have a limited grasp of their significance. These routines (e.g. prayers) can nonetheless be very comforting to young children, especially during stressful periods such as illness. Religious teaching such as right and wrong, reward or punishment, heaven or hell are understood, and wrong-doing provokes feelings of guilt in children. Because preschool children often misinterpret illness as punishment for real or imaginary transgressions, it is important to dismiss this idea and to emphasise the unconditional love of God rather than present God as a judge of good or bad behaviour.
- Young school-age children picture God as human, and they usually describe God in terms such as 'loving' and 'caring'. They are fascinated by the concepts of heaven and hell and are afraid to go to hell. These concepts should be dealt with and children should be assured that God loves children and doesn't expect them to be perfect. Children of this age are preoccupied with rules and regulations and expect to be appropriately punished for misbehaviour. Although they try to structure their lives in a logical and systematic way, they still find it difficult to distinguish between natural and supernatural phenomena. Because their understanding of symbols is limited, it is better to explain religion in more concrete terms to children of this age group. The young school-age child usually perceives illness as punishment. Religious acts such as prayers are important and the younger child expects them to be answered. As they grow older, children start to realise that prayers are not always answered and do not become so anxious when they are not.
- During the adolescent years beliefs become more principled and abstract, and less emphasis is placed on rituals and practice. Adolescents therefore emphasise the internal rather than the external aspects of commitment. At this stage children can understand and deal with most religious aspects of disease and illness. It is especially the fairness or unfairness of life that will be of great concern to the adolescent who is HIV positive or has lost a close relative to the disease.

because our culture is so materialistic that people find it difficult to believe in any kind of existence after death.

Dying is not unnatural – it is part of the cycle of life, but anxiety about what may be waiting after death is very real, even in the case of religious people. One can therefore expect people to engage in some kind of search for certainty, or attempt to contact the spiritual world – either in an attempt to link up with a loved one or to gain some certainty about life after death. A belief in an existence after death can make an approaching death more meaningful and bearable.

Regarding life after death, some people deny that there is any (the a-religious view) while at the other extreme are people who despise their earthly life and yearn only for the life hereafter. The latter view originated from Plato's philosophy which stated that the fleshly life represents all that is low and unacceptable, and that one's spirit should be relieved to get rid of its imprisoning body. Although this view is also common among Christians, it is (in its extreme form) more Platonic than biblical. The positive aspect of such a religious world-view is that it may be a big comfort to a person who is suffering and who needs to have some hope for a better future – albeit after death. The negative aspects of this world-view are that it may be escapist (although some escapism should not necessarily be denied an HIV-positive person) and that it sometimes fails to prepare people adequately for coping with the remainder of their lives. Why should they invest so much energy in the present life if it is so disappointing? Why not wait in anticipation for a better life to come? Such an attitude may cause a person to give up on this life long before death.

Most people occupy some middle position between totally denying an afterlife and living only for an afterlife. Religious counsellors should emphasise the importance of ensuring the quality of whatever life remains to the HIV-positive person – without denying the potential importance of life after death. Often a balanced view, emphasising the importance of both worlds, can offer comfort to religious people, and enhance the quality of their remaining life.

It is important for religious counsellors and their clients to talk about death, and for counsellors to attempt to strip the image of death of some of its horror and ugliness. The bereaved person is often comforted if one emphasises that death is a natural process and that it is not necessarily the end – it may in fact be the beginning of something new and wonderful. It should also be emphasised that it is only natural for a person to be uncertain about death. We don't know exactly *what* death will be like and ultimately we all have to face it on our own.

Ethical considerations

Ethical considerations are of the utmost importance when one counsels HIV-positive people within the community. Although one would expect religious communities and churches to be generally supportive and accepting of HIV-positive people, fears and unresolved complexes often override compassion and theological principles and bring out 'unexpected' negative reactions. In their mildest form such negative attitudes may be reflected by their indifference towards members of the community who are HIV positive. The more extreme forms include condemnation, stigmatisation, labelling of people, and a laager mentality.

Religious communities may have various responses to HIV/Aids. Some religious groups may state that the only effective way of stopping the spread of the disease is for people to adhere strictly to religious teachings about human sexuality and substance abuse (i.e. everyone should avoid sexual intercourse outside marriage, never be promiscuous and always abstain from drug abuse). Other groups might believe that, while religious teachings are very important, these should be supplemented with explicit information about methods known to be effective in reducing the risks of transmitting HIV (e.g. condom use) (Lyons, 1988). Experience has shown that the first type of idealistic view is not effective, and that the more realistic second option is probably a more honest and compassionate way of dealing with HIV/Aids within a religious context. This view accepts that although it is a realistic ideal to expect *some* people to adhere strictly to these higher religious ideals, it is NOT realistic in our world to expect it from *all* religious people.

The ethical principle of 'saving and sustaining life' should be emphasised within a religious context. In Jewish thought the saving of life takes precedence over all other considerations (Rose, 1988). *Reverence for life* plays an equally important role in Christianity and in religions such as Hinduism and Buddhism, and this principle should be emphasised as the basis for HIV/Aids prevention education.

Many Christian churches (and some other religions too) tend to judge people severely for sexual transgressions – often such judgements are based on double standards and a great deal of hypocrisy and self-righteousness (Sunderland & Shelp, 1987). These attitudes have no real connection with religious principles, and in fact contradict widely held religious principles of acceptance, compassionate care and forgiveness. Negative attitudes should therefore be exposed by religious counsellors for what they are – biased and unacceptable expressions of hatred. This should be emphasised not only when counselling HIV-positive clients who may have suffered because of such attitudes and behaviour, but also when training counsellors for dealing with members of the community.

For the same reasons it is hypocritical to keep on discussing the *morality* of teaching people safer sex practices while allowing people to die from Aids. *All human life is precious* and we cannot reject suffering people because they transgress *our* principles, moral standards, or religious beliefs. Although it may be important (and wise) within the framework of religious counselling to emphasise the value of sexual morality and promote the ideal of sexual abstinence outside marriage, churches and other religious organisations are avoiding their responsibility if they do not accept the realities of life. Those realities are that it is not easy to change behaviour and morals, and we should therefore also emphasise the importance of safer sex practices (Van Arkel, 1991). Even if a church does not condone the use of condoms (inside or outside marriage), it should not neglect to teach its members about the need for safer sexual practices (based on the principles of compassion and the reverence for life).

Religious counsellors should have an accommodating attitude towards gay people. Churches and religious institutions differ in their theological attitudes towards homosexuality, but many religions have begun to emphasise the importance of accommodating gay people within religious congregations without condemning them. In this regard – as in every other – it is the task of religious counsellors to avoid hypocrisy and refrain from judging other people, especially when it comes to sexual matters.

The labelling of people as *guilty* or *non-guilty* is rooted in a deep psychological need to create as much distance as possible between ourselves and a threatening disease such as HIV/Aids. It is therefore not surprising to learn that similar negative attitudes prevailed during the time of the Black Death. True believers should never be guilty of cruel labelling and lack of compassion. Their behaviour should be based on generally accepted principles of compassion and not on mindless fear, hypocrisy, denial and neurotic superstition.

Two of the most commonly expressed views about the Aids pandemic are firstly that it is God's punishment for a sinful and promiscuous lifestyle and secondly that it is nature's way of reducing the numbers of the human population. The first question can be answered by referring to the discussion above which outlines the invalid argument that sin directly causes all suffering and illness, and also by pointing out how many children, haemophiliacs and health care professionals (who have accidentally been exposed to HIV) have died as a result of being infected by the virus. To write off these so-called 'innocent' people as *the exception that proves the rule* is hypocritical and heartless in the extreme – and therefore incompatible with all compassionate expressions of religious dogma.

To view the Aids pandemic as a 'natural' way of 'culling' people may sound like a heartless but reasonable assumption – until a close family member or a friend gets culled. When confronted by this point of view, we should always question the true motives behind the question.

- What are the psychological reasons why anyone should express such a view? Is it an unconscious way of trying to deal with the tragedy of life by exposing the so-called ecological reasonableness of plagues? Or is it a way of withdrawing all emotional energy from the universal tragedy that is playing itself out in our midst?

- Is it a way of making the lack of compassion for HIV-positive people more acceptable by temporarily stepping outside of a religious or compassionate framework and resorting to natural and ecological explanations?
- Is it a mechanism used by people and counsellors to protect themselves emotionally?

The role of the church and other religious institutions

The church and other religious organisations should seriously consider their role in the HIV/Aids epidemic. Expressed hostility or indifference, which is even more common, should be exposed and condemned as heartlessness and should be opposed on all terrains. It should be affirmed that, because members of the church have Aids, the church has Aids, and so the church cannot ignore Aids (Anderson & Rüppell, 1999). We must educate and involve religious leaders and the faithful in the Aids field.

In the first place religious counsellors should become part of HIV/Aids counselling teams. Where possible, these religious counsellors should be members of the local clergy, and they should be adequately trained, and noted for their compassionate attitude towards suffering.

All religious institutions should be encouraged to become involved in an organised way in HIV/Aids care and counselling, for example by financially and physically supporting existing hospices or by founding such caring facilities. Research has shown that it is far more desirable in the long term to involve *local* agencies and religious institutions than to depend on often undependable foreign support. The World Council of Churches sees the role of the Church as providing a climate of love, acceptance and support in the everyday life of the church, reflecting on the theological and ethical issues raised by the pandemic, and physically taking care of the immediate and long-term effects of HIV/Aids (Anderson & Rüppell, 1999).

All religions emphasise that compassion should be expressed by actual physical help and the relief of pain, illness, hunger, poverty and other forms of suffering. In Africa poverty has had a huge impact on the spread of HIV/Aids and there can be no doubt that it also negatively affects the treatment and care of Aids patients. Aids patients often have barely enough food to keep them alive – expensive drugs and healthy food are too often beyond their grasp (UNAIDS, 2000a). Caregivers and volunteers themselves are often also hungry and needy. It very difficult to care for others if you are too weak to tend to your own physical needs.

In such circumstances churches, synagogues, temples, mosques and other religious organisations cannot sit back and remain unmoved by the tremendous suffering of infected people. In the face of the HIV/Aids pandemic, religious institutions will have to redefine their usual way of 'caring for the poor'. They will have to engage in prevention and education programmes and also pay attention to the spiritual and physical needs of people who are suffering from illnesses or who experience desperate poverty because of the loss to Aids of breadwinners and parents (in the case of the vast numbers of Aids orphans).

Above all, religious institutions should emphasise that all people are included in the pervasive love of God. Within the Judeo-Christian faith this fact is expressed by the belief that humans are created in the image of God and are therefore held within the scope of God's concern and faithful care (Anderson & Rüppell, 1999).

13.3 CONCLUSION

The Aids pandemic can be countered only if it is fought on all fronts – which includes the church and all other religious institutions being willing to preach publicly about behaviour change and to become actively involved in caring for sick and orphaned people. If they fail to do this, their failure will probably become one of the greatest failures of organised religion ever witnessed. If religious institutions fail us in this crisis, they will forever compromise their credibility and their relevance and role in society.

part 4

Care and Support

INTRODUCTION TO PART 4

The main theme of Part 4 is the care and support of individuals living with HIV/Aids. HIV/Aids makes demands on the community and society that cannot be met by hospitals alone. Families, loved ones and the community all have an indispensable role to play in the support and care of individuals with HIV/Aids. Part 4 concentrates on how to care for people with HIV infection and Aids in various health care settings such as hospitals, hospices and clinics – and in the patient's own home. Practical advice and solutions are offered about how to care for patients in health care settings with very limited resources, facilities and finances, such as we find in many rural clinics and homes.

The importance of family and community involvement in the care and support of people living with HIV/Aids is discussed in *Chapter 14*. The basic principles of home-based care programmes are presented, as well as guidelines and advice about how to start such programmes in your communities.

The plight of Africa's Aids orphans and other children made vulnerable by HIV/Aids, and strategies or models for the care of orphaned children, are discussed in *Chapter 15*.

The application of universal precautions to prevent HIV infection in various health care settings is discussed in *Chapter 16*. This chapter offers guidelines about infection control in hospitals, clinics, hospices, and homes in which family members have to care for a patient or patients with Aids.

Chapter 17 focuses on strengthening the immune system, the promotion of general health, nutrition, and the nursing care of general

Learning outcomes

After completing Part 4 you should be able to:

- develop a home-based care programme for the community in which you live
- devise a practical model for orphan care that will work in your community
- prepare and present a lecture to primary caregivers (involved in home-based care) about the basic principles of infection control at home
- prepare and present a lecture to professional nurses about universal precautions and infection control in the hospital
- advise HIV-positive individuals about a healthy diet and sound nutritional practices (remembering to take their personal circumstances into account)
- advise HIV-positive individuals on how to take care of their immune systems by living a healthy life
- teach volunteers the basic principles of caring for a patient with Aids in his or her home
- apply basic (or advanced) nursing principles in caring for patients with Aids who present with fever, diarrhoea, skin infections, problems with the mucous membranes (mouth and throat), respiratory problems, nausea and vomiting, genital problems, pain, weakness and mental confusion
- understand the principles of palliative care
- develop a programme to help caregivers who work in the HIV/Aids field care for themselves in such a way that they can prevent burnout

health problems and opportunistic infections. The principles of palliative (or terminal) care are also discussed. In the sections entitled *Home-based care*, the author offers practical advice about how to care for a patient with Aids with the minimal resources available in many homes.

In *Chapter 18*, the very important issue of care for the caregiver is discussed. Signs and symptoms of burnout are given for caregivers to use as a benchmark to evaluate their functioning, along with helpful hints on how to care for themselves to prevent burnout.

chapter

14 Home-based Care

A pool of light
In the silver morning,
when the land was still cool and windy,
only the village was a pool of light.

The magnitude of the HIV/Aids crisis has inevitably meant that the family and the community have had to become involved in most care programmes. Before the Aids pandemic it was not unreasonable to regard pandemics of this kind (such as the Black Death, the bubonic plague pandemic that killed over 50 million people in Europe and Asia in the 14th century) as tragic episodes from the distant past. We were complacent because we had become accustomed to the wonders of medical science and technology. Cures and treatments had been discovered (or were in the process of discovery) for most problems, illnesses and syndromes, and even death itself was considered an enemy that could be defeated or at least delayed. More and more hospitals and clinics were built, and wherever possible medical services such as vaccinations were extended to the majority of the population. And so we continued to be lulled into complacency by the advances and promise of modern medical science and scientific research.

But then HIV and Aids erupted onto the scene and everything changed. People are dying in their millions and medical science has no cure. Hospitals are overflowing with very sick and dying Aids patients, while people with curable diseases and conditions are being turned away. Many health care professionals find themselves unable to cope with the demands of the pandemic and begin to suffer from burnout because they can no longer heal and alleviate suffering as they were trained to do. Because we are a society in crisis, our only hope for coping effectively with HIV/Aids is to look beyond the crisis and to use the rich resources and strengths that have always resided in our family and community life.

HIV and Aids make tremendous new demands on health services that cannot be met by hospitals alone. Because HIV infection (and all its accompanying complications) can last for months or years, a person with HIV infection or Aids may move from the home to the hospital and back again several times. Hospital care is very expensive, and families can often not afford multiple admissions to hospital. Hospitals themselves do not have the personnel and resources to cope with the huge demands that Aids makes of them. The only practical and humane solutions are to care for patients in their own homes and communities for as long as possible; to develop an integrated home-based care service with professional, community and volunteer caregivers; and to use hospitals as a last resort when a patient's condition has deteriorated and professional help is needed.

But the demands on families and the community do not end with the death of the patient. The Aids epidemic has left behind millions of orphans and other children made vulnerable by HIV/Aids in Africa, and the conditions in which these children live are often appalling. If communities do not reach out to help these children, Aids will also kill our future.

> Every community must become involved in the fight against Aids, and they must be empowered to do so. Only through an enormous commitment of resources – within communities and between communities at an international, national and local scale – can the world hope to contain the HIV/Aids pandemic and care for those who are ill (WHO, 1993).

The basic principles of home-based care discussed in this chapter are based on the guidelines compiled by Fröhlich (1999), Marston (2003), Muchiru & Fröhlich (2001), Uys (2003) and the WHO (2000a).

14.1 DEFINITION OF HOME-BASED CARE

Home-based care is the care given in the home of the person living with HIV/Aids. It is usually given by a family member or friend (the primary caregiver), supported by a trained community caregiver. In ideal circumstances family and community caregivers are supported by a multidisciplinary team that can meet the specific needs of the individual and family. The team consists of all the people involved in care and support, and may include a medical practitioner or professional nurse, a social worker or trained counsellor, a pastor or spiritual leader, volunteers, a traditional healer, friends and neighbours, and community members.

For the purpose of this chapter, the term 'caregiver' will usually refer to professionals or volunteers trained in home-based care, and the term 'primary caregiver' will refer to the family or friend caregiver who looks after the patient most of the time, and who does not necessarily have any training to do so.

14.2 THE GOALS AND OBJECTIVES OF HOME-BASED CARE PROGRAMMES

The main goal of home-based care programmes is to provide the organisational structures, resources and framework that will enable the family to look after its own sick members. Important functions of home-based care programmes are:

- to *empower* the community and the family to cope effectively with the physical, psychosocial and spiritual needs of those living with HIV infection and Aids;
- to *educate* the community about the prevention of HIV transmission;
- to *support* family members in their care-giving roles; and
- to *reduce* the social and personal impact that living with HIV infection and Aids makes on all those concerned.

A very important function of home-based care programmes is to establish a well-functioning *referral system* to hospitals, hospices, clinics and other health care facilities in the community.

14.3 ADVANTAGES OF HOME-BASED CARE

Home-based care is often the best way to look after someone with Aids. Some of the reasons why home-based care is preferable to hospital care are listed below (Fröhlich, 1999; Uys, 2003; WHO, 1993):

- Good basic care can be successfully provided in the home.

- People who are very sick or dying often prefer to stay at home so that they can spend their last days in familiar surroundings – especially when they know they cannot be cured in a hospital.
- Sick people are comforted by being in their own homes and communities with family and friends around them. The ambience of home prevents the patient from feeling isolated and rejected.
- Home-based care allows the patient and the family time to come to grips with the illness, and to prepare for the impending death of the patient.
- Home-based care promotes a holistic approach to care. This means that the physical, social, cultural, psychological, emotional, religious and spiritual needs of a patient can all be fulfilled by the family and the health team.
- Home-based care can be comprehensive if it includes rehabilitative, preventive, promotive, curative and palliative care.
- It is usually less expensive for families to care for someone at home. The cost of hospitalisation and transportation to and from a hospital can be financially crippling.
- If the sick person is at home, family members can attend to their *other* responsibilities more easily. It can become very difficult to cope with one's own life if a loved one is in hospital and the caregiver has to make frequent trips to and from the hospital.
- Because the pressure on hospitals is reduced by home care, doctors, nurses and other health care professionals can use their time more effectively to care for other critically ill patients in hospitals.
- Home care reduces the enormous pressure on provincial and national health care budgets (which are already strained to breaking point).
- The network of health services available in the home-based care programme enables family members to gain access to counselling support for themselves.
- Family and community involvement in the care of their own members creates general Aids awareness in the community and this helps to break down fear, ignorance, prejudice and negative attitudes towards people with Aids.
- Home-based care is sensitive to the culture and value systems of the local community – a sensitivity that is often missing in clinical hospital settings.
- The intervention in home-based care is proactive rather than reactive.
- Home-based care puts Aids care providers in touch with potential orphans and people who really need help desperately.
- Home-based care is empowering. This means that people take responsibility for and control of their *own* lives and communities.
- Home-based caregivers are also in the ideal position to identify the needs of children who are affected by the illness of parents or siblings. They can assess issues such as whether the child is attending school or not; whether the child is involved in the care of the patient, and to what extent; whether the child is immunised; whether the child needs health care; and whether the child has time to play. The home-based caregiver is also in a position to know who supports the child psychologically and emotionally; whether the child understands what is going on in the family; and who will look after the child after the death of the parent (Marston, 2003; Uys, 2003:5).

14.4 POTENTIAL PROBLEMS ASSOCIATED WITH HOME-BASED CARE

The following potential problems associated with home-based care should be considered:

- Patients often feel isolated – especially when they are confined to the home or to bed.
- Many people in communities are not ready for home-based care because of ignorance, superstition and (mainly) the fear of being stigmatised by other members of the community. For these reasons people might reject the concept of home-based care. This increases the anguish, desperation and loneliness of those living with Aids. In a certain South African city with a high prevalence of HIV infection, a hospital offered a training programme for providers of home-based care for the dying *in which the word 'Aids' was never*

once mentioned (UNAIDS, 2000c). This situation expresses the extent of the prejudice, fear and ignorance that imprisons potential caregivers behind walls of silence and denial and so prevents them from giving the care and leadership they could offer.

- Non-compliance with treatment often occurs because the patient or primary caregivers do not know how or when to administer medication (because they are educationally disadvantaged) or because the medication they require is far too expensive and they do not know where to go for financial aid.
- A lack of knowledge about the disease, treatment, emergency situations and community resources often hampers home-based care, and many family caregivers are afraid that they themselves might become infected with HIV.
- One of the greatest drawbacks of home-based care is that the caregiver might give up because of exhaustion and burnout resulting from the extreme demands of caring for a terminally ill patient. It is absolutely vital for caregivers to have support systems and to know how to care for themselves, otherwise they will be overwhelmed by burnout (see Chapter 18, 'Care for the Caregiver' for more information about burnout). Home-based care can succeed only if caregivers are well trained and if ongoing support, advice, mentoring and supervision are available.

14.5 MODELS OF HOME-BASED CARE

Uys (2003:5–7) identified the following three home-based care models:

- The *integrated home-based care model* links all the service providers with patients and their families in a continuum of care. The patient and family are supported by a network of services, such as community caregivers, clinics, hospitals, support groups, non-governmental organisations (NGOs) and community-based organisations (CBOs), as well as by the larger community. This integrated model allows for referral between all partners as trust is built, and it ensures that community caregivers are trained, supported and supervised.
- In the *single-service home-based care model,* one service provider (usually a clinic, hospital, NGO or church) organises home-based care by recruiting and training volunteers, and brings them into contact with patients and their families at home. Many home-based care programmes start this way and build their way up to offer integrated care as they recruit other partners.
- In the *informal home-based care setting,* families care for their sick loved ones at home, with the informal assistance of their own social network. Nobody has any specific training or external support and there is no formal organisation or supervision of the care. Informal care can be very difficult because the primary caregiver often lacks the necessary knowledge, skills and emotional support needed to care for an Aids patient.

The integrated home-based care model is the ideal model for quality physical care and psychosocial support for the person living with Aids and his or her family. Figure 14.1 on page 263 gives an illustration of an integrated comprehensive home-based care model.

14.6 THE HOME-BASED CARE TEAM

The core of the integrated home-based care team consists of the following people:

- The individual living with HIV/Aids.
- The primary caregiver or informal caregiver who provides most of the care to the patient. This is usually the patient's mother, grandmother, partner, friend or a foster or adoptive parent.
- Community caregivers – people in the community trained to help the primary caregiver with direct care and support. Community caregivers may be professionals or volunteers.
- The family and/or significant others (in the home) who assist in various ways.

The core team is usually assisted by one or more of the following people or organisations:

- The programme coordinator – usually a professional person such as a nurse or social worker.

- Professional caregivers such as professional nurses, community health or TB workers, social workers, medical doctors, psychologists or counsellors, pharmacists, physiotherapists and occupational therapists.
- Trained volunteers and others who offer supportive services such as residential care, respite services, pastoral care, legal aid and advice, transport services, and the staff of various NGOs and CBOs.
- Complementary services such as those of traditional healers and herbalists.
- Community support from community leaders, traditional leaders, village committees, religious and spiritual leaders, teachers and youth groups.
- Friends and neighbours who can help the family with simple tasks and errands.

A well-functioning network and referral system should connect the home-based care team with hospitals, hospices, clinics and other community-based health care institutions. Government support in terms of recognition, education, financial support, supplies and staff is indispensable.

The role of volunteers in a home-based care programme

Local community volunteers play a very important role in home-based care programmes. Volunteers usually come from a variety of backgrounds and they may be trained and experienced professionals, trained community caregivers, family members, or compassionate community members who wish to help those in need (Marston, 2003). According to Fröhlich (1999), many of the perceived disadvantages of using volunteers can be

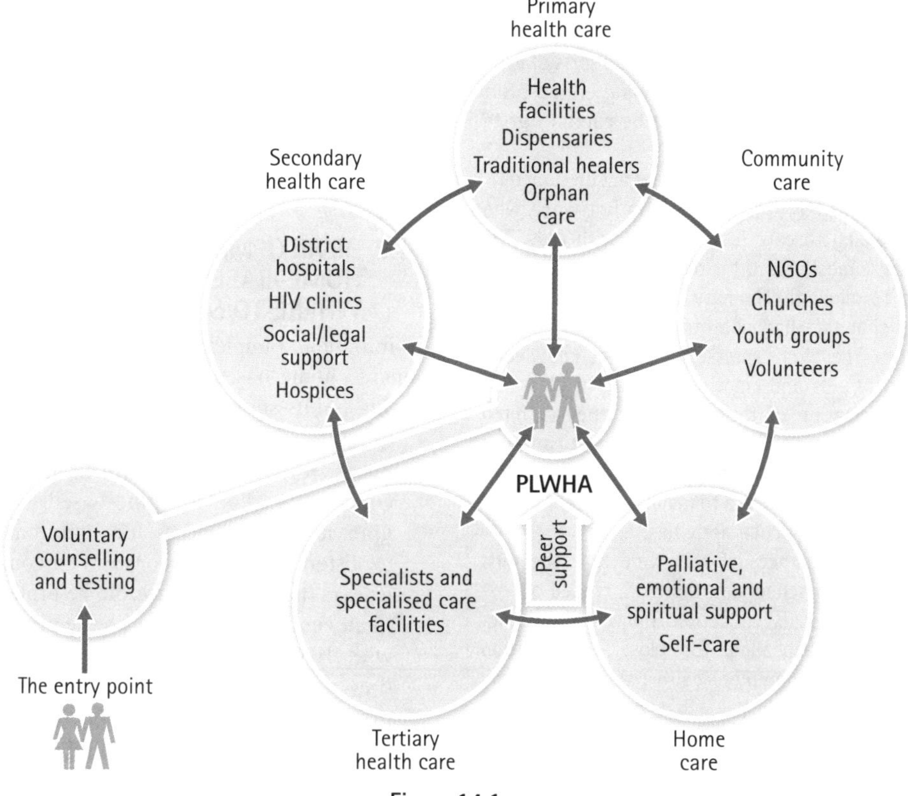

Figure 14.1
An integrated home-based care model
(Source: UNAIDS, 2002:155)

overcome if the volunteers are recognised as key workers in the programme; if they are chosen by members of the community; and if they are properly trained in basic home care. Volunteers should never be expected to offer home-based care without a good basic training and understanding of the physical, psychosocial, emotional and spiritual conditions that they may encounter and how to deal with these.

Some of the factors to be considered when selecting volunteers are age, gender, accessibility (do they live near the patient?), willingness, commitment, dedication, time (are they in full-time employment?), understanding of the problems involved, reliability, honesty, the ability to relate well to people, and the integrity to respect confidentiality and people's basic rights.

Enrichment

Using children in home-based care – a warning!

Children can be very helpful when there is a sick person in the home, and they can do all sorts of little things such as making tea or running errands. But the family and community must be careful not to misuse and exploit children.

Tlou (2000) investigated the impact on rural girls (aged between 11 and 16 years) in Botswana who were helping to care for a relative with Aids. The girls were mostly used for respite care after school hours to allow the primary caregiver a rest. Tlou found that this had potentially disastrous consequences. The girls expressed a lack of knowledge about HIV/Aids and emotions of fear, helplessness and anticipation of the worst, and they suffered from fatigue and lack of sleep because of caring at night. The schooling of the girls was also affected because they were forced to neglect their homework and skip extracurricular activities.

The consequences of this were that the girls dropped out of school and therefore missed opportunities for tertiary education. Tlou concluded her research by appealing for close collaboration between the community health team and primary caregivers in families so that home-based care would not become a process of merely 'dumping' patients on women and girls. If children have to care for adults, they need extra training, supervision and adult support (Marston, 2003).

Volunteers should be used wherever they fit best in terms of their personalities, qualities, expertise and interest. Volunteers directly involved in patient care should, for instance, be able to speak the language of the patient and his or her family, be able to read, write and calculate, have an interest (and preferably previous experience) in basic nursing care, and have good interpersonal and communication skills. There are also many tasks for other volunteers who are not interested in basic nursing care – tasks such as reading to patients, shopping, cooking and looking after children.

The issue of 'payment' for 'volunteer' services is a complex one. Many home-based care organisations realise that volunteers are often poor themselves, and remain active and function best if they are given incentives in the form of transportation reimbursement, uniforms or distinguishing attire, food, record-keeping materials and token payments (Smart, 2003). Some innovative volunteer programmes in South Africa reward volunteers by offering them some form of skills training programme that may generate work opportunities for them in future (e.g. computer or driving courses donated by companies in the community).

14.7 DEVELOPMENT OF AN INTEGRATED HOME-BASED CARE PROGRAMME: WHERE TO START

To initiate and implement an integrated comprehensive home-based care programme, the following points should be considered:

- Compile a community profile to establish the needs, resources and networks in a specific community. For a home-based care programme to be a success, it is important to talk to, listen to and collaborate with community leaders (because they are the key role players in any community) and with the people living with HIV/Aids and their families (because they are the people directly affected by the programme). A programme developed by outsiders without close consultation with the people in the community will fail. Establish programme objectives that meet the needs of the community.

- Establish a dedicated management team and appoint a programme coordinator.
- Recruit community caregivers and volunteers (preferably from the communities in which they will work) and train them thoroughly.
- Allocate community caregivers to specific areas and appoint a mentor (preferably a professional person) to supervise their work and to support them emotionally.
- Devise an HIV/Aids awareness programme that runs concurrently with the home-based care programme in the community to obtain the understanding, appreciation and support of the community for the home-based care programme.
- Make sure that the community knows how to access the services offered by the home-based care programme. Telephone numbers, a physical address, and the services offered should be widely publicised in places where potential patients and their families will see them.
- Make sure that all health-care services in the community know about the home-based care programme.
- Establish a care network and referral policies between service providers. Link up with a social welfare service to provide poverty relief where necessary to Aids patients and their families.
- Establish policies for the functioning of the home-based care service such as job descriptions for community caregivers, conditions of service, financial policy, policy on confidentiality and disclosure, and care policies (for example guidelines for dealing with specific symptoms) (Uys, 2003:9).
- Establish procedures, for example how to recruit patients, how often to visit them, how to visit them (public transport or dedicated vehicle), and how to prioritise work in the face of overwhelming demands.
- Access resources to support the care offered by the home-based care programme. Community caregivers are often paid a minimal salary or receive money for transport. Equipment might be needed to provide proper patient care, for example gloves, soap, towels and bedpans. Patients and their families might be so poor that caregivers have to take them food parcels or clothes.
- Monitor how well the home-based care programme works by keeping a record of all its activities. Teach community caregivers to keep record of all their visits and devise a patient assessment form that they can use to monitor the condition of the patient. They should also record patient or family needs such as spiritual support, the need to draw up a will, and future planning for children, and follow up with referral.
- According to Uys (2003), having access to the home and family provides caregivers with the opportunity to obtain valuable information that can influence local, provincial and national planning. The opportunity to network with researchers and academic institutions should therefore not be overlooked.
- Establish a support group for home-based caregivers where they can reflect on their work, share their problems and receive counselling and guidance. The support group can also provide educational talks, mentoring, supervision, socialising and participation in income-generating projects.
- Develop a standardised post-exposure management plan for incidents of caregiver exposure to HIV, hepatitis B or C, TB or any other transmissible disease (Ziady, 2003).

14.8 IMPLEMENTATION OF A HOME-BASED CARE PROGRAMME: WHAT THE CLIENT NEEDS

Those responsible for home-based care must find out what the patient's physical, psychosocial, emotional, spiritual and cultural needs are so that they can make informed decisions about the service to offer, the people to provide the service, and the kinds of referral to make. All the following factors need to be taken into account (Fröhlich, 1999; Marston, 2003):

- *Medical or nursing needs.* Does the client have medical or nursing problems requiring the attention of a nurse or referral to a clinic or hospital? Are there functional impairments, infections or disease of the cardiovascular, respiratory, neurological, digestive, or genito-urinary system? What is the general nutritional state of the patient? How is his or her general hygiene? Are there skin infections? Does the patient have wounds that should be treated or dressed? Does the patient have pain? Is the patient co-infected with TB and is it necessary for the community caregiver to supervise directly observed treatment (DOTS) as part of the home visit?

- *Basic needs.* Does the patient have food, shelter, clothes and blankets, electricity, water and sanitation? If the patient lacks these basic requirements, arrange for a social worker to visit him or her.
- *Activities of daily living.* Is the patient mobile, house-bound or confined to bed? Can the patient eat normally or does he or she require help to eat? Is the patient incontinent or is he or she able to use the toilet? Is there a toilet in the home, and if not, can a bedpan or commode be arranged for the patient? Who performs the following tasks for the patient: collecting water, cooking, bathing, washing clothes, shopping, collecting children from school, caring for pets, maintaining the house and garden? Volunteers can make an invaluable contribution by helping with these chores.
- *Social needs.* Who is the primary caregiver? How many people live in the house with the patient? Do friends, neighbours and family members offer their support?
- *Financial needs.* Does the household have any income? Does the patient receive a disability grant or pension? Possible sources of income (e.g. welfare departments, NGOs, help from the church, mosque, temple or other religious organisations) should be investigated and a list compiled.
- *Spiritual needs.* To what religious group does the patient belong? Does the patient have any spiritual needs that are not being attended to?
- *Legal needs.* Does the client need legal assistance? Does he or she need to draw up a will?
- *Psychosocial needs.* Are relationships in the home affected by the patient's HIV infection? Does it cause a lot of tension? Does the patient (or family) show any of the following psychosocial problems: denial of the infection, guilt, fear, anger, depression, suicidal thoughts, altered sleep patterns, uncertainty, anxiety, coping with multiple losses, coping with a changed body image, changes in relationships? Is the patient worried about what will happen to his or her children once he or she has died?
- *Sexual needs.* How does HIV infection impact on the patient's sexuality? How does the patient cope with changes in sexuality and sexual practices? How does the partner cope? Do they have the necessary information about safer sex practices? Do they have access to condoms?
- *Hospital, hospice and palliative care.* A time may come when the family is no longer able to cope with a critically ill patient. At this time it is important to refer the patient to a hospital or to ask for help from a hospice. If a patient prefers to die at home, counselling, palliative care (care that eases suffering) and practical support should be available to the patient and the caregivers.
- *Needs of the primary caregiver.* The primary caregiver (who is most often the mother or grandmother of the family) has to carry a huge load. She has to look after a sick and dying person, but life must go on for the young ones living in her home. Because this load can sometimes become overwhelming, it is vital for the primary caregiver to get time off from her duties. Volunteers can provide invaluable support by taking over the care of the patient for a few hours while the primary caregiver catches up on lost sleep, goes shopping, visits friends, or watches a movie.

14.9 TRAINING OF HOME-BASED CAREGIVERS

It is important to train home-based caregivers properly and thoroughly to provide a high standard of holistic care. The training provided will depend on the level of care required, but the following should be included in any training programme (based on Cameron, 2003:38–43):

- Background to home-based care (definition, purpose, team members and the health care system).

- Ethical principles of home-based care: confidentiality at all times; respect for the patient's wishes about disclosure; the autonomy of the patient to agree or disagree with treatment; and respect for the patient's choice on issues such as abortion.
- Basic facts about HIV/Aids and other sexually transmitted infections.
- Knowledge of the signs and symptoms of TB as well as an understanding of DOTS.
- Teaching and facilitation skills, especially adult education.

Home-care kits for caregivers
Home-care kits should be made available to community caregivers to provide them with the materials necessary to provide home-based care. A small backpack to carry the kit may be very useful for community caregivers who do home visits on foot. For caregivers using vehicles, a small suitcase might be useful, since it can also be used as a table to set out equipment while working.

The following items could be included in a home-care kit for caregivers (Marston, 2003): clinical (oral) thermometer, scissors, nail clippers, hand soap, plastic soap box, torch (penlight) with extra batteries, notebook, pen and patient evaluation forms, disposable paper towels, toilet paper, household bleach, disposable latex gloves, a plastic washable apron, black bags and plastic bags for waste and protection, aqueous cream or lotion for bed baths and skin massage, plastic straws (bending), linen savers, napkins (adult and child), sanitary pads, urine bags, uro-sheaths, syringe for feeding, newspaper, a large plastic sheet to protect bed linen, cotton wool and bandages, umbrella or raincoat and condoms.

Basic medication and nutritional support can also be included in the kit, e.g. calamine lotion, Vaseline, Valoid, paracetamol tablets and syrup, multivitamin syrup and tablets and Ensure.

The following items should be available as a resource bank should the caregiver need them for a particular client: bowl and equipment for dressings, bandages, kidney dish, foam mattress, bedpan, urinal, crutches, wheelchair, information brochures and washing detergents, as well as medications and nutritional support.

- Communication skills, including communication with children.
- Basic counselling skills (attending, listening, emotional support, how to deal with feelings, and problem solving skills).
- Promotion of positive living.
- Spiritual and religious issues.
- Gender and cultural issues.
- Infection control in the home-based care situation.
- Basic nursing care principles and the management of common illnesses.
- Practical procedures to help the patient, for example lifting, wound dressing, mouth care, feeding, bathing in bed, shaving, and using a bed pan.
- Nutrition and problems influencing nutrition.
- Incorporating palliative care principles into basic nursing care in the home.
- Social support, community support and referral possibilities.
- Care of the caregiver to cope with a very demanding task.

An assessment or evaluation process should be built into the training programme, and ongoing education, support and supervision should be offered.

Activity

- Develop a home-based care programme for the community in which you live. Make a list of the people in your community whom you would like to approach to help you with this programme (professional people as well as volunteers).
- Draw up your own Quick-Reference Guide, listing the resources and services available in your community. Use the following headings: Name; Service provided; Contact person; Address; Telephone number. If possible, visit some of these and see for yourself what they have to offer. Include the following services and people in your list: hospitals, clinics, hospices, crisis centres, government services, Aids clinics, NGOs, voluntary counselling and testing (VCT) services, nurses, community leaders, ministers, social workers, physiotherapists, occupational therapists, pharmacists, herbalists, traditional healers.

14.10 CONCLUSION

'Aids is not curable, but it is careable'. This quote from Thumi (UNAIDS, 2001:2) emphasises the invaluable role of home-based caregivers who take care of people in our communities living with HIV/Aids.

To fulfil and sustain this important role, caregivers need as much support and care as their patients. But 'home care can become home neglect' if appropriate planning, capacity building, community participation and support are not in place (Smart, 2001:74).

chapter

15 Support for Orphans and Other Vulnerable Children

The lonely children

Then they heard Raka from afar,
his cry like an animal, lost in the mist.
And the children sat wide-eyed, awake
silently clinging to each other
until the white ashes fell from the logs
and the fire died in the cold of the night.

> Neither words nor statistics can adequately capture the human tragedy of children grieving for dying or dead parents, stigmatised by society through association with HIV/Aids, plunged into economic crisis and insecurity by their parents' death, and struggling without services or support systems in impoverished communities.
>
> (UNICEF, 1999:8)

The Aids epidemic has created more than 15 million orphans worldwide (children under the age of 18 years who have lost a mother or both parents to Aids), and 80% (12 million) of these children live in sub-Saharan Africa (UNAIDS, 2004). By 2010, this number is expected to climb to more than 18 million in sub-Saharan Africa alone. In South Africa an estimated 2.2 million children (12% of all children) under the age of 18 years had lost one or both parents to Aids by the end of 2003. It is estimated that, without change in behaviour and interventions such as antiretroviral therapy, by 2015 there will be 3.1 million Aids orphans (18% of all children) under 18 in South Africa alone (Bradshaw et al., 2002).

Because the extended family system (which traditionally would have provided support for orphans) is greatly overextended in those communities most affected by Aids, it can often no longer take care of its orphaned children. Because of the stigma associated with Aids deaths in many communities, many families don't want to look after Aids orphans (UNAIDS, 2000c; 2004). As the number of adults dying of Aids rises over the next decade, increasing numbers of orphans will grow up without parental care and love, and be deprived of their basic rights to shelter, food, health and education.

After their parents' death, children often lose their rights to the family land or house. Relatives move in and often exploit the children by taking possession of their property but not providing support for them. Because these children no longer have access to education, and because they lack work skills and family support of any kind, they often end up living on the streets with no money whatsoever (except what they can raise from begging). Aids orphans suffer more frequently from malnutrition, illness, abuse and sexual exploitation than children who are orphaned by other causes. In most cases they live without basic human rights and dignity. They don't know how to protect themselves and they have no access to doctors, nurses, and other health care workers and facilities. Some studies have shown that death rates among Aids orphans are 2.5 to 3.5 times higher than those of children with a parent (HIV Infant Care Programme, 2000).

It is extremely important to identify orphans and other children made vulnerable by HIV/Aids in communities and provide support for them. Home-based care programmes can identify vulnerable children and launch orphan care in communities. Community caregivers must know what the needs and rights of orphans and other vulnerable children are; how these needs and rights can be disrupted by HIV/Aids; and what models of care and psychosocial support can be implemented to satisfy the needs.

Enrichment

Who is an orphan?

There are various definitions of what makes a child an orphan, and local ones should be used. UNAIDS (2004) defines an orphan as a child under the age of 18 who has lost at least one parent to death. A child whose mother has died is known as a maternal orphan, a child whose father has died is a paternal orphan, and a child who has lost both parents is a double orphan. The 2003 draft of the South African Children's Bill identifies an orphan as a child who has no surviving parent caring for him or her.

15.1 THE RIGHTS OF THE CHILD

Community caregivers are familiar with the actual living conditions of orphans and other vulnerable children in their communities, and it is therefore vital that they familiarise themselves with the rights of these children. Community caregivers have the capacity to be the guardians of children's rights, and they can integrate these rights into their intervention models.

The United Nations Convention on the Rights of the Child

In 1990 the United Nations adopted the Convention on the Rights of the Child, which sets out the social, economic, cultural, civil and political rights of children. The Convention on the Rights of the Child is a legal document that sets minimal acceptable standards for the well-being of all children. The South African government signed the Convention on the Rights of the Child in 1995, which means that it is legally bound to obey the rules as set out by the Convention.

There are four guiding principles upon which the Convention on the Rights of the Child is based:

- All children have the inherent right to life, survival and development.
- All children should be treated equally (non-discrimination).
- In all policies and decisions regarding children, the well-being of the child should be the primary consideration.
- The views of children should be respected and taken into account in all decisions concerning them.

The rights of the child as listed in the UN Convention on the Rights of the Child can be grouped into four main categories: survival, protection, development, and participation (De Villiers, undated; Kluckow, 2004; Smart, 2003).

- *Survival:* the provision of adequate food, shelter, clean water and primary health care. Children have a right to the highest level of health possible, which includes the right to health and medical services, with special emphasis on primary and preventive health care, public health education, and the reduction of infant mortality.
- *Protection:* from abuse, neglect, exploitation (sexual, labour and drug related) and war. (No child under fifteen may take a direct part in hostilities or be recruited into the armed forces.) Special protection should be provided to children deprived of their family environ-

ment. Appropriate, alternative family care or institutional placement should be made available to them, taking into account the child's cultural background. Children should also be protected from interference with their privacy regarding their families, homes and correspondence.

- *Development:* ensuring normal physical, emotional and psychological development through formal education, constructive play, leisure, art and culture, health care and a caring and nurturing environment. Children with disabilities have the right to special care, education and training designed to help them achieve their full potential and lead full active lives in society.
- *Participation:* being a part of a social environment and having some say in and access to information about issues that concern them, such as civil (a name and identity, non-discrimination and protection), economic (to participate in economic activities if desired), political (freedom of expression), cultural (freedom to participate in cultural activities), and religious (freedom to choose a religion).

Activity

How does HIV/Aids impact on the rights of children in your community? Give examples of the violation of the rights of the child (as listed in the UN Convention on the Rights of the Child) in the lives of Aids orphans or other children made vulnerable by HIV/Aids.

15.2 THE NEEDS OF THE CHILD

Manfred Max-Neef, who has worked extensively with the problems of development in the Third World, has co-developed a scale of human needs and a process by which individuals and communities can identify their 'wealth' and 'poverties' according to how these needs are satisfied (Kluckow, 2004; Max-Neef et al., 1991). According to Max-Neef, human needs (and therefore the needs of children) are few, finite and classifiable. These needs are constant in all cultures and all times. What does change over time and between cultures is the way in which these needs are satisfied.

According to the scale of human needs, all children have physical, emotional, social and intellectual needs that must be met if the children are to enjoy life, develop their full potential and develop into participating, contributing adults. Children's needs can be organised into the following ten fundamental categories. Within each category, each need occurs at four different levels of activity: of *being, having, doing* and *interacting* (Kluckow, 2004:7–8; Max-Neef et al., 1991:32–33).

- *Subsistence* needs concern the basic provision of food, water and shelter needed for survival.
- *Protection* is the provision of basic health, psychological and social safety and an infrastructure of protection against sickness, disease, violence, war and abuse.
- *Affection* refers to parental and family love and emotional nurturing, intimate relationships with others, friendships and peer support.
- *Understanding* refers to the need to develop the capacity for curiosity, intuition and critical thinking. This, in turn, will lead to the accumulation of knowledge and an understanding of how we fit into the world in general.
- *Participation* is the important process whereby we see ourselves as part of the bigger picture by taking part in it with family, friends, school community, church, or colleagues.
- *Leisure* is the opportunity to relax, rest and choose to be idle. We 'recharge' by playing, indulging in hobbies or sports, and spending time alone if we want to.
- *Creation* is being productive and having the capacity and skills to create something. The capacity for creation may refer to artistic creation, producing a crop or running a business.
- *Identity* is our sense of who we are; our self-esteem; the value we place on ourselves; and our sense of worth within our families, communities and peer groups.
- *Freedom* is the right of choice and autonomy, and freedom in a physical, emotional and social sense.

- *Transcendence* is the belief that we are part of something bigger than ourselves, and that the world is more than a physical reality. We have a need for spiritual awareness and connectedness.

15.3 SATISFIERS OF NEEDS

The above needs are satisfied at different levels, with different intensities and in different contexts (e.g. personal, social group and environment). Max-Neef believes that poverty should not be defined in terms of income threshold, but in terms of needs not satisfied: 'any fundamental human need that is not adequately satisfied reveals a human poverty' (Max-Neef et al., 1991:18).

The effects of satisfiers on the needs of people can be different. The following types of satisfiers can be identified to satisfy human needs (Max-Neef et al., 1991):

- *Destroyers* are satisfiers that address one need but end up destroying that need and others as well. Child labour (including prostitution) and child armies are examples of destroying satisfiers. They may provide a vocation and a certain type of identity for children, but they also stifle other needs such as *affection, participation* and *freedom* and they destroy the capacity for healthy development.
- *Pseudo-satisfiers* are appealing and promise to fulfil needs, but don't. They generate a false sense of satisfaction. Examples include the allure of the city and freedom, which pull many vulnerable children into prostitution, drugs and alcohol.
- *Inhibitors* satisfy one need but inhibit another. For example, an overprotective family provides *protection* but in various ways may inhibit *affection, understanding, participation, identity* and *recreation*. A refugee camp for displaced children is an example of an inhibitor that can seriously hamper a child's healthy psychological development because although it provides basic food and shelter it leaves most of the child's needs unsatisfied.
- *Singular satisfiers* satisfy one need in a child's life while ignoring others. The indiscriminate distribution of food to poor children is an example of a singular satisfier that satisfies the need for *subsistence* in a non-synergistic way.
- *Synergistic satisfiers* are those that satisfy a given need and stimulate and contribute to the fulfilment of others. Synergistic satisfiers therefore meet several different needs at once. Effective education, preventive medicine, educational or experiential games, music and art are examples of synergistic satisfiers. For example, an educational game that satisfies the need for leisure also stimulates and satisfies the needs for understanding and creation.

Max-Neef offers a practical framework for caregivers who are searching for a model to address the so-called 'orphan problem'. Rather than choosing between existing models, caregivers should use Max-Neef's framework to assess and analyse how to best meet the varied needs of children in ways that are both satisfying and sustainable. Care for orphans or other children made vulnerable by HIV/Aids should be based on the fulfilment of all the needs of the child by using synergistic satisfiers. To provide a child with food, clothing and shelter is very important to fulfil the basic need for subsistence, but the child needs much more to become a fulfilled and productive adult.

> Understanding the need to develop synergistic satisfiers is crucial for community caregivers who face on a daily basis a dizzying array of different strategies for solving 'the orphan problem', many of which are far from being synergistic.
>
> (Kluckow, 2004:7)

15.4 THE VULNERABILITY OF CHILDREN AFFECTED BY HIV/AIDS

Many children in Africa live in homes and in communities racked by the effects of HIV/Aids. These children often do not live within a loving family environment where they can receive support, nurturing and guidance to help them cope with life's challenges and to fulfil their needs. Kluckow (2004:24) identified the following challenges that children affected by HIV/Aids often have to face due to their parents' illness and death:

- *Role changes.* As their parents become more ill and dependent on them, children find their roles changing from child to primary caregiver as they have to care for their parents. Older siblings have to take on the parenting of younger siblings and the resultant loss of childhood has serious implications for normal childhood development.
- *Isolation from family and peer group.* Many children affected by HIV/Aids have to drop out of school because of financial problems or their new responsibilities as caregivers. This cuts them off from their peer group, robbing them of an influence crucial to their ongoing identity development. The loss of learning has equally serious implications for their development. Children who are responsible for their parents have little or no time to play or spend leisure time with same-age friends. These children are often further traumatised by stigmatisation and rejection, which leave them still more vulnerable and isolated.
- *Traumatic exposure to suffering, sickness and death.* Children who take care of their sick parents are faced with the trauma of nursing and watching their parents die of Aids. Even with help from outside agencies, it should be recognised that children are not emotionally equipped to deal with the roles they take on as caregivers to their dying parents. In some traditional cultures talk about death is taboo, and this further complicates the issue.
- *Physical poverty and deprivation.* Loss of parental income and changes in the family economy often spiral down into poverty and deprivation. It is also not uncommon for relatives to grab the deceased's property and leave the children destitute.
- *Multiple losses, emotional trauma and complicated grief.* Children affected by Aids start grieving in anticipation long before the parent's actual death. They often experience multiple losses after the death of their parents as they are caught up in inheritance squabbles and experience sibling separation (normally along gender lines) and eventual relocation that might result in separation anxiety. The child thus has little time to grieve for the death of the parent, and this can lead to a complicated form of grief. The resultant unresolved feelings of anger, sadness, guilt and fear, aggravated by the absence of empathy and opportunity for catharsis, shadow these children throughout their childhood years and into adulthood, with dire emotional and behavioural consequences (Kluckow, 2004:25).

According to Max-Neef's theory, a child whose needs are not fulfilled lives in poverty, and each poverty has the dire consequence of generating pathologies. Children made vulnerable by HIV/Aids who do not receive psychosocial support to fulfil all their basic needs may suffer long-term social and emotional impairment and may be at risk for developing depression, anxiety, suicidal thinking, behavioural disorders (school drop-out, delinquency, substance abuse,

Enrichment

Stigmatisation of Aids orphans

Stein (2003) voices her concern about the way in which the media and academics unwittingly add to the stigmatisation of children whose parents have died of Aids. Experts in the field often refer to 'Aids orphans' in the context of the possible threat they may pose to our economy and our social stability and security. Aids orphans are even sometimes labelled as delinquents and criminals in the making. There is no evidence to support these assumptions, and they may cause immeasurable harm to orphan care in general. Extensive research shows that stigma prevents governments and communities from responding effectively to the orphan problem, as well as hindering the emotional recovery of affected children themselves. Stigma and discrimination also intensify violations of these children's rights – in particular their access to education, social services, and community and familial support. According to Rachel Bray (Stein, 2003:2) 'it is not the fact of orphanhood which constitutes a threat but rather, the way in which we are choosing to deal with the many parentless children in our midst.' Owing to concerns about the consequences of stigmatising children whose parents have died of Aids, many organisations now avoid using the term 'Aids orphan'.

promiscuity, prostitution, criminal behaviour and violence), learning disorders, developmental delay and psychosomatic illnesses.

15.5 PSYCHOSOCIAL SUPPORT FOR ORPHANS AND OTHER VULNERABLE CHILDREN

In the care of orphans and other vulnerable children our first question should not be what model of care to use, but to what extent the existing models of care fulfil the ten human needs indicated by Max-Neef. Before we discuss the models of orphan care in Africa, it is important to look at the psychological and social support needed by orphans and other vulnerable children. Table 15.1 summarises the potential deprivation of the fundamental needs of the child due to HIV/Aids, and the psychosocial support needed to fulfil the child's needs in a synergistic way.

Table 15.1
Psychosocial support to fulfil fundamental needs of children
(Source: Adapted from Kluckow, 2004:25,35)

Fundamental human need	Potential deprivation due to HIV/Aids	Fulfilment of child's needs through psychosocial support from caring adults
Subsistence	• Loss of family home • Reduction or loss of the buying and production of food • Reduction or loss of monetary income • Deprivation of basic clothing needs • Deterioration of physical health • General decline into state of physical poverty	• Unconditional provision of adequate nutritious food • Provision of a family home providing adequate shelter • Provision of adequate and appropriate clothing • Provision of primary health care
Protection	• Loss of parental protection and guidance, leading to possible physical and sexual abuse • Loss of social security and protection from stigmatisation • Lack of protection from the elements due to physical poverty • Physical vulnerability	• Adult caregiver who promises to provide, and reliably provides, basic protection from illness, accident and danger in the form of neglect, abuse or abandonment, and who conveys a message of safety ('I am here for you and will keep you safe')
Affection	• Loss of physical and emotional parental and/or family love and nurturing • Loss of sibling and peer friendships and extended-family contact due to family break-up and relocation • Loss of environment for expressing emotions	• Familial and extended-family support and love • Stable, continuous, dependable and loving relationships • Unconditional love • Friendships and peer intimacy • Safe space for experimentation with expression of emotions
Identity	• Loss of cultural and family identity and normal childhood environment for healthy self-esteem development • Emotional trauma leading to identity crisis or developmental delay • Loss of sense of belonging	• Adult caregivers who create a sense of connectedness which stems from belonging to a family and having a past, present and future (see 'Memory projects' on page 277) • Adults who give plenty of encouragement, provide accurate empathy and build healthy self-esteem in children

Table 15.1 (continued)
Psychosocial support to fulfil fundamental needs of children
(Source: Adapted from Kluckow, 2004:25,35)

Fundamental human need	Potential deprivation due to HIV/Aids	Fulfilment of child's needs through psychosocial support from caring adults
Under-standing	• Understanding of self and environment impaired due to culture of secrecy, school drop-out, and extreme emotional and physical trauma • Loss of inquisitiveness and connection with wider world outside of immediate culture	• Adults who provide life skills, insight and guidance to build a child's knowledge and his or her world, community, family, culture and self • Teachers and schools to expand children's world-view and engender a sense of understanding and direction
Participation	• Loss of capacity for participation in family, community, school and peer group activities • Loss of participation in life in general due to heightened and continual state of emotional and physical trauma	• Adult caregivers who create environments where children can feel valued as significant contributors, and who acknowledge the existence of children and their rights • Adults who respect children and provide enriched environments for participation
Leisure	• Loss of free time due to adult responsibilities of sibling and self-care • Deprivation of playtime and idleness and pursuit of recreational pastimes due to new status of labourer in extended family, especially for girl child	• Caregivers who recognise the need children have to play, and who provide ample time, space and stimulation for play and leisure • Caregivers who see the importance of children spending time with friends and who encourage peer group participation
Freedom	• Loss of autonomy and control of one's destiny • Deprivation of human rights • Loss of freedom of speech and movement • Loss of choices regarding home, family structure and marital status for girl child	• Caregivers who honour the rights of children to experience and express freedom, thereby granting them appropriate status in their families, schools and communities • Allowing children to experience and express their independence
Creation	• Loss of capacity to nurture and express creative abilities, inventiveness, and curiosity due to removal from formal school setting or altered roles	• Families, schools and communities that stimulate and encourage creative expression in many forms, enabling children to utilise their creative abilities and talents in meaningful ways
Transcendence	• Confusion and dissonance or impairment of capacity to imagine one's place in the larger context of transcendent spirituality or religion	• Caregivers who inculcate in children a sense of wonder at the larger world and who acknowledge life's spiritual dimensions through cultural and religious practices

Many children in Africa who are made vulnerable by HIV and Aids do not have the psychosocial support, as outlined in Table 15.1, to fulfil their basic needs. Unless they are helped, these children face a very difficult future. Synergistic psychosocial support should preferably be provided by the child's own empowered community. Communities and governments could also address this very serious issue by establishing other resources such as:

- *Community-based caregivers* working within community-based initiatives.

- *Schools* in which life skills are developed in class and through extracurricular activities.
- *Youth camps* where the child's development can be aided by experiential learning programmes.
- *Youth clubs* offering day programmes and out-of-school activities such as social interaction, fun and growth activities.
- *Church youth groups* offering activities aimed at spiritual growth.
- *Vocational training projects* to equip children and youths with vocational skills to generate income when needed.
- *Self-help projects* designed to provide income-generating opportunities for young people.

A good example of youth camps offering synergistic experiential learning programmes is the programme for orphans offered by the Salvation Army in Zimbabwe. These life skills and coping capacity camps help children to overcome the loss of their parents and to rebuild their confidence. They also offer teenage parenting courses in which orphans looking after their siblings are taught parenting skills, children's rights, hygiene, nutrition and first aid. Vocational training programmes in arts, crafts, hospitality and catering management are also offered (Smart, 2003:189).

15.6 MODELS OF CARE AND SUPPORT

The following models of care and support for orphans and other vulnerable children that exist in South Africa were identified by the South African Law Commission (Smart, 2003):

- Independent living of orphans (including child-headed families).
- Independent living of orphans with external support and supervision (including child-headed families).
- Foster care including traditional family care, cluster care of multiple children, and collective care of individuals or multiple children.
- Adoption.
- Institutional care including places of safety, shelters, short-term infant homes, and traditional children's homes or orphanages.
- State- or NGO-sponsored community-based support structures including feeding posts and day-care facilities.

Experience with existing models has shown that family and community-based approaches to caring for orphans and other vulnerable children are the best way of meeting the child's physical, psychological, emotional, educational, spiritual and social needs in a synergistic way. But family- and community-based caregivers will require support and back-up by government or outside organisations to remain viable. They need access to functioning health, education, social and counselling services. And they should be supported with food, clothing and funding (e.g. for school fees) where necessary. Caregivers should contact the Department of Social Development to enquire about current social security provisions for children in the form of child support grants and foster child grants.

Every reasonable attempt should be made to trace the relatives of an orphaned child. If a child is placed in foster care with non-relatives, factors such as the traditional cultural background, norms and values of the child and the foster family should be taken into account when trying to make a match. Families who foster children usually receive a small foster grant from the government to help them with some of the costs involved in caring for another child. (See enrichment box 'Adoption may be problematic in traditional communities' on page 278, which explains why children in Africa are often *fostered* rather than *adopted*.)

Orphanages are not generally the most appropriate interventions for orphans and other vulnerable children, and should be seen as a last resort when all other options are inappropriate or unavailable. Although orphanages are doing the best they can, they often function as singular satisfiers or even as inhibitors, and a child's emotional and psychosocial needs can seldom be met in an orphanage. Orphanages should be used mainly to care for abandoned babies or very young children who need care for a short period until alternative solutions can be found for them.

Households headed by adolescents (sometimes as young as 12) who care for their younger siblings are not uncommon in our communities and will become more visible in future. If these children cannot be accommodated in foster care programmes, community (and governmental) support should be offered to help them cope with their plight. Religious organisations can play a very important role in providing them with necessary support. Social workers, counsellors and nurses should visit the child-headed households on a regular basis to provide psychosocial support and to check on their physical well-being. Students and other youth groups should get involved in supporting, educating and caring for these children in innovative ways to equip them with the skills to cope under difficult circumstances.

Enrichment

Memory projects

Children who have lost one or both parents to Aids are often saddled with a legacy of confusion and grief because many parents remain silent about their HIV status until they die. Although they hope that their silence will protect their children, it has the effect of leaving the children unprepared to face a future alone. The National Community of Women Living with HIV/Aids in Uganda initiated a highly innovative programme called the Memory Project to counteract this painful situation. The purpose of the Memory Project is to break the silence between infected parents and their children. Memory books are usually compiled by the mother, but in some cases the mother and child write the memory book together. The memory book takes children on a step-by-step journey through aspects of their own identity, their family history, their lifestyle, culture and beliefs. The mothers often explain their own HIV status to their children and introduce them to their future caregivers. The memory book consists of photographs, stories, anecdotes about the child and the mother's life, little lessons, and information that a child may need later on in life. 'The memory book embodies a treasure trove of childhood memories and family history for both parents and children. For the child, it reminds him or her of their roots, gives them a keen sense of belonging when orphaned, and provides answers to questions they would have asked their parents while growing up' ('Memory books', 2000:3). The memory book project in Uganda has stimulated children to take an active interest in the care of their sick parents, to ask questions about their own health and the health of their parents, and to take up the challenge of looking after themselves (as best they can) after their parents have died (Nyamayarwo, 2000). The memory book children will also probably be more careful and protect themselves from infection when they are older. Memory books, memory boxes, memory suitcases or other variations are now used in many countries in the world to give the child a sense of belonging.

Examples of innovative community-based foster care initiatives

There are many examples of innovative orphan care projects all over Africa – all of them characterised by the dedication, compassion, love and commitment of ordinary members of the community. One example of such a programme is a community-based foster care model for orphaned babies and children developed by Seepamore and Nkgatho (2000) in Alexandra township in South Africa. (Most of these orphaned babies are HIV-infected.) The Alexandra model is based on the premise that orphans and their foster parents should be actively supported by each other and by the community. Seepamore divided the Alexandra community into three wards. Each ward has its own pool of trained foster mothers, a social worker who is the coordinator, and a leader foster parent who networks with the foster mothers in her ward, with the social worker and with other informal community service providers. The foster mothers are trained in home-based care; they are visited each month by the social worker; they attend lectures; they know each other well; and they get lots of support and advice. The mothers are supported by a whole team of community workers such as students, volunteers, religious organisations and schools. A supervisor renders supportive services to all the social workers in the team. The Alexandra model has tremendous advantages for the child in terms of improved health, weight gain, psychological well-being and a longer life. The model also helps to promote acceptance of the children by the community and it changes the attitudes of some of the community members. Because they are well trained and supported, foster parents are often willing to look after more than one child, or to repeat the caring experience after a child's death.

The Alexandra Aids Orphans Project also hosts the 'Go-Go Grannies'. The Go-Go Grannies are a group of grandmothers who have lost their own children to Aids and who are now raising their orphaned grandchildren. They help and encourage each other to cope, both emotionally and physically, with this daunting task. They are also supported by the Alexandra Project, which provides psychosocial, financial and material support to the grandmothers. This includes one-time building grants to ensure adequate shelter for their growing families, as well as seeds and fertilisers so women can start their own gardens to bring in food and income for their families (UNAIDS, 2004).

An innovative group foster care model was initiated in Uganda to accommodate more children in foster care by using group foster care programmes. Older women ('grannies') were appointed and trained as foster parents. The grannies were then allocated various tasks. Some of them tended a food garden while other older, less agile grannies looked after the children. A third group worked in the kitchen where they did the cooking. All the caregivers received food from the kitchen to feed their own families. The granny project resulted in better care and nutrition for the orphans, better nutrition for the whole community (excess food was given to nearby squatters), improved community services (a crèche facility, a toy library and a resource centre were developed), job creation (vendors sold the excess food from the gardens), and a general alleviation of poverty in the community.

Enrichment

Adoption may be problematic in traditional communities

Adoption can be a problem in a traditional community if a child (especially a boy) is not of the same family lineage (clan) as the adopting family. If ancestors (and the honouring and continuation of their names) play an important role in the lives of the family, they may well be reluctant to introduce new ancestors – those of the orphaned child. Adopting a girl is less of a problem because a girl will usually adopt the ancestors of the new family – as happens in marriage (Seepamore, 2000).

Activity

- Devise a practical model for orphan care that will work in your community. Ensure that all the needs of the child are being met in a synergistic way.
- Read the enrichment box: 'Memory projects' on page 277. What advantages do you think this project holds for the HIV-positive mother? And for the child?

15.7 CONCLUSION

The orphans of Africa need all of us living in Africa to be their advocates – advocates who will plead for the recognition of their basic human rights and needs, their dignity and protection. As families and communities we need to get involved. For the sake of our future we cannot afford to look the other way. It seems appropriate to conclude this chapter with the following words from the musical *Miss Saigon* by Boubill and Schönberg:

We owe them fathers, and a family
and loving homes they never knew
because we know
deep in our hearts
that they are all
our children too.

chapter

16 Infection Control

Overcoming fear

And so he danced . . .
until one by one they dropped the blanket
of their fear.

The fear of infection should never prevent us from caring for people with HIV infection or Aids. The risk of contracting HIV while taking care of HIV-positive individuals is very low if caregivers follow a few basic rules to avoid accidental exposure to blood and certain other body fluids. (See 'How great is the risk of HIV transmission when a person has been accidentally exposed to the blood of an infected person?' on page 29 for details about risk of infection.) This chapter will concentrate on the application of universal precautions to prevent HIV infection in health care settings such as hospitals, clinics and hospices – as well as in homes in which family members look after a patient with Aids.

16.1 UNIVERSAL PRECAUTIONS TO PREVENT HIV INFECTION

In 1985 the Centers for Disease Control (CDC) in the USA developed a strategy of 'universal blood and body fluid precautions' to address concerns about the transmission of HIV in health care settings (CDC, 1989). Universal precautions are based on *risk of exposure to blood* (and other fluids) and *NOT* on a *positive diagnosis of HIV infection*. It is of the utmost importance to keep in mind that *any* patient who enters a hospital or clinic may potentially be infected with HIV. There is no way at all of telling *by merely looking at a person* ('by sight') whether or not he or she is infected with HIV. Believing that precautions should be applied *only* to a person who is known to be HIV positive gives a false sense of security and is a very dangerous attitude. So, instead of focusing on *individuals known to be infected with HIV*, it is much safer, more sensible and less prejudiced to concentrate on *all body fluids of all patients* and to observe universal blood and body fluid precautions for *all* patients.

HIV can be transmitted in the health care setting through:

- the skin being pierced with a needle or any other sharp instrument which has been contaminated with blood or other body fluids from an HIV-positive person;
- exposure to broken skin, open cuts or wounds of a person with HIV infection;
- exposure to blood or other body fluids from an HIV-positive person; and
- splashes of HIV-infected blood or body fluids onto the mucous membranes (eyes or mouth).

HIV can be transmitted to patients through:

- contaminated instruments that are re-used without adequate disinfection and sterilisation;
- transfusion of HIV-infected blood;
- organ transplants;
- skin grafts;
- HIV-infected donated semen; and
- contact with blood or other body fluids from an HIV-positive health care worker.

(WHO, 2000a:11-2)

Blood and body fluids requiring universal precautions

Because the following body fluids can be infectious when they are contaminated with HIV, the universal precautions should be strictly applied whenever there is any possibility of contact with them (these fluids should be considered to be *as likely* to transmit HIV infection as HIV-infected blood, i.e. they carry *the same risk factor* as HIV-infected blood):

- blood (including menstrual blood)
- semen
- vaginal secretions (including menstrual discharge)
- body tissue (or wound secretions)
- amniotic (pregnancy) fluid
- cerebrospinal (brain and backbone) fluid
- peritoneal (abdomen) fluid
- pericardial (heart) fluid
- pleural (chest) fluid
- synovial (joint) fluid
- any body fluids containing visible blood, semen, vaginal fluid, or any of the fluids mentioned above.

Body fluids not requiring universal precautions

Owing to the low concentration of the virus in the following body fluids, universal precautions are not required when handling these fluids – *unless visible blood is present*:

- faeces
- urine
- vomit
- nasal secretions
- saliva (spit)
- sputum (lung mucus)
- sweat
- tears.

Although universal precautions do not apply to body fluids such as faeces, saliva and urine, health care professionals and other caregivers should always use their common sense when deciding on how to handle these body fluids. Precautions should, for instance, be taken with saliva in a dental setting because such saliva is likely to be contaminated with blood. Care ought to be taken with the sputum of TB patients that contains blood. Nappies of HIV-positive babies with diarrhoea should also be handled with care when they contain blood.

Enrichment

Pregnant caregivers and HIV

Pregnant health care professionals are often very concerned about the possibility of an increased risk of contracting HIV in the health care situation, but no such increase in the risk has been found. A pregnant health care professional, for example, need not use any special precautions beyond those used by other health care professionals. Should a pregnant health care professional become infected, there is a risk of transmitting the virus to her baby before, during or after birth (exactly as in the case of any other woman who becomes infected during pregnancy). Since Aids patients often excrete CMV (cytomegalovirus), a virus found in the urine, saliva, semen, cervical secretions, faeces or breast milk of immune-depressed patients, a pregnant health care professional should wash her hands frequently and always wear gloves when in contact with any patient's body secretions. (CMV infection in pregnant women can lead to stillbirth.)

16.2 INFECTION CONTROL IN HOSPITALS, CLINICS, HOSPICES AND HOME-BASED CARE

The objective of HIV infection control measures is similar to that of all infection control: to prevent transmission of infection from one person to another. Infection control measures will also protect the patient against opportunistic infections such as diarrhoea and respiratory infections. It is important to remember that a patient with Aids is much more vulnerable to infections than the caregiver, because of the patient's depressed immune system.

Guidelines will now be given on how to prevent HIV infection in 'formal' as well as 'informal' health care settings. Practical solutions will be offered (where applicable) for infection control in the home-based care situation. These practical solutions can also be applied in rural clinics where there may be a lack of resources or modern facilities. These guidelines are based on those drawn up by the CDC (1989), the WHO (1988a, 1988b, 1990a, 1993) and the Department of National Health and Population Development (1989), as well as Hauman (1990), Lusby (1988), Pearse (1997), and Ziady (2003).

Basic hygiene principles: the first step to infection control

Adhering to basic hygienic principles such as washing your hands, covering all skin lesions and keeping the environment clean is the first step to infection control in any health care setting.

Hand washing

Hand washing is the most basic measure health care professionals can take to prevent the spread of infection. Hands should always be washed before and after contact with patients, especially when contact involves direct and prolonged physical care.

Hands should always be thoroughly washed:

- before and after prolonged physical contact with a patient;
- before eating, preparing food, or feeding patients;
- before care of severely immune-depressed patients (this means, for example, a patient with Aids – the last phase of HIV infection);
- before and after touching mucous membranes, broken skin, or moist body substances;
- immediately after contact with blood or body fluids;
- after contact with surfaces, equipment, linen, or rubbish contaminated with blood or body fluids;
- before invasive procedures in which the skin of the patient will be punctured, e.g. doing a blood glucose test;
- in nurseries or children's wards between touching infants, and after nappy changes;
- after gloves are removed – even if the gloves appear to be intact. Gloves do provide a protective barrier, but they do not necessarily provide enough protection to keep hands clean. Leakage of bacteria and viruses may occur in some cases. Even if no leakage takes place, the bacteria on the hands multiply rapidly inside the moist, warm environment of the gloves. The CDC has therefore emphasised that wearing gloves must not replace hand washing. Hands should be washed *on every occasion* after removal of gloves.

? What should we use for washing our hands: Plain (ordinary commercial) soap or an antimicrobial product?

The CDC recommends plain (ordinary commercial or toilet) soap for most general patient care situations in hospitals, clinics and hospices and in the home. Plain soap is adequate for *removing* dirt and transient organisms from the hands and is therefore sufficient and adequate for most situations. Ordinary hand washing with toilet or liquid soap should be done for at least thirty seconds.

Since plain soap however *does not kill* organisms, it is necessary to use a product that contains an antimicrobial ingredient in care settings where patients are at high risk of infection. Such settings include critical care units, emergency departments, settings where frequent exposure to blood and body fluids is likely, and sterile care procedures such as wound care.

For antimicrobial soap to be effective, it should remain in contact with the skin for at least 10 seconds. In addition, the hands should be thoroughly washed, especially between the fingers and under the fingernails.

Antiseptics such as Hibitane and alcohol or Hibiscrub, which is used in many hospitals, can kill HIV. Betadine and Savlon can also be used.

It is not enough merely to *wash* your hands with soap and water after contact with blood or other body fluids. Hands should be *decontaminated* with the above-mentioned antimicrobial products after contact with blood and body fluids.

Home-based care

Make your own 'waterless' hand antiseptic

Hand washing is your first line of defence against infections. It is best done with soap and clean running water. If clean running water is not available, you can make your own 'waterless' hand antiseptic by adding 1 part chlorine (household bleach) to 9 parts of boiled, cooled water in a spray bottle. Make a fresh solution every day as too much of the chlorine will evaporate within 24 hours to be an effective antiseptic. You can also add 1 part of spirit vinegar to 9 parts of boiled, cooled water in a spray bottle, but make a fresh solution every day. Community caregivers who do home visits should keep a spray bottle with this solution in their kits (Ziady, 2003:140).

Home-based care

The problem of water shortages and hand washing

Pearse (1997) believes that health care professionals working in rural areas should be challenged to use the available facilities to the best effect, and to use their imagination and creativity to improve hygienic standards and to create a safe working environment. 'To simply say "We do not have the facilities, therefore we cannot comply with basic standards" is a defeatist attitude' (p. 415).

When working in areas where water is in critically short supply and is therefore reserved only for drinking, a waterless antiseptic hand cleanser such as an alcoholic hand-rub could be used to clean hands. Alcoholic hand-rub is effective; it is easily used between patient contacts; it is transportable and relatively inexpensive (Pearse, 1997). Where there is a water shortage, do not pour water into a basin to wash and rinse your hands in the same water. It will be contaminated by the bacteria that were on the hands in the first place. Rather ask somebody to pour water over your hands while you wash and rinse them. Water in a 2-litre plastic milk bottle with holes in the cap works very well to pour water over hands.

Contaminated water should be decontaminated (cleaned) by using a cloth filter or a permanent sand filter, or by boiling the water for 10 minutes. Water can also be decontaminated by adding 2 to 4 drops of sodium hypochlorite (bleach or Jik) to 1 litre of water. Such solutions should stand for at least 20 minutes before they are used. Milton can also be used to decontaminate water, if available.

If only cake soap is available, it must be kept dry between uses. Keep the soap in a well-drained clean soap dish, or raise it off the surface with a bottle top. The cake of soap can also be hung from a piece of string (which should be changed daily) or a strip of plastic.

Wash the soap after every use, and use small rather than large cakes of soap. Carbolic soap is an inexpensive antiseptic soap. Traditional methods of boiling soap (fat, water and caustic soda or lye) should be used to make home-made soap if soap is not supplied. Spray bottles containing water and a fresh solution of either vinegar or bleach are relatively easy to transport for hand hygiene (Ziady, 2003).

Scrubbing hands for sterile care procedures such as wound dressings should be done with an antiseptic or antimicrobial soap. If no antiseptic soap is available, ordinary soap and water must be used and the hands must be washed twice. The second wash should last for two minutes.

Paper cloths for drying hands are usually not available in homes or in rural clinics. Nevertheless, it is not acceptable to use cloth towels that are constantly re-used all day long. Rather use small towels (such as face cloths) for each hand wash, and wash and dry them in the sun afterwards.

Disposable 'Daylee' cloths or Superwipes are reusable, provided that they are thoroughly washed and sun-dried.

Covering skin lesions

HIV can enter the bloodstream through broken skin. It is therefore important to ensure that your hands are always in good condition.

- Use hand lotion to prevent skin cracking, but do not apply the lotion just after washing your hands or immediately before giving direct care, because it might interfere with the action of the antimicrobial soap, and render it ineffective.
- Cover skin lesions on your hands with waterproof dressings until they are healed.
- Treat oozing lesions, weeping dermatitis (skin infections) or other breaks in the skin properly and cover (seal) them at all times.
- Health care professionals with serious oozing skin lesions *should refrain* from direct patient care and contact with patient care equipment until the condition has improved.

Ensure a clean and safe working environment

Ensure that your immediate environment is clean and safe to work in. Keep surfaces clean at all times. Disinfect and clean blood-stained equipment and body-fluid spills immediately (see 'Cleaning up blood and other body fluid spills' on page 290 for the relevant procedure). To prevent the risk of needle-stick injury, do not bend or re-sheath (or recap) needles. Always discard needles in a puncture-proof container for disposal, and never let needles or other sharp objects lie around where they could injure other people (for the proper handling of needles, see

Home-based care

Basic hygiene principles

If certain basic rules are followed, there is no risk of acquiring HIV infection from people with Aids in the home-based care situation. HIV is not easily transmitted except through unprotected sexual intercourse or close blood-to-blood contact. The following basic principles of hygiene should be applied in the home to protect the caregiver from HIV, as well as the immune-depressed Aids patient from opportunistic infections such as diarrhoea and respiratory infections:

- Wash your hands with soap and water before cooking, eating, feeding another person or giving medicine, after using a toilet or changing nappies, after changing soiled bed linen and clothing, and after having contact with body fluids.
- Use soap in a pump dispenser rather than bar soap, if possible, because soap in a dispenser cannot easily be contaminated.
- If soap is not available, boil your own soap or use herbal or traditional alternatives.
- Keep wounds covered with waterproof bandages or cloth. If these are not available, use a leaf or plastic wrap. Caregivers as well as Aids patients should cover cuts or wounds on their hands or other places that are likely to come into contact with other people, their bedding or their clothing.
- Keep kitchen and bathroom surfaces clean at all times so as to prevent fungal and bacterial growth. Household bleach (e.g. Jik) is an effective and cheap disinfectant to use for cleaning. Mix a quarter of a cup of Jik with two cups of water for cleaning purposes (see 'Disinfection' on page 292).
- Keep bedding and clothing clean. This will help to keep sick people comfortable and prevent skin problems.
- Don't share personal items such as make-up (sharing make-up can transmit skin infections) or anything that may pierce the skin, such as toothbrushes, razors, needles, or anything else that can cut or come into contact with blood. If any of these objects (e.g. a razor) *must* be shared, boil it in water for at least 30 minutes before use.
- Use clean water whenever possible and boil drinking water, especially water that is going to be given to young children.
- Store food properly to prevent it from spoiling and causing infection.
- When someone in the family is ill (e.g. with flu), wash drinking cups with water and soap before you share them.
- Cover your mouth and turn your head away when you sneeze or cough.
- Wash eating utensils, including items for babies, with soap and water.
- Wash all raw fruit and vegetables with clean water.
- Wash objects that a child or infant frequently puts in its mouth with soap and clean water.

'Precautions when giving injections and performing invasive procedures' on page 286).

Protective clothing

Protective clothing should be worn whenever there is a possibility of contact with blood or body fluids. What follows is a discussion about the universal infection control practices that apply to wearing gloves, eye shields, masks, aprons and footwear. Most of these precautions apply mainly to hospital settings, but their use in home-based care settings will be indicated where relevant. It is important to remember that workers such as cleaners must also wear protective clothing when they handle contaminated materials.

Gloves

Wearing gloves is not recommended for casual contact with a patient. It is not necessary to wear gloves when touching *intact* skin (such as when giving a back rub, bathing a patient, taking blood pressure or giving medication). If the administration of medication involves contact with mucous membranes, as is the case with rectal or vaginal suppositories, then gloves should obviously be worn.

Latex gloves should always be worn when touching blood and body fluids (to which universal precautions apply), mucous membranes, body tissue, or any compromised skin areas of all patients. Always wear gloves when handling items or surfaces soiled with blood or body fluids and when performing procedures during which hands are likely to be contaminated with blood. Always wear gloves in the following situations:

- when drawing blood;
- when starting IVs;
- while changing wound dressings;
- while changing drainage bags;
- while performing surgical procedures;
- while performing finger or heel pricks on babies and children;
- in emergency situations where tasks involve exposure to blood;
- while assisting with childbirth;
- whenever blood contamination is a possibility, for example while working with restless patients;
- for cleaning spills of blood and body fluids; and
- when you have open, weeping lesions or chronic dermatitis on your hands.

In emergency situations (such as car accidents) where large amounts of blood may be present, it is important that your gloves fit tightly around your wrists to prevent blood contamination of your wrists around the cuff. If there is more than one injured person, gloves must be changed between patient contacts. If it is not possible to change gloves, wash the gloved hands with an antiseptic product (not containing alcohol) between patients.

While you are wearing gloves, avoid handling personal items such as pens, watches and scissors that could become soiled or contaminated. Remove gloves that have become contaminated with blood or other body fluids as soon as possible. Do not use your teeth to put on or take off gloves. Avoid skin contact with the exterior surface of the gloves when removing them: peel the gloves off in such a way that the removed

Home-based care

Gloves

If gloves must be re-used, wash them in warm, soapy water, air dry them and re-powder them (with baby powder). Do not clean latex gloves with an alcohol solution because alcohol damages latex gloves. Some gloves can be boiled. While plastic disposable gloves are a poor substitute for latex gloves, they may be used if nothing else is available. Vinyl gloves (used in gardens) should preferably not be used. They are more expensive than latex gloves, and they have a larger pore size which allows viruses to penetrate (Pearse, 1997).

When gloves are not available at all, use other methods to prevent direct contact with blood and other body fluids (for example, an intact plastic bag, a towel, gauze, a piece of clothing, or any item that forms a barrier between blood or sharp instruments and the caregiver). If nothing else is available, even a big leaf can be used to remove soiled bandages or to hold a bloodstained needle or syringe (WHO, 1988b).

gloves turn inside out, thereby inverting the contaminated part so that it is not exposed. Place the used gloves in a plastic bag that doesn't leak. Reusable gloves should be changed, washed and disinfected after contact with each patient. Do not eat, drink or smoke while wearing gloves and do not touch any area of your face. Health care professionals and other caregivers who use gloves should always wash their hands immediately after removing their gloves.

Extra-heavy-duty gloves are recommended when there is a possibility of injury from sharp instruments (as, for instance, when sharp instruments are being cleaned).

Non-allergenic (latex-free, powder-free) *Nitrile* gloves are available for health care professionals who are allergic to latex gloves. Nitrile gloves are blue in colour to distinguish them from latex gloves. (Available from Levtrade International, Johannesburg, tel: 011 450-2288.)

Eye shields

The use of eye coverings (e.g. safety glasses or face shields) is recommended only for procedures during which there is a potential threat of blood or fluid splashes into the mucous membranes of the eyes. It is therefore advisable to wear eye-protecting glasses during procedures such as a bronchoscopy, and during certain surgical, dental and obstetric procedures, such as during childbirth. The CDC recommends, for example, that masks and eye wear should be worn together or that a face shield should be used by all personnel in any situation in which splashes of blood, or other body fluids to which universal precautions apply, are likely to occur.

Eye coverings are not required for fine, invisible, mist exposures, such as those produced by ventilators. Because the number of infective organisms in mists of that kind is low or absent, they do not cause transmission of blood-borne diseases (Lusby, 1988).

Masks

Masks, preferably surgical masks, and protective eye or face shields should be worn during any procedure likely to generate droplets of blood or body fluids. The inexpensive thin paper masks with elastic ear loops are useless and dangerous because they provide little protection for patients or staff (Pearse, 1997). When caring for TB patients, a mask that can filter particles that are one micron in size, and that has a filtration efficiency of 95%, should be worn.

Home-based care

Eye protection

Home-based caregivers may sometimes encounter situations where blood or body fluid splashes in the eyes are a possibility. A pair of clear glass spectacles will provide some protection against blood or other body fluid splashes. If the caregiver can afford them a pair of cheap glasses can be a good investment. Garden goggles or welding spectacles can also be used effectively.

Wear masks in the following situations:

- where there is extensive and productive (phlegm-producing) coughing;
- when a disease spread by the respiratory route (such as TB or meningococcal meningitis) is suspected;
- for suctioning an intubated patient;
- when a patient undergoes a surgical or other invasive procedure;
- when a procedure may splash blood or body fluids into the mucous membranes of the eyes, nose or mouth of the health care professional, for example, during bronchoscopy or deliveries; and
- when protection of the patient against infections is necessary (especially patients with depressed immune systems).

Containers with masks, as well as containers for the disposal of used masks, should be kept inside the patient's room, near the entrance. This will make it easier to put on a mask when entering the room and remove it before leaving. Hands should be washed thoroughly after removing a mask.

Aprons

It is not necessary to wear aprons or gowns for casual contact with patients or for routine care such as taking blood pressure or temperature or while administering medication. However, aprons must always be worn to protect clothing

Home-based care

Masks

If masks are not available, the home-based caregiver could buy the kind of dust-mist mask that is available at any hardware store. These masks are re-usable by the same person and they provide some protection. However, dust-mist masks do not fulfil the filter requirements for TB and will therefore not give protection against TB. A headscarf or large handkerchief can be used to cover the mouth and nose when a face shield or mask is needed and nothing else is available.

during procedures in which blood or body fluid splashes are likely to occur. A plastic, moisture-resistant, non-sterile apron is appropriate and adequate for protection, unless a sterile gown is required for patient protection.

Wear aprons in the following situations:

- whenever there is a threat of blood splashes or blood-contaminated secretions, for example during certain surgical or dental procedures, bronchoscopy, or vaginal deliveries;
- whenever splatter or heavy soiling is expected (for example, when lifting a patient with draining wounds);
- in reverse-barrier nursing when the patient is very ill, so as to protect the patient against further exposure to infections; and
- in children's wards, especially the gastroenteritis section.

Wear long-sleeved gowns in labour wards, theatres, burn units and gynaecological wards – all places where massive splashes of blood can be expected.

If a patient's care requires the frequent use of an apron, it is advisable to keep an apron inside the patient's room on a hook next to the bed. Mark the apron with the date and indicate the outside of the apron with a mark to ensure that you always wear the apron with the same side to your body. Spray the front side of a plastic apron with Hibitane and alcohol (or a similar disinfectant) before removing it from the hook. After every 24 hours aprons should be replaced (Hauman, 1990).

Home-based care

Aprons

Wear a plastic apron when handling a very sick patient to avoid staining your clothes with blood or other body fluids. Plastic aprons are not expensive and they can be re-used by the same person. If plastic aprons are not available, plastic rubbish bags can be cut to form a protective 'gown', or use a thin plastic raincoat.

Footwear

Wearing paper or plastic over-shoes is necessary only if there is a danger that the caregiver's shoes can become contaminated with blood or other body fluids.

Home-based care

Footwear

Recycled plastic shopping bags fastened with sticky-tape or string can be used to protect the caregiver's feet or shoes from body fluid splashes.

Examples of recommended protective clothing for various procedures in the hospital setting are given in Table 16.1 on page 287.

Precautions when giving injections and performing invasive procedures

Health care professionals can infect their patients with HIV if they use contaminated needles or other instruments on their patients.

- Never use the same needle, syringe or lancet on more than one patient.
- Never use the same immunisation needle on more than one child.
- Only use sterile instruments or equipment for all procedures on patients.

Needle sticks and other sharps injuries

One of the most important measures against injuries that may cause HIV or HBV (hepatitis B) infections is to learn how to handle needles and other sharp instruments. Although the chance of becoming infected is low, injuries with contaminated needles or other sharps are the most common way in which HIV and HBV are spread from an infected patient to the health care professional. The health care professional cannot afford to be lax or careless *for a single moment* when working with needles, scalpel blades or other sharp instruments during procedures; when cleaning used instruments; during disposal of used needles; and when handling sharp instruments after procedures.

Always observe the following guidelines:

- Do not resheath, bend or break needles or other sharp objects.
- Do not remove needles from disposable syringes. Rather discard the needle and syringe together.
- Do not manipulate a needle or other sharp instrument by hand.
- Do not remove scalpel blades by hand. Use artery forceps.
- Do not carry syringes with the needles exposed (use receivers or some other protection).
- Do not leave used sharp objects lying around.
- Do not dispose of needles or syringes in the rubbish bin.
- Discard used needles (without resheathing them) and other sharp instruments in puncture-proof containers immediately after use. A container should be available in every room in which sharps are used.

Table 16.1
Recommended protective clothing for hospital procedures
(Source: Adapted from CDC guidelines, 1989:35)

Task or activity	Disposable gloves	Plastic apron	Mask	Glasses or goggles
Bleeding control with spurting blood	Yes	Yes	Yes	Yes
Bleeding control with minimal bleeding	Yes	No	No	No
Childbirth (rupturing membranes)	Yes	Yes	Yes, because splashing is likely	Yes, because splashing is likely
Drawing blood	Yes	No	No	No
Lumbar puncture (CSF)	Yes	No	No	Yes, in case of splashing
Starting an intravenous line	Yes	No	No	No
Endotracheal intubation, oral/nasal suctioning, manually cleaning airway	Yes	No	No, unless splashing is likely	No, unless splashing is likely
Emptying blood-containing drains and other containers	Yes	No	Yes, in case of splashing	Yes, in case of splashing
Handling and cleaning instruments with microbial contamination	Yes	No, unless soiling is likely	No	No
Handling dressings and body fluids	Yes	No	No	No
Measuring blood pressure, or temperature	No	No	No	No
Giving an injection	No	No	No	No

- Puncture-proof containers should be located as near as is practically possible to where they are to be used. Make sure that the opening of the container is large enough not to obstruct disposal. Place the container below eye level for good visibility, but keep it out of reach of children. Cover and discard the container before the fill line is exceeded.
- Health care professionals who provide home-based care should take puncture-proof containers with them to dispose of needles they might use.
- Do not leave used discarded Jelcos (needles used to start IVs) lying around on the bed after an unsuccessful attempt to start an IV. Before using a new Jelco, dispose of the discarded Jelco safely.

The WHO recommends that injections and other skin-piercing procedures should be restricted to situations where they really are necessary. If a drug is equally effective when it is administered orally and the patient can take it in this manner, there is no reason at all to inject the medication. Reducing the number of unnecessary injections is important for protecting both the health care professional and the patient. Procedures for handling accidental exposure to blood and body fluids of infected patients are discussed under 'Management of accidental exposure to blood and other infectious body fluids' on page 347.

Enrichment

The safe use of Vacutainers when drawing blood

When Vacutainer systems are used to draw blood, the needle must, unfortunately, be disconnected because the Vacutainer barrels are re-used. An exception to the DO NOT RESHEATH rule may be made when you remove the needle from the Vacutainer barrel after the procedure. Extreme care should be taken when doing this:

- Do not hold the sheath in your hand when inserting the needle.
- Place the sheath on a flat surface or press it into a small block of polystyrene before introducing the tip of the needle into the sheath.
- Only when the whole needle is covered by the sheath should you handle the sheath to remove the needle from the Vacutainer barrel.
- An alternative technique to the above is to place an impenetrable cover or shield between your hand and the sheath so that it can protect your fingers while you insert the needle.

Home-based care

Disposal of syringes and needles

Use a rigid-walled container to dispose of used sharps (syringes). A coffee tin with a secure lid, a thick, non-penetrable plastic bottle with a screw cap, or a heavy plastic or cardboard box can be effectively used for disposal. If incineration is not possible, dispose of the container with sharps into a deep pit latrine. Do not dispose of sharps in refuse pits or landfills because children often play around these areas. If incinerated, the material should be heated to a temperature hot enough to melt the needles.

The second-person risk of sharps injuries

Health care professionals should be specifically aware of the second-person risk. One study on sharps injuries indicated that between 33% and 48% of all reported injuries involved a second person (Cope, 1994). In some of these cases the second person was the patient, who moved at a crucial moment – thereby accidentally pushing the needle into the health care professional. Good communication with a patient before a procedure and awareness of the risk when dealing with a child or a confused non-compliant patient will help to reduce the risk. Second-person risks also occur in the theatre or when commencing IV therapy or doing a lumbar puncture in the wards. Health care professionals should concentrate intensely and be alert at all times when working with sharps.

The most avoidable and most disturbing second-person injuries are those sustained by cleaning staff when emptying waste paper bins, handling soiled linen, or cleaning patient areas. Health care professionals should make sure that they remove all sharps used in a procedure and that they discard them into the correct container immediately after use.

Invasive procedures

Strict blood and body fluid precautions should be observed whenever a surgical entry into tissues, cavities or organs is made – whether for an operation or for the repair of an injury. In addition to this, bear the following points in mind (College of Medicine, 1991; WHO, 1988b):

- Wear gloves and a surgical mask for all invasive procedures.
- Wear double gloves or extra-heavy-duty gloves in operations where the risk of tearing gloves is high (as in orthopaedic procedures).
- Wear protective glasses or face shields and an apron if blood splashes are likely.
- Avoid unnecessary personnel, equipment or movement in the theatre during operations.
- Avoid the direct passing of sharp instruments between theatre personnel.
- Avoid, as far as possible, the use of unprotected sharp instruments. For example, use scissors instead of a knife, if possible.
- If a glove is torn, or any injury from a used sharp instrument occurs during invasive procedures, replace the glove with a new one as soon as possible. Remove the needle or instrument involved in the incident from the sterile field.
- Use a closed drainage system for wounds that require post-operative drainage, especially if the patient is known to be HIV positive.

Precautions during vaginal or caesarean deliveries

Health care professionals who perform or assist in vaginal or caesarean deliveries should wear gloves, aprons, masks and eye protection (if splashing is likely) in the following instances:

- while performing internal vaginal examinations on the mother;
- during artificial rupturing of the membranes (always wear eye protection);
- during the birth process and when cutting the umbilical cord;
- while handling the placenta during birth as well as during examination of the placenta;
- while suturing tears and episiotomies;
- while handling the baby until all the amniotic fluid and blood have been removed from the infant's skin;
- until post-delivery care of the umbilical cord is complete; and
- while caring for the mother and cleaning the environment until all blood and body fluids are removed.

If the mother is diagnosed as HIV positive, health care professionals in the maternity ward should observe the following precautions to keep the risk of transmitting the infection to the baby as low as possible:

- Avoid unnecessary rupture of the membranes.
- As far as possible, avoid intra-uterine catheterisation.
- Avoid invasive monitoring (such as the use of fetal scalp electrodes).
- Avoid an episiotomy whenever possible.
- Use chlorhexidine 0.25% for vaginal cleansing after vaginal examinations and during labour and delivery (see 'Childbirth' on page 32).
- If possible, avoid the use of forceps or vacuum delivery. If there is no alternative, use forceps rather than vacuum.
- If possible, avoid suctioning of the baby's nose and throat.
- Wipe blood and maternal secretions off the baby as soon as possible.

Home-based care

Childbirth at home

Home-based caregivers performing deliveries at home should be very careful not to come into contact with blood or other body fluids. Delivery in the home should not be done without latex gloves, a plastic apron and – if possible – eye protection. Protect the newborn baby from infection by wiping blood and other secretions from the baby as soon as possible. Wear gloves when you give the baby its first bath.

Post-partum care of mother and baby

One applies exactly the same post-partum (afterbirth) care to an HIV-positive mother and her baby as one would to other patients. Apply the same universal precaution measures. Wear gloves when handling the baby prior to its first bath, when changing meconium (first black stool after birth) nappies or diarrhoeal nappies and when providing umbilical cord care.

If a mother is breastfeeding her baby, make sure that good hygiene always prevails. Bleeding of cracked nipples should be prevented or treated immediately, as should mastitis (breast infections) and breast abscesses as well as any sores or thrush in the baby's mouth.

Cleaning up blood and other body fluid spills

It is important to remember that HI viruses can sometimes live for many hours outside the body *if they remain inside blood or body fluids.* It is vitally important to be extremely careful when cleaning up spilled blood or body fluids. An experienced person should clean blood and body fluid spills. Such tasks should *not* be given to a cleaner who does not know how to apply universal precautions. The following points should be borne in mind when cleaning blood and other body fluid spills:

- Wear latex gloves to avoid direct contact with spilled blood or body fluids.
- If splashes are anticipated, wear protective eye wear, a mask and a watertight apron. Where there is massive blood contamination on floors, wear disposable, impenetrable shoe coverings.
- Flood the spillage area with an appropriate disinfectant (preferably sodium hypochlorite or household bleach diluted 1:10 with water) and clean the mixed body fluid and disinfectant with absorbent, disposable towels or paper cloths. Or cover the spill with a towel or cloth soaked in a hypochlorite solution. Some sources recommend stronger solutions of bleach to clean up blood spills (see 'Disinfection' on page 292).
- Clean from the outside to the inside of the spillage area.
- Discard paper towels into a plastic bag immediately and then burn them in an incinerator (or bury them if there are no incinerator facilities).
- After removing the mixed body fluid and disinfectant, wipe the surface clean with more disinfectant – starting from a radius of one metre outside the spillage area.
- Remove gloves and place them in a plastic bag.
- Wash your hands *immediately* after you remove your gloves.
- If shoe coverings are worn, always remove them while still wearing gloves.
- If you have been wearing gloves, apron, mask, eye coverings and shoe coverings because of massive blood contamination, always take them off in the following order: first the shoe coverings, then the gloves, and finally the apron, mask and eye shield.
- Place re-usable items in a container with some disinfectant.

Home-based care

Cleaning up blood and body fluid spills

Household bleach or Jik will kill the HI virus. Mix 1 part of Jik with 10 parts of water (approximately a quarter of a cup of Jik with 2 cups of water), and pour onto the spilled blood or on the area after it is cleaned. If latex gloves are not available, use plastic bags as protection for your hands.

Precautions in resuscitation

Mouth-to-mouth resuscitation

HIV (or hepatitis B virus) transmission caused by mouth-to-mouth resuscitation has not been documented. Although HIV has been found in saliva, it is present in such small concentrations that the chance of transmission is extremely low. However, it is theoretically possible for the health care professional to become infected if he or she has a cut, sore or lesion in the mouth, and this comes into contact with a patient's infected blood and/or saliva containing infected blood.

Although HIV has rarely been detected in saliva, saliva can spread other infectious diseases such as herpes simplex, respiratory viruses, or bacteria that cause meningitis. It is therefore recommended that a device such as an Ambu Bag (a manual ventilator) or a mouthpiece be used for mouth-to-mouth resuscitation. The device not only protects the health care professional against infections but also gives him or her the assurance of being as safe as possible. It is important for hospitals to ensure that resuscitation devices are readily available in all patient care areas. Resuscitation equipment and devices should be used once only and then disposed of. If they are re-usable, they should be cleaned and disinfected thoroughly after each use.

Health care professionals frequently encounter emergency situations outside the hospital where their help is urgently needed. Even though resuscitation bags are usually not available at accident scenes, resuscitation should not be withheld because of a fear of contracting HIV. If the injured person is bleeding through the mouth, the health care professional should first wipe the blood out of the person's mouth with a clean cloth or handkerchief before proceeding with resuscitation. If it is possible, a thin cloth should be placed over the mouth to avoid any saliva or fluid exchange during mouth-to-mouth contact.

Resuscitation bags in the form of key-rings are available and these are valuable assets that health care professionals can easily carry with them at all times. The mouthpiece has a plastic cover to prevent contact with the patient's face as well as a one-way valve that allows the flow of air into the mouth of the patient while preventing fluids like vomit or blood from getting into the mouth of the helper. (Available from Levtrade International, Johannesburg, tel: 011 450-2288.)

Bleeding at accident scenes

Bleeding patients at accident scenes usually require immediate attention. If the person is conscious, the health care professional can instruct him or her to apply pressure to the wound himself or herself by using a thick cloth (use a T-shirt if nothing else is available). If the person is not able to help, the health care professional should stop the bleeding by applying pressure to the wound. If gloves are not available, use a barrier such as a thick cloth, several dressings or a piece of plastic wrap to prevent skin contact with the blood. Health care professionals should take special care to ensure that blood does not come into direct contact with their mucous membranes or any broken skin that they might have. Helpers should take care not to touch their own eyes or mouth, and they should wash their hands with soap and water as soon as possible after they have administered first aid.

It is a good idea to keep a pair of gloves in a *cool* place in the car at all times for use in emergencies.

Precautions that must be taken when handling laboratory specimens

- Health care professionals should always wear gloves when drawing blood and when handling any specimen of body fluid, regardless of the source (blood, cerebrospinal fluid, urine, sputum or faeces).
- Cover all open wounds on hands and arms with a waterproof dressing.
- Place all blood or body fluid specimens in firm, leak-proof, unbreakable plastic containers with secure lids to prevent leakage during transport.
- Avoid contaminating the outside of the container.
- Clean any contamination on the *outside* of the container with an antimicrobial solution before dispatching the specimen. Make sure that the forms accompanying a specimen are clean.
- No special precautionary labels are required on the container or form.
- Do not dispatch specimens in syringes with exposed needles.
- Hands must always be washed after accidental exposure to specimens.
- Cover working surfaces with a non-penetrative material (such as plastic film) that is easy to clean.
- Disinfect any spillage of blood or body fluid with an appropriate disinfectant before cleaning it. Wear gloves when cleaning up blood or body fluids.
- Dispose of specimens carefully by pouring them down a drain connected to a sewer. If this is not possible, decontaminate blood and body fluids with an appropriate disinfectant before disposal. Wear gloves during disposal.

Signs and labels identifying patients known to have infectious diseases such as HIV are unnecessary. They violate confidentiality and they may encourage a double standard of care. *All* body fluids should be viewed as potentially infected with HIV. Receptacles containing infected waste should however be marked with a *biohazard sign* to warn non-medical personnel (such as cleaners) to be careful.

Cleaning, sterilisation and disinfection of contaminated equipment

Efficient cleaning with soap and water removes a high proportion of any micro-organisms. Wear heavy-duty gloves while cleaning contaminated equipment, and if splashing with body fluids is likely, wear additional protective clothing. Dismantle all equipment before cleaning and wipe blood-stained equipment clean with paper towels which should then be discarded. Wipe equipment with a hypochlorite solution before sending it for normal sterilisation. If that is not possible, seal the equipment in a strong, clear and labelled plastic bag.

Since HIV is destroyed much more quickly than other organisms, routine sterilisation methods are appropriate for HIV. Table 16.2 gives an indication which methods to use for decontamination.

Sterilisation

All forms of sterilisation will destroy HIV. Methods of sterilisation recommended by the WHO (2000a) are steam (or moist heat) under pressure (e.g. autoclave or pressure cooker), dry heat (such as an oven), or gas sterilisation (with ethylene oxide) for non-heat-resistant equipment.

- Moist heat (autoclaving) readily kills the HI virus at 121 °C for 15 minutes, 126 °C for 10 minutes, or 134 °C for 3 to 5 minutes.
- Dry heat at 121 °C for 16 hours, 140 °C for 3 hours, 160 °C for 2 hours or 170 °C for 1 hour is sufficient to kill HIV.
- Exposure to ethylene oxide for between 4 and 16 hours, depending on the object and its volume, will be sufficient. The object must then be left for several days to allow the gas to evaporate.

Table 16.2
Decontamination methods
(Source: Adapted from WHO, 2000a:11-5)

Level of risk	Items	Decontamination method
High risk	Instruments that penetrate the skin or body	Sterilisation, or single use of disposables
Moderate risk	Instruments that come into contact with non-intact skin or mucous membrane	Sterilisation, boiling, or chemical disinfection
Low risk	Equipment that comes into contact with intact skin	Thorough washing with soap and hot water

Disinfection

Disinfection is a process that eliminates many or all growing micro-organisms (excluding bacterial spores) on inanimate objects. Examples of disinfection processes are pasteurisation, boiling and chemical soaking (WHO, 2000a; Ziady, 2003). HIV is easily destroyed by boiling for 20 minutes at sea level, and by boiling for at least 30 minutes at higher altitudes. Equipment should always be cleaned properly with soap and water before boiling and before using chemical disinfectants. Chemical disinfectants are diluted, neutralised or even de-activated by contamination or soiling (e.g. with organic residue) and will therefore not be effective if equipment is not cleaned properly first.

Enrichment

The difference between 'disinfectants' and 'antiseptics'

Disinfectants and antiseptics both kill micro-organisms (except bacterial spores). A disinfectant should be used only on inanimate objects and not on living tissue (people, animals or plants). Disinfectants will damage living tissue because of their chemical properties. Antiseptics are used on living tissue such as the skin and other delicate surfaces. Caregivers should never use products labelled 'disinfectants' on living tissue. Always use 'antiseptics' on skin or mucous membranes (Ziady, 2003:146).

Home-based care

Sterilisation and disinfection of instruments

Disinfection and sterilisation are two points on the continuum of cleanliness. Both processes easily kill HIV if the following steps are followed. Boil instruments for 30 minutes from the time when the water actually begins to boil. Don't add instruments after boiling has commenced. Domestic pressure cookers can also be used for 30 minutes at their highest pressure to sterilise equipment. Household bleach (chlorine) is effective for disinfecting equipment soaked in it for at least 30 minutes. Because disposable plastic instruments cannot be boiled, they should be soaked in household bleach or Milton for 30 minutes. Needles should *never* be re-used, and under *no* circumstances should they be sterilised with disinfectants such as household bleach (or any other disinfectant) because the disinfectants may not penetrate the bore of the needle.

Enrichment

The safety of hospital apparatus in everyday use

- *Blood pressure apparatus* and *stethoscopes* cannot contaminate health care professionals or patients – provided that they are used on intact skin. Clean the dome of stethoscopes with a 70% alcohol swab such as Preptic or Webcol if necessary.
- *Thermometers* used for routine observation rounds should be wiped with a 70% alcohol swab or placed into an alcohol solution after each use. If a patient's temperature needs to be taken more frequently, wipe the thermometer with a 70% alcohol swab and keep it in a dry container in the room.
- *Crockery and cutlery* such as cups, plates, knives, spoons and forks should be handled in a normal way. If the patient has bleeding mucous membranes (in the mouth, for example), disposable or exclusive cutlery is recommended.
- *Suction equipment* and *oxygen masks* should be handled in a normal way, conforming to the principles of universal precautions.
- *Bedpans or urine bottles* should be cleaned with an appropriate disinfectant.
- The HIV-positive patient may use the *ward bath* and *toilet* unless open bleeding perineal lesions are present.

Chemical disinfectants are not as reliable as sterilisation or boiling, but they can be used on heat-sensitive equipment or when other methods of decontamination are not available. Chemicals that are effective in destroying HIV include chlorine-based agents (such as bleach), 2% glutaraldehyde, 1% biodecyl, 70% ethyl alcohol, 70% isopropanol and 1% iodine.

Household bleaches (such as Jik) contain hypochlorite and may be effectively used for disinfection purposes. The hypochlorite concentrations vary from one product to another and should be diluted with water accordingly. When the concentration of hypochlorite in the product is 3.5%, a solution of 1:10 – approximately a quarter of a cup of bleach mixed with 2 cups of water – is usually sufficient to kill HIV. Some sources recommend a stronger solution of 1 cup of bleach mixed with 2 cups of water to clean blood spills (Evian, 2000:322). Used bleach solutions should be discarded and should never be re-used.

Disposal of infected waste, linen and rubbish

Infected waste

Adhere to the following WHO guidelines (1988b) for disposing of infected waste:

- Place needles and other sharp instruments or materials in a puncture-proof container immediately after use and incinerate them if possible.
- Prominently mark all containers containing infected waste with the word *BIOHAZARD* – *and* the biohazard logo (if possible).
- Carefully pour liquid wastes such as bulk blood, suction fluids, excretions and secretions down a drain connected to an adequately treated sewerage system, and if this is not available, dispose of the waste in a pit latrine.
- Regard solid wastes such as dressings and laboratory and pathology wastes as infectious and dispose of them by incineration, burning or autoclaving. Other solid wastes, such as excreta, may be disposed of in a hygienically controlled sanitary landfill or pit latrine.

Linen

Although soiled linen may be contaminated with pathogenic micro-organisms, the risk of actual disease transmission is very slim. Hygienic storage of clean linen and processing of soiled linen are adequate procedures for handling linen. When adhering to the following procedures, it is not even necessary to handle linen from 'known' infected patients separately:

- Sort linen into *used linen* and *soiled linen* at the patient's bedside. It is not necessary to wear gloves when handling used (but not soiled) linen, but you should wash your hands afterwards.

 Home-based care

Washing used and soiled linen

Keep sheets, towels and clothes stained with blood, diarrhoea, vomit or other body fluids separate from other household laundry. If washing machines are not available, used and soiled linen should be washed in the following ways:

Used linen (not soiled with blood or body fluids) can be washed by hand in a tub. Dissolve detergent in hot water, and add the linen. Soak the linen for one hour in hot water (to reduce the bacterial load). Stir the contents of the tub occasionally with a long stick to ensure that the water and detergent come into contact with all the linen. After this soaking period, the linen can be washed by hand. Rinse twice in clean water. Bleach can be added to the second-rinse water. Hang linen to dry in the sun as soon as possible. Iron with a hot iron.

Linen soiled with blood or other body fluids should be handled with care. While holding an unstained part, rinse off any blood or diarrhoea with water. *Soiled linen* should be soaked for a longer period than used linen – at least until no staining is visible. Soak linen soiled with blood in cold water. Add sodium hypochlorite (bleach) to the water. Use a stick to turn the linen in the soaking water. Use clean water and detergent after the soaking period. You can boil the linen on a stove or on a grid on the fire for 30 minutes if that is the method you prefer. Rinse twice. Add bleach to the second-rinse water to reduce the level of microbes. Dry in the sun and iron with a hot iron.

- Wear gloves and a protective apron when handling linen soiled with blood and other body fluids.
- Bag soiled linen at the location at which it was used.
- Do not rinse soiled linen in hospital wards.
- Place and transport linen soiled with blood or other body fluids in leak-proof (thick plastic) bags to prevent environmental contamination.
- If leak-proof bags are not available, fold the soiled parts of the linen towards the inside.
- Wash linen with detergent and water at a temperature of at least 71 °C for 25 minutes. If using low-temperature laundry cycles (i.e. with temperatures less than 70 °C), use chemicals suitable for low-temperature washing at the appropriate concentration.
- In the laundry, keep a strict separation between the pre-wash sorting area and the clean area.
- Laundry workers in the pre-wash area should wear protective clothes such as gloves, gowns, masks and caps.
- Workers in the 'soiled' laundry area should not work in the 'clean' area on the same day.

Protective clothing contaminated with blood or other body fluids should be handled in the same way as linen. Brush-scrub boots and leather goods with soap and hot water to remove dirt and micro-organisms.

Rubbish handling

Adhere to the following precautions when handling rubbish so that you can maintain a safe work environment and prevent accidents:

- Place all dressings and wet rubbish in plastic bags before placing them in holding containers.
- Place broken glass in separate puncture-proof containers.
- Line rubbish bins with strong plastic bags before disposing of rubbish.
- When plastic bags in bins are about two-thirds full, seal them and dispose of them.
- Use plastic bags instead of paper bags on the patient's bedside table.

Home-based care

Disposal of infected waste and rubbish

Handle soiled items such as wound dressings or menstrual pads with a piece of plastic, paper, gloves or a big leaf. Don't use your bare hands to touch items that are soiled with body fluids. Put soiled or dirty waste materials such as nappies, used menstrual pads, soiled dressings and used tissues out of the reach of children and animals until they can be removed from the home. Place them in a container that is hard to open until they can be cleaned or properly disposed of. Always double bag highly contagious waste (such as paper tissues used by a patient who has TB, or blood-soiled items of an Aids patient). It is preferable to burn menstrual pads and soiled dressings, but if this is not possible, dispose of them in tightly sealed double plastic bags in a domestic or public hygienically controlled sanitary landfill or pit latrine. Small amounts of infected waste can be burned in a metal drum or in a refuse pit. If infected waste is buried in a refuse pit, the pit should at least be 2 metres deep and 10 metres away from a water source. Refuse pits should be fenced off to prevent children, scavengers and animals from gaining access to the site. Avoid open piles of solid waste and never dump waste in rivers, lakes or areas where leaking can pollute water sources.

Home-based care

After the death of an Aids patient

Universal precautions should be adhered to after the death of an Aids patient. Hands should be protected when cleaning and laying out the body, or when performing cultural cleansing rituals, particularly if body fluids such as diarrhoea or blood are present. Hands should be thoroughly washed with soap and water afterwards. Wounds on the hands and arms of the caregiver, as well as wounds on the body of the deceased, should all be covered with a plaster or bandage. Patients who leak body fluid after death should be wrapped in plastic sheets, or placed in a plastic body-bag. Any traditional cleansing rites that may spread the infection should be avoided. Clean the room, especially the mattress and bed, with a disinfectant. No special precautions are necessary during the funeral because the HI virus can live and reproduce only inside a living person.

- Mark plastic bags containing rubbish of known Aids patients as *BIOHAZARD*. (Do *not* write 'Aids' on the bag!)
- If rubbish is not removed by local authorities, it should be burned.

Post-mortem procedures

Health care professionals performing post-mortem procedures should follow the normal local procedures and observe the following guidelines as precautions against infection:

- Keep universal precautions for blood and body fluids in mind at all times. For many hours after death, HI viruses can still be alive and active in the body fluids of a deceased patient.
- Handle bodies that have open wounds or are soiled with blood with gloves and plastic aprons.
- Cover leaking wounds on the body with waterproof dressings.
- If the patient has died of Aids, place the body in a plastic body-bag and seal it tightly.
- Wipe the outside of the body-bag with Biocide or an appropriate disinfectant before it leaves the room.
- If a body-bag is not available, wrap the body adequately so as to prevent contamination.
- After the death (or discharge) of a patient with Aids, disinfect the room in the routine way (HIV has no known environment-related transmission route). Because it is not possible for surfaces such as walls, ceilings or floors to transmit HIV, these may be cleaned in a routine household way.
- The mattress cover and bed can be cleaned with a disinfectant after the death of an Aids patient.

Activity

- Prepare a workshop for hospital cleaners on ways to avoid exposure to HIV in their workplace.
- Prepare a workshop for primary caregivers working in home-based care situations about the basic principles of infection control at home. Include aspects such as basic hygiene, when to wear gloves, the cleaning of body fluid spills, the handling of soiled linen and the disposal of rubbish.

16.3 CONCLUSION

Apart from adhering to the universal precautions discussed in this chapter, each hospital department, ward, speciality unit or clinic should identify those specific procedures that may increase the risk of exposure to blood or other body fluids in their particular environment.

In such cases, appropriate precautions should be developed and incorporated into routine practice. The best rule to remember is that *no rules and regulations can ever replace common sense*! If you feel uncomfortable in any situation, just use your common sense and err on the side of safety.

chapter

17 Care and Nursing Principles

Tending of Koki
One remained silently seated next to Koki.
With hands full of grass she cleansed his body
where it had been broken and soiled by Raka.
She did not cry but sang softly
about the holy, bright circle of birth and death . . .
and birth and death.

Patients with HIV infection and Aids need physical, emotional, psychological and spiritual care. Any care programme should be holistic, compassionate and person-centred, and it should always take place in a nurturing environment (Fahrner, 1988). Most of the difficulties of people with HIV/Aids are familiar to health care professionals because the physical and psychological needs of people with Aids are often similar to those of other terminally ill patients. But a much more holistic approach is required for people with HIV/Aids, because their immune systems are so depressed that they can contract virtually any disease (especially opportunistic infections). Because of this unique feature of HIV/Aids, it is impossible to recommend any *one* model of caring for those living with HIV or Aids. Caregivers should attend to a patient's physical, emotional, psychological or spiritual needs as they arise.

The current emphasis in the treatment and management of HIV infection and Aids is on: strengthening the immune system so that the infected person can be kept healthy for as long as possible; preventing opportunistic diseases (see 'The prevention of opportunistic infections' on page 47); treating opportunistic infections and addressing general health problems; and using antiretroviral therapy to suppress the viral load and to improve the general health of the patient (see chapter 5).

This chapter focuses on the promotion of general health, the strengthening of the immune system, the importance of good nutrition, and the care and treatment of general health problems and opportunistic infections. Practical advice will be offered on how to take care of patients with HIV/Aids in hospitals, hospices and clinics and at home.

17.1 THE PROMOTION OF HEALTH AND THE STRENGTHENING OF THE IMMUNE SYSTEM

One of the most important health measures that HIV-positive people can take is to do everything in their power to stay as healthy and fit as possible. A healthy lifestyle not only improves the quality of life, it also strengthens the immune system's capacity to combat infections. Some of the ways of promoting good health and strengthening the immune system are discussed below.

Rest, exercise and a healthy diet

HIV-positive people must get enough rest and sleep, and keep fit by exercising. Regular exercise can improve cardiovascular fitness and muscle function, increase the CD4 cell count, increase body weight, improve the mood, and help people cope better (La Perriere et al., 1997). HIV-positive people should start regular exercise programmes (at least three sessions a week) that include a balanced mix of cardiovascular (or aerobic) exercise, strength training and stretching. However, they should not do heavy exercise when they have symptoms such as fever, cough or diarrhoea.

A healthy, balanced diet can help keep the immune system healthy. Studies have shown that opportunistic infections are more common in people with gross nutritional depletion (Gwyther & Marston, 2003). (See 'Nutrition' on page 301.)

Avoidance of drug and alcohol abuse and smoking

Drinking alcohol, smoking, and taking substances such as amphetamines, nitrites (poppers), morphine, cocaine and heroin can suppress the immune system, lower the CD4 cell count, and increase secondary infections and illnesses such as *Pneumocystis carinii* pneumonia (Nyamathi & Flaskerud, 1989; Siegel, 1986). HIV-positive people who smoke heavily and who abuse alcohol or other drugs should be encouraged to stop these habits – or at least to use alcohol only very moderately.

Moderate drinking is not harmful, and many people find that it relieves stress and anxiety. But heavy drinking may harm the immune system, delay recovery from opportunistic diseases, interfere with the absorption of nutrients and negatively influence healthy decision making, and may also cause hepatitis and liver damage. Someone with hepatitis B or C as well as HIV should preferably not drink *any* alcohol, because even small amounts may then be harmful. Alcohol may also interact negatively with some medications.

Avoiding contact with illnesses or infections

People with depressed immune systems should avoid contact with infectious diseases. Diseases such as flu, and children's diseases such as measles or mumps, can have serious effects on someone with a depressed immune system. Large gatherings of people should also be avoided, especially in winter, and HIV-positive adults and children should be immunised against diseases such as flu.

Routine visits to the doctor or clinic

HIV-positive people should visit their doctors, hospitals or clinics regularly. Infections and illnesses must be treated as soon as possible. Warning signs should not be ignored. Advise HIV-positive people to seek professional help if any of the following symptoms appear: skin lesions; lesions of the mucous membranes of the mouth, anus or vagina; swollen lymph nodes; extreme fatigue or tiredness; nausea; vomiting; diarrhoea and weight loss; persistent fever; headaches; forgetfulness or dizziness; persistent coughing and shortness of breath; and unusual bleeding (Ungvarski, 1989).

Children with HIV infection can become ill very quickly, and caregivers should not wait too long before taking a sick child to a hospital or clinic, especially if the child has symptoms such as fever, vomiting and diarrhoea.

Infection control in the home

Although there have been no reported cases of HIV being transmitted through casual contact in the home, there needs to be strict infection control in the home to prevent transmission of other infections to the immune-depressed HIV-positive person.

Infection control in the home (discussed in chapter 16) includes basic hygiene principles such as regular hand washing, keeping the environment clean, and not sharing personal items such as toothbrushes, razors and make-up.

Pets in the home

Pets can be very rewarding and help people feel better, mentally and physically. There is no reason why HIV-positive people should not keep pets, so long as they refrain from cleaning cat litter boxes, bird cages, dog litter, and fish tanks. Serious opportunistic infections (such as toxoplasmosis, cryptosporidiosis and diarrhoeal illnesses caused by *Salmonella* or *Campylobacter* bacteria) can be transmitted through pet excreta. These diseases can cause severe diarrhoea, brain infections and skin lesions in people with depleted immune systems. If HIV-positive people have to care for their own pets, excreta must be handled with rubber or vinyl gloves and hands must be washed after removal of the gloves. HIV-positive people should avoid owning reptiles such as snakes, lizards and turtles, because many are carriers of *Salmonella.*

HIV-positive people can further protect themselves from infection by always washing their hands after playing with animals; never handling animals that have diarrhoea; never touching stray animals that might bite or scratch; asking a friend to take a sick animal to the veterinarian; and never allowing a pet to lick the person's mouth or any open cuts or wounds. Adults should be extra vigilant and always supervise an HIV-positive child's hand washing after he or she has been playing with pets.

HIV-positive people working with animals (e.g. in veterinary clinics, pet shops, farms and slaughterhouses) may run the risk of opportunistic infections, and they should take additional precautions such as wearing gloves, overalls and boots. They should avoid cleaning chicken coops and working with young farm animals with diarrhoea, because these can cause serious cryptosporidiosis and *Salmonella* infections.

Social and sexual life

HIV-positive people should be assured that social contact with friends and family members is perfectly safe. As long as there is no exchange of blood or any other body fluids to which universal precautions apply, people mixing socially with an infected person cannot become infected.

Being HIV positive does not necessarily mean the end of a person's sex life. Sex releases stress and provides much-needed human contact and intimacy. HIV-positive people should therefore learn to rediscover their enjoyment of sex. Safe sex should be practised at all times to protect sex partners from infection and themselves from re-infection with HIV and other sexually transmitted infections (see 'General safer sex rules' on page 136).

Stress management

Stress has a very negative effect on the immune system, and increased stress can decrease the number of CD4 cells. HIV-positive people must learn to cope with stress. To relieve stress, HIV-positive people should be encouraged to join support groups, practise relaxation techniques, visit friends, talk to people, obtain factual information about their condition from professional people, and ignore wild rumours and sensationalised anecdotal 'information' about Aids.

Positive living

HIV infection is an immune system disease, because the HI virus attacks the immune cells. The infected person can fight back by *living positively*, and by keeping the immune system as healthy as possible. Caregivers and counsellors should share the following helpful tips with their clients to help them on their road to positive living (Brouard et al., 2004):

- Follow a balanced diet with plenty of fruit, vegetables and whole-grains.
- Take a good quality anti-oxidant, multi-vitamin and immune booster.
- Avoid junk foods, caffeine, alcohol, smoking and drugs. (These things will suppress the immune system.)
- Get enough rest and sleep.

- Get regular exercise, preferably in the company of others.
- Keep yourself informed about HIV and Aids.
- Rediscover your enjoyment of sex. Always practise safer sex to protect sex partners, and to protect yourself against re-infection with another strain of the virus.
- Don't share needles.
- Join a support group and keep contact with friends and family. Research has shown that appropriate support combined with a positive attitude can raise T-cell counts, reduce symptoms and possibly prolong lifespan.
- Find a counsellor you can relate to, who understands HIV and Aids and who is prepared to be there for you and to support you.
- Find a doctor who is an expert in HIV management. Go for regular routine visits.
- Consider preventive treatment for infections such as TB and PCP.
- Get treatment for sexually transmitted infections immediately.
- Talk to your doctor about antiretroviral medications.
- If you use herbal medicine, discuss it with your doctor (some herbal remedies may interact negatively with antiretrovirals).
- Insist on good infection control from your dentist, dental hygienist, acupuncturist, tattooist, body piercer and traditional healer.
- If you are pregnant, consider the options to prevent transmission to your baby.
- Prevent stress. Find out what stresses you, be aware of the warning signs and listen to your body!
- Find a stress-management technique that works for you. Consider massage, meditation, acupuncture, yoga or deep breathing exercises.
- Manage your life better. Organise your time, set yourself realistic goals and accept change.
- Take good care of yourself. Love yourself, do fun things, surround yourself with people who are good for you, be optimistic and laugh a lot. (Laughter and optimism are natural immune boosters! Positive emotions have been linked with rises in antibody levels in saliva and in hormones that boost the immune system, increasing the activity of the natural killer cells that fight infection.)
- Become aware of your physical, psychological and spiritual needs, and nurture them.
- Music, art and dance can help you to express your emotions when talking about your feelings is difficult.
- Learn to communicate well, be more assertive, don't use negative self-talk, and act with self-assurance.

Enrichment

Psychoneuroimmunology

The field of psychoneuroimmunology (PNI) is concerned with the influence of psychological factors on the immune system. Research studies on PNI have found that psychological stressors such as anxiety, loneliness, helplessness, hopelessness, distress, rage, anger, depression, tension, tiredness, negativity and interpersonal problems all have an adverse effect on the immune system. Subjects with these negative emotions showed a decline in killer T cell activity and lower CD4 cell counts.

Personal coping style was shown to correlate to immunological reactions. Positive coping factors such as a fighting spirit, a sense of humour, the ability to relax, hope, social contact, social support, mothering and caring behaviour, as well as the emotional expression of traumatic experiences, all enhanced the immune system (Ader et al., 1991; O'Leary, 1990; Van Zyl, 1990).

PNI has very important implications for the management of HIV infection. Longo and his colleagues (in Van Zyl, 1990) found that subjects who were trained in relaxation, stress management and imagery techniques reported a significant reduction in the incidence of recurrent genital herpes activity when compared with the control group.

PNI therapists believe that interventions to reduce psychological distress (which can take many forms) may improve patients' health by strengthening immune functioning. HIV-positive people who practise PNI believe that self-efficacy, a positive self-image, a relaxed, positive attitude towards life, hope, humour and a healthy social support system enable their immune systems to fight HIV infection more effectively. (See 'The Caregiver's Bookshelf' on page 367 for further reading on positive living.)

Alternative therapies

HIV-positive people often use alternative therapies to relieve stress and improve general well-being. Alternative therapies should be integrated into the general health care plan of the patient to assure holistic care.

Many alternative therapies are based on the belief that a positive mind is the strongest weapon against HIV and Aids, and that the power of the mind can control what happens to the body. Alternative therapies are based on the premise that positive thinking can prolong and improve the quality of life. These include psychoneuroimmunology (see the enrichment box on page 300), meditation, mental imagery or visualisation therapy, positive mental reinforcement, reflexology, body massage, aromatherapy and visits to traditional healers. Many HIV-positive people also use acupuncture, homeopathy and hypnotherapy.

Activity

> Design an educational game (e.g. a computer game or a board game) for HIV-positive young people to help them 'strengthen their immune systems'. The game should involve players' defender cells (CD4 cells, macrophages, killer T cells, etc.) destroying the virus and the infected cells. Players should gain points (or CD4 cells) to strengthen their immune systems by doing the right things, such as eating nutritious foods, giving up smoking, using condoms, going for a jog, saying no to drugs, washing hands after playing with the dog, and so on.

17.2 NUTRITION

There is a strong correlation between malnutrition and immune depression. Research findings suggest that a healthy diet, vitamin and mineral supplementation and defensive eating (see page 303) may enhance the immune response to HIV infection and enhance resistance to opportunistic infections (Saunders, 1994).

Dietary recommendations

A healthy diet does not necessarily have to be expensive. Locally available, natural, unrefined and unprocessed foods are sufficient and adequate to protect the immune system and to keep a person healthy. What is really important is the *composition* of the meal. Food can be divided into three groups, and everyone should try to eat food from *each one* of these groups at *every meal.* A picture of a plate divided into five sections can be used to explain to clients what to eat at each meal of the day (see Figure 17.1).

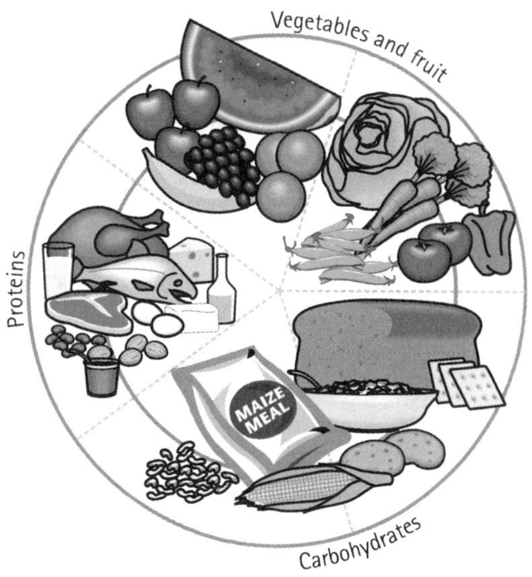

Figure 17.1
A healthy, balanced diet

Energy-giving foods: carbohydrates or starchy foods

Two fifths (2/5 or 40%) of a person's plate should consist of carbohydrates or energy-giving foods such as potatoes, yams and other sweet potatoes, wheat, samp, brown rice, maize meal (unsifted), maize rice, oats, mabela (ground sorghum), or rye, brown or wholewheat bread. Avoid refined starches such as white bread, white rice, white pasta, super maize meal or any foods made from white flour and refined cereals. Because sugar, animal fats and vegetable oils are also energy-giving foods, they are beneficial for patients who are trying to gain weight. However, anyone with thrush should avoid sugar, because it encourages the growth of the fungi that cause thrush.

Body-building foods: proteins

Proteins in the diet are important 'building blocks' for the development of muscles, immune cells such as T and B cells, teeth and bones. One fifth (1/5 or 20%) of a person's plate should consist of proteins such as dry peas or beans, soya, lentils, peanuts (or peanut butter), nuts, eggs, red meat, liver, chicken, fish, cheese and milk. Milk is an important source of protein, calcium and vitamins and one to two glasses of fresh pasteurised or boiled milk (or skimmed milk) should be drunk every day. Yoghurt or sour milk should also be used frequently. Since there are a number of good sources of high-grade protein other than meat, it is *not* necessary for people to eat meat every day. Excellent but far less expensive sources of protein (such as beans) can be substituted for meat. Mopani worms and flying ants are also good sources of protein.

Protective foods: vitamins and minerals

Two fifths (2/5 or 40%) of a person's plate should consist of vegetables and fruit. Vegetables and fruit contain important vitamins and minerals vital for fighting infections, recovering from infections and strengthening the immune system. Brightly coloured vegetables and fruit (dark green, dark yellow, orange and red) are the most nutritious. These include carrots, pumpkin, yellow sweet potatoes, pawpaws, marogo, cabbage, oranges, tomatoes, guavas, green beans and lettuce. Dark green leaves such as spinach, beetroot leaves and the outer leaves of cabbage and cauliflower are also very nutritious. Vegetables should be cooked or steamed lightly – cooking them for too long can destroy vitamins. Preferably at least one portion of vegetables should be eaten raw every day (they should be well washed or peeled). Don't throw nutritious foods away. The cooking water of vegetables, for example, can be re-used in a soup or sauce or as the basis for further cooking.

Specific dietary advice for sick patients who suffer from problems such as anorexia (loss of appetite), nausea, diarrhoea or fever is given in 'Care of general health problems and opportunistic infections' on page 304.

Activity

Teach children how to make and care for a vegetable garden. A patch of ground as big as a door (1 metre by 2 metres) can provide a constant supply of fresh vegetables!

Supplements

Many people with HIV infection decide to supplement their diet with additional vitamins, minerals, nutrients and herbs in order to protect or strengthen their immune systems and maintain or increase weight. Since the health benefits of dietary supplements are a matter of ongoing controversy in the scientific world, many HIV specialists recommend only a multivitamin supplement and a healthy, balanced diet. If HIV-positive individuals choose to supplement their diets, they should do so with caution and discuss the supplements they intend to take with their doctors. Megadoses (large doses) of any vitamin supplement are definitely not recommended because they may be toxic and harmful to health. Herbs should also be used with caution, because some herbs (e.g. St John's Wort) are implicated in rendering some antiretroviral medications ineffective (Piscitelli, 2000).

Vitamins and minerals that may enhance the immune system (when taken in moderation) include: beta carotene (boosts immune functioning), vitamin A (keeps lining of gut, lungs and skin healthy), vitamin E (boosts the immune system), vitamin B_6 (maintains immune and nervous systems), vitamin B_{12} (boosts production of T cells), calcium (strengthens bones), vitamin C (fights infections and helps recovery from infections), selenium (activates T cells), zinc (important for immune system), iron (builds blood supply), copper, magnesium, anti-oxidants (boost immune system), and pyridoxine. Most of these vitamins and minerals can be obtained through a healthy, balanced diet.

Studies have shown that there is an association between vitamin A deficiency in pregnant women and the transmission of the virus to the baby. Vitamin A supplementation may therefore be beneficial for pregnant HIV-positive women, but women should be warned that high doses of vitamin A may have harmful effects on both the baby and the mother.

Moducare or Immunoboost (natural plant sterols/sterolins extracted from the African potato plant) seems to be effective as an immune booster in HIV-positive individuals who have recently been infected, and in those with intact or healthy immune systems. A study by Bouic et al. (2000) found that patients (with a baseline CD4 cell count of more than 500 cells/mm^3) who took Moducare showed a significant increase in their CD4 cells and a significant decline in their viral loads. Within this group 15% showed undetectable viral loads within twelve months of starting the study. Moducare does not seem to work very well in people with already depleted immune systems.

The African potato plant is traditionally prepared by drying and powdering the bulb. The raw powdered substance should not be taken for longer than about three months at a time, because it contains small amounts of poisonous chemicals (alkaloids). These chemicals are removed from Moducare during the manufacturing process.

Eating defensively

People with HIV/Aids tend to be more vulnerable to food-borne illnesses because of their weakened immune systems. They should follow basic food safety guidelines and eat defensively.

- HIV-positive people should be aware that microbes in the food they eat can cause microbial infections (and food poisoning). They should always cook meat, chicken and fish very well (because heat kills bacteria) and should avoid products that contain any raw or underdone meat or dairy products. For the same reason they should avoid raw or soft-boiled eggs because these can be sources of *Salmonella* – as can biltong (dried meat), dried sausages and unpasteurised dairy products (milk and cheese). They should also avoid products that have passed their sell-by date. 'Raw' cow's milk or unpasteurised milk should be boiled and then kept in clean containers.
- Food should be handled and stored hygienically. Keeping shelves, counter tops, refrigerators, towels and utensils clean is important in preventing bacterial contamination of food. To prevent cross contamination (e.g. from raw meat to other foods), the food handler should wash his or her hands regularly and not use *wooden* chopping boards for cutting and chopping raw meat, fish or chicken. Uncooked food should be kept separate from cooked food. Food that is mouldy or about to go off should be avoided, and all previously cooked food should be re-heated at a high temperature for some time before it is eaten (heating can kill or neutralise dangerous organisms).
- Raw seafood (shellfish, oysters, clams, sushi and sashimi) poses a serious risk of food poisoning for people with Aids and should never be eaten. Lightly steamed seafood should also be avoided (Food and Drug Administration [FDA] brochure, 1992).
- Fruits and vegetables should always (if possible) be washed, scrubbed with a stiff brush, or peeled. Avoid fruit and vegetables that have been sprayed with pesticides. Canned fruits and vegetables could be used instead of fresh products if fresh products are contaminated. Raw alfalfa sprouts have been identified as carriers of food-borne diseases in the USA, and it is recommended that people with compromised immune systems should avoid eating raw sprouts (Kurtzweil, 1999).
- Water should be boiled if there is the slightest suspicion that the water source may be contaminated.
- Eat foods high in kilojoules and proteins, and avoid low-kilojoule or zero-kilojoule foods. Find out about ways of supplementing the nutritional value of meals. The addition of eggs, butter, margarine and milk to gravies, soups or milkshakes can provide additional kilojoules and protein.
- Avoid too many processed foods. Many of the nutrients in these foods have been destroyed during preparation. Avoid foods that contain

preservatives, artificial flavours and artificial colours. Avoid junk foods.
- Sugar is a good source of energy, but it can promote the growth of fungi and should be avoided if the patient has problems with oral or vaginal thrush. Foods containing yeasts should be avoided in patients with *Candida* infections.

Some HIV-positive people are on alternative diets. Health care professionals must make sure that these alternative diets are not harmful; provide adequate kilojoules and proteins; include a variety of nutritious foods; are not regarded as a substitute for general health care; do not contain substances in amounts that may be physically harmful to the person; and are not unnecessarily expensive (Pike, 1988).

Activity

- Devise a dietary plan for an HIV-positive man who lives alone and has to take care of himself. He is a very busy company executive and doesn't have much time to prepare food for himself.
- Devise a dietary plan for an HIV-positive woman with very limited financial means who has to care for her large family in a very poor rural part of the country. Because the kind of diet you devise would obviously be tailored to suit cultural tastes, decide on the woman's cultural group before you begin to draw up the dietary plan.

17.3 CARE OF GENERAL HEALTH PROBLEMS AND OPPORTUNISTIC INFECTIONS

We will now discuss the most common health problems of people with HIV infection or Aids, as well as general care principles to alleviate the symptoms associated with HIV infection and Aids. Because this discussion is by no means comprehensive, health care professionals and other caregivers are encouraged to use their own initiative and experience to supplement these care principles. If you don't have the equipment or material described in this chapter, just use your imagination and improvise!

The nursing care principles discussed in this chapter do not apply only to hospitals, hospices and clinics, but are equally important in home-based care. These principles should be taught on every possible occasion to patients and the primary caregivers (usually family) who care for them at home. Many health problems are recurrent, and it is important for people with HIV/Aids and their caregivers to know how to deal with these.

This chapter will give a brief description of the symptoms and possible causes of HIV/Aids-related illnesses, and will describe general care principles that can be applied to alleviate symptoms. In the 'Home-based care' boxes, additional practical advice will be given on how to prevent and treat symptoms at home with only the most basic and inexpensive commonly available resources. (See page 305 for an example of a home-based care box.) Each box has a section entitled 'Danger signs', in which caregivers at home are warned to look out for certain *changes* in the condition of the patient, and to seek professional medical help when these are encountered. Where the care of children differs from that of adults, it will be discussed separately (also see enrichment box 'General rules about caring for a child with HIV infection and Aids' on page 306). For additional information on the care of Aids patients, see 'The Caregiver's Bookshelf' on page 367. (The information provided in this chapter is based on Dickinson et al., 1988; Evian, 2000, 2003; Fahrner, 1988; Gwyther & Marston, 2003; Muchiru & Fröhlich, 2001; Reno & Walker, 1988; Ungvarski, 1989; Ungvarski & Flaskerud, 1999; and Van Dyk, 1999. Practical advice for home-based care is based on the WHO publication for Aids home care, 1993.)

Fever

Fever (high body temperature) is usually caused by the HIV infection itself, by diarrhoea and dehydration, by opportunistic infections such as TB, viral or bacterial infections, or by endemic diseases such as malaria. HIV infection itself can cause a low-grade fever (37–38 °C). A temperature of 38 °C or higher for a prolonged period may be caused by factors other than the HIV infection itself. Care for patients with fever includes the following measures:

- Encourage the patient to drink lots of fluid, especially cool fluids. Provide plenty of water, weak tea, broth or juice.
- Remove any unnecessary clothing or blankets.
- Give sponge baths or use a fan to keep the temperature down.

Home-based care

Fever

The best way to check whether someone has a fever is to measure his or her temperature with a thermometer. If a thermometer is not available, place the back of your hand on the patient's forehead, and the back of your other hand on your forehead. If the person has a fever, you will be able to feel the difference. If the patient has a fever, take the steps listed under 'Fever' on page 304 to lower his or her temperature. Keep the skin clean and dry in between bathing and cooling sessions to prevent skin problems such as rashes and sores.

Danger signs

Patients and caregivers at home should seek professional help:

- if the fever is very high and continues for a long time;
- if it is accompanied by coughing and weight loss (may be an indication of TB);
- if it is accompanied by symptoms such as stiff neck, severe pain, confusion, unconsciousness, a yellow colour in the eyes, sudden severe diarrhoea or convulsions;
- if the patient is pregnant or has recently had a baby; or
- if malaria is common in the area, or if the fever has not gone away after one treatment with antimalarial medicine.

Watch children with fever very carefully and take them to a clinic if you are unable to break the fever. Fever convulsions are common (and dangerous) in children with high fever. Use lukewarm water at room temperature to bathe babies or very young children. Never use cold water for this purpose because babies and very young children cannot yet tolerate temperatures that are too cold and may even go into shock when suddenly submerged in cold water.

- Pour water on the skin, or put cloths soaked in water on the forehead or chest and fan the body with wet cloths.
- Keep the room well ventilated and cool. Open the windows or doors to allow fresh air or a light breeze to penetrate.
- Use medicines that reduce fever (antipyretics) such as aspirin or paracetamol (two tablets every eight hours).
- Make sure that the patient eats nutritious foods (a high-kilojoule, high-protein diet).

(See the home-based care box 'Fever'.)

Diarrhoea

Diarrhoea is one of the most common problems in patients with HIV infection and Aids. A person has diarrhoea when he or she has three or more loose or watery stools per day. *Acute diarrhoea* lasts for less than two weeks; *persistent diarrhoea* usually lasts for more than two weeks.

The most common causes of diarrhoea in people with HIV infection are gastrointestinal infections from food and water that is not clean and fresh (e.g. *Salmonella* infections), opportunistic infections such as Kaposi's sarcoma in the gastrointestinal tract, the effect of HIV itself, inappropriate diet, and the side effects of medication.

Diarrhoea can lead to serious dehydration, electrolyte imbalance, malnutrition, weight loss, fatigue (tiredness), weakness and even death. Because diarrhoea is a common and recurrent problem for HIV-positive patients, they need to learn how to live with diarrhoea and to adjust their fluid and food intake appropriately. The following steps should be taken:

- Encourage the patient to drink lots of fluids (such as unsweetened juices, weak tea and food-based fluids such as gruel, soup or rice water) so that he or she remains well hydrated all the time.
- Encourage the patient to consume a bland but nutritionally balanced low-fat, low-sucrose, low-fibre and lactose-free diet. Include foods such as mashed potatoes (not chips), white rice and maize meal, meat, poultry and fish, cooked (scrambled) eggs, mashed bananas, apple juice, peeled (and preferably cooked)

apples, grape juice, avocados, white bread or crackers made from refined (white) flour, noodles and pasta made from (white) refined flour, cooked vegetables such as carrots or potatoes, and soups *without* whole-grain thickeners such as barley. Marmite or Bovril as a soup (a few teaspoons dissolved in boiling water) or spread very thinly on dry toast also helps to restore electrolyte balance. If the patient can tolerate lactose, include *small* amounts of milk, cottage cheese, cream cheese and yoghurt in the diet. Try to make food (such as rice or mashed potatoes) more appetising by making gravies from the juice of vegetables and meat and thickening them with Bisto or small amounts of Maizena. Remove excessive fat from meat juice before making the gravy.

- Avoid all foods that may aggravate diarrhoea, especially foods high in fibre. Such foods include (for example) All Bran flakes and all other wholewheat or whole-grain products (such as muesli bars), whole-grain cereals (especially if, like muesli, they contain raw ingredients), wholewheat bread (use white bread instead), brown rice (white rice is ideal), unpeeled or fibrous fruit and vegetables (rather have bland fruits such as mashed bananas or very finely grated apple), nuts, seeds, popcorn, fried foods, raw vegetables, green vegetables, raisins, currants, dried fruit, foods that are difficult to digest (this will vary

Enrichment

General rules about caring for a child with HIV infection and Aids

Children have the same symptoms as adults, and are usually treated in the same way. The situations in which they do have to be treated differently will be emphasised. The following general rules apply when caring for a child with HIV infection and Aids (WHO, 1993, 2000a):

- *Maintain good nutrition.* In most countries in the developing world, HIV-positive mothers are still breastfeeding their babies. The health care professional should help the HIV-positive mother to make an informed decision about whether to breastfeed or bottle-feed her baby. This advice should be based on facts and on the circumstances of the mother and the availability of resources. (See 'Breastfeeding' on page 32.) The growth of the baby should be regularly monitored (preferably at least once a month) to ensure that the baby is being adequately fed.
- *Provide early treatment for infections.* Children should be treated early and vigorously for infections such as measles, ear infections (otitis media), oral thrush, skin infections, STIs in the newborn, unexplained fever, diarrhoea or vomiting. Because the immune systems of children with HIV infection are often impaired, and presenting symptoms of these diseases may be more persistent and more severe, these children may respond poorly to treatment, develop severe complications and die.
- *Diagnose and treat TB early.* TB is one of the most common and deadly opportunistic infections, and the HIV-positive child is very susceptible to it. TB prevention and treatment should be available to all family members.
- *Treat the child as normal and ensure a good quality of life.* Many HIV-positive children remain relatively symptom-free for months or even years, and they should be treated as normal. Let them play with other kids, go to school and do normal 'kid stuff'. Make sure, however, that they always maintain high standards of hygiene. This will help prevent infections.
- *Hospitalisation of children should be avoided if possible.* The hospital environment exposes children to many harmful germs that can be particularly dangerous if the immune system is depressed. Hospitalisation of HIV-positive children should be considered only if they are seriously ill and need special care not available at home (Evian, 2000).
- *Immunise according to standard schedules.* All children, including those with HIV infection and Aids, should be given all the standard vaccinations (e.g. DPT, polio, measles and Hib). The only exception is that while BCG (the TB vaccine) should be given to all healthy HIV-positive children at birth, it should NOT be given to infants with clinical symptoms of HIV infection. (See 'Immunising children and adults with HIV infection' on page 86.)

from patient to patient), heavily spiced foods, very rich foods, dairy products, foods that contain excessive amounts of sugar, oil, alcohol, nicotine or caffeine. Also avoid foods that increase flatus (gas), coffee, very strong tea (rooibos tea is acceptable), commercial aerated colas, chocolate and smoking. Every patient reacts differently to foods, and it is always a good idea to question the patient about his or her needs and then experiment cautiously with *small* amounts of desired foods to establish an optimal dietary regimen.

- Small, frequent meals will help prevent stomach distension.
- Make food easier to digest by mashing or grinding it.
- Foods at room temperature may be better tolerated than very hot or cold foods.
- Relieve dryness of the mouth with frequent sips of water or ice chips and apply lip cream or Vaseline.
- Absorb unpleasant odours by placing a small bowl of vanilla essence or charcoal under the bed, or by using air-freshener, a bunch of lavender or aromatic herbs.
- Medical treatment of diarrhoea involves an appropriate antibiotic or anti-protozoal where indicated, loperamide or codeine phosphate.

To prevent secondary infections, the skin in the rectal area should be kept very clean and dry. The skin should be washed with mild soap and

Home-based care

Diarrhoea

Prevent diarrhoea by boiling water from an unsafe water supply (e.g. a dirty well or container) before using it in food or drinks. Eat only clean and safe food and make sure that stored food is reheated thoroughly at a high temperature. Avoid raw or uncooked meat, and peel fruit or wash it well before eating. Always wash your hands before preparing or eating food.

There are three basic rules for treating diarrhoea:

1. Drink more fluids than usual. Drink something after every stool.
2. Continue to eat, even if you only consume small amounts of nutritious foods at a time.
3. Recognise and treat dehydration early. Watch out for the following signs of dehydration: severe thirst, dry mouth, sunken eyes, sunken fontanelle in young children, rapid pulse and breathing, irritability, lethargy (lack of vitality), poor urine output and a dry skin (skin going back slowly when pinched). Treat with an oral rehydration solution such as Oral Rehydration Salts mixed with water. Or use the following home-made oral rehydration fluid:

   Home-made oral rehydration fluid

   Mix 1 litre (4 big cups) of boiled and cooled water with 8 teaspoons of sugar and half a teaspoon of salt. If available, add fresh orange juice for taste and potassium replacement. Adults should take 1 to 2 cups of this fluid after every diarrhoeal stool. (To make 1 cup of rehydration fluid, mix 1 cup of water with 2 teaspoons of sugar and a pinch of salt.)

Danger signs

Patients and caregivers should seek professional medical help if patients have diarrhoea and if they:

- are very thirsty;
- have a fever;
- cannot eat or drink properly;
- do not seem to be getting better;
- pass many watery stools;
- have blood in the stools;
- are vomiting and cannot keep fluids down;
- are irritable, confused or lethargic; or
- have a very dry skin.

It is very important to encourage children with diarrhoea to drink. Children under two years old should drink about a quarter to half a cup of fluid (e.g. the home-made rehydration fluid given above, rice-water, porridge-water, soup or tea) after each loose stool. Older children should drink half a cup to one cup of fluid after each loose stool. In the case of breast-fed infants with diarrhoea, the mother should continue to breastfeed and try to do so more often than normal (at least every three hours.) Watch children very carefully for signs of dehydration and take them to the nearest hospital or clinic if necessary. Severely dehydrated children can easily go into shock and coma.

water after each bowel movement and patted dry. Broken skin can be dried with a cool hair-dryer. A protective lotion can be applied to relieve discomfort, such as zinc ointment, and the patient can sit in warm water containing a pinch of salt or Savlon three to four times a day. Diarrhoea may cause painful and bleeding haemorrhoids. A block of ice wrapped in a soft cloth can be put against the anus to control the bleeding and reduce the swelling.

Observe babies and young children very carefully for signs of dehydration such as a dry mouth, eyes and skin, poor skin elasticity, poor urine output, sunken fontanelle and eyes, and rapid pulse and breathing.

(See the home-based care box 'Diarrhoea' on page 307.)

Anorexia, nausea and vomiting

Patients with HIV/Aids often experience anorexia (lack of appetite), nausea and vomiting as a result of gastrointestinal problems, infections such as *Candida*, side effects of medication, constipation, Kaposi's sarcoma in the intestines and HIV infection itself. In some people with Aids, nausea and vomiting are short-lived and usually disappear after treatment. In others it may persist and become a part of daily life. This may cause weight loss and fluid and electrolyte imbalance. In such cases, apply the following care principles:

- Stop the intake of food and fluids for 1–2 hours if the patient is vomiting. Then gradually introduce clear fluids such as water or flat Coke. To maintain or restore the fluid balance, increase the amount of fluids as soon as the patient can tolerate it. Later the patient may eat dry toast or crackers.
- Use the appropriate anti-nausea medication based on the cause of the problem (is the nausea induced by gastrointestinal problems, by medication, by anxiety, or by intracranial pressure?)
- Anti-nausea medicine should be taken 30–60 minutes before meals (or as prescribed).
- Sit patients upright while eating or drinking, and keep them in an upright position for 20–30 minutes after meals.
- If the patient needs to lie down, ensure that he or she lies on the side with the head slightly raised, to prevent aspiration of vomit.
- Keep a kidney dish or other container within reach of the patient.
- Advise nauseous patients not to take liquids before, during or immediately after meals.
- Give hourly sips of cold water or ice chips.
- Rooibos tea, herbal tea, or weak black Ceylon tea may be tolerated well. Rooibos tea can stimulate the appetite.
- Low-fat foods and dry, salty foods should be introduced. Avoid gas-producing, greasy, spicy foods.
- Present food in an attractive and appetising way. Keep the windows open to eliminate food odours that may nauseate the patient.

 Home-based care

Nausea and vomiting

Apply the principles listed under 'Anorexia, nausea and vomiting'. Avoid cooking smells. Watch out for signs of dehydration and start giving oral rehydration solution, weak tea or other clear liquids to the patient an hour or two after severe vomiting has stopped. Start with about two tablespoons of liquid an hour for one to three hours. Increase this to four to six tablespoons an hour for the next hour or two. If the patient feels up to it, he or she should begin to eat small quantities of dry, plain foods such as bread or rice. Keep the mouth clean and fresh by rinsing it with water or diluted lemon juice.

Danger signs

Advise caregivers to seek professional help:

- if vomiting occurs repeatedly and fluids cannot be kept down;
- if regular vomiting lasts more than 24 hours, particularly if it is accompanied by pain in the abdomen;
- if there is fever in addition to the vomiting;
- if the vomiting is violent, especially if the vomit is dark green, brown, or smells like faeces; or
- if the vomit contains blood.

Note: Be very careful with vomiting children and watch them carefully for signs of dehydration. Babies can dehydrate and die within hours if vomiting (and diarrhoea) are neglected.

- Serve food cold or at room temperature. Patients should eat slowly in a relaxed atmosphere.
- In order to increase appetite, encourage patients to take small, frequent meals high in protein and kilojoules throughout the day, rather than three larger meals. Kilojoule intake can be increased by using extra peanut butter, sugar, honey, ice cream, milk shakes and sweets. Patients should be encouraged to eat all their favourite foods and to drink lots of fluids.
- Encourage the use of nutritional supplements such as Ensure, Complan, PVM and vitamin supplements.
- Teach patients relaxation and breathing techniques and encourage them to use these techniques when they are nauseous.
- Thorough oral care should be encouraged to prevent thrush (because thrush makes eating difficult).

Fluid and electrolyte imbalance

Fluid and electrolyte status should be continually monitored. Assess the skin for dryness and turgor. Measure fluid intake and output daily. Monitor the patient for decreases in systolic blood pressure or increases in pulse associated with sitting or standing. Look out for the signs and symptoms of electrolyte disturbances such as muscle cramping, weakness, irregular pulse, altered mental status (e.g. confusion), nausea and vomiting. Monitor serum electrolyte values and report abnormalities to the doctor.

- Help the patient select foods that will replenish electrolytes, for example oranges and bananas (potassium), cheese and soups (sodium).
- Encourage a fluid intake of 2 500 ml or more per day (unless contra-indicated) in order to regain fluid lost from diarrhoea or vomiting.
- Start measures to control diarrhoea.
- If fluid and electrolyte imbalances persist in a hospitalised patient, administer intravenous fluid and electrolytes as prescribed by a doctor.

Constipation

If patients with HIV/Aids become constipated, the following measures can be taken:

- Encourage the intake of fluids such as water and fruit juices, as well as fresh fruits and vegetables.
- Constipation can be prevented by using honey, molasses, stewed prunes and grated beetroot.
- Give the patient high-fibre foods if he or she can tolerate them. Add extra fibre to cereals, porridge or soup. If extra fibre is added, the patient must be able to drink extra fluids.
- Encourage mobility and exercise.
- Certain medications (e.g. codeine) can cause constipation, and a stool stimulant and softener should be prescribed to prevent constipation.
- Ask the patient what he or she usually uses to prevent constipation and keep to familiar remedies (e.g. Black Forest tea or marula jam). Senekot, Lactulose or glycerine suppositories can also be used.
- Check stools for blood.

Incontinence

Incontinence (loss of control over the bladder or bowels) needs careful nursing care. Keep the patient clean and dry and protect the skin with creams such as Vaseline and Fissan paste. Use adult disposable nappies if available, or large towelling nappies. Incinerate or burn disposable nappies. Protect the bed with a plastic sheet, or with newspapers if there is no other form of mattress protection. Get rid of unpleasant odours, and help the patient and family emotionally.

Skin problems

The skin is an important barrier against infections. It must be kept intact, and skin problems must be treated immediately. The following skin problems occur more often in people with Aids than in healthy people: rashes, itching skin, increased dryness of the skin, painful sores, boils and abscesses, and slow healing of wounds. These skin problems may be caused by genital or oral herpes, thrush, other fungal infections (e.g. ringworm or tinea), bacterial infections, shingles (herpes zoster) (see the home-based care box

'How to care for a patient with shingles' on page 311), allergies, Kaposi's sarcoma, poor hygiene, immobility, malnutriti)on, dehydration or prolonged pressure (bed sores).

Wear gloves when caring for lesions, rashes or weeping skin. The patient's skin can be protected in the following ways:

- Inspect the patient's skin thoroughly every morning and afternoon for redness, lesions or excessive moisture.
- If lesions are present, assess daily for changes in appearance, location and size of lesions.
- Maintain thorough foot and skin care. Skin breakdown can be prevented by stimulating the circulation through frequent massaging with lotions, oils or creams. Pay special attention to areas over bony prominences.
- Advise patients with foot lesions to wear white cotton socks and shoes that do not cause the feet to perspire.
- If the patient has a wound on his or her foot or leg, raise the affected area (e.g. on a pillow) as high as possible and as often as possible. Make sure that circulation is not restricted in any way, especially in the area behind the knee.
- Keep the skin clean by washing with a mild soap and water. Add a spoon of aqueous cream to soften the water. Pat dry gently.
- Encourage the use of non-perfumed skin moisturisers on a dry skin.
- Avoid the use of strong soaps on the skin.
- Avoid scratching itchy skin. This may lead to broken skin and infections.
- Encourage mobile patients to change their positions at least every two hours and to get out of bed as often as possible.
- Turn bedridden patients from side to side every two hours, repositioning their pillows.

Home-based care

Skin problems

As a general rule, cleaning the skin frequently with soap and water and keeping it dry between washing will prevent the most common problems. Itching can be reduced by cooling the skin with water, by applying lotions such as calamine, and by using effective traditional remedies that are usually available from local herbalists. A very dry skin can be treated by avoiding soap and by applying aqueous cream, Vaseline, glycerine, and vegetable or plant oils (or by applying the more expensive oils and creams available in shops). To prevent babies (and confused adults) from scratching themselves, gloves or socks can be put over their hands, and fingernails can be kept short.

The buttock area of babies with diarrhoea, nappy rash or yeast infections needs the following special care: leave the baby's bottom exposed to air as much as possible; soak the baby's bottom with warm water between nappy changes; change wet and soiled nappies immediately, and avoid wiping the buttock area (rather squeeze water from a cloth or pour water over the area and pat dry); and apply lotions supplied by the local clinic, or use Fissan paste.

Wash open sores with clean water (cooled boiled water if necessary) mixed with salt (1 teaspoon of salt to 1 litre of clean water) or with a gentian violet solution (1 teaspoon of gentian violet crystals in half a litre of clean water). Protect the area by covering it with clean gauze bandages or cloths.

Don't touch soiled (bloody) bandages or dressings with your bare hands: use gloves, plastic bags, or a big leaf to handle the dressings, and always wash your hands afterwards. If the sore is on the feet or legs, raise the affected area as high and as often as possible.

Boils and abscesses should be washed with salt water and a hot compress should be placed over the abscess four times a day (take care not to burn the patient).

Danger signs

Seek professional help at the clinic or hospital when the skin problem is associated with any of the following symptoms:

- pus, redness or fever (indicating infection);
- severe pain, difficulty in sleeping and eye problems such as blurred vision (which is often a symptom of shingles);
- allergic reactions to medication; or
- a bad smell, oozing of a grey or brown liquid, blackening of the skin around a wound with air bubbles or blisters (an indication of gangrene).

- Use pressure-relieving devices such as sheepskin and foam heel and elbow protectors. Heel and elbow protectors can be made out of cloth or bandages.
- Kaposi's sarcoma lesions (a purplish skin lesion) usually require no care unless they are open and draining. Always report open, draining lesions to the doctor for possible chemotherapy. Open lesions should be thoroughly cleaned and left open to air.
- In hospitalised incontinent patients, use condom catheters and faecal incontinence bags to prevent skin irritation and lesions caused by wet skin. For incontinent patients at home, keep the skin and linen dry and clean at all times. Use plastic sheeting, undercovers or nappies (for adults) to keep linen clean.
- Clean the perineal area (between the anus and the scrotum or vulva) after each bowel movement with non-irritating soap and water to prevent breakage of the skin and infection.
- Wash genital or rectal herpes with warm water and non-irritating soap, and pat dry or dry with a cool hair-dryer two to four times per day.
- Discourage patients with genital or rectal abrasions from using toilet paper as this may worsen the condition. Soft disposable cloths such as Wet Ones or cotton wool should be used instead.
- A separate wash cloth should be used to wash areas with infectious lesions.
- Discomfort caused by genital herpes can be relieved by Savlon or salt baths and pain medication.
- Protect skin surfaces from friction and rubbing by keeping bed linen free from wrinkles and by avoiding tight or restrictive clothing.

Home-based care

How to care for a patient with shingles

Patients with Aids often develop shingles. Shingles is characterised by a rash (blisters or sores), usually on the chest or back. It is very painful and itchy. The following points are important in caring for a patient with shingles (Muchiru & Fröhlich, 2001:34):

- Keep sores dry and do not let clothing rub against them.
- Let the patient wear clean, loose-fitting clothing.
- Bathe sores with clean water three times a day, or apply a gentian violet solution.
- Apply calamine lotion twice a day to relieve pain and itching.
- Relieve pain with aspirin or paracetamol.
- Watch for signs of infected sores, such as redness or pus, and seek medical help if necessary.

Problems with the oral mucous membranes (mouth and throat)

Oral mucous membranes are often dry or painful because of secondary infections such as thrush (white patches and redness), oral herpes simplex (blisters and sores on the lips), malnutrition (cracks and sores on the mouth), dehydration, inadequate oral hygiene, Kaposi's sarcoma of the mouth or throat, hairy leukoplakia, drug therapy, dental problems, and poorly fitting dentures (caused by weight loss). It is important to ensure that a patient's mouth remains in a healthy condition so that he or she can swallow, eat and drink properly.

- Inspect the inside of the mouth (preferably with a light) every day before breakfast.
- Give adequate fluids to prevent dehydration and encourage the patient to eat a healthy diet.
- Treat oral thrush or lesions immediately.
- Thorough mouth hygiene should be observed at all times. Patients should have mouthwashes after every meal. If the tongue is coated, it should be cleaned at least two to three times a day by gently scrubbing with a soft toothbrush.
- Encourage patients with oral thrush to suck a lemon (if it is not too painful). The acid in the lemon juice slows the rate at which the fungus grows. Follow the 'candida diet': avoid foods containing yeast and sugar and don't drink beer until the oral thrush has been absent (cleared up) for at least three weeks.
- Teeth should be brushed with a soft toothbrush and non-abrasive toothpaste or sodium bicarbonate (baking soda) to avoid injuries.

- Give soft or pureed bland foods to a patient having difficulty in eating.
- Serve moist foods and avoid spicy and acid foods.
- Use a straw for liquids and soups to prevent the food from touching the sore areas.
- Cold foods and drinks or ice may help to numb the mouth and relieve discomfort.

Home-based care

Mouth and throat problems

To prevent problems in the mouth and throat, rinse the mouth with warm salt water (half a teaspoon of salt in a cup of water) or with a mouthwash solution after eating and between meals. (Do not allow the patient to swallow the mouthwash because it may cause diarrhoea and nausea.)

Thrush can be treated by gently scrubbing the tongue and gums with a soft toothbrush; by rinsing the mouth with a mouthwash, salt water or lemon water; and by applying a gentian violet solution three to four times a day (1 teaspoon of gentian violet crystals in half a litre of water). The gentian violet solution can also be applied to herpes simplex sores (or blisters) on the lips.

A patient who does not have a toothbrush can use a tooth-cleaning stick (a stick with one end sharpened to clean between the teeth, and the other end chewed to use the fibres as a brush), or tie a piece of rough towel around the end of a stick and use it as a toothbrush (WHO, 1993). If toothpaste is not available, a tooth-cleaning powder can be made by mixing salt and bicarbonate of soda (or ashes) in equal amounts. Wet the toothbrush before dipping it into the powder so that the powder sticks.

Danger signs

Seek professional help if:

- the patient becomes dehydrated or unable to swallow properly; or
- there are symptoms of oesophageal thrush, such as a burning pain in the chest or a deep pain on swallowing.

Respiratory problems

Respiratory problems such as shortness of breath, difficulty in breathing, chronic coughing, chest pains and an increased production of mucus are the most common problems of people with Aids. These problems may be caused by colds and flu, bronchitis, TB, pneumonia (e.g. PCP), respiratory tract invasions by Kaposi's sarcoma or lymphomas, or by anaemia. The following nursing care principles apply in such situations:

- Administer medication for the cough or control pulmonary secretions as prescribed.
- Ensure that the patient takes medication regularly in the case of TB. With the help of the patient, identify a family member or friend who will assume the responsibility of ensuring that the patient will take every dose, and complete *the whole course* of TB medication.
- Provide PCP prophylaxis if the patient's CD4 count is lower than 200.
- If the patient is hospitalised, give oxygen when needed.
- Give a bronchodilator for bronchospasm.
- Apply nasopharyngeal or tracheal suction if necessary while the patient is hospitalised.
- Give physiotherapy.
- Encourage patients to drink lots of fluids to dilute secretions.
- Teach patients deep breathing and productive coughing techniques (to drain the lungs of accumulated mucus and bacteria) and encourage them to rest between activities.
- Patients with respiratory problems can breathe more freely when sitting upright in bed (the high or semi-Fowler's position). Help the patient to find the most comfortable position that allows him or her to breathe freely, and use pillows to support the patient in that position.
- Vaporisers and humidifiers can provide symptomatic relief for coughs, and are especially helpful when treating children.
- Alleviate factors such as anxiety that may aggravate respiratory problems.
- Discourage smoking. If a patient insists on smoking, discourage smoking before eating and before, during and immediately after performing activities.

(See the home-based care box 'Respiratory problems' on page 313.)

Home-based care

Respiratory problems

Help patients to cough (and drain the lungs) by massaging or patting the back of the chest over the lungs. Teach patients to hold a pillow or hand tightly over the painful chest or rib area while coughing if they find it painful to cough. Teach them to cover their mouths with a clean cloth when coughing, because many disease-causing agents (e.g. TB bacilli) can be passed on to others through the air. Keep sputum in a covered container and dispose of it safely. If nothing else is available, give the patient a tin containing sand to spit into, and close the tin tightly with a lid.

Soothe an irritating cough with remedies such as tea with sugar or honey, or use safe home-made cough syrups (e.g. three drops of eucalyptus oil on a teaspoon of sugar). If a constant cough interferes with sleep, a cough suppressant can be prescribed for night-time, but not during the day, because it is important to cough and get rid of mucus and disease-causing bacteria.

The following measures might alleviate the distress of respiratory problems:

- Lie with pillows under the head, or with the head of the bed raised on blocks.
- Sit leaning forward with the elbows on the knees or on a low table.
- Make sure that there is always someone with the patient. Difficulty in breathing can be very frightening and distressing.
- Keep the patient in a clear, open space. Ideally, the patient should be near an open window so that he or she does not feel closed in and therefore more anxious.
- Keep the area dust free.
- If a child finds it difficult to breathe, clean the nose if it is congested.
- Don't let people smoke in the patient's room and take care that paraffin stoves do not release fumes into the area.

Danger signs

Advise people to seek help if the sick person has a cough or difficulty in breathing, and if:

- sudden high fever develops;
- the person is in severe pain or discomfort;
- the colour of the sputum changes to grey, yellow or green;
- the sputum has blood in it; or
- the cough persists for more than three weeks, especially if accompanied by the spitting up of blood, pain in the chest, difficulty in breathing, and night sweats (TB may be the cause and should be treated immediately).

In children (particularly those younger than five) respiratory infections can be very serious. Children should be brought to a clinic or health care professional immediately if they are:

- breathing with difficulty through the mouth or wheezing audibly;
- breathing faster than usual; or
- unable to drink because of their breathing problems.

Circulatory impairment

Circulatory impairment may be caused by factors such as pressure on body parts or by immobility. Circulation problems should be suspected if any of the following signs are visible: oedema or swelling of extremities, ulceration or skin breakdown, weak pulses and a cool skin temperature.

- Stimulate circulation by massaging the skin regularly with lotion.
- Encourage the patient to be active. If the patient is bedridden, passive exercises should be performed and the patient should be turned every two hours.
- Elevate the extremities (e.g. the legs).
- Avoid pressure on the extremities from cushions, heavy blankets or tight-fitting clothes.
- A bedridden child who has a severe chronic illness should be held in someone's lap as often as possible. Not only does this improve circulation and avoid bedsores, it also gives the child the love and attention that he or she needs.

Oedema (swelling)

HIV-positive people often have symptoms of oedema because of HIV infection, Kaposi's sarcoma, or other opportunistic infections. Intervention and health teaching should include compliance with the following measures:

- Avoid excessive sodium (salt) intake. Read the labels on canned products and substitute other (non-salt) spices for salt. Salt substitutes that do not contain salt are sold in most health shops.
- Keep the swollen areas (e.g. the legs) above the level of the heart, but take care not to restrict blood flow by placing pillows at pressure points such as those behind the knees.
- Avoid tight-fitting clothes and discourage the patient from crossing his or her ankles or knees.
- Examine the skin over the swollen areas regularly for circulation and skin discolorations or breakdown.

Home-based care

Swelling

If a person experiences swelling of the legs, raise the legs or other swollen parts on pillows, or raise the foot of the bed on blocks. Take care not to restrict blood flow.

Genital problems and sexually transmitted infections

Opportunistic infections of the genital area, including certain sexually transmitted infections, are common in both men and women with Aids. These infections can cause pain and discomfort. Genital problems can present as an unusual discharge (mucus or a pus-like substance) from the vagina, the urethral opening or the penis; open sores or ulcers in the genital, groin or rectal areas (which sometimes start as blisters or a rash in or around the genital area); warts in the genital area or around the anus; and swollen glands in the groin. (For more information on STIs see 'Sexually transmitted infections and HIV: a deadly combination' on page 53.) People with STIs are usually not hospitalised. The home-based caregiver should follow the principles and advice listed below when looking after a patient with an STI (WHO, 1993):

- Seek treatment for STIs from a health care professional or clinic immediately. Antibiotics can cure most STIs completely.
- The patient should abstain from sex until the STI is healed. Thereafter a condom should be used for every sexual contact. It is dangerous for someone who is already infected with HIV to be exposed to other sexually transmitted infections.
- Women with an abnormal vaginal discharge should keep the vulva and anal area clean by washing with water and a mild, non-abrasive soap. The affected area should be kept dry between washings.
- Women should avoid washing out or flushing the vagina (douche), or putting anything (e.g. antiseptics, leaves, herbs) inside the vagina, unless advised to do so by a health care professional. The practice of dry sex should be avoided.
- Open genital sores should be washed with soap and water and they should be kept dry between washings.
- If herpes is diagnosed, advise the person to bathe the affected area with a salt solution (one teaspoon of ordinary cooking salt in half a litre of clean water) every two or three hours. Keep the area dry between bathing, and apply calamine lotion, talcum or starch powder.
- For candidiasis (vaginal thrush), apply gentian violet (one or two teaspoons of gentian violet crystals dissolved in a litre of clean water) to the affected areas.
- Plain yoghurt is very effective in the treatment of vaginal thrush. Rub plain yoghurt on any red areas or dip a tampon in the yoghurt and insert it in the vagina twice a day.
- Women with vaginal thrush should follow the 'candida diet' and avoid all foods and beverages containing yeast (e.g. bread and beer) and sugar.
- Women with vaginal thrush should not wear tights or nylon panties, only cotton panties.
- A rash on the penis or under the foreskin can be treated by soaking the penis in a dilute salt and water solution. Dissolve a teaspoon of salt in a glass or jam jar of water; pull back the foreskin; put the penis in the water and soak for five minutes. Repeat two or three times a day. If the salt solution does not work, repeat the procedure with a gentian violet

solution. Ask for advice from a health care professional if the condition does not clear up in three or four days.
- Loss of menstruation and irregular bleeding are common in women with Aids. If a woman misses one or two periods she should go to the clinic to be examined to establish the cause. Women who have stopped menstruating should be supported emotionally, because the loss of menstruation often represents a loss of femininity, of motherhood, of a sense of meaning and of self-esteem. This may cause a woman to feel sad and depressed.

Home-based care

Sexually transmitted infections (STIs)

People with HIV/Aids and their families should seek professional medical help when they suspect that they may have an STI; if they experience difficulty or pain in passing urine; if they have genital warts, genital ulcers, unusual vaginal discharge that is foul-smelling, itchy, green, yellow or grey in colour; if a woman develops pain in her lower abdomen (particularly if it is accompanied by a fever); if a woman's periods stop or become irregular; if there is a discharge from the penis; and if there is swelling and/or pain in the scrotum. Most STIs (except those caused by viruses) can be cured with antibiotics and should be treated as soon as possible. Take the steps listed on page 314 to manage sexually transmitted infections in home-based care.

Pain

Some people in the later stages of Aids may have continuous pain, and others may have pain only occasionally. Pain may have many causes, including immobility, infections such as herpes zoster (shingles), swelling of the extremities (caused by Kaposi's sarcoma or heart problems), headaches (sometimes associated with encephalitis or meningitis), lesions caused by Kaposi's sarcoma, pain of the oral, rectal or vaginal mucous membranes due to opportunistic infections such as herpes simplex or thrush, muscle aches, chest and abdominal conditions, ulcerations and surgical wounds, and peripheral neuropathy. This last condition is caused when the HI virus infects the nerve cells and causes extreme pain in the lower extremities. Depression and anxiety often accompany a patient's physical pain. Counselling and exploring fears, worries or concerns with the patient may help relieve pain. Pain should be dealt with in the following ways:

- Attempt to diagnose and treat the actual cause of the pain (e.g. abdominal cramps, constipation, headache, sleep problems). Don't assume that all pain is due to the HIV infection alone.
- Pain management should follow the following guidelines: by mouth, by the clock and by the ladder (Evian, 2003):
  - *By mouth*: Pain medication should be given orally if possible, because good absorption is assured and it avoids the complications of injections.
  - *By the clock*: Pain medication should be given regularly as prescribed (e.g. every 4, 6 or 8 hours) to prevent the pain, and not only when the patient is complaining of pain. Regular pain treatment can help people feel that they have control over their pain, and they will feel reassured if they take the medicine before the pain becomes too great.
  - *By the ladder*: Pain medication should be increased in a step-by-step manner. Start with the mildest non-opioid drugs first: for example, aspirin, paracetamol or ibuprofen. If these do not relieve the pain, go up the ladder to moderate medication, or to the weaker opioids such as codeine and aspirin (Codis), codeine and paracetamol (Paracodol), codeine by itself or dihydrocodeine (DF118). If the pain persists, try the stronger opioids, such as dextropropoxyphene (Doloxene). Finally move to the top step of the ladder and ease the patient's pain with the strongest opioids such as morphine. Morphine is the most commonly used strong opioid analgesic and it should not be withheld from Aids patients with pain. This is not the time to debate possible addiction! Also note that therapeutic dosages of morphine do not cause respiratory depression. The correct mor-

Enrichment

Notes on the use of medication

Home-based caregivers should make sure that their clients know how to take their medication. It is always a good idea to give clients and their families written instructions on how to take the medication. If they cannot read, someone can always be found to read it for them. Pictures can also be used to remind people who cannot read when to take their medication. The World Health Organization, for example, recommends the following format (WHO, 1993:34–135):

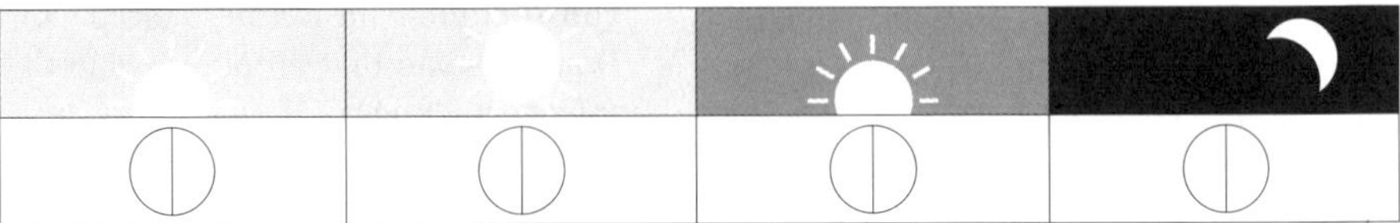

This picture means one tablet four times a day: one at sunrise, one at noon, one at sunset, and one in the middle of the night.

This picture means half a tablet three times a day: one at sunrise, one at noon, and one in the middle of the night.

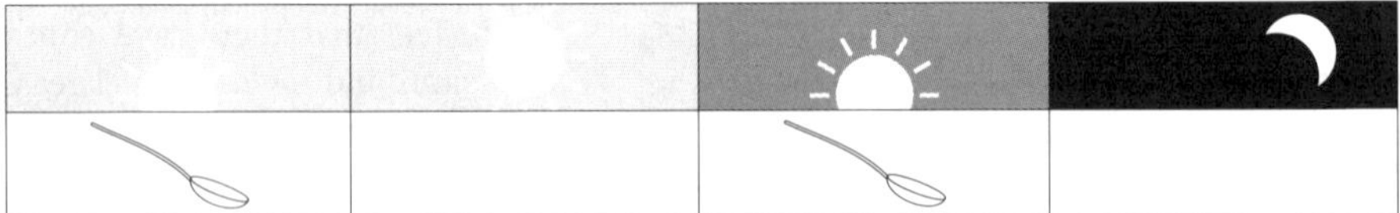

This picture means one teaspoonful twice a day: one at sunrise and one at sunset.

Advice for giving medication to children:

- Liquid medicines can be squirted slowly into the side of the child's mouth with a dropper or syringe, or poured from a spoon.
- Always praise a child after he or she has taken medicine.
- If the medicine tastes unpleasant, warn the child in advance.
- Coat the child's mouth with peanut butter or use chocolate milk if he or she has to swallow a bitter medication.
- If a pill cannot be swallowed whole, crush it and mix it with the smallest possible amount of something the child likes to eat. Do not hide medicine in food, because the child may begin to refuse food.
- If the child vomits immediately after taking a medicine, give the dose again. But if vomiting occurs twenty minutes or longer after taking the medicine, do not repeat the dose.

(Evian, 2000; WHO, 1993:136)

phine dose is the dose that relieves the pain and gives the patient the best quality of life.

- Keep in mind that some pain medications, such as codeine- and morphine-containing drugs, cause constipation. Laxatives must be given along with these medications.
- Antiretroviral therapy (ART) may improve the immune status and reverse various HIV-related conditions that cause pain.
- Support a painful joint or limb or immobilise it with a splint such as a plaster slab, wooden plank or rolled up newspaper.
- Give pain medication thirty minutes before carrying out a procedure that may be painful.
- Provide a soft, soothing diet when the patient has oral candidiasis.

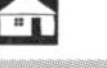

Home-based care

Pain

Keep the environment as calm as possible, talk calmly and in gentle tones to the sick person, avoid bright lights, play soft music, read to the person, apply a cool cloth on the forehead or give a light massage. Ask the patient what you can do to ease the pain. Some patients prefer to be wrapped in a blanket to ease the pain. A child who is in pain should be lifted with the palms of the hands rather than with the fingertips (which may feel like a pinch for a child in pain). Give pain medication regularly as prescribed – even if the patient does not have pain at that stage. If movement of a limb causes pain, make a home-made splint from a plank or a rolled up newspaper to immobilise the limb.

Danger signs

Professional advice should be sought:

- if the pain becomes unbearable or if it is associated with new symptoms such as severe headache or weakness;
- if there is a sudden or recent occurrence of pain in the hands or feet; or
- if there is a persistent headache lasting more than two weeks, a severe headache getting rapidly worse and not relieved by the usual methods of dealing with pain, a headache associated with vomiting or a headache that affects the sick person's ability to think or move.

- Offer comfort measures such as massages and back rubs; warm soaks for painful muscles, joints, feet or legs; ice packs for headaches; and soothing music of the patient's choice.
- Encourage relaxation exercises and teach deep and regular breathing techniques.
- Maintain a quiet and restful environment, and limit the number of visitors.
- Keep the patient company, listen attentively and provide verbal support. Remember that pain is influenced by the patient's emotional and psychological state.
- Identify factors that aggravate the patient's pain and try to eliminate them.
- Encourage mental imagery (the formation of mental pictures). Encourage the patient to imagine or remember a favourite place or event.
- Practise aromatherapy or reflexology.

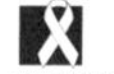

Enrichment

Aspirin, Reye's syndrome and children

Aspirin has been implicated in Reye's syndrome, a rare but serious illness in children and teenagers with chickenpox and flu. Reye's syndrome is triggered by viral infections (such as flu) and it seems that aspirin (which is taken to alleviate the symptoms of the viral infections) plays a role in turning these viral infections into Reye's syndrome. Reye's syndrome is characterised by symptoms such as encephalitis, headache, fever, nausea, vomiting and convulsions (brain and liver cells are attacked). Children and adolescents should take paracetamol rather than aspirin if they have flu or a cold.

Impaired vision

One of the symptoms of Aids is impaired vision or blindness due to eye infections caused by the cytomegalovirus (CMV), Kaposi's sarcoma or lymphoma. The following principles and procedures should be included in a nursing care plan designed to assist patients with impaired vision:

- Orientate patients to their surroundings.
- Do not change the environment.
- Assist patients with feeding; cut up their food and describe the various foods on the plate.
- Do not leave the patient unattended with hot foods, hot plates or hot liquids.

- Do not speak more loudly than you normally do – the patient is not deaf.
- Do not leave patients unattended if they are smoking.
- If the patient is in the hospital, keep the bed in the lowest position, make sure that the patient can use the call system and keep a night light on at night for the convenience of patients with impaired vision.
- Apply general safety measures in the home (do not change the position of furniture, and remove loose rugs and exposed sharp objects).
- Promote independence and help the patient to relearn daily activities such as bathing, dressing and feeding.

General fatigue (tiredness) and weakness

Aids can make a person feel very tired and weak, especially in the later stages. Feelings of fatigue and weakness can be caused by chronic HIV infection, opportunistic infections (particularly respiratory illnesses), diarrhoea and anaemia, and prolonged immobility, poor nutrition and depression.

- Help the patient adjust to his or her limited ability.
- Help patients with their personal hygiene and daily activities such as bathing, dressing and feeding.
- Encourage regular rest.
- Adequate nutrition and nutritional supplements may help fight fatigue. High-energy drinks used by athletes and cyclists may boost energy for short periods of time.
- Encourage frequent repositioning and massage the patient's body with lotion to stimulate circulation (this prevents bedsores).
- If necessary, encourage the use of devices such as a walking stick, crutches, a walker or a wheelchair to prevent injuries from falling.
- Find ways of making activities easier, for example sitting down while washing, dressing or preparing food, and using a bedpan rather than walking to the toilet.
- Keep frequently used personal items within the patient's reach so that the patient does not have to walk to get them.
- If the patient is depressed, get a prescription for appropriate antidepressant medication and counsel the patient.
- Relaxation techniques and guided imagery may decrease anxiety that contributes to weakness and fatigue. Keep the environment safe if the person is weak but moving about, and try not to leave the person alone for long periods.

Home-based care

Tiredness and weakness

Involve the whole family in the care of the patient. Make a list of what the sick person can still do alone in the home, and of those activities for which he or she needs assistance. Ask family members to help with the things that the patient cannot do. Help the patient to learn to accept (and ask for) the help of others. Keep the person involved in the activities and decisions of everyday family life (even though he or she may be very weak). This will give the patient a sense of belonging and being needed.

Danger signs

Professional help should be sought if the patient suddenly becomes very weak (e.g. unable to walk), particularly if there are other symptoms such as high fever, headache or confusion.

The risk of falling

Aids patients can be prone to falling because of factors such as sedation, weakness, mental confusion, severe diarrhoea and hypotension (low blood pressure). Because Aids patients are usually young and accustomed to independence and self-care, they do not always remain aware of their new limitations. Follow the guidelines listed below to limit the risk of falling:

- Ensure that items used regularly are within reach.
- Severe diarrhoea can considerably weaken patients, so persuade patients with diarrhoea not to walk to the toilet but rather to use a bedpan (or a bedside commode if the patient is in a hospital).
- Encourage the use of devices such as a cane (walking stick), crutches or wheelchair to prevent falling injuries.

- Caregivers and patients should be warned that certain medications (such as IV pentamidine, which is used to treat *Pneumocystis carinii* pneumonia) can cause hypotension (low blood pressure). Low blood pressure can lead to serious falls.
- Use bedside rails to protect delirious or weak patients from falling out of bed in the hospital. If it is impossible to safeguard a patient all the time at home, nurse the patient on a mattress on the floor.

Activity

Devise a commode (or portable toilet) for a very weak patient who can get out of bed, but can no longer walk to the outside toilet. Use the following materials to construct your portable toilet: an old chair, a piece of wood, a bucket with a lid, a saw, nails and paint.

Alteration of mental status: confusion and dementia

Some degree of mental confusion (or dementia) is common in people with Aids because of the effect of HIV on the brain. The mental changes can vary from scarcely noticeable to a serious and obvious disability. These may include: an *inability to think clearly* (problems with concentration, memory loss, losing track of conversations or tasks); *changed behaviour* (irritable and uninterested, confused, disorientated, unpredictable, delusional), *loss of strength or coordination* (dropping things, loss of balance and falling, slow movements, shakiness, difficulty in swallowing) and *personality changes* (withdrawal or combativeness and irrational aggression). The care and treatment of a patient with an altered mental state will depend on the problem, and could include any of the following:

- Reassure the patient of your presence, *especially at night*, so as to alleviate fears.
- Modify the home environment for safety and convenience. Remove dangerous objects and medications from the patient's reach.
- Keep the patient orientated with respect to time, place and people by using clocks, a calendar, photographs, night lights, and written schedules of daily routine, dates of appointments and telephone numbers of friends.
- Keep the environment structured. Avoid unnecessary changes in the patient's room or home and keep only familiar objects around the patient.
- Use signs to orientate patients to their surroundings: identify the patient's bedroom, the bathroom and the kitchen with name plates if necessary.
- Try to keep the environment quiet, without sudden loud noises that can startle the patient.
- Explain the changes in the patient's behaviour or cognitive functioning to the patient's family and involve them in his or her care.
- Give the patient only one instruction at a time, and speak in a slow, simple and clear way when giving instructions.
- Ask questions that can be answered with yes or no. Be concrete and specific, and give the patient enough time to respond to questions, directions or conversations.
- Try to interpret the *feelings* the person is trying to express rather than just the words.
- Distract upset or angry patients by changing the subject, switching on the radio, giving them manual tasks (such as folding clothes) or removing them from the upsetting environment. Soft music can be very calming.
- Ensure that the patient gets enough food and fluids, and is kept clean and dry.
- Zidovudine (AZT) is very effective in reversing Aids dementia for a period of time.
- Talk about the distant past. Every person should have *some* happy memories of things that happened long ago. Help the patient recall these happy memories by skilful questioning. Such memories should give the patient some pleasure. (Do *not* allow the patient to dwell on traumatic, upsetting or disconcerting memories from the past.) When the patient is hospitalised, encourage the family and friends to bring favourite objects from home to the hospital. These will make the environment more familiar and less threatening.
- Protect the patient from injury during hospitalisation. Put the bell within easy reach; keep

side rails up and the bed in a low position; instruct the patient to wear shoes and slippers with non-skid soles; and keep an eye on a patient who is smoking or shaving.

Don'ts

- Don't expect patients to perform complex or demanding tasks. (Give them one thing at a time to do.)
- Don't argue with patients when they are confused. You will *not* convince them and they will only become even more upset.
- Don't challenge delusions or fantasies; they are usually harmless. If, for some practical reason, you have to cast doubt on fantasies, do so kindly and reassuringly.
- Don't talk to the person as though he or she were a child.
- Don't give the person choices, because having to make decisions can be very confusing for people in this state.

Home-based care

Confusion and dementia

Take measures to prevent accidents in the home. Pay careful attention to open fires or boiling water; provide walking sticks or walkers for people who are weak or who tend to lose their balance when they walk; remove loose and potentially dangerous objects in the home; keep walkways clear; do not rearrange the furniture; store poisonous or toxic substances safely out of reach; keep medicines out of reach and give them according to the prescribed schedule only; install handrails or put a securely positioned and stabilised chair in a shower or bath; store sharp objects such as knives, scissors, razors and saws safely and out of reach; and try not to leave the sick person unattended for long periods.

Danger signs

Pay careful attention to the following danger signs and take appropriate action if:

- there are sudden changes in the ability to move or think, especially when accompanied by a high fever, headache or difficulty in breathing;
- the patient begins to manifest serious mental or personality changes; or
- the patient becomes unmanageable at home.

Activity

Develop a weekly practical session to teach volunteers involved in home-based care to become skilled in the following activities:

- bed-bathing a bedridden patient;
- bathing a baby;
- positioning and lifting a patient in bed; and
- positioning a patient in the semi-Fowler's position.

17.4 CARE OF PATIENTS WITH A SENSE OF SOCIAL ISOLATION

Patients with HIV infection and Aids face many problems and stressors, and these may cause them to withdraw physically and emotionally from social contact. People with HIV/Aids are often stigmatised by society; they may be forced to reveal hidden lifestyles to family, friends and co-workers; they may be rejected by loved ones; and they may have to face and cope with many serious losses.

Because of these unfortunate experiences, HIV-positive people commonly experience emotions such as anxiety, anger, shame, fear, depression, loneliness and a desire to withdraw from social interaction. The infection control measures at home or in the hospital may further contribute to the patient's feelings of isolation. Health care professionals and other caregivers should be sensitive to the HIV-positive person's needs, and they should be able to notice when the person's social interactions deteriorate. The following ways of decreasing the patient's sense of social isolation should be applied whenever possible (Smeltzer & Bare, 1992):

- Assess the patient's usual (currently normal) levels of social interaction as early as possible so as to provide a baseline for monitoring changes in behaviour.
- Obtain an understanding from the patient of how he or she coped with illnesses and major life stressors in the past.
- Encourage patients to *express* their feelings of isolation and aloneness. Assure them that such feelings are not unique or abnormal, and certainly nothing to feel guilty or ashamed about.

- Provide information about how to protect themselves as well as others from HIV infection and re-infection. This may give patients the kind of confidence they need to stop avoiding social contact.
- Assure patients, family and friends that HIV cannot be spread through casual contact.
- Help the patient to explore and identify resources for support and mechanisms for coping.
- Encourage the patient to telephone family, friends and Aids support groups.
- If possible, identify and eliminate specific barriers to social contact.
- Encourage social interaction with family, friends and co-workers.
- Encourage patients to keep themselves occupied with their usual day-to-day activities.

17.5 PALLIATIVE CARE OF AIDS PATIENTS

Palliative care is active, compassionate and comprehensive care that comforts and supports patients whose disease is no longer responsive to curative treatment. The purpose of palliative care is to meet the physical, psychological, emotional, social and spiritual needs of the individual and family while remaining sensitive to personal, cultural and religious values, beliefs and practices.

Palliative care is planned and delivered by a multidisciplinary team that includes the patient, the family, the caregivers and other health and social service providers, and it should always take into account the needs of the *whole* person. Palliative care includes medical and nursing care, social and emotional support, counselling and spiritual care. It emphasises living, encourages hope, and helps people to make the most of each day.

Palliative caregivers must treat patients with respect and acceptance, acknowledge their right to privacy and confidentiality, and respond caringly to their individual needs. An important part of palliative care is giving the family and caregivers the opportunity, support and encouragement to work through their own emotions and grief (Canadian Palliative Care Association, 1995: 12; WHO, 2000a:8–1).

Enrichment

Should Aids patients be isolated in a special room?

Patients with HIV infection or Aids should never be isolated in a special room merely because they are HIV positive. There is no way in which an HIV-positive patient can infect other people in the house, or other patients in the hospital ward, if the prescribed universal precautions are observed. Isolation of a patient with HIV/Aids *is*, however, appropriate if large-scale contamination by blood and body fluids is expected, if the patient is severely immune-depressed and needs to be isolated to protect him or her against secondary infections, if privacy is needed or preferred for one reason or another, or if the patient has another communicable disease such as TB. If the patient has pulmonary (lung) TB or multi-drug-resistant TB, he or she should be accommodated in a single room in the hospital or at home until the TB is no longer transmissible. If a patient with HIV infection or Aids is placed in a room or ward with other patients, the health care professional or home-based caregiver should ensure that the other patients in the room are not suffering from immune depression (because this will make them more susceptible to opportunistic infections). They should also ensure that the other patients do not have any infections or diseases that can be transmitted to the patient with Aids. Isolation of an Aids patient in the home should be very carefully considered because it may seriously impact on the person's quality of life.

The purpose of palliative care is to:

- affirm the right of the patient and the family to participate in informed discussions and make treatment choices;
- affirm life while regarding dying as a normal process;
- neither hasten nor postpone death;
- provide relief from pain and other distressing symptoms;
- treat opportunistic infections and provide antiretroviral therapy if possible;
- integrate the psychological and the spiritual aspects of care;
- provide a support system to help patients live as actively and meaningfully as possible until death;
- provide a support system to help the family and loved ones cope during the patient's illness and during their own bereavement; and

- help patients die in comfort, with dignity and in keeping with their expressed wishes (WHO, 2000a:8–2).

It is very difficult to decide when to stop active treatment and begin preparing the patient and his or her family for dying. This decision should never be taken by the health care professional alone, but always in collaboration with the patient (if possible), the family and the loved ones. Palliative care takes over when there is no reasonable chance of improvement; when medical treatment is no longer effective; when the side effects of treatment outweigh the benefits; when the patient does not want to continue with treatment; when a child's condition becomes unbearable for the child and for the family; or when the body's vital organs begin to fail.

If possible, the patient should make a choice about where to die. While many people prefer to die at home, others might choose a hospice or terminal care facility. Many hospices can provide trained staff to care for dying patients and their families at home. The support of the local community should be mobilised to help the caregivers (usually the women in the family) to cope with the pressure of caring for a dying patient in the home. (The spiritual, emotional and psychological support of the dying patient and his or her family are discussed in chapter 13.)

17.6 CONCLUSION

Tristano Palermino, a patient with Aids, gave the following advice to health care professionals who care for patients dying with Aids:

> As in life, people facing death have a right to do it their own way. Do not pry or force patients to feel feelings or 'face' death. It's a disservice to force patients to give up their denial or to give cheery false hopes. Sometimes I just want someone to listen. Sometimes I do not want to talk about my medical treatments. Sometimes I do not want to talk at all. If you stay in the moment, contribute what you can, and permit the patient to do the same, you cannot fail. I thank you for your commitment to helping all sick people.
>
> (Palermino, 1988)

chapter 18 Care for the Caregiver

And who will heal my wounds?

And when the morning was white in the east –
the morning star a faint ghost above the trees
he stood up and laid down the heavy fear of death
like one, cured from a wound, still trembling . . .
rising from his fire to engage the beast.

I often have to give eight HIV-positive results in one day. I know most of these people. They are my neighbours or go to the same church. Some days it becomes so hard, that I send people away by telling them that their results are not yet back – in the hope that they will come back another day when I am off duty . . .

(A 45-year-old nurse working in a community clinic in the Free State province, South Africa.)

Nothing can be more stressful and draining on the caregiver's resources than caring for or counselling patients or clients with HIV infection or Aids. Caregivers and patients are faced with frightening issues such as the vulnerability of youth, continuous physical and psychological deterioration, their own mortality, the fear of contagion and death. If caregivers do not also learn how to care for *themselves*, they will not survive the onslaught of the Aids pandemic.

18.1 WHO ARE THE CAREGIVERS?

A caregiver in the HIV/Aids context is anyone (professional, lay or family) involved in taking care of the physical, psychological, emotional and/or spiritual needs of a person infected or affected by HIV/Aids. In the formal health sector, caregivers are usually nurses, counsellors and social workers, but Africa has so many Aids patients that hospitalisation or formal care is not always an option. The enormous need for care leaves the community with no choice but to care for its own sick members. A UNAIDS (2000a) study carried out in Uganda and in South Africa found that the caregivers who battle with HIV/Aids in their communities comprise the following groups and individuals:

- At the family level, the burden of care is predominantly borne by *women and girls*. Men are also increasingly willing (or forced) to care for sick partners. However, the least acknowledged caregivers within the home are *children*. When one parent dies, there is often no one else to look after the other parent when he or she falls ill.

- The backbone of community care programmes for people with Aids are *volunteers*. Some are informal volunteers such as friends, neighbours and church members, but most are formal volunteers working for Aids care programmes, recruited, trained and supervised by the organisations they work for.
- *Health care professionals* (mostly nurses and welfare workers) work with Aids patients in hospitals and clinics and on a home-based care basis. One of their responsibilities is to recruit, train and support volunteer caregivers in the community.
- Voluntary counselling and testing (VCT) services have drawn many health care professionals and lay counsellors to the field of HIV/Aids, and they find it a heavy burden to have to tell clients that they are HIV positive.
- *Traditional healers* are widely consulted throughout Africa. But because their importance within communities is often not officially recognised, they care for people with HIV/Aids without training or support from the formal health services.

Caregivers are often not trained to care for patients with Aids, and those who are trained carry a very heavy load. Because society cannot afford to lose its caregivers to stress and burnout, it is important for us to take good care of our caregivers.

18.2 STRESS WITHIN THE CONTEXT OF HIV/AIDS

The word 'stress' is derived from the Latin verb *stringere*, meaning to 'tighten up' (Weybrew, 1992). While a certain amount of stress is necessary for us to function, too much stress can have a negative impact on our lives, our work and our relationships. Although there are many different definitions of 'stress', it can broadly be defined as the perception of being unable to cope with an internal or external expectation or demand (Huxley Consulting, 2001). Caring for people living with HIV/Aids can be extremely stressful, and caregivers and counsellors must recognise their own stress factors and deal with them in a self-caring way to prevent burnout.

Causes of stress

Much of the stress experienced by caregivers is inherent in the nature of the work itself – dealing with an incurable and extremely cruel disease that kills mostly young people and causes terrible suffering. The following causes of stress and burnout in health care professionals, counsellors and volunteers caring for Aids patients in Africa can be identified (Miller, 2000; UNAIDS report, 2000a):

- *Financial hardship.* Aids in Africa is often concentrated among the very poor. A training officer in Uganda said the following: 'The messages about living positively, eating well, looking after your health, can seem cruel when people are struggling to bring in *any* food to the home' (UNAIDS, 2000a:28). The caregivers themselves are often in a similar position. 'We go to see hungry people and we are hungry too,' said a volunteer in KwaZulu-Natal.
- *Stigma associated with HIV and Aids.* HIV/Aids stigmatises infected people *and* uninfected people working in the field. This 'secondary stigma' can have a powerful effect on the caregiver's status with family, friends and the public at large. Being avoided because he or she works with people with Aids can be very stressful for a caregiver. Ostracism of this kind can deprive the caregiver of much-needed support.
- *Secrecy and fear of disclosure* among people with Aids make the task of caring for Aids patients very difficult. If the diagnosis has to be kept secret, it is difficult or impossible to get outside help. Caregivers from outside cannot easily pass on knowledge or health care skills to family members if the family members don't know that the patient has Aids. So the caregiver has to carry the responsibility alone. It is also impossible for the caregiver to prepare the family for death if the Aids diagnosis is a secret.

- *Over-involvement with people with Aids and their families.* Caregivers often experience stress because they are unable to be there for their clients when needed; because they can't provide needs such as food; because they feel inadequate and guilty when they can do no more to help; because of feelings of loss and sadness after the death of a client; and because of a lasting anxiety about the family left behind, especially if these are children.
- *Setting professional boundaries* is often difficult in traditional communities where the extended family system means that a person is rarely a stranger in a village or community. 'From your name people can see what clan you are from, and there is always someone to whom you are related by clan.' It is not always possible to maintain clear boundaries in a traditional setting where people are very poor; where they may not have medical, financial or social support; and where they may be rejected by loved ones. In her study on the needs of HIV/Aids lay counsellors within economically disadvantaged communities, Nefale (2004) found that counsellors often had to get involved with funeral arrangements of clients; care for orphaned children; and fill other unforeseen practical roles. Involvement in these activities constitutes the 'bending of the frame', which emotionally burdens the caregiver and can lead to emotional distancing or over-identification.
- *Personal identification with the suffering of people with Aids.* Because many caregivers are HIV positive themselves, they observe at first hand while caring for people with Aids how they too will become sick and die.
- *Bereavement overload and grief.* Caregivers seldom allow themselves time to grieve for their patients when they die. There is usually no time to work through a patient's death because the caregiver has to move on to care for another critically sick patient.
- *Difficult patients.* Many caregivers who look after sick family members experience stress because the sick family member may often be moody, uncooperative, and hostile. On the other hand, patients may feel hurt, angry, dependent and vulnerable because Aids has put them in this vulnerable position.
- *The terrible plight of children.* Caregivers often do not know how to care for or talk to the children who are left behind.
- The *workload* may be very demanding, and caregivers may experience stress because of a lack of 'space' and privacy in their work.
- *Professional and role* issues may frustrate health care professionals and volunteers. These include the following:
    - They do not get the necessary support from superiors.
    - They experience role ambiguity due to role expansion: they now have to counsel or care for Aids patients although this was not previously part of their duties.
    - They feel that they work in isolation.
    - They don't have a voice in decisions that affect them and their work.
    - Finances for volunteer workers and important prevention projects are often drastically cut.
    - Creativity is discouraged because innovative ideas and suggestions are not implemented.
    - They have too little autonomy and responsibility.
    - The necessary supportive infrastructures and supervision are not always in place.
    - There is not enough time to do what needs to be done.
    - Training, skills and preparation for the work are often inadequate.
    - They do not feel comfortable in addressing issues of patient sexuality.
    - They might fear HIV contagion due to occupational exposure.
    - There may be a lack of medication and health care material, or of the resources for observing universal precautions.
    - Referral mechanisms are not available.
    - Valuable workers resign out of frustration, leaving those who stay behind with a bigger burden.
- *Family caregivers* also suffer from isolation, the effect of HIV and Aids on their personal relationships and family dynamics, insecurity

and fear about the future, difficulty in disclosing to or in communicating with children, and difficulty in facing bereavement.

18.3 BURNOUT

Burnout or role stress may be defined as 'a syndrome of physical and emotional exhaustion, involving the development of a negative self-concept, negative job attitudes, and loss of concern and feelings for clients' (Pines & Maslach, 1978:233). The common approach to an understanding of burnout is that it is an end stage in the stress cycle (Oosthuizen, 2002). A person usually progresses through various stages, starting with idealistic enthusiasm and ending with frustration, apathy and emotional exhaustion, due to the pressures that a disease such as Aids places on them. Because of their personalities (a sense of commitment to the well-being of others), health care workers tend to have high expectations of themselves: they find it difficult to set limits to the demands placed upon them, and they are inclined to lose themselves in their work. Confronted by the realities of Aids, health care workers can become disillusioned, which is often the first step to burnout.

Burnout usually has three components: emotional exhaustion (characterised by a lack of energy and the feeling that emotional resources have been depleted), depersonalisation (treating patients or clients as if they were objects), and feelings of low personal accomplishment and negativity. Stress and burnout in the workplace and in the personal lives of caregivers manifests in the following ways:

- loss of interest in and commitment to work, and a lack of job satisfaction;
- unpunctuality and neglect of duties;
- feelings of inadequacy, helplessness and guilt;
- loss of confidence, diminished self-esteem;
- a tendency to withdraw from clients and from colleagues;
- loss of sensitivity in dealing with clients or patients; referring to clients in a dehumanised or impersonal way (which may include sick humour);
- avoidance of clients or limiting the time spent with them, and frequent and earlier-than-necessary referral of clients to other health care professionals;
- indifference to the suffering of others; experiencing boredom with clients, and seeing all clients as being alike;
- loss of quality work – working harder but accomplishing less;
- irritability, tension, tearfulness, loss of concentration, sleeplessness, chronic exhaustion, depression and feelings of distress;
- vulnerability to all kinds of illnesses and psychosomatic symptoms;
- deteriorating relationships with colleagues and friends; tensions and distress in personal life; difficulty in getting on with people;
- feeling isolated from colleagues;
- feelings of being oppressed by the system or institution;
- increased use of alcohol or drugs in order to cope at home or at work;
- feelings that the work lacks meaning and that efforts are wasted; and
- the decision to leave the job or profession.

Recovery from burnout is a process that could last for a number of years, and it is therefore important for caregivers to recognise the symptoms of burnout and to take steps to protect themselves from its debilitating effects. The enrichment box 'Burnout checklist' on page 327 lists the most common symptoms associated with burnout (based on Miller, 2000:51). If you experience a significant number of these symptoms it may be an indication that you should slow down a bit.

The burnout checklist is a helpful tool for caregivers to assess themselves for signs of exhaustion and to find ways to alleviate the pressure before it results in burnout. It is also a useful benchmark for caregivers whose energy levels are still high. They can compare their functioning six months to a year later. We also have to look out for our colleagues, and it may be helpful to point out the symptoms to them if we see changes in their behaviour.

Enrichment

Burnout checklist

Which (if any) of the following are you currently experiencing, or have you experienced in the past?

Physical
- [ ] Frequent headaches
- [ ] Change in appetite
- [ ] Feelings of exhaustion or fatigue
- [ ] Insomnia or sleeplessness
- [ ] Muscle aches or general aches and pains
- [ ] Unable to shake off colds or bronchial complaints
- [ ] Gastrointestinal disturbances
- [ ] Shortness of breath
- [ ] Skin complaints

Emotional
- [ ] Anxiety
- [ ] Frustration
- [ ] Discouragement
- [ ] Touchy and irritable
- [ ] Bad temper
- [ ] Easily moved to tears
- [ ] Marked sadness
- [ ] Screaming and shouting
- [ ] Unwarranted suspicion and paranoia
- [ ] Avoiding commitment to caring
- [ ] Lethargic
- [ ] Pessimism and hopelessness
- [ ] Boredom and cynicism

Behavioural
- [ ] Increased alcohol and/or drug use
- [ ] Inflexibility in problem-solving
- [ ] Impulsivity and acting out
- [ ] Self-righteousness
- [ ] Withdrawal from non-colleagues
- [ ] Decrease in libido

Spiritual
- [ ] Emptiness
- [ ] Loss of meaning
- [ ] Doubt (of self and/or life)
- [ ] Need to prove yourself
- [ ] Lack of forgiveness (from others and/or for others)

Mental
- [ ] Dull senses
- [ ] Forgetfulness
- [ ] Confusion
- [ ] Poor concentration
- [ ] Negative attitude

Relational
- [ ] Isolation
- [ ] Resentment
- [ ] Distrust
- [ ] Loneliness
- [ ] Hiding
- [ ] Marital and relationship problems

18.4 MANAGING STRESS AND BURNOUT

It is important for the self-preservation of caregivers and for their emotional survival that they should take care of themselves. Employers should also do everything possible to support their employees in the fulfilment of their duties. A first requirement in supporting caregivers is to formally acknowledge that their work is inherently stressful and that feelings of distress are a legitimate reaction to their experiences rather than signs of personal weakness or lack of professionalism. Bottled-up feelings almost inevitably lead to burnout, and caregivers need to feel confident and free to express doubts and distress, and to seek timely help. The following skills may help caregivers and counsellors to cope with the pressure of working with HIV-positive people (Brouard, 2002; Oosthuizen, 2002; Skovholt, 2001;* UNAIDS, 2000a; Van Dyk, 1999).

Re-evaluation of expectations and performance goals

It is important for caregivers and counsellors to know themselves. They should take time to think

* Material in this chapter credited to Skovholt, 2001 is based on material from Thomas M. Skovholt, *The Resilient Practitioner: Burnout Prevention and Self-Care Strategies for Counselors, Therapists, Teachers,* published by Allyn and Bacon, Boston, MA. Copyright © 2001 by Pearson Education. Reprinted by permission of the publisher.

about what they can realistically expect from themselves and their clients, and re-evaluate their performance goals accordingly. If they feel that they do not reach these goals, they should establish new, more obtainable goals. Caregivers should, for example, accept that the emphasis in caring for Aids patients is on *caring* and not on *curing*. Caregivers should learn not to take responsibility for things they cannot help or alter. They should know that they can only do their best, and no more, and that they are not perfect. The message that 'bad things happen and it is not your fault' is very important. Skovholt (2001) gives the following tips in this regard:

- Relish the small '*I made a difference*' victories. Sometimes, if we expect less in terms of a client's gain, we can be more satisfied. This does not mean becoming mediocre, but ensuring that your expectations are realistic.
- Ensure that you have both long-term and short-term goals in your work with clients. In this manner, you may feel rewarded or have a sense that progress is being made along the way towards achieving your long-term vision.
- Learn how to work for self-confirmation rather than relying on external forms of validation.
- Be the '*good enough practitioner'*. Accept the fact that you cannot give your clients or patients 100% of your effort 100% of the time. It may be a wonderful fantasy, but it will lead only to exhaustion and burnout. Rather follow the style of the veteran athlete in knowing when to sprint and when to jog. In the words of Kushner (cited in Skovholt, 2001:140): 'If we are afraid to make a mistake because we have to maintain the pretence of perfection . . . we will never be brave enough to try anything new or anything challenging. We will never learn; we will never grow.'

Development of self-awareness

Know yourself and critically evaluate yourself and your motives from time to time. Ask yourself why you are in the helping profession. We often enter into the caring role because of our own needs for appreciation and worth. While the interaction with clients and patients may contribute to the satisfaction of our own needs, they may also frustrate our needs at times. This dynamic will have a negative impact on the relationship with the client. We therefore need to explore our own needs in becoming caregivers. Personal therapy and supervision provide valuable contexts for exploring these issues.

Self-care

Caregivers are responsible for their own physical and mental health, and they should look after themselves in the following ways:

- Develop and maintain *a healthy lifestyle* in order to build up physical resistance to stress. A balanced diet and sufficient exercise, rest and sleep are important. Also try to change harmful habits such as smoking and heavy drinking.
- *Nurture yourself* and take time out to do things that you enjoy, like walking, listening to music, or reading.
- Actively search for ways to *cope with stress* that work for you, and use these methods of coping. Relaxation exercises, breathing exercises, visualisation, imagery and meditation work very well in coping with stress.
- *Set a strict boundary between your professional and your personal life.* Force yourself to forget the suffering of your patients when you close the door to go home. Spend time with your family and try not to think of Aids at all.
- Maintain a balance between *identification* with a patient and *over-identification*: empathise but do not lose objectivity. Of course this cannot apply to family caregivers who look after their own sick loved ones, or to professionals who close the door after a patient only to go to somebody at home who is also HIV positive.
- *Work on your relationships.* Learn to be assertive but not aggressive, communicate effectively, resolve conflict and solve problems constructively.
- *Learn how to be professional, but also how to be playful, have fun, tell jokes and laugh.* This helps to introduce positive emotions into an

environment filled with heavy or negative emotion, and it brings emotional balance.

- *Understand the reality of early anxiety.* If you are new to the counselling relationship, accept that feeling anxious is natural to all of us when we start out on any new venture. It is not because you are incapable. Be kind to yourself and give yourself time.
- *Learn to set boundaries, create limits and say no to unreasonable helping requests.* To really take care of yourself and your clients or patients, you have to learn how to pace yourself so that you can be there at the critical moments. Find your own balance in knowing how much to give. If it is hard for you to say no, explore the reasons for it. Do you fear not being liked if you are not being all things for all people?
- *Invest constantly in a Personal Renewal Process.* The feelings of sadness and loss that you may encounter in your work with HIV/Aids patients or clients must be balanced with experiences in your personal life that generate feelings of happiness and peace. It becomes a necessary process of self-renewal to create these experiences in your personal life.
- Keep a *stress diary* to find out what causes your stress; to gain insight into the level that is optimal for you; to see how you function under pressure; and to test the effectiveness of your stress management strategies.
- *Manage your environment* in such a way that it does not cause undue stress. If you feel overwhelmed by what has to be done, make a list of chores that must be done and prioritise them. Amend the list as needed.
- Do not be afraid to *accept the offers of others to help.* They may need to do this for themselves.
- *Take care of your soul.* Meditate and pray, nurture your spirit and stay connected to yourself and to others.
- *Express your grief.* Some of the most difficult times emotionally for caregivers is when patients or clients die. The death of a patient evokes a sense of personal loss in the caregiver. Grieve and cry without shame if you need to. Explore your personal and cultural mechanisms and rituals for dealing with death, and use them.
- Take an *Aids holiday* during which you do not think about HIV/Aids at all.

Using support systems

Caregivers cannot cope with the tremendous burden of HIV/Aids unless they have personal and organisational support. Caregivers should create and use personal support systems, for example a spouse or partner to whom they can talk. Caregivers should also be encouraged to talk and listen to each other. The following tips may be helpful:

- Make use of *professional venting.* Venting to a colleague about your frustrating experiences is cathartic and can cleanse or purge your emotions. You can 'sweep clean' and continue your work. Note that professional venting differs from complaining or negativity which, in time, will leave you feeling unmotivated. Venting also does not mean gossiping about patients or colleagues. Ensure that confidentiality is never violated in the process of venting.
- *Group support* can be very powerful, and allow colleagues to share concerns, problems and fears. A social support system relieves stress, loneliness, depression and anxiety, and it strengthens the sense of self-worth, trust and life direction. If support groups do not exist, take the initiative and form groups.
- *Support systems* should be put in place for caregivers who look after their own families – a task which is impossible if secrecy and non-disclosure is the norm in a community.
- Be aware of the danger of *one-way caring relationships* in your own personal life. To what extent do you continue to fulfil the role of caregiver in your personal relationships as well? How much (or rather how little) care for your own needs do you ask in return from friends, family or partners? Changing the balance may be difficult and painful, but a greater awareness that you also need support and care is a start.
- Learn to ask for support and assistance when necessary.

Activity

Draw a map of your caring network with yourself at the centre. Draw a solid line to all those relationships and connections in which you are the caregiver personally and professionally. Draw a dotted line to those relationships in which you receive care in return. What are the similarities and differences between the relationships in which you give and receive care? Is there a balance between the care you give and the care you receive?

Organisational support

Managers should consciously try to ensure that every effort is made to keep the stress of their staff within reasonable limits. Volunteer and home-based care organisations, hospitals and clinics cannot afford to lose the caregivers caring for people with Aids. For the sake of their morale and self-confidence, caregivers at every level need to know that their work is recognised and valued, and that they are supported. To support caregivers, the following should be kept in mind.

- Words of praise and thanks from superiors are important to let caregivers know that they are appreciated.
- Frequent meetings between caregivers and supervisors are important to discuss policy and share problems. Management should involve caregivers in decisions, and ask their opinions – they are after all the people working in the field.
- Caregivers should be allowed flexibility and scope to use their own initiative in caring for patients, while having a clear understanding of their duties and the limits of their responsibilities for any client.
- Managers should create a supportive environment for the caregiver to work in by assuring that a good network system is in place. Caregivers should know when and where to refer a client to at all times, and where to go for help themselves.
- The appointment of mentors with counselling skills (e.g. volunteer psychologists) to look after the caregivers working in the front line is very helpful. These mentors should be responsible for the *welfare* of the caregivers, and not for the quality or style of their work.
- Managers of HIV/Aids programmes should ensure that their caregivers receive good salaries and that their weekends and annual leave are respected. In regions where caregivers and their clients are poor, income-generating activities (such as food gardens) should be financed and supported to ensure that caregivers and their clients have food.
- Working in a multidisciplinary team is an effective way of protecting staff from undue stress because it spreads the burden of care and responsibility. For example, it is very helpful to disperse the emotional burden when a patient is dying by extending the team of caregivers who sit with the patient. Family, extended family and volunteers from the church can take turns to sit with and comfort the dying patient. Share the workload, work cooperatively and not competitively, and delegate where you can.
- Training plays a central role in the management of stress and burnout in caregivers. Refresher courses for caregivers and upgrading of skills are very important. Issues of stress, burnout and coping skills should be directly addressed in training sessions. The training needs of caregivers should be identified.

Mentoring and supervision

The term 'mentoring' is sometimes used synonymously with 'supervision', but there are important differences. Supervision refers to a hierarchical managerial situation that implies evaluation of the caregiver. Mentoring involves a supportive and equal relationship without evaluation or assessment. It is strongly recommended that all caregivers and counsellors, whether professional or lay, are mentored by appropriate professional mentors.

The mentor discusses the counsellor's cases with him or her; observes the counsellor in a counselling setting; resolves problems encountered in the counselling setting; assesses situations and issues raised by clients; and applies relevant counselling interventions as required. The South African Department of Health offers the following guidelines for mentors (Guidelines for the care and support of health care workers, 2000).

- Guide the process of case management and ensure that counselling is helpful and not harmful to the client.
- Correct misperceptions and misinterpretations by the counsellor of the problems and issues presented by the client, and give guidance to the counsellor as and when necessary.
- Give specific input around counselling issues and problems encountered.
- Provide the counsellor with continuing education, updates and input relevant to counselling by introducing journal articles, techniques and strategies related to HIV/Aids/STIs and TB.
- Provide input about appropriate interventions as requested by the group.
- Act as a sounding board for the counsellor in terms of perceptions, interpretations and understanding of the issues and problems presented by the client and how these should be addressed.
- Recommend sources of referral to the counsellor and advise the counsellor on when to employ these.

Caregivers and their mentors should ideally get together every second week, or at least once a month. Individual mentoring or exploring counselling experiences in a group is a very important tool in the care for caregivers for the following reasons:

- Mentoring gives *constructive feedback* from peers and mentor(s) by which you can measure your effectiveness as a caregiver or counsellor. This is extremely important, because relying on client improvement in the HIV/Aids context may lead to feelings of defeat and futility.
- Mentoring provides a *safe and holding context* in which to explore personal *growth in self-awareness*. The perspectives of colleagues and mentors can help caregivers to understand why they must care for one another, and how these needs function in their relationships with their clients and patients.
- The dynamics of the care or counselling relationship in the HIV/Aids context are difficult to explain to others who are not involved. Confidentiality requirements also limit the number of people you can talk to. Mentoring is a context in which you can *debrief* yourself (and in so doing *moderate your stress*) with others who share similar experiences to your own and can therefore listen to you in a *supportive* way. In addition, it provides a protected environment in which to discuss your caseload without violating your clients' *confidentiality*.
- Mentoring creates a *context of learning and cross-pollination of ideas*. In sharing your feelings and listening to others' experiences you may learn how to deal with similar situations when confronted with them. If your group includes practitioners from other disciplines you may also *broaden your understanding*.
- Mentoring has a *nurturing* element. Having an hour or more a week during which you take *time out* to reflect and focus allows you to de-stress and re-energise. If self-care is about preventing burnout, then this medium is an important remedy.

18.5 CONCLUSION

It is important for caregivers – nurses, social workers, psychologists, counsellors, volunteer workers and family caregivers – to know themselves; to understand the burden that HIV/Aids places on them; to recognise the signs when they are in psychological trouble; and to know where to find help and how to care for themselves. Only when they can care for themselves will caregivers be able to give quality time to those in their care.

part

5

Legal, Ethical and Policy Issues

INTRODUCTION TO PART 5

South Africa's Constitution guarantees people living with HIV and Aids the same basic human rights and responsibilities as all other citizens of this country. Under no circumstances may employers, health care professionals, teachers or any other person discriminate against people on the grounds of their HIV status.

Chapter 19 discusses the basic rights of people living with HIV/Aids. It examines specific applications of the law in the workplace, in medical settings and in schools and tertiary institutions. The National Policy on Testing for HIV, the Health Professions Council Guidelines on the management of patients with HIV infection or Aids, the Code of Good Practice on key aspects of HIV/Aids in the workplace and employment, and the National Policy on HIV/Aids for Learners and Educators are summarised in this chapter. Questions frequently asked by caregivers and counsellors and other relevant comments are highlighted. Recommendations are made on how to develop effective management and policy plans that take the needs of HIV-positive people into account.

Learning outcomes

After completing Part 5, you should:

- understand what basic rights the South African Constitution guarantees to people living with HIV/Aids
- be able to give an informed and considered answer to the legal and ethical questions that you might encounter in your work as a caregiver or counsellor
- be able to contribute to the development and evaluation of HIV/Aids policies in the workplace, hospitals, schools or tertiary institutions
- be able to develop a personal ethical credo that will guide you in your work with people who live with HIV or who have Aids

chapter 19 Legal, Ethical and Policy Issues

The law
Has he learnt to live under the laws?
Those about which our elders sing.
Words – finely woven like a net.

No more complex challenge could ever have been devised to test our moral fibre than HIV/Aids. The pandemic has given rise to a vast array of ethical, moral and legal issues, many of them previously unknown. If we can't address these issues, we may well slip back into the ignorance, irrational fear and inhumane conduct that characterised the dark years of the Black Death in late medieval Europe. If that happens history will judge us harshly, because it will prove that the *great cruel beast* alluded to at the beginning of each of the chapters was, after all, not HIV/Aids, but *us*.

We need laws and policies, but we should be guided not so much by those laws (however valuable they may be) as by our common sense, our ethical and moral values, our compassion and our basic respect for the human rights and dignity of all people.

19.1 THE CONSTITUTION AND THE LEGAL FRAMEWORK

This chapter discusses South African legislation and policies. These are based on the *basic human rights* that apply to all citizens and that should not be denied people with HIV infection or Aids.

The South African Constitution (Act 108 of 1996) is the supreme law of the country and all other laws must comply with its provisions. The Constitution includes a Bill of Rights which lists basic human rights that apply to all citizens and therefore also to people living with HIV/Aids. According to the Constitution, people have the following rights:

- the right not to be unfairly discriminated against, either by the state or by another person;
- the right to bodily and psychological integrity, which includes the right to security and control over the body;

- the right not to be subjected to medical or scientific experiments without the person's own informed consent;
- the right of access to health care services, including reproductive health care;
- the right not to be refused emergency medical treatment;
- the right to information and a basic education;
- the right to privacy; and
- the right not to have the privacy of one's communications infringed.

The information in this chapter on the rights of people with HIV/Aids in the workplace, in medical settings, in schools and in higher-education settings is based on the following legislation, policies, proposals and common-law rights (Barrett-Grant et al., 2003; Van Wyk, 2000; Whiteside & Sunter, 2000):

- the Employment Equity Act 55 of 1998;
- the Promotion of Equality and Prevention of Unfair Discrimination Act 4 of 2000;
- the Labour Relations Act 66 of 1995;
- the Occupational Health and Safety Act 85 of 1993;
- the Mines Health and Safety Act 29 of 1996;
- the Compensation for Occupational Injuries and Diseases Act 130 of 1993;
- the Basic Conditions of Employment Act 75 of 1997;
- the National Education Policy Act 27 of 1996;
- the National Policy on HIV/Aids for Learners and Educators in Public Schools and Students and Educators in Further Education and Training Institutions (Notice 1926 of 1999, *Government Gazette* 410 of 10 August 1999);
- the Medical Schemes Act 131 of 1998;
- the National Policy on Testing for HIV (Department of Health, August 2000);
- the Health Professions Council Guidelines on the Management of Patients with HIV Infection or Aids; and
- common-law protection of the right to privacy and dignity.

19.2 THE BASIC RIGHTS OF PEOPLE LIVING WITH HIV/AIDS

People living with HIV or Aids have the same basic rights and responsibilities as all other citizens. The *Charter of Rights on Aids and HIV* which was launched in 1992 is the Bill of Rights of people living with HIV or Aids. The human rights principles in the Charter are essential to ensure non-discrimination and public health in South Africa.

Liberty, autonomy, security of the person and freedom of movement

People living with HIV or Aids have the same rights to liberty and autonomy, security of the person and freedom of movement as all others. No restrictions should be placed on the free movement of HIV-positive people, and they may not be segregated, isolated or quarantined in prisons, schools, hospitals or elsewhere merely because of their HIV-positive status. People with HIV infection or Aids are entitled to maintain *personal autonomy* (i.e. the right to make their *own* decisions) about any matter that affects marriage and child-bearing, but counselling about the consequences of their decisions should be provided.

Confidentiality and privacy

People with HIV infection and Aids have the right to confidentiality and privacy about their health and HIV status. Health care professionals are ethically and legally required to keep all information about clients or patients confidential. Information about a person's HIV status may not be disclosed to anyone without that person's fully informed consent. After death, the HIV status of the deceased person may not be disclosed without the consent of the deceased's family or partner, except when required by law.

HIV testing

No person may be tested for HIV infection without his or her free and *informed consent,* except in the case of *unlinked, anonymous* epidemiological screening programmes undertaken by authorised agencies such as the national, provincial or local health authorities. In all *other* cases, including HIV testing for research purposes or screening of donated blood, the informed consent of the individual is required by law. Anonymous and confidential HIV antibody testing with pre- and post-test counselling should be available to all. Those who test HIV positive should have access to continuing support and health services.

Education on HIV and Aids

All people have the right to proper education and full information about HIV and Aids, as well as the right to full access to and information about prevention methods. Public education with the specific objective of eliminating discrimination against people with HIV or Aids should also be provided.

Employment

HIV testing should not be included in any pre-employment policy or used as grounds for refusing employment. HIV or Aids do not, by themselves, justify termination of employment or demotion, transfer or discrimination in employment. The mere fact that an employee is HIV positive or has Aids does not have to be disclosed to the employer. There is no warrant for requiring existing employees to undergo testing for HIV.

Health and support services

People with HIV/Aids have the same rights to housing, food, social security, medical assistance and welfare as all other members of society. Reasonable accommodation in public services and facilities should be provided for those affected by HIV or Aids. The source of a person's infection should not be grounds for discrimination in the provision of health services, facilities or medication. *Medical schemes* may not discriminate unfairly – directly or indirectly – against any person on the basis of his or her state of health.

Insurance

People with HIV infection or Aids (and those suspected of being at risk of having HIV or Aids) should be protected from arbitrary discrimination in insurance. Insurance companies may not unfairly refuse insurance to any person solely on the basis of HIV/Aids status.

The responsibilities of the media

People with HIV infection or Aids have the right to fair treatment by the media and to observance of their rights to privacy and confidentiality. The public has the right to informed and balanced coverage and presentation of information and education on HIV and Aids.

The right to safer sex

All people have the right to insist that they or their sexual partners take appropriate precautionary measures to prevent the transmission of HIV. The especially vulnerable position of women in this regard should be recognised and addressed, as should the vulnerable position of youths and children.

The rights of prisoners

Prisoners with HIV infection or Aids should enjoy the same standards of care and treatment as other prisoners. Prisoners with HIV/Aids should have access to the kind of special care that is equivalent to that provided to other prisoners with other serious illnesses. Prisoners should have the same access to education, information and preventive measures as the general population.

Equal protection under the law, and access to public benefits

People with HIV or Aids have the right to equal access to public benefits and opportunities, and HIV testing should not be required as a precondition for eligibility to such advantages. Public measures should be adopted to protect people with HIV or Aids from discrimination in employment, housing, education, child care and custody and the provision of medical, social and welfare services.

Duties of people with HIV or Aids

People with HIV or Aids have the duty to respect the rights, health and physical integrity of others, and to take appropriate steps to ensure this when necessary.

Caregivers and counsellors in the HIV/Aids field must heed the national policies, laws and guidelines relevant to their work. Knowledge of these policies and guidelines is required to advise and assist clients who may be unfairly discriminated against. The following policies and guidelines will be discussed in more detail: the National Policy on Testing for HIV, the Health Professions Council Guidelines on the Management of Patients with HIV Infection or Aids, the Code of Good Practice on Key Aspects of HIV/Aids and Employment, and the National Policy on HIV/Aids for Learners and Educators. (The information concerning these policies is based on the *HIV/Aids and the Law Resource Manual* compiled by Barrett-Grant et al. and published by the Aids Law Project and the Aids Legal Network in 2003). Questions frequently asked by health care professionals, along with relevant comments and notes, are included where applicable. Special attention is given to the rights of women and of children.

19.3 NATIONAL POLICY ON TESTING FOR HIV

Background

The Department of Health published the National Policy on Testing for HIV in August 2000. It is a guideline on how and when HIV testing should take place. It gives guidelines on the duties of health care workers and the rights of people considering HIV testing. The National Policy should be read with other guidelines such as the Health Professions Council Guidelines on the Management of Patients with HIV Infection or Aids (see section 19.4 on page 339). Note that some parts of the National Policy are already law, e.g. rules on HIV testing with informed consent.

Caregivers and counsellors can use the National Policy:

- to understand their own rights when considering HIV testing; and
- to help patients, clients and people in their communities understand their rights around testing.

Guidelines

In accordance with the constitutional guarantees of freedom and security of the person, and the right to privacy and dignity, the following HIV testing policy constitutes national policy. This policy applies to persons who can give consent, as well as to those legally entitled to give proxy consent to HIV testing in terms of the law.*

1. *Circumstances under which HIV testing may be conducted*

1.1 Testing for human immunodeficiency virus (HIV) may be done only in the following circumstances:

- Upon individual request, for diagnostic and treatment purposes, with the informed consent of that individual.
- On the recommendation of a medical doctor that such testing is clinically indicated, with the informed consent of the individual.
- As part of HIV testing for research purposes, with the informed consent of the individual and in accordance with national legal and ethical provisions regarding research.
- As part of screening blood donations, with the informed consent of the individual and in accordance with statutory provisions regarding blood donations (see enrichment box 'Point of controversy: Testing and blood donations' on page 339).
- As part of unlinked and anonymous testing for epidemiological purposes undertaken by the national, provincial or local health authority or an agency authorised by any of these bodies, without informed consent, provided that HIV testing for epidemiological purposes is carried out in accordance with national legal and ethical provisions regarding such testing.†

* *Proxy consent* is consent by a person legally entitled to grant consent on behalf of another individual. For example, a parent or guardian of a child below the age of consent to medical treatment may give proxy consent to HIV testing of the child.

†Anonymous, unlinked testing means that no names are used, and that the results cannot be traced back to the person who was tested. The annual survey of the number of pregnant women who are HIV positive is an example of anonymous, unlinked testing that can be done without informed consent.

- Where an existing blood sample is available, and an emergency situation necessitates testing the source patient's blood (e.g. when a health care worker has sustained a risk-bearing accident such as a needlestick injury), HIV testing may be undertaken without informed consent but only after informing the source patient that the test will be performed, and only after providing for the protection of privacy. The information regarding the result may be disclosed to the health care worker concerned but must otherwise remain confidential and may be disclosed to the source patient only with his or her informed consent. (An existing blood sample may be available in cases where the patient's blood was drawn previously and sent to the laboratory for other purposes.)
- Where statutory provision or other legal authorisation exists for testing without informed consent.

1.2 Routine testing of patients for HIV infection to protect health care workers from infection is not allowed, regardless of consent.

1.3 HIV testing of an employee in the workplace is prohibited unless justified by an order of the Labour Court.

1.4 Proxy consent may be given where the individual is unable to give consent.

2. *Informed consent, pre-test counselling and post-test counselling*

2.1 Testing for HIV infection at all health care facilities will be carried out with informed consent, which includes pre-test counselling. The result of the test must remain fully confidential, and may not be disclosed without the individual's fully informed consent unless there is an overriding legal or ethical reason.

2.2 In the context of HIV/Aids, testing with informed consent means that the individual has been made aware of and understands the implications of the test.

Must a person sign a written consent form before an HIV test?

2.3 Consent means giving express agreement to HIV testing in a situation devoid of coercion, in which the individual should feel equally free to grant or withhold consent. Written consent should be obtained where possible. (The law does not say consent must be in writing, but it is preferable to obtain written proof that the person has received pre-test counselling and has agreed to be tested.)

2.4 Pre-test counselling should be given before an HIV test. It should be a confidential dialogue with a suitably qualified person such as a doctor, nurse or trained HIV counsellor, undertaken as a means of passing on information and gaining consent.

2.5 Posters, pamphlets and other media (including videos) may be used in making information on HIV/Aids available, but cannot be regarded as a general substitute for pre-test counselling.

What if a person refuses pre-HIV test counselling (and HIV testing)?

2.6 A doctor, nurse or trained HIV counsellor should accept, after personal consultation, an individual's decision to refuse pre-test counselling and/or HIV testing. Try to find out *why* a person refuses to receive pre-HIV test counselling and attempt if possible to rectify the person's preconceptions. (He or she might have had a previous traumatic or negative experience with an inadequate or unsympathetic counsellor.) Record the person's decision in writing.

2.7 A doctor, nurse or trained HIV counsellor should ensure that post-test counselling takes place as part of a process of informing an individual of an HIV test result.

2.8 If a health care facility lacks the capacity to provide pre- or post-test counselling, the client should be referred for counselling to a counselling agency or other facility for pre- and post-test counselling.

2.9 Where a patient presents with recognisable HIV/Aids specific symptoms but no facilities exist for pre-test counselling, then treatment for the specific symptom or illness should proceed without an HIV test. Referral for pre-test counselling with a view to a possible HIV test must occur at the earliest opportunity.

Enrichment

Point of controversy: Testing and blood donations

The voluntary donation of blood at a Blood Transfusion Service Centre is controlled by the *Human Tissue Act*. The Human Tissue Act says that blood can be donated only with informed consent, but it doesn't say anything about the consent for an HIV test. The National Policy on Testing, on the other hand, recommends that blood donors should give informed consent for their blood to be tested for HIV. Blood donation services only require the filling in of a form where the person answers questions, which are used to find out if the person's blood is likely to have any viruses or infections. The blood is then screened for HIV (without consent or pre-test counselling), other STIs and hepatitis B and C. If any of these tests are positive, the blood donor is informed of the results.

19.4 HEALTH PROFESSIONS COUNCIL GUIDELINES ON THE MANAGEMENT OF PATIENTS WITH HIV INFECTION OR AIDS

Background

The *Health Professions Council of South Africa* (HPCSA) Guidelines of 2001 replace the *South African Medical and Dental Council* (SAMDC) Guidelines of 1994. The HPCSA guidelines are in keeping with international best practice and reflect to a large extent, if not fully, the views of organisations such as the United Nations Joint Programme on HIV/Aids (UNAIDS) and the World Health Organization (WHO).

Caregivers and counsellors can use the Guidelines:

- to claim their rights when interacting with health professionals; and
- to help clients or patients understand their rights when dealing with health professionals.

Guidelines

1. *Occupational transmission of HIV*

1.1 The risk of transmission of HIV infection in the health care area from patient to patient, from patient to health care worker, and from health care worker to patient through inoculation of infected blood or other body fluids has been shown scientifically to be very small. Fears, which are not always based on reality, have thus tended to exaggerate the risks out of all proportion.

1.2 Health care workers and patients are not only exposed to HIV. It should be recognised that at present infection by the hepatitis B virus poses a far greater risk. Universal precautions against blood-borne infections should therefore be adhered to in all health care encounters to minimise exposure of health care workers and their patients.

1.3 Post-exposure treatment of health care workers in whom inoculation or significant contamination might have occurred, may be beneficial and should be considered in consultation with the Infection Control Medical Officer of the institution, or other designated person. When there has been a risk of contamination, PEP (post-exposure prophylaxis) should also be strongly recommended and the health care worker should receive thorough counselling about the possible benefits of PEP in reducing the risk of seroconversion.

2. *Limiting the spread of HIV*

2.1 The medical fraternity supports all efforts to keep the spread of HIV infection in the community as low as possible. Such measures include appropriate education regarding the infection, alteration of lifestyle, improved management of predisposing and aggravating factors, including other sexually transmitted diseases, mobilising support from the community, and disseminating information regarding preventive measures.

2.2 Since the guidelines were first published, there have been very significant advances in the treatment of opportunistic infections and in the use of antiretroviral drugs. The medical fraternity is committed to improved access to medical care and treatment for patients, whatever disease they are suffering from.

3. *Education*

3.1 Education and training are essential components of the successful implementation of universal precautions, i.e. those precautions that should be universally applied to prevent transmission of HIV and other diseases in the health care setting (see Chapter 16). These precautions have been proven to be the most effective measures to protect health care workers.

3.2 These and all other measures instituted to prevent the transmission of infections in the health care setting will probably fail if they are not supported by an ongoing educational programme. Such educational programmes should be:

- structured and preferably assessed by formal examinations;
- ongoing throughout the period of employment; and
- continuously evaluated and monitored.

4. *The doctor's (and other health care professional's) duty towards HIV-positive patients*

4.1 In the management of the HIV-positive patient, the health care worker has a primary responsibility to the patient. The health care worker also has certain responsibilities to other health care workers and other parties that might be in danger of contracting the disease from the patient.

May a doctor or other health care professional refuse to treat an HIV-positive patient?

4.2 No doctor (or other health care professional) may ethically refuse to treat any patient solely on the grounds that the patient is, or may be, HIV seropositive.

4.3 No doctor (or other health care professional) may withhold normal standards of treatment from any patient solely on the grounds that the patient is HIV seropositive, unless such variation of treatment is determined to be in the patient's interest.

4.4 Treatment should not be suboptimal because of a perceived potential risk to the health care workers.

4.5 It is accepted that a health care worker will examine or treat a patient only with the informed consent of the patient.

4.6 Health care professionals are reminded that an HIV-positive diagnosis, without further examination (such as measuring viral load or CD4 cell count), provides no information about a person's prognosis or actual state of health. Unilateral decisions not to resuscitate people with HIV are a violation of fundamental rights and may lead to disciplinary action being taken against a health care professional guilty of such action.

5. *Obligations of employers*

What are employers' obligations to employees who get infected with HIV?

5.1 An employer should have a clear-cut policy statement that declares the responsibility of the employer towards employees who become infected while performing official duties.

5.2 This policy should state the procedures the employee should follow after occupational exposure, which should include guidelines with regard to the reporting of the incident for purposes of compensation, the HIV testing of the health care worker and, where informed consent can be obtained, of the source patient, and access to post-exposure prophylaxis (see 'Management of accidental exposure to blood and other infectious body fluids' on page 347).

5.3 Employers should ensure that all employees are insured against the consequences of infections such as HIV. This insurance may be under the Workmen's Compensation Act, and/or a private insurance scheme.

May health care professionals apply for compensation if they become infected with HIV in their workplace?

5.4 Although HIV/Aids is not a listed occupational disease in terms of the Workmen's Compensation Act, an employee who can show that he or she was infected as a result of an exposure during the course of carrying out his or her occupational duties, may claim compensation. (Also see 'Compensation for occupationally acquired HIV' on page 351.)

5.5 Medical students who are not legally recognised employees should also be insured against such incidents, either by their university or by the hospital where they undergo their practical training.

5.6 There is consensus that adherence to universal precautions is the most important and possibly the only action that will significantly protect health care workers against infection by HIV and other blood-borne pathogens. (The exception is immunisation against hepatitis B.) Therefore:

- All employers must make facilities to institute universal precautions available to health care workers.
- Such facilities should be provided to the full spectrum of health care workers and should include those paramedical personnel who initially come into contact with the patient, as well as auxiliary and unskilled workers who handle patients or could be exposed to contaminated materials. Such facilities should also be available to medical students, who are particularly vulnerable because they are technically inexperienced and not recognised as official employees.
- The facilities available should include the additional sophisticated precautionary measures that may have to be instituted to protect professional personnel who perform invasive procedures known to be associated with a high risk of inoculation with patients' blood.

6. *Knowledge of the HIV status of patients*

6.1 There is persuasive scientific evidence that knowledge of the HIV status of a patient does not provide additional protection to the doctor or other health care worker treating the patient.

6.2 Nevertheless, there is a perception amongst some doctors that under exceptional circumstances the knowledge of the HIV status of a patient may be useful in order to ensure the use of 'extended' universal precautionary measures such as special gloves, clothing and face masks; and that inexperienced personnel should not be allowed to perform the surgery. It is argued that selective use of such expensive measures will be cost-effective. Exceptional circumstances are defined as palpation of a needle-tip in a body cavity, or the simultaneous presence of the health care worker's fingers and a needle or other sharp object or instrument in a poorly visualised or highly confined anatomical cavity. Orthopaedic and other procedures where there is an aerosol of blood, bone fragments or bloody fluids also qualify.

6.3 Where certain well-defined high-risk or exposure-prone procedures are contemplated, the patient should be informed of the concerns and asked to consent to HIV testing. It should be emphasised that the condoning of pre- operative or pre-treatment HIV testing when high-risk procedures are contemplated should not be abused to justify routine HIV testing of all patients, nor should patients be told that pre-HIV testing is mandatory in such circumstances. All patients have a right to refuse testing, and if a patient refuses to be tested for HIV under such circumstances, he or she may not be refused treatment on this basis. A patient who declines to be tested for HIV should be managed by health care professionals as if HIV positive.

6.4 Health care workers should realise that there are factors that make it unrealistic to rely on HIV testing of patients to protect themselves against occupational exposure. Health care workers must appreciate the significance of the window period of infectivity; the ever-increasing prevalence of HIV infection, especially among hospital patients; the time required for a reliable HIV test result; and the need to treat, under less than ideal conditions, patients outside hospitals and in emergency care units.

6.5 The factors mentioned in 6.4 are not under the control of the health care worker and strengthen the view that to minimise the risk of infection, health care workers should adopt appropriate universal precautions in all clinical situations rather than rely on knowledge of the HIV status of patients.

7. *Testing patients for HIV antibodies/antigens*

7.1 HIV testing should take place only with the voluntary, informed consent of the individual. (See 'National Policy on Testing for HIV' on page 337.)

Can a hospital or health care facility routinely test patients before admission?

7.2 Requirements of routine or universal testing of patients in the health care setting are unjustifiable and undesirable (also see paragraph 6.4). However, patients may be requested to consider HIV testing when certain well-defined high-risk procedures are to be undertaken as set out in paragraph 6.2.

7.3 As part of informed consent, the patient should be given information regarding the purpose of the laboratory test; what advantages or disadvantages testing may hold for him or her as patient; why the surgeon or physician wants this information; what influence the result of such a test will have on his or her treatment; and how his or her medical protocol will be altered by this information. The psychosocial impact of a positive test result should also be addressed. All such communication should be conducted in a language that is easily understood by the patient.

If a hospital has a wall poster saying that they do HIV testing on all patients, does this mean that all patients automatically give their consent to be tested?

7.4 If posters are displayed in an attempt to inform patients that testing for HIV may be undertaken, these must be supplemented by verbal pre-test counselling of the patient by the doctor or other health care professional in order to appropriately obtain the patient's informed consent. (Remember that not all patients can read, and even if they can, it does not necessarily mean that they really understand.)

7.5 The principle of informed consent further entails that the health care worker accepts that if the patient is HIV-positive, appropriate counselling will follow. The health care worker must therefore ensure that the patient is directed to appropriate facilities that will oversee his or her further care and, if possible, counsel his or her family and/or sexual partners.

7.6 The attention of patients should be drawn to the potential abuse of HIV test kits that are available on the market nowadays. Any person who wishes to use such a kit should ascertain from his or her doctor or another credible source whether the kit is reliable and safe. New forms of HIV testing should be adopted only if they conform with the guidelines set out in this policy document.

Is it ever justifiable to test for HIV without the patient's consent?

7.7 It is justifiable to test for HIV without the patient's consent ONLY in the circumstances set out in the National Policy on Testing for HIV. Of relevance in the medical context is testing in emergency situations.

7.7.1 An emergency situation is generally considered to be a situation where a patient's health is in serious danger, and immediate treatment is necessary. In terms of HIV testing, it is generally argued that there are few, if any, situations where in order to provide for the immediate care of a patient who is unable to consent, it would be necessary to determine the patient's HIV status.

What happens if a health care worker has sustained a needle-stick injury, and the source patient refuses to be tested?

7.7.2 A risk-bearing incident such as a needle-stick injury may be considered as an emergency situation in which immediate post-exposure measures may benefit the health care worker, and under such circumstances information as to the HIV status of the source patient may be obtained in the following ways:

(*a*) Testing any existing blood specimen. This should be done with the source patient's consent, but if consent is withheld, the specimen may nevertheless be tested, but only after informing the source patient that the test will be performed, and providing for the protection of privacy. The information regarding the result may be disclosed to the health care worker but must otherwise remain confidential and may be disclosed to the source patient only with his or her informed consent.

(*b*) If the patient is unable to give informed consent, and is likely to remain unable to do so for a significant time in relation to the prophylactic needs of the health care worker or other patients, then every reasonable attempt should be made to obtain appropriate vicarious consent. Vicarious consent means the consent of the patient's closest relative or, in the case of a minor, the consent of the medical superintendent in the absence of a parent or other guardian.

(c) If consent for testing cannot be obtained from the source patient, the health care worker should consider taking antiretroviral medication (after baseline testing to indicate that he or she is HIV negative).

Can a mentally ill patient be tested or treated without his or her consent?

7.8 According to the Mental Health Act, if a mentally ill patient is unable to consent to treatment or testing, consent can be obtained from the patient's curator (a person appointed by law to look after him or her), spouse (husband or wife), parent, child (if the child is 21 years or older), or brother or sister. If the patient is in a mental institution, the medical superintendent can, in serious cases, consent on behalf of the patient if the next-of-kin cannot be found. Note, however, that the patient can only be tested for HIV if this information is necessary for his or her medical treatment.

8. *Confidentiality*

8.1 There is no persuasive evidence that knowledge of a patient's HIV status diminishes the incidence of exposure incidents. In fact, our law has recognised the important public health benefits of maintaining patient confidentiality regarding HIV status, in order to encourage patients with HIV to be tested and treated.

8.2 The results of HIV testing should be treated at the highest possible level of confidentiality.

May doctors keep the diagnosis of their patients secret from the nursing staff or other doctors?

8.3 Our courts have recognised that confidentiality regarding HIV status extends to other medical colleagues and health care workers, and other health care workers may not be informed of a patient's HIV status without that patient's consent. If there is a need to share clinical data with medical colleagues and health care workers directly involved with the care of the patient, it should be discussed with the patient in order to obtain his or her consent. Disclosures (with the patient's consent) should be considered only if they are in the patient's best interest in terms of treatment and care.

If a patient's consent cannot be obtained, may the caregiver divulge the information to other parties who are at clear risk of danger?

8.4 If the patient's consent cannot be obtained, ethical guidelines recommend that the health care worker should use his or her discretion whether or not to divulge the information to other parties involved who are *at clear risk of danger*. There is, to date, no legal clarity regarding whether this situation is an acceptable limitation of the right to confidentiality. The decision to disclose a patient's HIV status to, say, the sex partner, must be made with the greatest care, after explanation to the patient and with acceptance of full responsibility at all times. The sex partner should be clearly known and identifiable (e.g as the patient's wife, Susan) and not vaguely known (e.g. as 'all the girls at the club'). The following steps are recommended:

- Counsel the patient on the importance of disclosing to his or her sexual partner and discuss measures to prevent HIV transmission.
- Provide support to the patient to make this disclosure him- or herself with or without the help of the counsellor.
- If the patient still refuses to disclose his or her HIV status to the sex partner or refuses to consider other measures to prevent infection, counsel the patient on the health care worker's ethical obligation to disclose such information and request consent to do so.
- If none of the above succeed, and a health care professional discloses a client's HIV-positive status without the client's consent, he or she must also be prepared to accept full responsibility for the decision, as well as the possible legal consequences.

8.5 When informing the patient about the importance of disclosure, the attention of the patient should be drawn to the possibility of violence and other adverse consequences that such disclosure may hold in store for him or her. HIV-positive women in particular are very vulnerable to violence and even murder, and health care professionals should take this into account. (Also see 'Confidentiality' on page 184.)

8.6 Reports of HIV test results from laboratories (like all other laboratory test results) should be considered confidential information. Breach of confidentiality is more likely to occur in the ward, hospital or doctor's reception area than in the laboratory. It is therefore essential that health care institutions, pathologists and doctors formulate clear policies on how such laboratory results will be communicated and how confidentiality of the results will be maintained.

9. *Doctors (and other health care workers) infected with HIV*

Should HIV-positive doctors and other health care professionals inform their employers about their HIV-positive status?

9.1 No doctor or health care worker is obliged to disclose his or her HIV status to an employer, nor may any employee be unfairly discriminated against or dismissed as a result of HIV status.

9.2 The benefits of voluntary HIV testing should be explained to all health care workers and they should be encouraged to consider HIV testing. Any doctor or health care worker who finds him- or herself to be HIV positive should be encouraged to seek counselling from an appropriate professional source, preferably one designated for this purpose by a medical academic institution. Counsellors must of course be familiar with recommendations such as those of the Centers for Disease Control so that unnecessary, onerous, and scientifically unjustifiable restrictions are not placed on the professional activities of an HIV-positive health care professional.

Should an HIV-positive doctor continue to practise, and should HIV-positive nurses be allowed to care for patients?

9.3 Infected doctors and nurses may continue to practise and care for patients. They must, however, seek and implement a counsellor's advice on the extent to which they should limit or adjust their professional practice in order to protect their patients. HIV-positive nurses with oozing lesions or weeping dermatitis should *under no circumstances* be allowed to perform or assist in direct patient care activities until such conditions heal. It is the responsibility of the employer and of the health care professional to make sure that safe procedures are followed at all times and to be aware of any changes in the mental or physical abilities of employees (Expert Advisory Group on Aids, 1988; WHO, 1988b). If a patient is infected by an HIV-positive health care professional, both the health care professional and the employer may face civil claims. Liability would depend on proof of either *negligence* or *intent* on the part of the nurse or employer (Strauss, 1989).

? Should an HIV-positive health care professional be allowed to perform or assist in invasive procedures?

9.4 Invasive procedures in which possible injury to the health care professional may cause accidental contamination of the patient may be an area of concern for patient safety. The type of invasive procedure should, however, be kept in mind before making any decisions. Invasive procedures such as injections and starting of intravenous lines carry very little risk of exposing the patient to the health care professional's blood. It is, however, recommended that HIV-positive health care professionals should seek expert advice if they perform or assist in surgical invasive procedures where blood-to-tissue contact could occur. It may be necessary for them to modify or limit their duties to protect patients.

10. Notifiability, sick and death certificates

? What should be written on a sick certificate?

10.1 A sick certificate gives an employer confidential information on the employee's medical condition. The patient or the employee may therefore ask the doctor to leave private information off the certificate. Health care professionals should discuss with their patients what information to give on medical sick certificates.

? What should be written on a death certificate?

10.2 In terms of regulations published in July 1998 under the Birth and Death Registration Act, death certificates must have two pages:

- Page 1 is for the registration of the death with the Department of Home Affairs so that it can issue a burial order. This page has to state only whether the cause of the death was natural (e.g. illness or old age) or unnatural (e.g. murder).
- Page 2 is a confidential document used only for data collection. It is not a public record. This page contains information about the deceased (for instance, the deceased's occupation) and the medical cause of death (the underlying illness or condition, such as an Aids-related illness). This page of the death certificate will be given only to the family of the deceased on their specific request, for example when they need it to make a legal claim.

? Why is it not feasible to make HIV infection and Aids a notifiable disease?

10.3 Regulations on the notification of Aids disease and death were published for public comment by the South African Department of Health in 1999. Because of widespread resistance to such a step, and fears for the safety of HIV-positive people, the Government decided in January 2001 to abandon the notification proposal ('Vigs-aanmeldingsplan laat vaar', 2001).

The reasons for and implications of classifying a disease as notifiable are to give medical and health care professionals the opportunity to:

- positively identify the disease as soon as possible;
- treat patients; and
- attempt to prevent the disease from spreading to other members of the community.

In the case of notifiable diseases such as malaria, tetanus, TB, typhoid, cholera, viral hepatitis and meningococcal infections, all three of the above reasons for notifiability are present. In each of these diseases, infection can be positively diagnosed *as soon as* the first symptoms appear; treatment can start immediately; and the spread of the disease (which is usually transmitted by mosquitoes, through direct contact with urine and faeces, in respiratory droplets and by means of contaminated food) can be prevented if specific preventive measures are taken by those who are at risk.

In the case of HIV infection, none of the justifiable reasons for notifiability apply unambiguously. Swift identification of the infection is impossible because of the long period between infection with HIV and the appearance of definite signs of Aids. During this period people may show no symptoms and are frequently not even aware that they are infected. This long period between infection and visible serious illness and the fact that HIV does not spread through casual contact, renders notification an impractical and unjustifiable procedure.

Some say that notifiability will give health authorities the opportunity to suggest to infected people that they seek treatment for opportunistic infections and educate themselves about necessary sexual behavioural changes (such as safer sex). However, people should rather be motivated to go for voluntary HIV counselling and testing to establish their status and to take the necessary steps to prevent further transmission and care for themselves.

11. Creating a safe working environment

The Occupational Health and Safety Act of 1993 requires that employers (as far as it is reasonably practicable) create a safe working environment. It is also the responsibility of employers to develop policies and programmes to educate and protect their employees. This is not only a legal obligation; it is also an ethical obligation.

What are employers' obligations in terms of creating a safe working environment?

Fine et al. (1997) recommend that employers integrate the following steps, plans and procedures into their management and policy plans:

- Universal precautions should be applied in every workplace.
- Employers should classify activities in terms of the potential risk of exposure to blood and body fluids.
- Employers should make protective equipment and clothes available to all workers who come into contact with blood or body fluids.
- Matters and issues relating to the occupational transmission of HIV/Aids should be placed on the agenda of companies' health and safety committees so that appropriate controls can be instituted.
- Employers should ensure that appropriate protective equipment and clothing are used and worn by workers when they perform activities involving blood and body fluids.
- Employers should ensure that appropriate first-aid equipment is always readily available for dealing with spilt blood and body fluids, and that staff are trained to institute safety precautions after accidents.
- Employers should develop standard procedures for all activities in which people may be exposed to blood and body fluids.
- Procedures should be instituted for ensuring and monitoring compliance with safety measures.
- If personnel are not complying with safety measures, they should be subjected to appropriate counselling, re-education and training.
- Employers should make certain that workers who might be exposed to infection are well trained and educated in appropriate preventive measures. No health care professional should be allowed to perform a duty that may involve exposure to blood or body fluids without having had the necessary training and education to do so.
- All employees should be taught the correct methods of cleaning up blood and body fluid spills.
- If necessary, the workplace should be redesigned so that it becomes a safer place.
- All accidents that result in blood and body fluid exposure should be investigated. Counselling should be made available to all health care professionals who need it, including HIV-positive personnel and all health care professionals who work with HIV-positive patients.
- If employees feel that their work environment is not safe, they have the right to refuse to work and to request an inspector from the Department of Labour to look into the matter. Nurses and doctors may also refuse to carry out certain tasks (such as drawing blood or

surgical operations) if proper personal protective equipment is not supplied.

12. *Management of accidental exposure to blood and other infectious body fluids*

It is highly advisable for management to institute strict procedures governing the accidental exposure of employees to HIV so that their employees' rights will be secured and so that they can protect themselves against unfounded and punitive legal actions.

What precautions should be applied after accidental exposure to blood and other infectious body fluids?

If a health care professional is exposed to blood and/or other body fluids (through a needle stick or injury with a contaminated sharp instrument), or if infected blood or body fluid comes into contact with open wounds and cuts, or the mucous membranes of the mouth or eyes, the following precautions should be applied immediately (CDC, 1989; Hauman, 1990; WHO, 1988b):

- Immediately rinse blood and body fluid splashes from the skin, eyes and mouth with water or (preferably) with an antimicrobial solution.
- Encourage bleeding in the case of accidental penetrating injuries (such as those resulting from needle sticks) and then wash the area thoroughly with an antimicrobial product (or if that is not available, with soap and water).
- Report all accidents through the same channel that you would use to report other on-duty accidents (such reports would usually be made to the medical officer or nursing manager of a hospital). The employer should report the injury to a central committee for possible compensation. The following circumstances of the exposure should be recorded: the nature of the activity in which the health care professional was engaged at the time of exposure; a precise description of the injured area; the extent to which appropriate work practices and protective equipment were used; and a description of the source of exposure.
- After exposure, a blood sample should be drawn from the *source individual* (the patient to whom the health care professional was exposed) as well as from the health care professional. (Note that the source patient must give his or her informed consent for the blood to be drawn and the test to be done. Also see section 7.7.2 on page 343 about testing an existing blood sample.) The blood sample taken from the health care professional at the time of exposure serves as a *baseline specimen* and can be used later to compare future test results.
- If the source individual turns out to be HIV positive, or if it is impossible to determine the serostatus of the source individual (for example if he or she refuses to be tested), the health care professional should be tested again after 6 weeks, 12 weeks and 6 months. This retesting procedure is essential to make allowance for the window period. A PCR test (see 'The PCR technique' on page 67) is preferable, because it can prove or disprove HIV infection much sooner than HIV antibody tests.
- If the source patient refuses to be tested, report in writing the requests made to the source patient to be tested.
- If the health care professional's subsequent test is HIV positive, the baseline specimen taken at the time of the injury should also be tested. If this baseline specimen is HIV positive, it indicates that the health care professional was infected with HIV some time *prior* to the injury. If, however, the baseline specimen is negative, it is highly probable (provided that one can rule out sexual transmission) that the seroconversion was a direct consequence of the injury involving infected blood.
- If the source individual is seronegative, baseline testing of the exposed health care professional as well as follow-up testing after 6 weeks, 12 weeks and 6 months may be performed (if desired) by the health care professional or if recommended by the doctor. This makes allowance for the possibility that the source individual might have been in the window period at the time of testing.

- If the source individual cannot be identified, testing should still be made available to all health care professionals who are concerned about the possibility of having been infected with HIV because of an occupational exposure.
- The health care professional should report any signs of acute seroconversion illness that occur within 12 weeks after exposure to blood or body fluids. Illnesses characterised by fever, rash or lymphadenopathy (swelling of the glands) may indicate recent HIV infection.
- Testing of the source individual (as well as the health care professional) should not be performed without informed consent and thorough pre-test counselling. Post-test counselling and referral for treatment should also be provided if necessary.
- In the period after exposure but before the results have been confirmed, health care professionals should modify their sexual behaviour to prevent possible transmission of HIV to sex partners. Safer sex (such as using condoms) should be practised, and health care professionals should refrain from donating blood.
- During all the phases of follow-up testing and counselling it is vital to protect the health care professional's confidentiality.
- Post-exposure antiretroviral treatment should be made available to the health care professional, to be started as soon as possible after the injury. (See the note on post-exposure prophylaxis on page 84.)
- Provide counselling to support the health care professional.

19.5 HIV/AIDS AND EMPLOYMENT: CODE OF GOOD PRACTICE

Background

The Code of Good Practice on Key Aspects of HIV/Aids and Employment was published on 1 December 2000 under the Labour Relations Act and the Employment Equity Act. The Code is a guide for employers and employees. It is not legally binding on all employers and its adoption in the workplace is voluntary. However, parts of the Code are already law, e.g. those sections dealing with non-discrimination, pre-employment testing and confidentiality.

Caregivers and counsellors can use the Code:

- to discuss issues around HIV/Aids in the workplace;
- to campaign for the implementation of the Code in the workplace; and
- to develop workplace policies on HIV/Aids.

Guidelines

1. Introduction

The Code of Good Practice recognises that the HIV/Aids epidemic will affect every workplace with prolonged staff illness, absenteeism and death, impacting on productivity, employee benefits, occupational health and safety, production costs and workplace morale. Furthermore, it recognises that, in the workplace, unfair discrimination against people living with HIV and Aids has been perpetuated through practices such as pre-employment HIV testing, dismissals for being HIV positive, and the denial of employee benefits.

2. Objectives

The Code's primary objective is to set out guidelines for employers and trade unions to ensure that people with HIV are not unfairly discriminated against in the workplace. A secondary objective is to provide guidelines for employers, employees and trade unions on how to manage HIV/Aids within the workplace. In addition, the Code promotes the establishment of mechanisms to foster cooperation between employers, employees and trade unions in the workplace, as well as between the workplace and other stakeholders at a sectoral, local, provincial and national level.

3. Policy principles

3.1 The promotion of equality and non-discrimination between people with HIV infection and those without, and between HIV/Aids and other comparable health/medical conditions.

3.2 The creation of a supportive environment so that HIV-positive employees can continue working under normal conditions in their current employment for as long as they are medically fit to do so.

3.3 The protection of the human rights and dignity of people living with HIV or Aids is essential to the prevention and control of HIV/Aids.

3.4 HIV/Aids impacts disproportionately on women, and this should be taken into account in the development of workplace policies and programmes.

3.5 Consultation, inclusivity and encouraging full participation of all stakeholders are key principles that should underpin every HIV/Aids policy and programme.

4. *Applications and scope*

4.1 All employers and employees and their respective organisations are encouraged to use the Code to develop, implement and refine their HIV/Aids policies and programmes to suit the needs of their workplaces.

4.2 For the purposes of this code, the term 'workplace' should be interpreted more broadly to include the working environment of persons not necessarily in an employer–employee relationship, those working in the informal sector, and the self-employed.

5. *Legal framework*

The Code should be read in conjunction with the Constitution of South Africa as well as with the relevant legislation (see 'The Constitution and the legal framework' on page 334).

6. *Promoting a non-discriminatory work environment*

6.1 No person with HIV or Aids shall be unfairly discriminated against within the employment relationship or within any employment policies or practices, including with regard to:

- o recruitment procedures, advertising and selection criteria;
- o appointments and the appointment process, including job placement;
- o job classification or grading;
- o remuneration, employment benefits and terms and conditions of employment;
- o employee assistance programmes;
- o job assignments;
- o training and development;
- o performance evaluation systems;
- o promotion, transfer and demotion; and
- o termination of services.

6.2 To promote a non-discriminatory work environment based on the principle of equality, employers and trade unions should adopt appropriate measures to ensure that employees with HIV and Aids are not unfairly discriminated against and are protected from victimisation through positive measures such as:

- o preventing unfair discrimination and stigmatisation of people living with HIV or Aids through the development of HIV/Aids policies and programmes for the workplace;
- o awareness, education and training on the rights of all persons with regard to HIV and Aids;
- o mechanisms to promote acceptance and openness around HIV/Aids in the workplace;
- o providing support for all employees infected or affected by HIV and Aids; and
- o grievance procedures and disciplinary measures to deal with HIV-related complaints in the workplace.

7. *HIV testing, confidentiality and disclosure*

7.1 *HIV testing*

Can an employer force a job applicant to have an HIV test?

7.1.1 No employer may require an employee or an applicant for employment to undertake an HIV test in order to ascertain that employee's HIV status. (The Labour Court may be approached to obtain authorisation for testing under very special circumstances.)

7.1.2 It has not yet been established by the courts whether, in the case of an employee requesting a test from an employer who provides health services, that employer may provide the test and whether the employee then waives the protection discussed in 7.1.1 above.

7.1.3 In implementing the guidelines below, the position set out in item 7.1.2 should be taken into account.

7.1.4 Authorised testing
The following are some of the circumstances under which employers must approach the Labour Court for authorisation if they want to test employees:
- During an application for employment.
- As a condition of employment.
- During procedures related to termination of employment.
- As an eligibility requirement for training or staff development programmes.
- As an access requirement to obtain employee benefits.

7.1.5 Permissible testing
- An employer may provide testing to an employee who has requested a test in the following circumstances:
  - As part of a health care service provided in the workplace.
  - In the event of an occupational accident carrying a risk of exposure to blood or other body fluids.
  - For the purposes of applying for compensation following an occupational accident involving a risk of exposure to blood or other body fluids.
- Furthermore, such testing may take place only within the following defined conditions:
  - At the initiative of an employee.
  - Within a health care worker and employee–patient relationship.
  - With informed consent and pre- and post-test counselling.
  - With strict procedures relating to confidentiality of an employee's HIV status.

7.1.6 All testing, including both authorised and permissible testing, should be conducted in accordance with the Department of Health's National Policy on Testing for HIV (see 'National Policy on Testing for HIV' on page 337).

7.1.7 Informed consent means that the individual has been provided with information, understands it, and on this basis has agreed to undertake the HIV test. It implies that the individual understands what the test is, why it is necessary, and what the benefits, risks, alternatives and possible social implications of the outcome are.

7.1.8 Anonymous, unlinked surveillance or epidemiological HIV testing in the workplace may occur provided it is undertaken in accordance with the ethical and legal principles of such research. Where such research is done, the information obtained may not be used to unfairly discriminate against individuals or groups of persons. Testing will not be considered anonymous if there is a reasonable possibility that a specific person's HIV status can be deduced from the results.

? Can an employer refuse to employ a person on the grounds of an HIV-positive diagnosis?

No. An employer may refuse to employ a person who is clearly too ill to work, but to refuse to employ a person simply because he or she is known or suspected to be HIV positive, is unfair discrimination.

7.2 *Confidentiality and disclosure*

? Can an employer demand to know if the cause of an illness is HIV infection?

7.2.1 All persons with HIV or Aids have the legal right to privacy. Employees are not required by law to disclose their HIV status to their employers or to other employees.

7.2.2 If an employee chooses voluntarily to disclose his or her HIV status to the employer or to other employees, this information may not be disclosed to others without the employee's express written consent. Where written consent is not possible, steps must be taken to confirm that the employee wishes to disclose his or her status.

7.2.3 Mechanisms should be created to encourage openness, acceptance and support for those employers and employees who voluntarily disclose their HIV status within the workplace, including:
- encouraging persons openly living with HIV or Aids to conduct or participate in education, prevention and awareness programmes;
- encouraging the development of support groups for employees living with HIV or Aids; and
- ensuring that persons who are open about their HIV or Aids status are not unfairly discriminated against or stigmatised.

8. *Promoting a safe workplace*

8.1 An employer is obliged to provide and maintain, as far as is reasonably practicable, a workplace that is safe and without risk to the health of its employees.

8.2 The risk of HIV transmission in the workplace is minimal. However, occupational accidents involving bodily fluids may occur, particularly in the health care professions. Every workplace should ensure that it complies with the provisions of the Occupational Health and Safety Act, including the Regulations on Hazardous Biological Agents, and the Mine Health and Safety Act, and that its policy deals with:
- the risk, if any, of occupational transmission within the particular workplace;
- appropriate training, awareness and education on the use of universal infection control measures so as to identify, deal with and reduce the risk of HIV transmission in the workplace;
- providing appropriate equipment and materials to protect employees from the risk of exposure to HIV;
- the steps to be taken following an occupational accident, and the appropriate management of occupational exposure to HIV and other blood-borne pathogens, including access to post-exposure prophylaxis;
- the procedures to be followed in applying for compensation for occupational infection;
- the reporting of all occupational accidents; and
- adequate monitoring of occupational exposure to HIV to ensure that the requirements of possible compensation claims are being met.

9. *Compensation for occupationally acquired HIV*

9.1 In terms of the Compensation for Occupational Injuries and Diseases Act, an employee may be compensated if he or she becomes infected with HIV as a result of an occupational accident. Employers should take reasonable steps to assist employees with the application for benefits, including:
- providing information to affected employees on the procedures that should be followed in order to qualify for a compensation claim;
- helping to collect information proving that the employee was occupationally exposed to HIV; and
- advising the employee that if an accident is not reported to an employer or the Compensation Commissioner within 12 months, the employee loses the right to claim compensation.

9.2 Occupational exposure should be dealt with in terms of the Compensation for Occupational Injuries and Diseases Act. Employers should ensure that they comply with the provisions of this Act and with the procedures or guideline issued in terms thereof.

10. *Employee benefits*

Can an employer refuse to give an employee who has HIV or Aids employee benefits?

10.1 Employees with HIV or Aids may not be unfairly discriminated against in the allocation of employee benefits.

10.2 With regard to access to employee benefits, an employee who becomes ill with Aids should be treated like any other employee with a comparable life-threatening illness.

10.3 Information from benefit schemes on the medical status of an employee should be kept confidential and should not be used to discriminate unfairly.

10.4 Employers offering medical schemes as part of their employee benefit packages must ensure that these schemes do not discriminate unfairly on the basis of HIV status.

Can medical schemes discriminate against people with HIV/Aids?

According to the Medical Schemes Act of 1999, registered medical schemes may not discriminate directly or indirectly against any person on the basis of their health status.

- A medical scheme is not allowed to exclude from membership people living with HIV or Aids.
- Every scheme must provide minimum benefits, including for people living with HIV/Aids. At the moment, minimum benefits include treatment for all opportunistic infections of HIV or Aids. However, medical schemes do not have to provide for antiretroviral treatment.
- There is no waiting period for getting minimum benefits. If a person already has HIV when he or she joins the scheme, there may be a waiting period of twelve months before the person can claim any extra benefits that the scheme has for HIV/Aids.

11. Dismissal

May an employer dismiss an HIV-positive person? And if so, when?

11.1 Employees with HIV/Aids may not be dismissed solely on the basis of their HIV/Aids status.

11.2 If an employee becomes too ill to perform his or her current work, the employer is obliged to follow accepted guidelines regarding dismissal for incapacity before terminating an employee's services (as set out in the Labour Relations Act).

11.3 The employer should ensure that, as far as possible, the employee's right to confidentiality regarding his or her HIV status is maintained during any incapacity proceedings. An employee cannot be compelled to undergo an HIV test or to disclose his or her HIV status as part of such proceedings unless the Labour Court authorises such a test.

What are the duties of an employer to make a dismissal for incapacity fair?

11.4 The employer should investigate the extent of the incapacity or injury, and should decide whether the incapacity is likely to be permanent or temporary. Alternatives to dismissal should be investigated, and possible ways of adapting the duties or work circumstances of the employee should be considered to accommodate the employee's disability.

11.5 An employer may dismiss an employee on the grounds of incapacity and poor work performance after all steps have been taken to accommodate the person's disability.

Are employers legally permitted to dismiss HIV-positive employees if the colleagues of such people refuse to work with them?

It is an unfair labour practice and therefore unlawful to dismiss infected employees simply because other employees refuse to work with them (Fine et al., 1997). Employers should take extraordinary measures to persuade unwilling co-workers that they are unreasonable in their attitudes and to assure them that the risk of HIV infection within any normal work situation is extremely limited. The employees who refuse to work with the HIV-positive person should furthermore be made aware that their refusal may be the grounds for disciplinary action against them. It is vitally important to prevent such unpleasant situations from arising by educating all employees about all aspects of HIV infection and Aids. Health care professionals should also be assured that preventive equipment is available and that everything possible will be done to protect them as employees (Strauss, 1989).

12. Grievance procedures

12.1 Employers should ensure that the rights of employees with regard to HIV/Aids, and the remedies available to them in the event of a breach of such rights, become integrated into existing grievance procedures.

12.2 Employers should create an awareness and understanding of the grievance procedures and how employees can utilise them.

12.3 Employers should develop special measures to ensure the confidentiality of the complainant during such proceedings, including ensuring that such proceedings are held in private.

13. Management of HIV in the workplace

The effective management of HIV/Aids in the workplace requires an integrated strategy that includes an understanding and assessment of the impact of HIV/Aids on the workplace and long- and short-term measures to deal with and reduce this impact. These measures include an HIV/Aids policy for the workplace; HIV/Aids programmes aimed at preventing the spread of HIV among employees and their communities; to manage employees with HIV so that they can work productively for as long as possible; and dealing with the direct and indirect costs of HIV/Aids in the workplace.

14. Assessing the impact of HIV/Aids on the workplace

Employers and trade unions should develop appropriate strategies to understand, assess and respond to the impact of HIV/Aids in their particular workplace and sector. Impact assessments should include:

- *Risk profiles.* How vulnerable are employees to HIV infection? Does the nature and operations of the organisation (e.g. migrancy or hostel dwellings) increase susceptibility to HIV infection? What is the profile of the communities from which the organisation draws its employees? What is the profile of the communities surrounding the organisation's place of operation? What is the impact of HIV/Aids upon the target markets and client base?
- *Assessment of the direct and indirect costs of HIV/Aids.* What are the direct costs, such as employee benefits, medical costs, training and recruitment costs, and the costs of implementing an HIV/Aids programme? What are the indirect costs such as the cost of increased absenteeism, employee morbidity, loss of productivity, a general decline in workplace morale and possible workplace disruption?

15. Measures to deal with HIV/Aids within the workplace

15.1 *A workplace HIV/Aids policy*

This policy could be a specific policy on HIV/Aids, or be incorporated in a policy on life-threatening illness.

? Should every workplace have an HIV/Aids policy?

15.1.1 Every workplace should develop an HIV/Aids policy to ensure that employees affected by HIV/Aids are not unfairly discriminated against in employment policies and practices. This policy should cover:

- o the organisation's position on HIV/Aids;
- o an outline of the HIV/Aids programme;
- o details on employment policies (e.g. position regarding HIV testing, employee benefits, performance management and procedures to be followed to determine medical incapacity and dismissal);
- o standards of behaviour expected of employers and employees, and appropriate measures for dealing with deviations from these standards;
- o grievance procedures in line with item 12 on page 353;
- o the means of communication within the organisation on HIV/Aids issues;

- o details of employee assistance available to persons affected by HIV/Aids;
- o details of implementation and coordination responsibilities; and
- o monitoring and evaluation mechanisms.

15.1.2 All policies should be developed in consultation with key stakeholders within the workplace including trade unions, employee representatives, occupational health staff and the human resources department.

15.1.3 The policy should reflect the nature and needs of the particular workplace.

15.1.4 Policy development and implementation is a dynamic process, so the workplace policy should be communicated to all concerned; routinely reviewed in light of epidemiological and scientific information; monitored for its successful implementation; and evaluated for its effectiveness.

15.2 *Developing workplace HIV/Aids programmes*

15.2.1 It is recommended that every workplace works towards developing and implementing a workplace HIV/Aids programme aimed at preventing new infections, providing care and support for employees who are infected or affected, and managing the impact of the epidemic in the organisation.

15.2.2 The nature and extent of a workplace programme should be guided by the needs and capacity of each individual workplace. However, it is recommended that every workplace programme should attempt to address the following in cooperation with the sectoral, local, provincial and national initiatives:

- o hold regular HIV/Aids awareness programmes;
- o encourage voluntary testing;
- o conduct education and training on HIV/Aids;
- o promote condom distribution and use;
- o encourage health seeking behaviour for STIs;
- o enforce the use of universal infection control measures;
- o create an environment that is conducive to openness, disclosure and acceptance amongst all staff;
- o endeavour to establish a wellness programme for employees affected by HIV/Aids;
- o provide access to counselling and other forms of social support for people affected by HIV/Aids;
- o maximise the performance of affected employees through reasonable accommodation, such as investigations into alternative sick leave allocation;
- o develop strategies to address direct and indirect costs associated with HIV/Aids in the workplace, as outlined under item 14 on page 353; and
- o regularly monitor, evaluate and review the programme.

15.2.3 Employers should take all reasonable steps to assist employees with referrals to appropriate health, welfare and psychosocial facilities within the community, if such services are not provided at the workplace.

19.6 NATIONAL POLICY ON HIV/AIDS FOR LEARNERS AND EDUCATORS

Background

In August 1999 the Minister of Education launched the National Policy on HIV/Aids for Learners and Educators in Public Schools, and Students and Educators in Further Education and Training Institutions. The National Policy emphasises the vulnerability of young people to HIV infection, and is aimed at educators and learners. The National Policy is a voluntary guideline for schools, but many parts of the policy have already become law, e.g. protection of rights to privacy.

Caregivers, counsellors and teachers can use the National Policy:

- to discuss managing HIV and Aids in the school environment; and
- to support learners and educators living with or affected by HIV or Aids.

Guidelines

1. Introduction: some of the premises regarding HIV/Aids in schools

1.1 Although there are no known cases of the transmission of HIV in schools or institutions, there are learners with HIV/Aids in schools. More and more children who acquire HIV prenatally will, with adequate medical care, reach school-going age and attend school.

1.2 Because of the increase in infection rates, learners, students and educators with HIV/Aids will increasingly form part of the population of schools and institutions. Since many young people are sexually active, increasing numbers of learners at primary and secondary schools as well as students attending higher education institutions might be infected. There are additional risks of HIV transmission among learners and students due to sexual abuse and intravenous drug use. Although the possibility is remote, recipients of infected blood products during blood transfusions (for instance haemophiliacs) may also be present at schools and institutions. Because of the increasing prevalence of HIV/Aids in schools, it is imperative for each school to have a planned strategy to cope with the epidemic.

1.3 Compulsory disclosure of a learner's, student's or educator's HIV/Aids status to school or institution authorities is not advocated as this would serve no meaningful purpose. In cases of disclosure, educators should be prepared to handle such disclosures and be given support to handle confidentiality issues.

1.4 A learner or student with HIV/Aids should lead as full a life as possible and should not be denied the opportunity of receiving an education to the maximum of his or her ability. Likewise, an educator with HIV/Aids should lead as full a professional life as possible, with the same rights and opportunities as other educators and with no unfair discrimination against him or her.

1.5 Infection control measures and adaptations must be universally applied and carried out regardless of the known or unknown HIV status of the individuals concerned. Current scientific evidence suggests that the risk of HIV transmission during teaching, sport and play activities is insignificant. There is no risk of transmission from saliva, sweat, tears, urine, respiratory droplets, handshaking, swimming-pool water, communal bath water, toilets, food or drinking water. Adequate wound management must take place if an open, bleeding wound is sustained in the classroom or laboratory, or on the sports field or playground. Contact sports such as boxing and rugby could probably be regarded as posing a higher risk of HIV transmission than other sports, but the inherent risk of transmission during any sport is very low.

1.6 Within the context of sexual relations, the risk of contracting HIV is significant. The school-going population includes many sexually active people. This considerably increases the risk of HIV transmission in schools and institutions for further education and training. Educators should provide sexuality, morality and life-skills education, and parents should be encouraged to instil healthy morals in their children, as well as providing sexuality education and guidance on sexual abstinence and faithfulness. Sexually active persons should be advised to practise safe sex and to use condoms. Learners and students should be educated about their rights concerning their own bodies, and taught to protect themselves against rape, violence, inappropriate sexual behaviour and contracting HIV.

1.7 The constitutional rights of all learners, students and educators must be protected on an equal basis. If a learner, student or educator poses a medically recognised significant health risk to others, appropriate measures should be taken (e.g. the presence of untreatable contagious or highly communicable diseases, uncontrollable bleeding, unmanageable wounds, or sexual or physically aggressive behaviour, which may create the risk of HIV transmission).

1.8 Learners and students with infectious illnesses such as measles, German measles, chickenpox, whooping cough and mumps should be kept away from the school or institution to protect all its other members, especially those whose immune systems may be impaired by HIV/Aids.

1.9 Schools and institutions should inform parents of vaccination/inoculation programmes and of their possible significance for the well-being of learners and students with HIV/Aids. Local health clinics could be approached to assist with immunisation.

Do children have the right to sexuality education?

1.10 The United Nations Convention on the Rights of the Child, and the National Policy on HIV/Aids state that children should have access to information that will help them develop their physical and emotional well-being. This includes information about HIV/Aids.

1.11 Learners and students must receive ongoing education about HIV/Aids and abstinence in the context of life-skills. Life-skills and HIV/Aids education should not be presented as isolated learning content, but should be integrated in the curriculum. It should be presented in a scientific but understandable way. Appropriate course content should be available for the pre-service and in-service training of educators to cope with HIV/Aids in schools. Sufficient educators should be available to educate learners about the epidemic.

1.11.1 The purpose of education about HIV/Aids is to prevent the spread of HIV infection; to allay excessive fears of the epidemic; to reduce the stigma attached to it; and to instil non-discriminatory attitudes towards persons with HIV/Aids. Education should ensure that learners and students acquire age- and context-appropriate knowledge and skills so that they may adopt and maintain behaviour that will protect them from HIV infection.

Who should provide HIV/Aids education in schools?

1.11.2 In the primary grades, the regular educator should provide education about HIV/Aids. In secondary grades a guidance counsellor would be the appropriate educator. Because of the sensitive nature of the learning content, the educators selected to offer this education should be specifically trained and supported by the support staff responsible for life-skills and HIV/Aids education in the school and province. The educators should feel at ease with the content and should be role models with whom learners and students can easily identify. Educators should be informed by the principal and educator unions of courses for educators where they can increase their knowledge of and skills in dealing with HIV/Aids.

1.11.3 All educators should be trained to give guidance on HIV/Aids. Educators should respect their position of trust and the constitutional rights of all learners and students in the context of HIV/Aids.

2. *Non-discrimination and equality with regard to learners, students and educators with HIV/Aids*

2.1 No learner, student or educator with HIV/Aids may be unfairly discriminated against, directly or indirectly. Educators should be alert to unfair accusations against any person suspected of having HIV/Aids.

2.2 Learners, students, educators and other staff with HIV/Aids should be treated in a just, humane and life-affirming way.

2.3 Any special measures in respect of a learner, student or educator with HIV should be fair and justifiable in the light of medical facts, established legal rules and principles, ethical guidelines, the best interests of the person with HIV/Aids, school or institution conditions, and the best interests of other learners, students and educators.

2.4 To prevent discrimination, all learners, students and educators should be educated about the fundamental human rights listed in the South African Constitution (see 'The Constitution and the legal framework' on page 334).

3. HIV/Aids testing and the admission of learners and students, or the appointment of educators

3.1 No learner or student may be denied admission to or continued attendance at a school or institution on account of his or her HIV/Aids status or perceived HIV/Aids status.

3.2 No educator may be denied the right to be appointed, to teach or to be promoted on account of his or her HIV/Aids status or perceived HIV/Aids status. HIV/Aids status may not be a reason for dismissal of an educator, or for refusing to conclude, or continue, or renew an educator's employment contract, or for treating him or her in any unfair discriminatory manner.

Can a school or other institution require an HIV test as prerequisite for admission?

3.3 There is no medical justification for routine testing of learners, students or educators for evidence of HIV infection. The testing of learners or students for HIV/Aids as a prerequisite for admission to a school or institution, or to continue attendance at a school or institution, or to determine the incidence of HIV/Aids at schools or institutions, is prohibited. The testing of educators for HIV/Aids as a prerequisite for appointment or continued service is prohibited.

4. Attendance at schools and institutions by learners or students with HIV/Aids

Can a child with HIV be excluded from a school?

4.1 Learners and students with HIV have the right to attend any school or institution. The needs of learners and students with HIV/Aids with regard to their right to basic education should, as far as is reasonably practicable, be accommodated in the school or institution.

4.2 Learners and students with HIV/Aids are expected to attend classes in accordance with statutory requirements for as long as they can do so effectively.

What should schools or institutions do to assist learners or students who are unable to attend classes?

4.3 In terms of section 4(1) of the South African Schools Act of 1996, learners of compulsory school-going age with HIV/Aids who are unable to benefit from attendance at school or home education, may be granted exemption from attendance by the head of the department, after consultation with the principal, the parent and the medical practitioner, where possible.

4.4 If and when learners and students with HIV/Aids become incapacitated through illness, the school or institution should make work available to them for study at home and should support continued learning where possible. Parents should, where practically possible, be allowed to educate their children at home in accordance with the policy for home education in terms of section 51 of the South African Schools Act of 1996, or provide older learners with distance education.

4.5 Learners and students who cannot be accommodated in this way or who develop HIV/Aids-related behavioural problems or neurological damage should be accommodated, as far as is practically possible, within the education system in special schools or specialised residential institutions for learners with special education needs. Educators in these institutions must be empowered to take care of and support HIV-positive learners.

However, placement in special schools should not be used as an excuse to remove HIV-positive learners from mainstream schools.

5. *Disclosure of HIV/Aids-related information and confidentiality*

Must a learner, student or educator disclose his or her HIV-positive status to the school, institution or employer?

5.1 No learner or student (or parent on behalf of a learner or student) or educator is compelled to disclose his or her HIV/Aids status to the school or institution or employer.

5.2 Voluntary disclosure of a learner's, student's or educator's HIV/Aids status to the appropriate authority should be welcomed and an enabling environment should be cultivated in which the confidentiality of such information is ensured and in which unfair discrimination is not tolerated. In terms of section 39 of the Child Care Act 74 of 1983 learners or students older than 14 (or the parents of those under 14) are free to disclose such information voluntarily.

5.3 A holistic programme for life-skills and HIV/Aids education should encourage disclosure. In the event of voluntary disclosure, it may be in the best interests of a learner or student with HIV/Aids if a member of the staff of the school or institution directly involved with the care of the learner or student is informed of his or her HIV/Aids status. An educator may disclose his or her HIV/Aids status to the principal of the school or institution.

5.4 Any person to whom any information about the medical condition of a learner, student or educator with HIV/Aids has been divulged, must keep this information confidential.

5.5 Unauthorised disclosure of HIV/Aids-related information could give rise to legal liability.

5.6 No employer can require an applicant for a job to undergo an HIV test before he or she is considered for employment. An employee cannot be dismissed, retrenched or refused a job simply because he or she is HIV positive.

6. *A safe school and institutional environment*

What precautions should be taken to provide a safe school environment?

6.1 The MEC (member of executive council) should make provision for all schools and institutions to implement universal precautions for effective elimination of the risk of transmission of all blood-borne pathogens, including HIV, in the school or institutional environment. Universal precautions are discussed in chapter 16, and these principles also apply to the school or institutional environment. Universal precautions specific to the school situation include the following:

6.1.1 All open wounds, sores, breaks in the skin, grazes and open skin lesions should be cleaned immediately with running water and/or antiseptics, and should at all times be covered completely and securely with non-porous or waterproof dressings or plaster so that there is no risk of exposure to blood.

6.1.2 Blood, especially in large spills, such as from nosebleeds, and old blood or blood stains, should be handled with extreme caution. Always wear latex gloves and flood spilled blood with a hypochlorite solution such as household bleach before cleaning it.

6.1.3 Skin accidentally exposed to blood should be washed immediately with soap and running water. (Schools without running water should keep a supply on hand (e.g. in a 25-litre drum) specifically for use in emergencies. This water can be kept fresh for a long time by adding a disinfectant such as Milton to it.) Pour the water over the area to be cleaned, don't soak the area in the container.

6.1.4 If there is a biting or scratching incident where the skin is broken, the wound should be washed and cleansed under running water, dried, treated with antiseptic and covered with a waterproof dressing.

6.1.5 Blood splashes to the face (mucous membranes of eyes, nose or mouth) should be flushed with running water for at least three minutes.

6.1.6 Disposable bags and incinerators must be made available to dispose of sanitary wear.

6.1.7 All persons attending to blood spills, open wounds, sores, breaks in the skin, grazes, open skin lesions, body fluids and excretions should wear protective latex gloves or plastic bags over their hands to eliminate the risk of HIV transmission effectively. Bleeding can be managed by compression with material that will absorb the blood, e.g. a towel.

6.2 All schools and institutions should train learners, students, educators and staff in first aid. At all school events and outings, at least two first-aid kits should be available and accessible at all times, and the contents should be checked every week. Each first-aid kit should contain:

- two large and two medium pairs of disposable latex gloves;
- two large and two medium pairs of household rubber gloves for handling blood-soaked material in specific instances (for example when broken glass makes the use of latex gloves inappropriate);
- absorbent material, waterproof plasters, disinfectant (such as hypochlorite), scissors, cotton wool, gauze tape, tissues, containers for water and a resuscitation mouthpiece or similar device with which mouth-to-mouth resuscitation can be applied without any contact being made with blood or other body fluids;
- protective eye wear; and
- a protective face mask to cover the nose and mouth.

6.3 Universal precautions are essentially barriers to prevent contact with blood or body fluids. Adequate barriers can also be established by using less sophisticated devices than those described in 6.2, such as unbroken plastic bags on hands, household bleach for use as disinfectant (one part bleach to ten parts water), spectacles and a scarf.

6.4 Each classroom or other teaching area should preferably have a pair of latex or household rubber gloves, and gloves should be available at every sports event and should also be carried by the playground supervisor.

6.5 Learners, students, educators and other staff members should be trained to manage their own bleeding or injuries and to assist and protect others.

6.6 Learners (especially those in pre-primary and primary schools) and students should be instructed never to touch blood, open wounds, sores, breaks in the skin, grazes and open skin lesions of others, or to handle emergencies such as nosebleeds, cuts and scrapes of friends on their own. They should be taught to call for the assistance of an educator or other staff member immediately.

6.7 All cleaning staff, learners, students, educators and parents should be informed about the universal precautions that will be adhered to at a school or institution.

7. *Prevention of HIV transmission during play and sport*

How big is the risk of HIV transmission during contact sport?

The risk of HIV transmission as a result of contact play and contact sport is generally insignificant. The risk increases where open wounds, sores, breaks in the skin, grazes, open skin lesions or mucous membranes of learners, students and educators are exposed to infected blood. Certain contact sports may represent an increased risk of HIV transmission. Adequate wound management, in the form of the application of universal precautions is essential to contain the risk of HIV transmission during contact play and contact sport. The following guidelines apply:

7.1 No learner, student or educator may participate in contact play or contact sport with an open wound, sore, break in the skin, graze or open skin lesion.

7.2 If bleeding occurs during contact play or contact sport, the injured player should be removed from the playground or sports field immediately and treated appropriately. Only then may the player resume playing and only for as long as any open wound, sore, break in the skin, graze or open skin lesion remains completely and securely covered.

7.3 Blood-stained clothes must be changed.

7.4 A fully equipped first-aid kit should be available wherever contact play or contact sport takes place.

7.5 Sports participants (including coaches) with HIV/Aids should seek medical counselling before participating in sport, in order to assess risks to their own health as well as the risk of HIV transmission to other participants.

7.6 Staff members acting as sports administrators, managers and coaches should ensure the availability of first-aid kits and the adherence to universal precautions in the event of bleeding during participation in sport.

8. *Education on HIV/Aids*

8.1 A continuing life-skills and HIV/Aids education programme must be implemented at all schools and institutions for all learners, students, educators and other staff members. Measures must also be implemented at hostels.

8.2 Age-appropriate education on HIV/Aids must form part of the curriculum for all learners and students, and should be integrated in the life-skills education programme for pre-primary, primary and secondary school learners. (See Chapter 9 for age-appropriate education on HIV/Aids.) Education should include information and life skills necessary to prevent HIV transmission; basic first-aid principles; and the role of drugs, sexual abuse, violence and sexually transmitted infections in the transmission of HIV. It should empower learners and students to deal with these situations; encourage them to make use of health care, counselling and support services offered by community service organisations and other disciplines; raise awareness of prejudice and stereotypes about HIV/Aids; cultivate a culture of non-discrimination towards persons with HIV/Aids; and provide information on appropriate prevention and avoidance measures, including abstinence, the use of condoms, faithfulness and obtaining prompt medical treatment for sexually transmitted diseases and TB.

8.3 Parents of learners and students must be informed about all life-skills and HIV/Aids education offered at the school and institution; the learning content and methodology to be used; and the values that will be imparted. They should be invited to participate in parental guidance sessions and should be made aware of their role as sexuality educators and imparters of values at home.

8.4 Educators may not have sexual relations with learners or students. Should this happen, the matter has to be handled in terms of the Employment of Educators Act of 1998.

8.5 If learners, students or educators are infected with HIV, they should be informed that they can still lead normal, healthy lives for many years by taking care of their health.

9. *Duties and responsibilities of learners, students, educators and parents*

9.1 All learners, students and educators should respect the rights of other learners, students and educators.

9.2 The Code of Conduct adopted for learners or students should include provisions regarding the unacceptability of behaviour that may create the risk of HIV transmission.

9.3 The ultimate responsibility for the behaviour of a learner or a student rests with his or her parents. Parents of all learners and students are:

- expected to require learners or students to observe all rules aimed at preventing behaviour that may create a risk of HIV transmission; and
- encouraged to take an active interest in acquiring any information or knowledge on HIV/Aids supplied by the school or institution, and to attend meetings convened for them by the governing body or council.

9.4 It is recommended that a learner, student or educator with HIV/Aids (and parents in the case of learners or students) should consult medical opinion to assess whether the person poses a medically recognised significant health risk to others. If so, the principal of the school or institution must take the necessary steps to ensure the health and safety of other learners, students, educators and staff members.

9.5 Educators have a particular duty to ensure that the rights and dignity of all learners, students and educators are respected and protected.

10. Refusal to study with or teach a learner or student with HIV/Aids or to work with or be taught by an educator with HIV/Aids

May a learner refuse to study with another learner who has HIV/Aids? Or may a learner refuse to be taught by an HIV-positive educator?

Refusal to study with a learner or student, or to work with or be taught by an educator or other staff member who has, or is perceived to have, HIV/Aids should be pre-empted by providing accurate and understandable information on HIV/Aids to all educators, staff members, learners, students and their parents. Learners or educators who refuse to be taught by or to work with people with HIV/Aids should be counselled, and if they still refuse, disciplinary steps may be taken.

11. Health advisory committee

Where community resources make this possible, it is recommended that each school and institution should establish its own Health Advisory Committee with a chairperson with knowledge in the field of HIV/Aids and health care. The function of a health advisory committee should be to advise the governing body or council on all health matters, including HIV/Aids, and to be responsible for developing, promoting, reviewing and implementing a school or institution policy on HIV/Aids.

12. Implementation of the National Policy on HIV/Aids

Who is responsible for the implementation of the policy on HIV/Aids?

12.1 The Director-General of Education and the heads of provincial departments of education are responsible for the implementation of this policy. Every education department must designate an HIV/Aids Programme Manager and a working group to communicate the policy to all staff; to implement, monitor and evaluate the Department's HIV/Aids programme; to advise management on programme implementation and progress; and to create a supportive and non-discriminatory environment.

12.2 The principal or the head of a hostel is responsible for the practical implementation of this policy at school, institutional or hostel level, and for maintaining an adequate standard of safety according to this policy.

12.3 It is recommended that a school governing body or the council of an institution should take all reasonable measures to provide adequate barriers to prevent contact with blood or body fluids.

12.4 Strict adherence to universal precautions under all circumstances (including play and sports activities) is advised, as the State will be liable for any damage or loss caused as a result of any act or omission in connection with any educational activity conducted by a public school or institution.

19.7 WOMEN'S RIGHTS

The Bill of Rights gives all women the right to equality. The Equality clause in the Bill of Rights lists grounds on which people may not be discriminated against. These include sex and gender. This section will give special attention to the rights of women in the HIV/Aids context (based on Barrett-Grant et al., 2003). Women in Africa are seriously affected by HIV/Aids, and a large percentage of people living with HIV in South Africa are women. For various biological, socio-economic and sexual reasons, women are especially vulnerable to HIV infection. (See 'Why are women more easily infected by HIV than men?' on page 24.)

Termination of pregnancy

The Choice on Termination of Pregnancy Act gives a woman the right to have a safe and legal termination of pregnancy. An abortion can only take place with the *informed consent* of the woman, and she cannot be forced to have an abortion because she is HIV positive. Every woman has the right to have a family as well as the right to reproductive care and counselling (e.g. that with proper management and access to antiretroviral drugs, the possibility of mother-to-child transmission can be greatly reduced). The Department of Health should provide counselling both before and after the termination. (See 'Counselling HIV-positive pregnant women' on page 231.)

In terms of time periods, when does a woman have the right to terminate her pregnancy?

- A woman is entitled to the termination of her pregnancy upon request during the first 12 weeks of pregnancy. Up to 3 months into the pregnancy, she is not required to give a reason why she wants to terminate the pregnancy.
- Between 13 and 20 months of pregnancy a woman may still have the pregnancy terminated if:
  - the continued pregnancy poses a physical or mental risk to her or to her baby;
  - the pregnancy resulted from rape or incest; or
  - the continued pregnancy would significantly affect her social and economic circumstances, for example, if she will not be able to care for the baby financially.
- After the 20th week a woman can have her pregnancy terminated only if a doctor, after consultation with another doctor or midwife, believes that the pregnancy could be dangerous for the woman or could result in a deformed baby.

Where does a woman go for the termination of her pregnancy?

Termination of pregnancies takes place at hospitals or clinics that have been authorised to do terminations by the Minister of Health. Doctors, nurses, social workers, and midwives will be able to advise a woman where the nearest designated hospital or clinic is.

Does a woman need her husband's consent to terminate a pregnancy?

No. The Termination of Pregnancy Act does not require a woman to get her husband's consent to end her pregnancy. Health care workers cannot refuse to terminate a pregnancy because a woman has not told her husband. Only the pregnant woman's consent is required for the termination of the pregnancy.

Can a girl under 18 years of age consent to termination of pregnancy?

Yes. A girl of any age can consent to terminate her pregnancy. The Choice on Termination of Pregnancy Act says that if the person wanting an abortion is under 18, the doctor or midwife must advise her to speak to her parents or other family members before having the abortion. The girl does not have to follow the advice and she does not need to have the consent of her parents or guardian for the procedure. Health care workers cannot refuse to terminate her pregnancy if she does not want to discuss her decision with her parents.

Sterilisation

All women, including women with HIV, have the right to bear children. A woman with HIV cannot be sterilised without her consent. A woman of 18 years or older can consent to sterilisation. Sterilisation is a medical operation, and a woman under 18 years of age must have the consent of a parent or legal guardian before a hospital will agree to the sterilisation. The husband's consent is not required.

Rape

Rape is an act of violence against women and it increases a woman's risk of being infected with HIV. A woman may want to be tested for HIV to find out whether she was HIV negative at the time of the rape, and to follow up with more tests in case she was infected with HIV as a result of the rape. Pre-test counselling should be done before HIV testing. The following guidelines may be helpful:

- If possible, rape survivors should ask for the PCR test, which will indicate HIV infection much sooner than HIV antibody tests. The PCR test is, however, very expensive.
- Antiretroviral therapy should be given as soon as possible after the rape – within 72 hours.

Must a rape survivor pay for prophylactic antiretroviral drugs?

In April 2002 the South African cabinet decided that government should provide antiretroviral drugs free of charge to rape survivors. Some provinces or hospitals have unfortunately been slow to carry out the decision.

If a rape survivor has been infected with HIV by the rapist, she can make a civil claim against him for the cost of her medical expenses.

Rape survivors should tell the prosecutor if they believe that they have been infected with HIV as a result of rape. The law was changed in 1997 to create tougher penalties for rapists infected with HIV. If a person accused of rape knew that he had HIV, he is automatically denied bail. If a person convicted of rape knew that he had HIV at the time of the rape, by law he will receive a minimum sentence of life.

Can a rapist's blood be tested without his consent?

The South African Law Commission recommended in 2001 that the law be amended so that a person accused of a sexual offence in which there is a risk of HIV transmission (e.g. a person accused of rape) can be tested without his permission, and that his HIV status can be disclosed to the victim. A rape survivor will then have the option of requesting a magistrate to order HIV testing of the rapist. However, until that law is passed, a rapist still has the right to refuse an HIV test.

Virginity testing: a women's rights issue

Virginity testing is a traditional practice usually carried out on girls (in some cases boys are also tested). People in favour of testing believe that it is a valuable cultural practice that should be preserved, and that it is also a way to prevent the spread of HIV. Most gender activists believe the following (Barrett-Grant et al., 2003:202):

- Virginity testing is a violation of a woman's rights to privacy and dignity under the Constitution.
- Virginity testing does not help to stop the spread of HIV/Aids. It might even cause an increase in HIV infection because girls and young women are having anal sex to avoid vaginal penetration.
- People with no medical training often do the tests – if they don't do it correctly, it can cause serious infections.
- Virginity testing may stigmatise young women who are not virgins, without recognising that many young women are not in a position to choose whether or not to have sex, and may be forced to have sex.
- The practice can be dangerous because it identifies the virgins in a community, and this may expose them to rape and sexual abuse.

Commercial sex work

In South Africa it is a crime to be a commercial sex worker, and it is also a crime to solicit or to get customers. Sex workers are extremely vulnerable to violence, abuse and HIV infection. Sex workers are not always able to insist that their customers use condoms, and the sex is often violent. Because sex work is still illegal, it is difficult for sex workers to get information about HIV and safer practices. They are also afraid to openly say that they are sex workers and they are often not able to go to organisations where they could get help and information. It is difficult for them to report rape and abuse to the police without disclosing the illegal nature of their work. There is currently much discussion in women's organisations about the need to *decriminalise* sex work.

19.8 THE RIGHTS OF CHILDREN

Children are protected by the Constitution of South Africa and by the United Nations Convention on the Rights of the Child (to which South Africa became a signatory on 16 June 1995). (Also see 'The rights of the child' on page 270.) According to the Constitution, children have the right to equality and non-discrimination; the right to privacy and dignity; the right to appropriate parental or alternative care, basic health care and social services; and the right to special protection against abuse, bad treatment, and child labour. The following HIV/Aids-related questions on the rights of children are relevant for health care professionals and counsellors.

What is the legal age for giving permission to be tested for HIV?

Under the Child Care Act, children who are 14 years or older can consent on their own to *medical treatment*. This means that a child of 14 can consent to an HIV test and to treatment for an STI. Children and youths of 18 and older can consent to an *operation*. When a child is too young to consent, consent must be given by the child's parent or guardian (Barrett-Grant et al., 2003:142).

Who may give permission for medical treatment or for an operation if a child under 14 does not have a parent or guardian?

If a child does not have parents or a guardian, or if the parents or guardian are not available or cannot be found in time, consent to general medical treatment or an operation (which is not risky to the child's life or health) can be given by:

- a person with parental power over the child (e.g. a teacher or relative);
- a person who has custody of the child (e.g. a foster parent or the head of a children's home); or
- the Minister of Social Development.

In an emergency in which the child's life or health is in serious danger (and the parents or guardian cannot be reached) a person with parental power or custody, or the medical superintendent of the hospital, may consent to treatment or an operation. Note that there will seldom be a necessity to know a child's HIV status before emergency treatment can be given.

Are children tested for HIV before being placed in foster care?

No, children are not tested for HIV before being placed in foster care. When a child's HIV status is known and the child is under 14, this may be told to the foster parents if it is in the best interests of the child, for example, if the child needs special medical care.

Does a child have to be tested for HIV before he or she is adopted?

The Child Care Act does not say whether or not HIV testing should take place before an adoption. This means that various welfare organisations may have different HIV testing policies. Child Welfare's policy is that everyone involved in an adoption arranged through a Child Welfare agency is tested for HIV, including the adoptive parent or parents, the child and the natural parents, where possible. According to the Aids Law Project the practice of compulsory HIV testing of parents and children before an adoption violates the right to privacy, and the results of the HIV test can be used to discriminate against the adoptive parents or against the child to be adopted.

Who should know the HIV results of a child who is 14 or older?

If a child is 14 years or older, the child has the same rights to confidentiality as an adult. A child of 14 years or older who consents to an HIV test has the right to keep the results private. Nobody is allowed to disclose the HIV status of someone aged 14 years or older without that person's consent.

Activity

The ethical and legal implications of HIV/Aids

Carry out the following exercise with a group of people, and follow it up with either a lecture or a handout about the ethical and legal issues of HIV and Aids.

Draw three big faces on three separate flipchart papers: (1) a smiling face (with 'agree' written underneath), (2) an unhappy face (with 'disagree' written underneath) and (3) a neutral face (with 'don't know', 'neutral', and 'two sides of the story' written underneath).

Stick each face up in a different corner of the room.

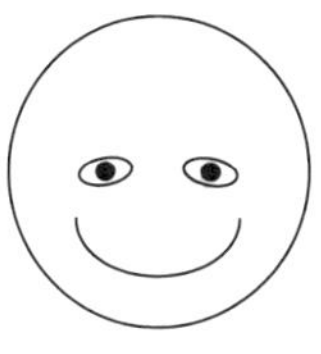

Agree

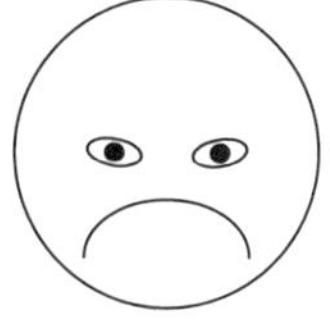

Disagree

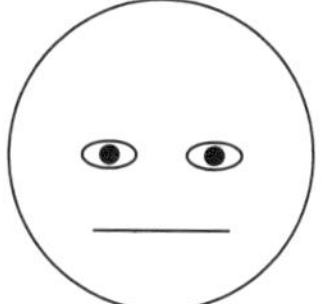

Neutral/Don't know/
Two sides to the story

Explain to the group that you will read a statement. The whole group must then get up and walk to one of the faces (either the agree face, or the disagree face, or the don't know/neutral/two sides to the story face). Ask two or three participants from each group to explain why they made the choice they did. Then encourage all three groups to debate with each other about the issue.

Encourage everyone to listen attentively and respectfully to every opinion that is expressed. (You may have to intervene tactfully but firmly to ensure that this happens.) Allow members to walk over to other groups if they change their minds as a result of the discussion. You should also draw up your own list of ethical and legal issues. Here are a few statements that will stimulate discussion (credit to Ilse Bence and Emmi Bootha):

- People who are HIV positive should abstain from sexual intercourse.
- Fellow employees have the right to know if someone in their workplace is HIV positive.
- The media has the right to publish the HIV status of any celebrity who has died.
- Pregnant women who are HIV positive should be encouraged to have an abortion.
- Homosexual men should not be allowed to donate blood.
- All domestic workers should be tested for HIV because they are in close contact with children.
- If an HIV-positive person refuses to tell his or her sexual partner about the infection, the counsellor should inform the partner.
- Children who are HIV positive should not be admitted to crèches and pre-school centres.
- Commercial sex work (prostitution) should be legalised.
- Clinics should refuse to give condoms to children younger than 16 years.

Who should know the HIV results of a child who is younger than 14?

When a child is younger than 14 years, the child cannot consent to an HIV test alone. The consent of a parent or guardian is necessary. The parent or guardian has the right to decide whether to disclose the results of the test to the child. Disclosure to the child will depend on whether the child is old enough to understand the results, as well as on what is in the child's best interests. (Also see 'How to tell a child that he or she is HIV positive' on page 222.)

Should a children's home or place of safety have information on a child's HIV status?

A children's home or place of safety does not have a right to information on a child's HIV status. Children with HIV/Aids often face discrimination, and some children are even excluded from children's homes because of their HIV status. If a child is older than 14, the child can decide who to tell about his or her HIV status. For children younger than 14 it is recommended that a children's home or place of safety be informed of the child's HIV status if:

- the child's HIV status is already known because of previous testing;
- it is in the best interests of the child;
- the children's home or place of safety does not discriminate on the basis of HIV; and
- the children's home or place of safety has policies on confidentiality.

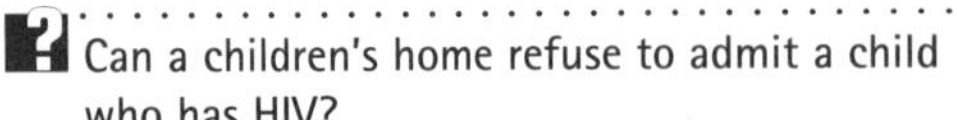

Can a children's home refuse to admit a child who has HIV?

A children's home, place of safety or any other institution (including schools and pre-schools) may not refuse to admit a child simply because of the child's HIV status, because it is unfair discrimination.

Can a child ask for contraceptives such as condoms or the pill at clinics or family planning centres?

The Child Care Act states that a child of 14 or older can consent to medical treatment. This means that a 14-year-old girl can decide to take an oral contraceptive (the pill) to control her reproductive system. Contraceptives like the male or female condom are not considered to be 'medical treatment'. This means that a child of under 14 can ask for condoms at a clinic or family planning centre.

Who may consent to termination of pregnancy?

A girl of any age can consent to the termination of her pregnancy. The Choice on Termination of Pregnancy Act says that if a person wanting an abortion is under 18, the doctor or midwife must advise her to speak to her parents or other family members before having the abortion. But she is not required to follow this advice, nor does she require anyone else's consent for the procedure.

19.9 CONCLUSION

Employers, schools and institutions should have a responsible attitude towards the legal and ethical implications of HIV/Aids and use the information provided in this chapter to draw up a detailed policy about HIV/Aids. This policy should include basic principles that acknowledge the rights of all people; create a safe working or school environment; specify detailed procedures for handling and coping with accidents and accidental exposure to blood and body fluids (see 'Management of accidental exposure to blood and other infectious body fluids' on page 347); and provide adequate education about HIV and Aids. Management should ensure that its HIV/Aids policy is properly implemented.

The Caregiver's Bookshelf

Suggestions for Further Reading

HIV and Aids in perspective

- Schoub, B.D. 1999. *Aids and HIV in perspective. A guide to understanding the virus and its consequences*, 2nd edn. Cambridge: Cambridge University Press.

The search for the virus: history and interesting theories

- Connor, S. & Kingman, S. 1988. *The search for the virus: the scientific discovery of Aids and the quest for a cure.* London: Penguin.
- Garrett, L. 1995. *The coming plague: newly emerging diseases in a world out of balance.* New York: Penguin.
- Hooper, E. 1999. *The river. A journey back to the source of HIV and Aids.* London: Penguin.
- Shilts, A. 1987. *And the band played on.* London: Penguin.

Traditional African beliefs and customs

- Hammond-Tooke, D. 1989. *Rituals and medicines.* Johannesburg: A.D. Donker.
- Mbiti, J.S. 1969. *African religions and philosophy.* London: Heinemann.

Sexuality, HIV/Aids education and lifeskills training for school children

- Edwards, D. & Louw, N. 1998. *Outcomes-based sexuality education.* Pretoria: Kagiso.
- Greathead, E. 1998. *Responsible teenage sexuality.* Planned Parenthood Association of South Africa. Pretoria: J.L. van Schaik.
- Norton, J. & Dawson, C. (written for PPSASA). 2000. *Life skills and HIV/Aids education. A manual and resource guide for intermediate phase school teachers.* Johannesburg: Heinemann.
- Rooth, E. 1995. *Life skills: a resource book for facilitators.* Pietermaritzburg: Macmillan.
- Von Mollendorf, J.W., Kekana, M.M., Froneman, T. & Kekana, L.T. 2000. *Reach Out life orientation.* Pietermaritzburg: Reach Out Publishers. (This series includes educator guides as well as learner books.)

Counselling skills

- Egan, G. 1998. *The skilled helper: a problem-management approach to helping*, 6th edn. Pacific Grove: Brooks/Cole.
- Gilles, H. 1994. *Counselling young people. A practical guide for parents, teachers and those in the helping professions.* Pretoria: Kagiso.
- Gladding, S.T. 2004. *Counseling: A comprehensive profession*, 5th edn. Columbus: Merrill Prentice Hall.
- Goldenberg, I. & Goldenberg, H. 1985. *Family therapy: an overview*, 2nd edn. Belmont: Wadsworth.
- Okun, B.F. 1997. *Effective helping: interviewing and counselling techniques*, 5th edn. Pacific Grove: Brooks/Cole.

Case studies and stories

- Morgan, I. 2003. *LongLife. Positive HIV stories.* Cape Town: Double Storey.
- Rasebotsa, N., Samuelson, M. & Thomas, K. 2004. *Nobody ever said Aids: Poems and stories from Southern Africa.* Cape Town: Kwela.

Positive living

- Orr, N., & Patient, D. 2004. *The healer inside you.* Cape Town: Double Storey.

Death and dying

- Kübler-Ross, E.C. 1969. *On death and dying.* New York: Macmillan.
- Kübler-Ross, E.C. 1997. *The wheel of life.* London: Bantam.

Primary care and home-based care for the patient with HIV/Aids

- Evian, C. 2003. *Primary HIV/Aids care*, 4th edn. Houghton: Jacana.
- Muchiru, S. & Fröhlich, J. 2001. *HIV/Aids: home-based care. A guide for caregivers.* Manzini: Macmillan Boleswa.
- Ungvarski, P.J. & Flaskerud, J.H. 1999. *HIV/Aids. A guide to primary care management*, 4th edn. Philadelphia: Saunders.
- Uys, L. & Cameron, S. (Eds.). 2003. *Home-based HIV/Aids care.* Cape Town: Oxford University Press.

Care for the caregiver

- Miller, D. 2000. *Dying to care: work, stress and burnout in HIV/Aids.* London: Routledge.
- Skovholt, T.M. 2001. *The resilient practitioner: burnout prevention and self-care strategies for counsellors, therapists, teachers and health professionals.* USA: Pearson Education.

HIV/Aids and the law

- Barrett-Grant, K., Fine, D., Heywood, M. & Strode, A. 2003. *HIV/Aids and the law. A resource manual*, 3rd edn. Johannesburg: Aids Law Project, University of the Witwatersrand.

Websites and Toll-free Helplines

- AEGIS HIV Daily Briefing: http://www.aegis.org
- Aids Law Project (University of the Witwatersrand, South Africa): http://www.hri.ca/partners/alp
- Antiretroviral therapy guidelines: http://www.aidsinfo.nih.gov
- Antiretroviral therapy guidelines (South African): http://www.afroaidsinfo.org http://www.sahivcliniciansociety.org Email address: sahivsoc@sahivsoc.org
- Beyond Awareness Campaign (South Africa): http://www.aidsinfo.co.za
- CDC (Centers for Disease Control, Division of HIV/Aids Prevention): http://www.cdc.gov/hiv/dhap.htm
- Body database: http://www.thebody.com
- Harvard Aids Institute: http://www.hsph.harvard.edu/organizations/hai
- Health, South African Department of (AfriHealth): http://www.health.gov.za
- Internet Resources on HIV/Aids : http://www2.wn.apc.org/sahiv/link.htm
- Johns Hopkins Aids Service (see the HIV life cycle animation): http://www.hopkins-aids.edu
- National policy on HIV/Aids in South Africa (for learners, students and educators): http://education.pwv.gov.za
- UNAIDS (Joint United Nations Programme on HIV/Aids) for the latest statistics on HIV/Aids: http://www.unaids.org
- WHO (World Health Organization): http://www.who.int/healthtopics/hiv.htm
- World Bank – Aids in Africa: http://www.worldbank.org/afr/aids
- Child and rape websites http://www.childline.org.za http://www.rapcan.org.za http://www.rapecrisis.org.za http://www.speakout.org.za (where to get PEP in South Africa)

Toll-free helplines

- Aids helpline: 0800-012-322
- Life Line: 0861-322-322
- Childline: 0800-055-555
- Stop Women Abuse: 0800-150-150

References*

- Ader, R., Felten, D.L. & Cohen, N. (Eds.). 1991. *Psychoneuroimmunology*, 2nd edn. San Diego: Academic Press.
- Adler, M.W. 1988. Development of the epidemic. In *The Aids reader: documentary history of a modern epidemic*, eds. L.K. Clarke & M. Potts, pp. 84–88. Boston: Branden Publishing Company.
- Ahlberg, B.M. 1994. Is there a distinct African sexuality? A critical response to Caldwell. *Africa* 64(2): 220–241.
- Airhihenbuwa, C.O. 1989. Perspectives on Aids in Africa: strategies for prevention and control. *Aids Education and Prevention* 1(1): 57–69.
- Ajzen, I. 1991. The theory of planned behaviour. *Organizational Behaviour and Human Decision Processes* 50: 179–211.
- Albers, G.R. 1990. *Counselling and Aids*. Dallas: Word Publishing.
- An open letter from an Aids patient. September 1988. *Cosmopolitan*.
- Anderson, K. & Rüppell, G. 1999. *Facing Aids: education in the context of vulnerability to HIV/Aids*. Geneva: World Council of Churches.
- Baldwin, J.D. & Baldwin, J.I. 1988. Factors affecting Aids-related sexual risk-taking behaviour among college students. *Journal of Sex Research* 25(2): 181–196.
- Ballard, R., Htun, Y., Fehler, G. & Neilsen, G. 2000. *The diagnosis and management of sexually transmitted infections in South Africa*. Johannesburg: South African Institute for Medical Research.
- Bandura, A. 1977. Self-efficacy: toward a unifying theory of behavioural change. *Psychological Review* 84(2): 191–215.
- Bandura, A. 1989. Perceived self-efficacy in the exercise of control over Aids infection. In *Primary prevention of Aids: psychological approaches*, eds. V.M. Mays, G.W. Albee & S.F. Schneider, pp. 128–141. Newbury Park: Sage.
- Bandura, A. 1991. Social cognitive theory of self-regulation. *Organizational Behaviour and Human Decision Processes* 50: 248–287.

* Every effort has been made to trace copyright holders. We, the publishers, apologise for any errors or omissions, and invite copyright holders to contact us if any have occurred, so that they can be rectified.

- Baron, R.A. & Byrne, D. (Eds.). 1994. *Social psychology: understanding human interaction,* 7th edn. Boston: Allyn and Bacon.
- Barrett-Grant, K., Fine, D., Heywood, M. & Strode, A. 2003. *HIV/Aids and the law: a resource manual,* 3rd edn. Johannesburg: Aids Law Project, University of the Witwatersrand.
- Becker, M.H. & Maiman, L.A. 1975. Socio-behavioural determinants of compliance with health and medical care recommendations. *Medical Care* 13(1): 10–24.
- Beuster, J. 1997. Psychopathology from a traditional Southern African perspective. *UNISA Psychologia* 24(2): 4–16.
- Blom, S. 2001. *Pre- and post-test counselling and testing.* Unpublished workshop notes, CAPE Consultancy, Cape Town.
- Boahene, K. 1996. The IXth International Conference on Aids and STD in Africa. *Aids Care* 8(5): 609–616.
- Bodibe, R.C. 1992. Traditional healing: an indigenous approach to mental health problems. In *Psychological counselling in the South African context,* ed. J. Uys, pp. 149–165. Cape Town: Maskew Miller Longman.
- Bodibe, R.C. & Sodi, T. 1997. Indigenous healing. In *Mental health policy issues for South Africa,* eds. D. Foster, M. Freeman & Y. Pillay, pp. 181–192. Pinelands: Medical Association of South Africa.
- Bond, G. 1993. *Death, dysentery and drought: coping capacities of households in Chiawa.* Paper presented at the Institute of Africa Studies, Lusaka, Zambia.
- Botha, A., Van Ede, D.M., Louw, A.E., Louw, D.A. & Ferns, I. 1998. Early childhood. In *Human development,* eds. D.A. Louw, D.M. van Ede & A.E. Louw, 2nd edn., pp. 233–318. Pretoria: Kagiso.
- Bouic, P., Lamprecht, J. & Freestone, M. July 2000. *Use of the plant E-sitosterol/E-sitosterol glucoside mixture (Moducare) for the management of South African HIV-infected individuals: an open labelled study over 40 months* (Abstract No. WeOrB538). Paper presented at the XIIIth International Aids Conference, Durban.
- Bowlby, J. 1977. The making and breaking of affectional bonds, I and II. *British Journal of Psychiatry* 130: 201–210.
- Bradshaw, D., Johnson, L., Schneider, H., Bourne, D. & Dorrington, R. 2002. The time to act is now. *Aids Bulletin* 11(4): 20-23.
- Brave Gugu hasn't died in vain. 2 January 1999. *The Independent on Saturday,* 3.
- Brouard, P. 2002. *HIV/AIDS counselling course trainer's manual.* Unpublished trainer's manual, Centre for the Study of AIDS, University of Pretoria, Pretoria.
- Brouard, P., Maritz, J., Van Wyk, B. & Zuberi, F. 2004. *HIV/AIDS in South Africa. Course Companion to the CSA Entry Level Volunteer Course.* University of Pretoria: Centre for the Study of Aids.
- Brown, L.K., Nassau, J.H. & Barone, V.J. 1990. Differences in Aids knowledge and attitudes by grade level. *Journal of School Health* 60(6): 270–275.
- Bührmann, M.V. 1986. *Living in two worlds.* Illinois: Chiron.
- Caesar, M. 2002. Everything you ever wanted to know about microbicides. *Aids Bulletin* 11(1): 17-18.
- Caldwell, J.C., Caldwell, P. & Quiggin, P. 1989. The social context of Aids in sub-Saharan Africa. *Population and Development Review* 15(2): 185–233.
- Cameron, S. 2003. Training community caregivers for a home-based care programme. In *Home-based HIV/Aids care,* eds. L. Uys & S. Cameron, pp. 33–49. Cape Town: Oxford University Press.
- Campbell, T. & Kelly, M. 1995. Women and Aids in Zambia: a review of the psychosocial factors implicated in the transmission of HIV. *Aids Care* 7(3): 365–373.
- Canadian Palliative Care Association. 1995. *Palliative care: towards a consensus in standardised principles of practice.* Toronto: Palliative Care Association.
- Carbello, M. 1988. *Introduction in Aids prevention and control.* Invited presentations and papers from the World Summit of Ministers of Health on programmes for Aids prevention, pp. 77–81. Oxford: Pergamon.
- Carpenter, C.C.J., Cooper, D.A., Fischl, M.A., Gatell, J.M., Gazzard, B.G., Hammer, S.M., et al. 2000. Antiretroviral therapy in adults: updated recommendations of the International Aids Society – USA Panel. *Journal of the American Medical Association* 283: 381–390.
- Carson, R.C., Butcher, J.N. & Mineka, S. 1998. *Abnormal psychology and modern life,* 10th edn. New York: Longman.
- Catania, J., Kegeles, S. & Coates, T. 1990. Towards an understanding of risk behaviour: an Aids Risk Reduction Model (ARRM). *Health Education Quarterly* 17: 53–72.
- Centers for Disease Control (CDC). 1988. Guidelines for effective school health education to prevent the spread of Aids. *Journal of School Health* 58(4): 142–148.
- Centers for Disease Control. 1989. Guidelines for prevention of the transmission of human immunodeficiency virus and hepatitis B virus to health-care and public-safety workers. *Morbidity and Mortality Weekly Report* 38: S-6.
- Centers for Disease Control. 2000. *HIV/Aids resources: frequently asked questions about HIV and Aids.* Retrieved 25 November 2000, from the World Wide Web: http://www.cdcnpin.org/hiv/faq/prevention.htm

- Centers for Disease Control Prevention Messages. 2002. *Condoms and sexually transmitted infection.* Atlanta: Centers for Disease Control.
- Chipfakacha, V.G. 1997. STD/HIV/Aids knowledge, beliefs and practices of traditional healers in Botswana. *Aids Care* 9(4): 417–425.
- Coates, T.J. 22 June 1990. HIV testing only part of the answer. *Aids Conference Bulletin*: 1.
- Coates, T.J. & Collins, C. 1998. Preventing HIV infection. *Scientific American* 279(1): 76–77.
- Cochrane, S.D., Mays, V.M. & Roberts, V. 1988. Ethnic minorities and Aids. In *Nursing care of the person with Aids/ARC*, ed. A. Lewis, pp. 17–24. Rockville, Maryland: Aspen.
- Coker, R. & Miller, R. 1997. HIV associated tuberculosis: a barometer for wider tuberculosis control and prevention. *British Medical Journal* 314: 1847.
- Cole, S.W., Kemeny, M.E. & Taylor, S.E. 1997. Social identity and physical health: accelerated HIV progression in rejection-sensitive gay men. *Journal of Personality and Social Psychology* 72: 320–335.
- College of Medicine of South Africa. 1991. Management of HIV-positive patients. *South African Medical Journal* 79: 688–690.
- Connor, S. & Kingman, S. 1988. *The search for the virus: the scientific discovery of Aids and the quest for a cure.* London: Penguin.
- Coombe, C. June 2000. *HIV/Aids and the education sector: the foundations of a control and management strategy in South Africa.* A briefing paper for the United Nations Economic Commission for Africa (UNECA).
- Coopersmith, S. 1967. *The antecedents of self-esteem.* San Francisco: W.H. Freeman.
- Cope, F. June 1994. Sharp management. *Hospital Supplies*: 3–4.
- Davidson, D. 1988. National coalition of advocates for students: guidelines for selecting teaching materials. In *The Aids challenge: prevention education for young people*, eds. M. Quackenbush & M. Nelson, pp. 447–461. Santa Cruz: Network.
- Department of National Health and Population Development. 1989. *Aids information and guidelines for nurses.* Pretoria: Department of National Health and Population Development.
- De Villiers, F.M.J. 1988. *Care of the dying. A Christian perspective.* Pretoria: NG Kerkboekhandel.
- De Villiers, S. Undated. *These are your rights. The United Nations Convention on the rights of the child.* Department of Justice and Constitutional Development.
- Dickinson, D., Clark, C.M.F. & Swafford, M.J. 1988. Aids nursing care in the home. In *Nursing care of the person with Aids/ARC*, ed. A. Lewis, pp. 215–237. Rockville, Maryland: Aspen.
- Du Toit, A.S., Grobler, H.D. & Schenck, C.J. 1998. *Person-centred communication: theory and practice.* Halfway House: Thomson.
- Eastaugh, A.N. 1997. Breaking bad news. *Update: The Journal of Continuing Education for General Practitioners* 12(5): 90–93.
- Edhonu-Elyetu, M. 1997. The significance of herpes zoster in HIV/Aids in Kweneng District, Botswana. *Update: The Journal of Continuing Education for General Practitioners* 12(5): 116–120.
- Edwards, D. & Louw, N. 1998. *Outcomes-based sexuality education.* Pretoria: Kagiso.
- Egan, G. 1998. *The skilled helper: a problem-management approach to helping*, 6th edn. Pacific Grove: Brooks/Cole.
- Elkind, D. 1978. Understanding the young adolescent. *Adolescence* 13(49): 127–134.
- Erikson, E.H. 1968. *Identity, youth and crisis.* New York: Norton.
- Evian, C. 2000. *Primary Aids care*, 2nd edn. Houghton: Jacana.
- Evian, C. 2003. *Primary HIV/Aids care*, 4th edn. Houghton: Jacana.
- Expert Advisory Group on Aids. March 1988. *Aids: HIV-infected health care workers.* London: Her Majesty's Stationery Office.
- Fahrner, R. 1988. Nursing interventions. In *Nursing care of the person with Aids/ARC*, ed. A. Lewis, pp. 115–130. Rockville, Maryland: Aspen.
- Feldman, D.A. 1985. Aids and social change. *Human Organization* 44(4): 343–348.
- Felhaber, T. (Ed.). 1997. *South African traditional healers' primary health care handbook.* Cape Town: Kagiso.
- Fine, D., Heywood, M. & Strode, A. (Eds.). 1997. *HIV/Aids and the law: a resource manual.* Johannesburg: Aids Law Project.
- Fishbein, M. & Ajzen, I. 1975. *Belief, attitude, intention and behaviour: an introduction of theory and research.* Reading, Mass: Addison-Wesley.
- Fishbein, M. & Middlestadt, S.E. 1989. Using the theory of reasoned action as a framework for understanding and changing Aids-related behaviours. In *Primary prevention of Aids: psychological approaches*, eds. V.M. Mays, G.W. Albee & S. F. Schneider, pp. 93–110. Newbury Park: Sage.
- Food and Drug Administration brochure. 1992. *Eating defensively: food safety advice for persons living with Aids.* Retrieved 22 October 2000, from the World Wide Web: http://vm.cfsan.fda.gov/~dms/aidseat.html
- Franzini, L.R., Sideman, L.M., Dexter, K.E. & Elder, J.P. 1990. Promoting Aids risk reduction via behavioural training. *Aids Education and Prevention* 2(4): 313–321.
- Friesen, H., Ekpini, E., Sibailly, T. & De Cock, K. 1997. Diagnosing symptomatic HIV infection and Aids in adults. *Update: The Journal of Continuing Education for General Practitioners* 12(3): 102–104.
- Fröhlich, J. 1999. *Draft guidelines for community home based care and palliative care for people living*

with Aids. Pretoria: Department of Health – Directorate: STDs and HIV/Aids.

- Galloway, M.R. 2002a. Microbicides – where are we now? *Aids Bulletin* 11(4): 15-17.
- Galloway, M.R. 2002b. Rape in schools a 'substantial public health problem' in South Africa. *Aids Bulletin* 11(1): 4-5.
- Galloway, M.R. 2003. Medicines Control Council approves first HIV vaccine trial in South Africa. *Aids Bulletin* 12(2): 4-5.
- Garcia, R., Klaskala, W., Pena, Y. & Baum, M.K. July 2000. *Behavioural change intervention for women at low and high risk for STD/HIV in Columbia* (Abstract No. ThPeC5347). Poster presented at the XIIIth International Aids Conference, Durban.
- Garrett, L. 1995. *The coming plague: newly emerging diseases in a world out of balance*. New York: Penguin.
- Gayle, H.D. 2000. Letter to colleagues from Helene D. Gayle, M.D., M.P.H., director, National Center for HIV, STD and TB Prevention, U.S. Centers for Disease Control and Prevention, 4 August 2000.
- Gayton, A.C. 1971. *Textbook of medical physiology*, 4th edn. Philadelphia: W.B. Saunders.
- Gelatt, H.B. 1989. Positive uncertainty: a new decision-making framework for counselling. *Journal of Counselling Psychology* 36: 252–256.
- Gillis, H. 1994. *Counselling young people*, 2nd edn. Pretoria: Kagiso.
- Gladding, S.T. 1996. *Counselling: a comprehensive profession*. London: Merrill Prentice Hall.
- Goss, E. 1989. Living and dying with Aids. *Journal of Pastoral Care* 43: 297–308.
- Gray, G. & McIntyre, J. 2002. *Adherence*. Notes taken from a therapeutic counselling research proposal at the Perinatal HIV Research Unit, Chris Hani Baragwanath Hospital, Johannesburg.
- Gray, G.E., McIntyre, J.A., Jivkov, B. & Violari, A. 2001. Preventing mother-to-child transmission of HIV-1 in South Africa. Recommendations for best practice. *Southern African Journal of HIV Medicine* 4: 15-26.
- Greathead, E. 1998. *Responsible teenage sexuality*. Planned Parenthood Association of South Africa. Pretoria: J.L. van Schaik.
- Green, E.C. 1988. Can collaborative programmes between biomedical and African indigenous health practitioners succeed? *Social Science and Medicine* 27(11): 1125–1130.
- Green, E.C. 1994. *Aids and STDs in Africa. Bridging the gap between traditional healing and modern medicine*. Pietermaritzburg: University of Natal Press.
- Green, E.C., Jurg, A. & Dgedge, A. 1993. Sexually-transmitted diseases, Aids and traditional healers in Mozambique. *Medical Anthropology* 15: 261–281.
- Green, E.C., Zokwe, B. & Dupree, J.D. 1995. The experience of an Aids prevention programme focused on South African traditional healers. *Social Science and Medicine* 40(4): 503–515.
- Gwyther, L. & Marston, J. 2003. Dealing with the symptoms of Aids. In *Home-based HIV/Aids care*, eds. L. Uys & S. Cameron, pp. 94–113. Cape Town: Oxford University Press.
- Gyeke, K. 1987. *An essay on African philosophical thought: the Akan conceptual scheme*. Cambridge: Cambridge University Press.
- Halperin, D. July 2000. *Neglected risk factors for heterosexual HIV infection and prevention programmes: anal intercourse, male circumcision and dry sex* (Abstract No. TuPeC3477). Poster presented at the XIIIth International Aids Conference, Durban.
- Hammond-Tooke, D. 1989. *Rituals and medicines*. Johannesburg: A.D. Donker.
- Harrison, A., Smit, J.A. & Myer, L. 2000. Prevention of HIV/Aids in South Africa: a review of behaviour change interventions, evidence and options for the future. *South African Journal of Science* 96(6): 285–290.
- Hauman, L. 1990. *Voorkoming van die oordrag en verspreiding van HBV (hepatitis B) en HIV (VIGS) in die hospitaal*. Unpublished protocol for nurses, Bloemfontein.
- Hauser, J. 1981. Adolescents and religion. *Adolescence* 16: 309–320.
- Heald, S. 1995. The power of sex: some reflections on the Caldwells' African sexuality thesis. *Africa* 65(4): 489–505.
- Herselman, S. 1997. A multicultural perspective on health care. In *Contemporary trends in community nursing*, eds. M. Bouwer, M. Dreyer, S. Herselman, M. Lock & S. Zeelie, pp. 28- 53. Johannesburg: Thomson.
- Hickson, J. & Mokhobo, D. 1992. Combating Aids in Africa: cultural barriers to effective prevention and treatment. *Journal of Multicultural Counselling and Development* 20(1): 11–22.
- HIV Infant Care Programme. 2000. *The impact of HIV/Aids on families and children*. Johannesburg: Cotlands.
- Holdstock, T.L. 1979. Indigenous healing in South Africa: a neglected potential. *South African Journal of Psychology* 9: 118–124.
- Hooper, E. 1999. *The river. A journey back to the source of HIV and Aids*. London: Penguin.
- Huxley Consulting. October 2001. *Managing Stress Workbook*. Johannesburg: Huxley Consulting.
- Inhelder, B. & Piaget, J. 1964. *The early growth of logic in the child: classification and serialization*. London: Routledge & Kegan Paul.
- Introducing HIV/Aids vaccines. 2002. Brochure developed by the South African HIV Vaccine Action Campaign (SA HIVAC).
- Irion, P.E. 1985. The grief continuum and the alternation of denial and acceptance. In *Loss, grief,*

and bereavement, eds. O.S. Margolis et al., pp. 9–15. New York: Praeger.

- Janz, N.K. & Becker, M.H. 1984. The health belief model: a decade later. *Health Education Quarterly* 11(1): 1–47.
- Jaret, P. June 1986. Our immune system: the wars within. *National Geographic*: 702–734.
- Jeffery, B., Webber, L. & Mokhondo, R. July 2000. *Determination of the effectiveness of inactivation of HIV in human breast milk by Pretoria pasteurisation* (Abstract No. MoPeB2201). Poster presented at the XIIIth International Aids Conference, Durban.
- Johnson, P. 2000. *Basic counselling skills: applications in HIV/Aids counselling.* Unpublished manuscript, Unisa Centre for Applied Psychology, Pretoria.
- Kalichman, S.C. 1996. *Answering your questions about Aids.* Washington: American Psychological Association.
- Kluckow, M. 2004. *Psychological support of orphans and vulnerable children.* Study guide for DYD218-4. Pretoria: University of South Africa.
- Kohlberg, L. 1978. Revision in the theory and practice of moral development. In *Moral development: new directions for child development*, ed. W. Damon. San Francisco: Jossey-Bass.
- Kohlberg, L. 1985. *The psychology of moral development.* San Francisco: Harper & Row.
- Korber, B. February 2000. *Timing the origin of the HIV-1 pandemic.* Paper presented at the 7th Annual Conference on Retroviruses and Opportunistic Infections, San Francisco.
- Krog, A. 2003. *A change of tongue.* Johannesburg: Random House.
- Kübler-Ross, E.C. 1969. *On death and dying.* New York: Macmillan.
- Kurtzweil, P. 1999. *Questions keep sprouting about sprouts.* U.S. Food and Drug Administration. Retrieved 22 October 2000, from: http://www.fda.gov/fdac/features/1999/199_sprt.html
- La Perriere, A., Klimas, N., Fletcher, M.A., Perry, A., Ironson, G., Perna, F., et al. 1997. Change in CD4+ cell enumeration following aerobic exercise training in HIV-1 disease: possible mechanisms and practical applications (Supplement 1). *International Journal of Sports Medicine* 18: S56–61.
- Larson, E. 1989. Handwashing: it's essential – even when you use gloves. *American Journal of Nursing* 89: 934–939.
- Leclerc-Madlala, S. 2002. On the virgin cleansing myth: gendered bodies, Aids and ethno-medicine. *African Journal of Aids Research* 1(2): 87-95.
- Levy, J. 21 June 1990. Levy discusses changing concepts in research. *Aids Conference Bulletin*: 1.
- Lie, G.T. & Biswalo, P.M. 1994. Perceptions of the appropriate HIV/Aids counsellor in Arusha and Kilimanjaro regions of Tanzania: implications for hospital counselling. *Aids Care* 6(2): 139–151.
- Life Line. 1997. *Counselling course – skills manual.* Pretoria: Life Line.
- Long, V.O. 1996. *Facilitating personal growth in self and others.* Pacific Grove: Brooks/Cole.
- Louw, D.A., Van Ede, D.M. & Ferns, I. 1998. Middle childhood. In *Human development,* eds. D.A. Louw, D.M. van Ede & A.E. Louw, 2nd edn., pp. 321–379. Pretoria: Kagiso.
- Lowell, W.E. 1980. The development of hierarchical classification skills in science. *Journal of Research in Science Teaching* 17(5): 425–433.
- Lusby, G. 1988. Infection control. In *Nursing care of the person with Aids/ARC*, ed. A. Lewis, pp. 191–202. Rockville, Maryland: Aspen.
- Lyons, C. 1988. The religious setting: a natural place for learning. In *The Aids challenge: prevention education for young people,* eds. M. Quackenbush & M. Nelson, pp. 207–210. Santa Cruz, CA: Network.
- Maartens, G. 2003. *Antiretroviral management of HIV infection.* The Foundation for Professional Development.
- Macfie, C. 1997. Loss, grief and mourning. *The Journal of Clinical Medicine: Modern Medicine* 22(9): 36–41.
- Mader, S.S. 1998. *Biology,* 3rd edn. Boston: McGraw-Hill.
- Marston, J. 2003. Doing a home visit. In *Home-based HIV/Aids care*, eds. L. Uys & S. Cameron, pp. 115–131. Cape Town: Oxford University Press.
- Max-Neef, M.A., Elizalde, A. & Hopenhayn, M. 1991. *Human scale development: conception, application and further reflections.* New York: Apex Press.
- Mbiti, J.S. 1969. *African religions and philosophy.* London: Heinemann.
- McCall, J.C. 1995. Rethinking ancestors in Africa. *Africa* 65(2): 256–270.
- McIntosh, E. 2004. *What you should know about oral sex.* Unpublished document. Johannesburg: DISA.
- Memory books. 3 June 2000. *Sukuma Newsletter* (p. 3), XIIIth International Aids Conference, Durban.
- Meyer, W.F. 1997. The ego psychological theory of Erik Erikson. In *Personology: from individual to ecosystem*, eds. W.F. Meyer, C. Moore & H.G. Viljoen, pp. 203–228. Johannesburg: Heinemann.
- Meyer, W.F. 1998. Basic concepts of developmental psychology. In *Human development*, eds. D.A. Louw, D.M. van Ede & A.E. Louw, 2nd edn., pp. 3–38. Pretoria: Kagiso.
- Meyer, W.F. & Van Ede, D.M. 1998. Theories of development. In *Human development*, eds. D.A. Louw, D.M. van Ede & A.E. Louw, 2nd edn., pp. 41–96. Pretoria: Kagiso.
- Miller, D. 1988. *Counselling of persons with Aids.* Invited presentations and papers from the World Summit of Ministers of Health on programmes for Aids prevention, pp. 90–94. Oxford: Pergamon.

- Miller, D. 2000. *Dying to care: work, stress and burnout in HIV/Aids.* London: Routledge.
- Miller, R. & Bor, R. 1988. *Aids: a guide to clinical counselling.* London: Science Press.
- Mkaya-Mwamburi, D., Qwana, E., Williams, B. & Lurie, M. July 2000. *HIV status in South Africa: who wants to know and why?* (Abstract No. MoPeC2376). Poster presented at the XIIIth International Aids Conference, Durban.
- Montauk, S.L. & Scoggin, D.M. 1989. Aids: questions from fifth and sixth grade students. *Journal of School Health* 59(7): 291–295.
- Montgomery, S.B., Joseph, J.G., Becker, M.H., Ostrow, D.G., Kessler, R.C. & Kirscht, J.P. 1989. The Health Belief Model in understanding compliance with preventive recommendations for Aids: how useful? *Aids Education and Prevention* 1(4): 303–323.
- Moses, S. & Plummer, F.A. 1994. Health education, counselling and the underlying causes of the HIV epidemic in sub-Saharan Africa. *Aids Care* 6(2): 123–127.
- Muchiru, S. & Fröhlich, J. 2001. *HIV/Aids: home-based care. A guide for caregivers.* Manzini: Macmillan Boleswa.
- National Department of Health. 1997. *Protocol for the management of a person with a sexually transmitted disease.* Marshalltown: Gauteng Directorate for Aids and Communicable Diseases.
- Nefale, M. 2000. *Bereavement counselling.* Unpublished manuscript, Unisa Centre for Applied Psychology, Pretoria.
- Nefale, M. 2004. HIV/Aids counselling and psychotherapy – challenges to the traditional psychotherapeutic framework. *Journal of Psychology in Africa* 14(1): 61-76.
- Nel, J.A. 2000. *Facilitation skills.* Unpublished manuscript, Unisa Centre for Applied Psychology, Pretoria.
- Ngubane, H.S. 1977. *Body and mind in Zulu medicine.* London: Academic Press.
- Norton, J. & Dawson, C. 2000. *Life skills and HIV/Aids education. A manual and resource guide for intermediate phase school teachers.* Johannesburg: Heinemann.
- Nyamathi, A.M. & Flaskerud, J.H. 1989. Risk factors and HIV infection. In *Aids/HIV infection: a reference guide for nursing professionals*, ed. J. H. Flaskerud, pp. 169–197. Philadelphia: W.B. Saunders.
- Nyamayarwo, A. July 2000. *The dilemma of HIV positive parents revealing serostatus to their children* (Abstract No. MoOrD250). Paper presented at the XIIIth International Aids Conference, Durban.
- Okun, B.F. 1997. *Effective helping: interviewing and counselling techniques*, 5th ed. Pacific Grove: Brooks/Cole.
- Okwu, A. November 1978. *Dying, death, reincarnation and traditional healing in Africa.* Paper presented at the 21st Annual Meeting of the African Studies Association, Baltimore, Maryland.
- O'Leary, A. 1990. Stress, emotion and human immune function. *Psychological Bulletin* 108(3): 363–382.
- Oosthuizen, P. 2002. *Care for the caregiver.* Unpublished workshop notes. Pretoria: Unisa Centre for Applied Psychology.
- Osborne, J. June 1990. Science can provide the light. *Aids Conference Bulletin*, 3.
- Paediatric HIV Working Group. 1997. *Guidelines for the management of HIV positive children.* Marshalltown: Gauteng Directorate for Aids and Communicable Diseases.
- Palermino, T. 1988. Psychosocial issues: one man's experience. In *Nursing care of the person with Aids/ARC*, ed. A. Lewis, 3rd edn., pp. 63–69. Rockville, Maryland: Aspen.
- Pando, M., de Los A., Gianni, S., Salomon, H., Negrete, M., Russell, K.L., et al. July 2000. *Risk behaviour of HIV-1 infected maternity patients and their sexual partners in Buenos Aires, Argentina* (Abstract No. TuPeC3471). Poster presented at the XIIIth International Aids Conference, Durban.
- Parkes, C.M. 1972. *Bereavement: studies of grief in adult life.* New York: International Universities Press.
- Paterson, D.L., Swindells, S., Mohr, J., Brester, M., Vergis, E.N., Squier, C., et al. 2000. Adherence to protease inhibitor therapy and outcomes in patients with HIV infection. *Annals of Internal Medicine* 133: 21-30.
- Pasteur, A.B. & Toldson, I.L. 1982. *Roots of soul. The psychology of black expressiveness.* New York: Anchor Press.
- Pearce, B. 1997. Counselling skills in the context of professional and organizational growth. In *Handbook of counselling*, ed. S. Palmer, 2nd edn., pp. 230-251. London: Routledge.
- Pearse, J. 1997. *Infection control manual. A practical guide for the prevention and control of infection in the health care setting.* Houghton: Jacana.
- Perelli, R.J. 1991. *Ministry to persons with Aids. A family systems approach.* Augsburg: Fortress.
- Petty, R.E. 1995. Attitude change. In *Advanced social psychology*, ed. A. Tesser, pp. 195–255. New York: McGraw-Hill.
- Piaget, J. 1932. *The moral judgement of the child.* London: Routledge & Kegan Paul.
- Piaget, J. 1970. *The child's conception of physical causality.* London: Routledge & Kegan Paul.
- Piaget, J. 1971. *The psychology of intelligence.* London: Routledge & Kegan Paul.
- Piaget, J. 1972. Intellectual evolution from adolescence to adulthood. *Human Development* 15: 1–12.
- Piaget, J. 1973. *The child's conception of the world.* London: Paladin.

- Piaget, J. & Inhelder, B. 1969. *The psychology of the child.* London: Routledge & Kegan Paul.
- Pies, C. 1988. Aids education in school settings: Grades 7–9. In *The Aids challenge: prevention education for young people*, eds. M. Quackenbush & M. Nelson, pp. 185–193. Santa Cruz, CA: Network.
- Pike, J.T. 1988. Nutritional support. In *Nursing care of the person with Aids/ARC*, ed. A. Lewis, pp. 159–174. Rockville, Maryland: Aspen.
- Pilot Project on Life Skills and HIV/Aids Education in Primary Schools. December 1999. *Final report for the Department of Education.* Pretoria.
- Pines, A. & Maslach, C. 1978. Characteristics of staff burnout in mental health settings. *Hospital and Community Psychiatry* 29: 233–237.
- Piscitelli, S. 2000. Indinavir concentrations and St John's wort. *Lancet* 355: 547–548.
- Post, J. 1988. Aids education in school settings: Grades 4–6. In *The Aids challenge: prevention education for young people*, eds. M. Quackenbush & M. Nelson, pp. 177–183. Santa Cruz: Network.
- Prevention of mother-to-child HIV transmission and management of HIV positive pregnant women. May 2000. HIV/Aids policy guidelines. South African Department of Health.
- Prochaska, J.O. & Di Clemente, C.C. 1984. *The trans-theoretical approach: crossing traditional boundaries of therapy.* Malabar: Krieger.
- Project Inform. 2002. Adherence: keeping up with your meds. Retrieved 3 May 2002, from the World Wide Web: http://www.projectinform.org
- Pugh, K. 1995. Suicide in patients with HIV infection and Aids. In *Grief and Aids*, ed. L. Sherr, pp. 45–58. Chichester: John Wiley.
- Quackenbush, M. 1988. Aids education in school settings: preschool – Grade 3. In *The Aids challenge: prevention education for young people*, eds. M. Quackenbush & M. Nelson, pp. 169–176. Santa Cruz: Network.
- Quackenbush, M. & Villarreal, S. 1988. *Does Aids hurt? Educating young children about Aids.* Santa Cruz: Network.
- Reno, C.L. & Walker, A.P. 1988. Providing direct nursing care in the adult inpatient setting. In *Nursing care of the person with Aids/ARC,* ed. A. Lewis, pp. 73–94. Rockville, Maryland: Aspen.
- Roddy, R.E., Zekeng, L., Ryan, K.A., Tamoufe, U. & Tweedy, K.G. 2002. Effect of nonoxynol-9 gel on urogenital gonorrhea and chlamydial infection. A randomized controlled trial. *Journal of the American Medical Association* 287: 1117-1122.
- Rogers, C.R. 1980. *A way of being.* Boston: Houghton Mifflin.
- Rooth, E. 1995. *Lifeskills: a resource book for facilitators.* Manzini: Macmillan Boleswa.
- Rose, A. 1988. Educating for life: Aids and teens in the Jewish community. In *The Aids challenge: prevention education for young people,* eds. M. Quackenbush & M. Nelson, pp. 219–226. Santa Cruz, CA: Network.
- Rosenheim, E. & Reicher, R. 1985. Informing children about a parent's terminal illness. *Journal of Child Psychology and Psychiatry* 26: 995-998.
- Rosenstock, I.M. 1966. Why people use health services. *Milbank Memorial Fund Quarterly* 44: 94–127.
- Rosenstock, I.M. 1974. The health belief model and preventive health behavior. *Health Education Monographs* 2(4): 354–386.
- Rotter, J.B. 1966. Generalized expectancies for internal versus external control of reinforcement. *Psychological Monographs* 80(1): 1–28.
- Runganga, A.O. & Kasule, J. 1995. The vaginal use of herbs/substances: an HIV transmission facilitatory factor? *Aids Care* 7(5): 639–645.
- Saunders, L. 1994. *Nutrition in Aids.* Paper presented at the South African Nutritional Congress, Durban.
- Schoepf, B.G. 1992. Aids, sex and condoms: African healers and the reinvention of tradition in Zaire. *Medical Anthropology* 14: 225–242.
- Schoub, B.D. 1997a. Guidelines to the management of occupational exposure to HIV. *Virus SA* 6(3): 5–7.
- Schoub, B.D. 1997b. Management of HIV in general practice. *Virus SA* 6(2): 3–7.
- Schoub, B.D. 1999. *Aids and HIV in perspective. A guide to understanding the virus and its consequences*, 2nd edn. Cambridge: Cambridge University Press.
- Schurink, E. & Schurink, W.J. 1990. *Aids: lay perceptions of a group of gay men.* Pretoria: Human Sciences Research Council.
- Scott, S.J. & Mercer, M.A. 1994. Understanding cultural obstacles to HIV/Aids prevention in Africa. *Aids Education and Prevention* 6(1): 81–89.
- Seeley, J., Wagner, U., Mulemwa, J., Kengeya-Kayondo, J. & Mulder, D. 1991. The development of a community-based HIV/Aids counselling service in a rural area in Uganda. *Aids Care* 3(2): 207–217.
- Seepamore, N. October 2000. *Counselling in the traditional African context.* Paper presented at the Unisa Centre for Applied Psychology, Pretoria.
- Seepamore, N. & Nkgatho, E. 2000. *Social work: working model for Alexandra township.* Report for the Gauteng Department of Social Services and Population Development, Johannesburg.
- Selwyn, P.A. 1986. Aids: what is now known: history and immuno-virology. *Hospital Practice* 21(5): 67–82.
- Serima, E. & Manyenna, S.B. July 2000. *VCT a new HIV prevention strategy* (Abstract No. TuPeD3767). Poster presented at the XIIIth International Aids Conference, Durban.
- Sherman, J.B. & Bassett, M.T. 1999. Adolescents and Aids prevention: a school-based approach in

Zimbabwe. *Applied Psychology: An International Review* 48(2): 109–124.

- Sherr, L. 1995. The experience of grief: psychological aspects of grief in Aids and HIV infection. In *Grief and Aids*, ed. L. Sherr, pp. 1–27. Chichester: John Wiley.
- Sidje, G., Foua Bi, K. & Aguirre, M. July 2000. *The involvement of PLHAs in reducing young women's vulnerability and socio-cultural determinants to the HIV/Aids epidemic in Vavoua (Côte d'Ivoire)* (Abstract No. ThPeD5808). Poster presented at the XIIIth International Aids Conference, Durban.
- Siecus Fact Sheet. November 2002. *The truth about condoms.*
- Siegel, D., Lazarus, N., Krasnovsky, F., Durbin, M. & Chesney, M. 1991. Aids knowledge, attitudes, and behavior among inner city, junior high school students. *Journal of School Health* 61(4): 160–165.
- Siegel, L. 1986. Aids: relationship to alcohol and other drugs. *Journal of Substance Abuse Treatment* 3: 271–274.
- Sikkema, K.J. & Bissett, R.T. 1997. Concepts, goals, and techniques of counselling: review and implications for HIV counselling and testing. *Aids Education and Prevention* 9 (Supplement B): 14-26.
- Skovholt, T.M. 2001. *The resilient practitioner: burnout prevention and self-care strategies for counsellors, therapists, teachers and health professionals.* USA: Pearson Education.
- Smart, R. 2003. Planning for orphans and HIV/Aids affected children. In *Home-based HIV/Aids care*, ed. L. Uys & S. Cameron, pp. 174–191. Cape Town: Oxford University Press.
- Smeltzer, S.C. & Bare, B.G. 1992. *Medical surgical nursing*, 7th edn. Philadelphia: J.B. Lippincott.
- South African Department of Health. 2000. *HIV/Aids policy guideline. Guidelines for the care and support of health care workers.* Pretoria: Department of Health.
- South African Tuberculosis Control Programme – Practical guidelines. 2000. South African Department of Health.
- Southern African AIDS Trust. The case studies on pages 220-221 are reproduced with the permission of Southern African AIDS Trust (SAT), PO Box 390, Kopje, Harare, Zimbabwe, www.satregional.org, from *Counselling Series No. 1: Counselling Guidelines on Disclosure of HIV Status*, June 2000.
- Southern African HIV Clinicians Society. 2002a. SA HIV Clinicians Society clinical guidelines: antiretroviral therapy in adults.
- Southern African HIV Clinicians Society. 2002b. SA HIV Clinicians Society clinical guidelines: antiretroviral therapy in children.
- Sow, I. 1980. *Anthropological structures of madness in Black Africa.* New York: International Universities Press.
- Spielman, A. & D'Antonio, M. 2002. *Mosquito.* London: Faber and Faber.
- Stein, J. 2004. HIV/Aids and the culture of silence. Disclosure to children. *Aids Bulletin* 13(1): 15-19.
- Strauss, S.A. 1989. *The nurse and Aids: legal issues.* Pretoria: SA Nursing Association.
- Sue, David, Derald Sue and Stanley Sue. 2000. *Understanding abnormal behaviour*, 6th edn. Boston: Houghton Mifflin. Copyright © 2000 by Houghton Mifflin Company. Used with permission.
- Sue, D.W. & Sue, D. 1999. *Counselling the culturally different: theory and practice,* 3rd edn. New York: John Wiley. Copyright © 1999 John Wiley & Sons, Inc. Reprinted with permission of John Wiley & Sons, Inc.
- Sunderland, R.H. & Shelp, E.E. 1987. *Aids: a manual for pastoral care.* Philadelphia: Westminster Press.
- Sy, F.S., Richter, D.L. & Copello, A.G. 1989. Innovative educational strategies and recommendations for Aids prevention and control. *Aids Education and Prevention* 1(1): 53–56.
- Taylor, C.C. 1990. Condoms and cosmology: the 'fractal' person and sexual risk in Rwanda. *Social Science and Medicine* 31(9): 1023–1028.
- Thom, D.P., Louw, A.E., Van Ede, D.M. & Ferns, I. 1998. Adolescence. In *Human development*, eds. D.A. Louw, D.M. van Ede & A.E. Louw, 2nd edn., pp. 383–468. Pretoria: Kagiso.
- Tlou, S. July 2000. *The girl child and Aids: The impact of secondary care-giving in rural girls in Botswana* (Abstract No. ThOrD690). Paper presented at the XIIIth International Aids Conference, Durban.
- True terror of Aids. 1997. *Update: The Journal of Continuing Education for General Practitioners* 12(7): 152.
- Ulin, P.R. 1992. African women and Aids: negotiating behavioural change. *Social Science and Medicine* 34(1): 63–73.
- Ungvarski, P.J. 1989. Nursing management of the adult client. In *Aids/HIV infection: a reference guide for nursing professionals*, ed. J.H. Flaskerud, pp. 74–110. Philadelphia: W.B. Saunders.
- UNICEF. 1999. *Children orphaned by Aids: front-line responses from Eastern and Southern Africa.* Geneva: UNICEF.
- United Nations Programme on HIV/Aids. October 1997. *Tuberculosis and Aids.* Geneva: Joint United Nations Programme on HIV/Aids.
- United Nations Programme on HIV/Aids. May 2000a. *Caring for carers: managing stress in those who care for people with HIV and Aids.* Geneva: Joint United Nations Programme on HIV/Aids.
- United Nations Programme on HIV/Aids. September 2000b. *Collaboration with traditional healers in HIV/Aids prevention and care in sub-Saharan Africa: a literature review.* Geneva: Joint United Nations Programme on HIV/Aids.
- United Nations Programme on HIV/Aids. June 2000c. *Report on the global HIV/Aids epidemic.*

Geneva: Joint United Nations Programme on HIV/Aids.

- United Nations Programme on HIV/Aids. July 2002. *Report on the global HIV/Aids epidemic*. Geneva: Joint United Nations Programme on HIV/Aids.
- United Nations Programme on HIV/Aids. July 2004. *2004 Report on the global HIV/Aids epidemic*, 4th global report. Geneva: Joint United Nations Programme on HIV/Aids.
- United Nations Programme on HIV/Aids (UNAIDS) and World Health Organization (WHO). 2003. *Aids epidemic update: December 2003*. Geneva: Joint United Nations Programme on HIV/Aids.
- Update. June 1996. Provisional public health service recommendations for chemoprophylaxis after occupational exposure to HIV. *Morbidity and Mortality Weekly Report* 45(22): 463–467.
- Uys, L. 2003. A model for home-based care. In *Home-based HIV/Aids care*, eds. L. Uys & S. Cameron, pp. 3–15. Cape Town: Oxford University Press.
- Van Arkel, J. de J. (Ed.). 1991. *Living in an Aids culture*. Pretoria: University of South Africa.
- Van den Boom, F.M. 1995. The death of a parent. In *Grief and Aids*, ed. L. Sherr, pp. 145- 160. Chichester: John Wiley.
- Van Dyk, A.C. 1991. *Voorkoming van VIGS: psigo-sosiale voorspellers van houdings, gedrag en gedragsverandering*. Unpublished doctoral thesis, University of South Africa, Pretoria.
- Van Dyk, A.C. 1999. *Aids care and counselling*. Cape Town: Maskew Miller Longman.
- Van Dyk, A.C. 2001a. Traditional African beliefs and customs: implications for Aids education and prevention in Africa. *SA Journal of Psychology* 31(2): 60-66.
- Van Dyk, A.C. 2001b. 'Why me and not my neighbour?' HIV/Aids care and counselling in a traditional African context. *Curationis* 24(3): 4-9.
- Van Dyk, A.C., Johnson, P., Nefale, M. & Nel, J.A. 2000. *HIV/Aids management and counselling: a training manual for the Gauteng Department of Social Services and Population Development*. Pretoria: Unisa Centre for Applied Psychology.
- Van Dyk, A.C. & Van Dyk, P.J. 2003a. 'To know or not to know': service-related barriers to voluntary HIV counselling and testing (VCT) in South Africa. *Curationis* 26(1): 4-10.
- Van Dyk, A.C. & Van Dyk, P.J. 2003b. 'What is the point of knowing?' Psycho-social barriers to HIV/Aids voluntary counselling and testing programmes in South Africa. *SA Journal of Psychology* 33(2): 118-125.
- Van Dyk, P.J. 2000. *A brief history of creation*. Pretoria: University of South Africa.
- Van Wyk, C. March 2000. *The legal aspects of Aids*. Paper presented at the Unisa Centre for Applied Psychology, Pretoria.
- Van Zyl, D.A. 1990. Psychoneuroimmunology. In *Health psychology in South Africa*, ed. M. Visser, pp. 59–62. Pretoria: HSRC.
- Verkragters 'is in ons skole'. 7 October 2000. *Beeld*, 2.
- Vigs-aanmeldingsplan laat vaar. 12 January 2001. *Beeld*, 4.
- Viljoen, H.G. 1997. Eastern and African perspectives. In *Personology: from individual to ecosystem*, eds. W.F. Meyer, C. Moore & H.G. Viljoen, pp. 591–627. Johannesburg: Heinemann.
- Visagie, C.J. 1999. *HIV/Aids: the complete story of HIV and Aids*. Pretoria: J.L. van Schaik.
- Wallston, K.A., Wallston, B.S. & De Vellis, R. 1978. Development of the multidimensional health locus of control (MHLC) scales. *Health Education Monographs* 6(2): 160–170.
- Walsh, M.E. & Bibace, R. 1990. Developmentally-based Aids/HIV education. *Journal of School Health* 60(6): 256–261.
- Walters, J.L., Canady, R. & Stein, T. 1994. Evaluating multicultural approaches in HIV/Aids education material. *Aids Education and Prevention* 6(5): 446–453.
- Watts, J. 1988. Breaking the Aids taboo. *The Illustrated London News* 7082(276): 26–32.
- Weber, J.N. & Weiss, R.A. 1988. HIV infection: the cellular picture. *Scientific American* 259(4): 81–87.
- Weybrew, B.B. 1992. *The abc's of stress: a submarine psychologist's perspective*. USA: Praeger.
- Whiteside, A. & Sunter, C. 2000. *Aids: the challenge for South Africa*. Cape Town: Human & Rousseau Tafelberg.
- Williams, A.F. 1972. Factors associated with seat belt use in families. *Journal of Safety Research* 4(3): 133–138.
- Wong, D.L., Hockenberry-Eaton, M., Wilson, D., Winkelstein, M.L., Ahmann, E. & DiVito-Thomas, P.A. 1999. *Whaley & Wong's nursing care of infants and children*, 6th edn. St Louis: Mosby.
- Worden, J.W. 1982. *Grief counselling and grief therapy*. New York: Springer. Copyright Springer Publishing Company, Inc., New York 10012. Used by permission.
- World Health Organization (WHO). 1988a. *Guidelines on sterilization and high-level disinfection methods effective against human immunodeficiency virus (HIV)* (Aids Series No. 2). Geneva: World Health Organization.
- World Health Organization. 1988b. *Guidelines for nursing management of people infected with human immunodeficiency virus (HIV)* (Aids Series No. 3). Geneva: World Health Organization.
- World Health Organization. 1990a. *Guidelines on Aids and first aid in the workplace* (Aids Series No. 7). Geneva: World Health Organization.
- World Health Organization. 1990b. *Guidelines for counselling about HIV infection and disease* (Aids Series No. 8). Geneva: World Health Organization.

- World Health Organization. 1993. *Aids home care handbook*. Geneva: World Health Organization.
- World Health Organization. 2000a. *Fact sheets on HIV/Aids: a desktop reference*. Geneva: World Health Organization.
- World Health Organization. 2000b. *Principles of antiretroviral therapy*. Retrieved 20 September 2000, from the World Wide Web: http://www.who.int/HIV_AIDS/WHO_HSI_2000.04_1.04/001.htm
- Wyatt, H.V. 1989. Ambiguities and scares in education material about Aids. *Aids Education and Prevention* 1(2): 119–125.
- Yamba, C.B. 1997. Cosmologies in turmoil: witchfinding and Aids in Chiawa, Zambia. *Africa* 67(2): 200–223.
- Zazayokwe, M. 1989. *Some barriers to education about Aids in the black community*. Paper presented at an Aids training course of the South African Institute for Medical Research, Johannesburg.
- Ziady, L. 2003. Infection prevention and control aspects in home-based health care. In *Home-based HIV/Aids care*, eds. L. Uys & S. Cameron, pp. 133–160. Cape Town: Oxford University Press.

Glossary

- **Aids** Acquired Immune Deficiency Syndrome. This acronym emphasises that the disease is *acquired* and not inherited. It is caused by a virus that invades the body. This virus then attacks the body's immune system and makes it so weak and ineffectual that it is unable to protect the body from both serious and common infections and pathogens.
- **Aids-defining disease** Specific diseases or conditions which indicate the clinical development of Aids in a person who is HIV positive.
- **Antibodies.** Special protein complexes produced by the immune system that attack and neutralise specific disease-causing organisms. The antibodies which the body creates in response to the HI virus are unfortunately powerless to protect the body against the long-term destructive effects of the HI virus.
- **Antiretroviral therapy** Drugs which suppress or prevent the replication of HIV in cells.
- **ART** See **Antiretroviral therapy**.
- **AZT** The antiretroviral drug azidothymidine – which is also called zidovudine or Retrovir.
- **BCG** The vaccine against tuberculosis.
- **CD4 cells** T helper lymphocytes (a type of white blood cell). These cells play an important role in keeping the immune system healthy. The HI virus attaches itself to the CD4 receptors on the outer layer of the CD4 cells. They are also called T4 helper cells.
- **CD4 count** The laboratory test most commonly used to estimate the level of immune deficiency in HIV-infected individuals by 'counting' the CD4 cells.
- **CMV** The cytomegalovirus. This virus is often excreted in the urine, saliva, semen, cervical secretions, faeces or breast milk of immune-depressed patients. CMV may cause infections of the retinas of the eyes. (Such infections may ultimately cause blindness in the person thus infected.)
- **d4T** Stavudine – an antiretroviral drug.
- **ELISA test** ELISA stands for 'enzyme-linked immunosorbent assay'. This is a laboratory test (technique) to detect antibodies in the blood.
- **Epidemiology** The study of the determinants, distribution, prevalence and control of disease.
- **Episiotomy** Incision of the vulva to avoid lacerations of the perineum (the region between the vagina and the anus) as the baby is delivered.

- **False negative** A test result that is HIV negative when the person is actually HIV positive.
- **False positive** A test result that is HIV positive when the person is actually HIV negative.
- **HBV** The hepatitis B virus.
- **Herpes zoster** (also known as **shingles**) A condition characterised by an extremely painful skin rash or tiny blisters on the face, limbs or body. Shingles is caused by a virus, and it affects nerve cells.
- **HIV** The human immunodeficiency virus – the virus which causes Aids.
- **HIV antibody positive** This phrase means the antibodies to HIV are present in the bloodstream – an indication that the person concerned has been exposed to (and is therefore infected with) the HI virus.
- **HIV P24 antigen** A core protein found in the HI virus. The presence of this antigen in the blood is evidence that the HI virus is present in the body. These antigens are usually detectable in the early and very late stages of HIV infection.
- **Home-based care** Home-based care is the care given to individuals in their own homes by their families, their extended families or any other available and concerned helpers, when such home-based caregivers are supported in a systematic and organised way by a multi-disciplinary team, and by complementary caregivers who have the ability to meet the specific needs of the individual and family.
- **Immune deficiency** A weakening or deficiency in the immune system.
- **Informed consent** The kind of consent to medical testing or treatment that is accompanied by *information* and *permission*. Before an HIV test can be done, the client must understand the nature of the test *and* he/she must also give verbal or written permission to be tested. A client may never be misled or deceived into consenting to an HIV test.
- **Kaposi's sarcoma** A rare form of skin cancer, characterised by a painless reddish-brown or bluish-purple swelling on the skin and mucous membranes.
- **Lymphoid interstitial pneumonia (LIP)** A rare respiratory or lung disease found in HIV-infected children which is characterised by continuous coughing and mild wheezing.
- **MTCT** Mother-to-child transmission of the HI virus.
- **Nevirapine** An antiretroviral drug which is often administered to pregnant women to prevent mother-to-child transmission of the HI virus.
- **NNRTI** Non-nucleoside reverse transcriptase inhibitor – a class of antiretroviral medications that includes drugs such as nevirapine. NNRTIs disturb the life cycle of the HIV virus by directly inhibiting the reverse transcriptase enzyme.
- **NRTI** Nucleoside reverse transcriptase inhibitor – a class of antiretroviral medications that includes drugs such as zidovudine (AZT), lamivudine (3TC) and stavudine (d4T). NRTIs disturb the life cycle of the HIV virus through interference with the reverse transcriptase enzyme by mimicking the normal building blocks of HIV DNA.
- **Opportunistic infections** Infections that would not normally cause disease in a healthy body but which exploit the *opportunity* presented by an infected person's weakened immune system to attack the body.
- **Oral hairy leukoplakia** Thickened white patches on the side of the tongue.
- **Palliative care** is the terminal care of patients dying of Aids (or any other disease).
- **PCP** See *Pneumocystis carinii pneumonia.*
- **PCR** Polymerase chain reaction technique, a method of testing for the presence of HIV in the body. The PCR technique does not have to rely on the formation of antibodies in order to diagnose HIV infection – it detects the virus itself in the blood.
- **Persistent generalised lymphadenopathy (PGL)** Swollen lymph nodes that are wider than 1 centimetre in diameter in areas such as the groin, the neck and the armpits and that have been present continuously for a period of at least 3 months.
- **PI** Protease inhibitor. A class of antiretroviral drugs which includes drugs such as saquinavir and indinavir. PIs inhibit the late stages of HIV replication by inhibiting the protease enzyme.
- ***Pneumocystis carinii* pneumonia (PCP)** A parasitic infection of the lungs caused by a protozoan. PCP is often seen in patients with severe immune deficiency (such as patients in the last stages of Aids).
- **Post-exposure prophylaxis (PEP)** Methods of attempting to prevent HIV infection in a person who has been exposed to infected blood or other body fluids as in the case of, for example, accidental exposure or rape.
- **Rapid HIV antibody test** An HIV antibody test that produces rapid or fast results. Rapid HIV tests are relatively easy to use (they involve pricking a finger with a lancet), and the results are usually available within 10 to 30 minutes.
- **Retrovirus** A type of virus (of which HIV is one) that replicates by changing its genetic RNA into DNA by using the host's cells.
- **Reverse transcriptase** An enzyme which retroviruses produce and use to transform their viral RNA into viral DNA in the replication process.
- **Seroconversion** The point at which a person's HIV status converts or changes from being HIV negative to HIV positive. This coincides with the time when an HIV test will show that a person is HIV positive. Sero-conversion usually occurs 4 to 8 weeks after an individual has been infected with the HI virus.
- **Seroconversion illness** Some individuals who sero-convert may show flu-like symptoms such as fever, tiredness, rash, sore throat, muscle pains and swollen lymph glands.
- **Shingles** See Herpes zoster.

- **STI** Sexually transmitted infections are infections transmitted primarily through sexual intercourse. These include (for example) syphilis, gonorrhoea, candidiasis, genital herpes and HIV infection.
- **Syndrome** A collection of specific signs, indicators and symptoms that characteristically occur together and that are indicative of the presence of a particular pathological condition.
- **T4 cell** See CD4 cells.
- **3TC/lamivudine** An antiretroviral drug.
- **T helper cells** See CD4 cells.
- **Universal precautions** are a variety of precautions that any person who comes into contact with blood and certain other body fluids or products in a health care setting should always apply so as to prevent himself or herself from being infected by the HI virus (or any other dangerous pathogen such as the highly infectious hepatitis B virus).
- **Virus** A microbiological organism which is the smallest and most basic of all known biological organisms.
- **Western Blot test** A blood test that detects the antibodies to HIV infection. It is sometimes used to confirm an ELISA test that has produced a (HIV) positive result.
- **Window period** The time between infection with HIV and the development of detectable HIV antibodies. Any HIV test done during this time will render false negative results (see **False negative** above) – even though the person is actually already infected with HIV.

Index

A

I

Q

R

WHO 2012 Service delivery approaches to HIV testing & counselling; a strategic HTC programme framework